W9-ATO-009

Stuttering

An Integrated Approach to its Nature and Treatment

FIFTH EDITION

Stuttering

An Integrated Approach to Its Nature and Treatment

FIFTH EDITION

BARRY GUITAR, PhD

Professor
Department of Communication Sciences
University of Vermont
Burlington, Vermont

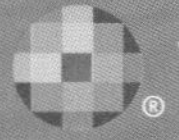

Wolters Kluwer

Philadelphia • Baltimore • New York • London
Buenos Aires • Hong Kong • Sydney • Tokyo

Acquisitions Editor: Matt Hauber
Development Editor: Amy Millholen
Editorial Coordinators: Andrea Klingler and Kerry McShane
Editorial Assistant: Parisa Saranj
Production Project Manager: Kim Cox
Marketing Manager: Jason Oberacker
Designer: Stephen Druding
Artist: Bot Roda
Compositor: SPi Global

5th Edition

Copyright © 2019 Wolters Kluwer

Copyright © 2014 Lippincott Williams & Wilkins, a Wolters Kluwer business. Copyright © 2006 by Lippincott Williams & Wilkins. Copyright © 1999, 1991 by Williams & Wilkins. All rights reserved. This book is protected by copyright. No part of this book may be reproduced or transmitted in any form or by any means, including as photocopies or scanned-in or other electronic copies, or utilized by any information storage and retrieval system without written permission from the copyright owner, except for brief quotations embodied in critical articles and reviews. Materials appearing in this book prepared by individuals as part of their official duties as U.S. government employees are not covered by the above-mentioned copyright. To request permission, please contact Wolters Kluwer at Two Commerce Square, 2001 Market Street, Philadelphia, PA 19103, via email at permissions@lww.com, or via our website at shop.lww.com (products and services).

9 8 7 6 5 4 3 2 1

Printed in China

Library of Congress Cataloging-in-Publication Data
Names: Guitar, Barry, author.
Title: Stuttering : an integrated approach to its nature and treatment / Barry Guitar.
Description: Fifth edition. | Philadelphia : Wolters Kluwer, [2019] | Includes bibliographical references and index.
Identifiers: LCCN 2018049600 | ISBN 9781496346124 (paperback)
Subjects: | MESH: Stuttering—therapy | Stuttering—etiology | Stuttering—diagnosis
Classification: LCC RC424 | NLM WM 475.7 | DDC 616.85/54—dc23 LC record available at https://lccn.loc.gov/2018049600

This work is provided "as is," and the publisher disclaims any and all warranties, express or implied, including any warranties as to accuracy, comprehensiveness, or currency of the content of this work.

This work is no substitute for individual patient assessment based upon healthcare professionals' examination of each patient and consideration of, among other things, age, weight, gender, current or prior medical conditions, medication history, laboratory data and other factors unique to the patient. The publisher does not provide medical advice or guidance and this work is merely a reference tool. Healthcare professionals, and not the publisher, are solely responsible for the use of this work including all medical judgments and for any resulting diagnosis and treatments.

Given continuous, rapid advances in medical science and health information, independent professional verification of medical diagnoses, indications, appropriate pharmaceutical selections and dosages, and treatment options should be made and healthcare professionals should consult a variety of sources. When prescribing medication, healthcare professionals are advised to consult the product information sheet (the manufacturer's package insert) accompanying each drug to verify, among other things, conditions of use, warnings and side effects and identify any changes in dosage schedule or contraindications, particularly if the medication to be administered is new, infrequently used or has a narrow therapeutic range. To the maximum extent permitted under applicable law, no responsibility is assumed by the publisher for any injury and/or damage to persons or property, as a matter of products liability, negligence law or otherwise, or from any reference to or use by any person of this work.

shop.lww.com

CCS1218

Preface

Stuttering is an intriguing and mysterious disorder. In the past 50 years, we have learned many secrets about what is different in the brains of those of us who stutter. Yet many unanswered questions remain. For example, we don't know exactly how these brain differences result in the speech disfluencies that we see in the onset of stuttering in children. We also don't know how the usually mild beginnings of stuttering become—for some children—severe, struggled behaviors accompanied by avoidance and emotional turmoil.

This book is an attempt to present the latest scientific findings and theoretical perspectives and integrate them with the best clinical approaches for evaluating and treating stuttering. As I worked on this new edition, I realized that my current thinking has been influenced deeply by my own stuttering therapist, Charles Van Riper, who summarized his final thoughts (1990) about stuttering in this way:

- Stuttering begins when the brain mistimes the complex movements required for fluent speech.
- The child's responses to these mistimings are the repetitions and prolongations that we observe as stuttering begins.
- Most children recover from stuttering "because of maturation or because *they do not react* to their lags, repetitions, or prolongations by struggle or avoidance" (Van Riper, 1990, 317 [italics mine]).
- The struggle and avoidance are learned and can be modified, although the mistimings are always there.

Some of my thinking in this edition focuses on the children who do not recover because they *do* react to their repetitions and prolongations. I view our therapies for preschool children as *preventing* these struggle and avoidance reactions and *minimizing the stuttering* they would be reacting to. We do this by helping them feel ok about their stuttering and teaching them how to talk more fluently. I also think that once the struggle and avoidance reactions are learned, they can be modified by *reducing* the (nonconscious) *threat* and (conscious) *fear* of stuttering that trigger these reactions. A combination of a strong, supportive client-clinician relationship and a program of reducing fear and shame, and confronting and tolerating the moment of stuttering to reduce tension, and then easing out of it will diminish struggle and avoidance. The resulting experience of feeling in control of stutters will further reduce maladaptive behaviors and negative feelings.

Have I anything more to say? Yes. I hope if you have suggestions for improving the next edition of this text, you'll let me know.

— Barry Guitar
bguitar@med.uvm.edu

Acknowledgments

Thank you to all my clients and students. You taught me as much as I taught you.

And thanks to my colleagues in Communication Sciences and Disorders and in Psychological Sciences whose writings and conversations, in person and via e-mail, have helped me become woke.

A round of applause for Andrea Klingler, Mike Nobel, Kerry McShane, and Amy Millholen, whose editorial talents made this book what it is.

Cheers for Bot Roda—the talented illustrator who gave life to all my notions about what might be helpful to put in visual form.

Kudos to Adinarayanan Lakshmanan Sivakumar (Siva) and his team who have done a wonderfully thorough job of compositing my manuscript into the printed page.

Hooray! Rebecca McCauley and Charlie Barasch, who have edited each chapter, making them more readable, updated, and cogent than my original drafts.

As with all the earlier editions, I bestow love and appreciation to my wife, Carroll. She has used her librarian and literary skills to edit, find references, keep databases, get permissions, help with videos, and keep me moving so this edition will finally see the light of day.

Contents

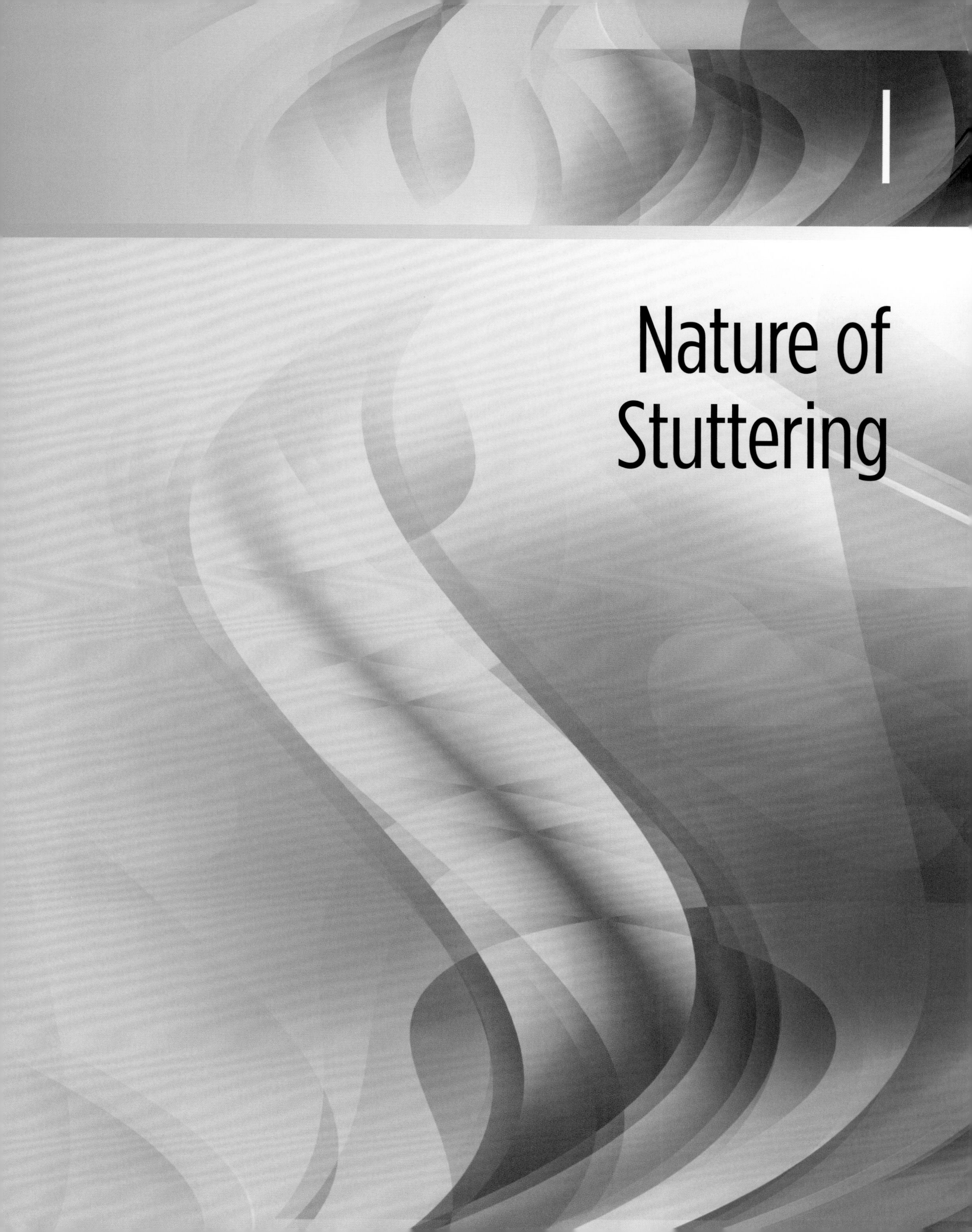

I

Nature of Stuttering

1

Introduction to Stuttering

Chapter Objectives

After studying this chapter, readers should be able to:

- Explain why it is good practice to use the term "person who stutters" rather than "stutterer"
- Describe factors that may (1) predispose a child to stutter, (2) precipitate stuttering, and (3) make stuttering persistent
- Name and describe the core behaviors of stuttering
- Name and describe the two major categories of secondary stuttering behaviors
- Name and describe different feelings and attitudes that can accompany stuttering
- Describe the elements of the new International Classification of Functioning, Disability, and Health (ICF) system that are most relevant to stuttering
- Discuss the age range of stuttering onset and the types of onset, and explain why the onset of stuttering is often difficult to pinpoint
- Describe the meanings of the terms "prevalence" and "incidence," and give current best estimates of each of these characteristics for stuttering
- Give an estimate of the number of children who recover without treatment, and describe factors that predict this recovery

- Give an estimate of the sex ratio in stuttering at onset and in the school-age population
- Explain what is meant by "anticipation," "consistency," and "adaptation" in stuttering
- Explain some relationships between stuttering and language, and suggest what they mean about the nature of the disorder
- Describe several conditions under which stuttering is usually reduced or absent, and suggest why this may be so

Key Terms

Adaptation: The tendency for speakers to stutter less and less (up to a point) when repeatedly reading a passage

Anticipation: An individual's ability to predict on which words or sounds he or she will stutter

Attitude: A feeling that has become a pervasive part of a person's beliefs

Avoidance behavior: A speaker's attempt to prevent stuttering when he or she anticipates stuttering on a word or in a situation. Word-based avoidances are commonly interjections of extra sounds, like "uh," said before the word on which stuttering is expected.

Block: A disfluency that is an inappropriate stoppage of the flow of air or voice and often the movement of articulators as well

Consistency: The tendency for speakers to stutter on the same words when reading a passage several times

Core behaviors: The basic speech behaviors of stuttering—repetition, prolongation, and block

Developmental stuttering: A term used to denote the most common form of stuttering that develops during childhood (in contrast to stuttering that develops in response to a neurological event or trauma or emotional stress)

Disfluency: An interruption of speech—such as a repetition, hesitancy, or prolongation of sound—that may occur in both individuals who are developing typically and those who stutter

Escape behavior: A speaker's attempts to terminate a stutter and finish the word. This occurs when the speaker is already in a moment of stuttering.

Fluency: The effortless flow of speech

Heterogeneity: Differences among various types of a disorder

Incidence: An index of how many people have stuttered at some time in their lives

Normal disfluency: An interruption of speech in a typically developing individual

Prevalence: A term used to indicate how widespread a disorder is over a relatively limited period of time

Prolongation: A disfluency in which sound or air flow continues but movement of the articulators is stopped

Repetition: A sound, syllable, or single-syllable word that is repeated several times. The speaker is apparently "stuck" on that sound or syllable and continues repeating it until the following sound can be produced.

Secondary behaviors: A speaker's reactions to his or her repetitions, prolongations, and blocks in an attempt to end them quickly or avoid them altogether. Such reactions may begin as random struggle but soon turn into well-learned patterns. Secondary behaviors can be divided into two broad classes: escape and avoidance behaviors.

PERSPECTIVE

No one is sure what causes stuttering, but it is an age-old problem that may have its origins in the way our brains evolved to produce speech and language. Its sudden appearance in some children is triggered when they try to talk using their just-emerging speech and language skills. Its many variations and manifestations are determined by individual brain structure and function, learning patterns, personality, and temperament. It also provides lessons about human nature: the variety of responses that stuttering provokes in cultures around the world is a reflection of the many ways in which humans deal with individual differences.

This description of stuttering makes it seem like a very complicated problem—one that will take a long time to learn about. It's true that you could spend a lifetime and still not know everything there is to know about stuttering. But you don't need to understand everything in order to help people who stutter. If you read this book critically and carefully, you will get a basic understanding of stuttering and a foundation for evaluating and treating people who stutter and their families. And once you start working with people who stutter, your understanding and ability will expand exponentially.

If you continue to work with stuttering, you will soon outgrow this book and begin to make your own discoveries. You will experience the satisfaction of helping children, adolescents, and adults regain an ability to communicate easily. Someday you may even write about your therapy procedures and measure their effectiveness. Those of us who have spent many years engaged in stuttering research and treatment all began where you are right now, at the threshold of an exciting and rewarding profession that can have a major impact on others' lives.

The Words We Use

In any field—whether it's education, medicine, or speech-language pathology—words may be used in specific ways. Definitions of many of the specialized terms used in our field are provided in the Key Terms list at the beginning of each chapter. But some words and phrases deserve to be discussed at the beginning.

People Who Stutter

Until recently, it was common practice to refer to people who stutter as "stutterers." In fact, some of us who stutter refer to ourselves as stutterers and feel some pride in this term. It reminds me that a friend of mine who has Parkinson's disease is happy to call himself a "parkie" and even "a mover and shaker." However, many people prefer not to be labeled "a stutterer" and prefer instead to be called "a person who stutters." They feel, and rightly so, that stuttering is only a small part of who they are.

Adults who stutter often say that changing the way they think of themselves—as people who happen to stutter but with many more important attributes—was one of the most significant things they did to break free of the bonds of stuttering. Such reports remind us that clients are far more than people who stutter. They are people, each with a huge array of characteristics, only one of which happens to be that they stutter. This way of thinking enables us to help both our clients and their families. When we use the phrase "child who stutters" rather than "stutterer," families listen beyond the sounds of stuttering to the thoughts and feelings that their children are communicating. It helps everyone view disfluencies in perspective as only a small part of the whole child.

Some authors abbreviate "people who stutter" as "PWS." Personally, I feel that substituting an acronym that highlights stuttering is not really different from using "stutterer." In fact it may be even more demeaning. So I won't employ "PWS" as an acronym. However, I know that the language in this book would grow stale and cumbersome if I were to use "person who stutters" over and over. So I often refer to the "adult . . .," "child . . .," or "adolescent you are working with."

Disfluency

In our literature, "**disfluency**" is used to denote interruptions of speech that may be either normal or abnormal. That is, it can apply to pauses, repetitions, and other hesitancies in individuals who are typical speakers. It can also apply to moments of stuttering. This makes it a handy term to use when describing the speech of young children whose diagnosis is unclear.

When someone's speech hesitancies are unequivocally not stuttering, I'll use the term "typical disfluency." I won't use the older term for the abnormal hesitations in stuttering—"dysfluency" with a "y"—because it can easily be mistaken for "disfluency" when you see it on the page and because the two are indistinguishable when spoken.

OVERVIEW OF THE DISORDER

This section previews the next few chapters on the nature of stuttering and gives me a chance to reveal my own slant on the disorder. I think this may be helpful for anyone, but especially for those readers who have not had a course in stuttering and who may, therefore, know few details of its nature.

Do All Cultures Have Stuttering?

Stuttering is found in all parts of the world and in all cultures and races. It is indiscriminate of occupation, intelligence, and income; it affects both sexes and people of all ages, from toddlers to the elderly. It is an old curse, and there is evidence that it was present in Chinese, Egyptian, and Mesopotamian cultures more than 40 centuries ago (Van Riper, 1982). Moses was said to have stuttered (Garfinkel, 1995) and to have used a trick typical of many of us who stutter—getting his brother to speak for him. I did something similar when I was asked to read a prayer aloud in Sunday school.

What Causes People to Stutter?

The cause of stuttering is still something of a mystery. Scientists have yet to discover what causes stuttering, but they have many clues. First, there is strong evidence that stuttering often has a genetic basis—that is, something is inherited that makes it more likely a child will stutter. This genetic "something" has to do with the way a child's brain develops its neural pathways for speech and language. For example, the neural pathways for talking may be less dense and less well developed in those who stutter. This could impede the rapid flow of information needed to precisely sequence the movements of many muscles needed for fluent speech. What's more, the commands to muscles must be coordinated with the many components of language, including word choice, syntax, and semantics. The pathways may also be vulnerable to disruption by other brain activity, such as emotions. Isn't it amazing that many of us learn to talk at 200 syllables per minute, using huge vocabularies and complicated syntax and suiting what we say to every particular situation!

Another clue about the nature of stuttering is that most stuttering begins in children between ages 2 and 5. Thus, the onset of stuttering occurs at about the same time that many typical stresses of early childhood are occurring. One child may begin to stutter during a dramatic growth in vocabulary and syntax. Another's stuttering may first appear when the family moves to a new home. Still another child may start soon after a baby brother or sister is born. Many different factors, acting singly or in combination, may precipitate the onset of stuttering in a child who has a neurophysiological predisposition, or inborn tendency, for stuttering.

Once stuttering starts, it may disappear within a few months, or it may get gradually worse. When it gets worse, learned reactions may be an important factor in its severity. Playmates at school or adults who don't know how to correctly respond may cause a child to become highly self-conscious about his stuttering. The child will quickly learn that by pushing hard, he can get traction on a word that has been stuck. He may find that an eye blink or an "um" said quickly before trying to say a hard word may avoid stuttering temporarily. By the time a child is a teenager, learned reactions influence many of the symptoms. He has learned to anticipate stuttering and may thrash around in a panic when he speaks, trying to escape or avoid it. By adulthood, his fear of stuttering and his desire to avoid it can permeate his lifestyle. An adult who stutters often copes with it by limiting his work, friends, and fun to those situations and people that put few demands on speech. Figure 1.1 provides an

Repeated embarrassment with stuttering leads to negative feelings and attitudes about communication
I wish talking were easier
Hey... uh...l-l-lets go... uh... p-p-play v...v...v... well... uh... video games
Yo! B-B-BILLY! how cccome you talk so f-f-funny?
Age 18
Age 8
Now stop and start over
Environmental influences such as criticism of speech or stressful events combine with neurodevelopmental factors to make stuttering more severe and chronic
I wo... wo... wonder what sssschool will be... be... like
Billy, we're going to be moving tomorrow!
Age 6
Mmm... mommy's sock
Speech and language acquisition and other developmental influences precipitate disfluencies
Age 3
Genetic and congenital influences predispose the child to stuttering
Mommy's sock
Mommy sock
Sock
Start

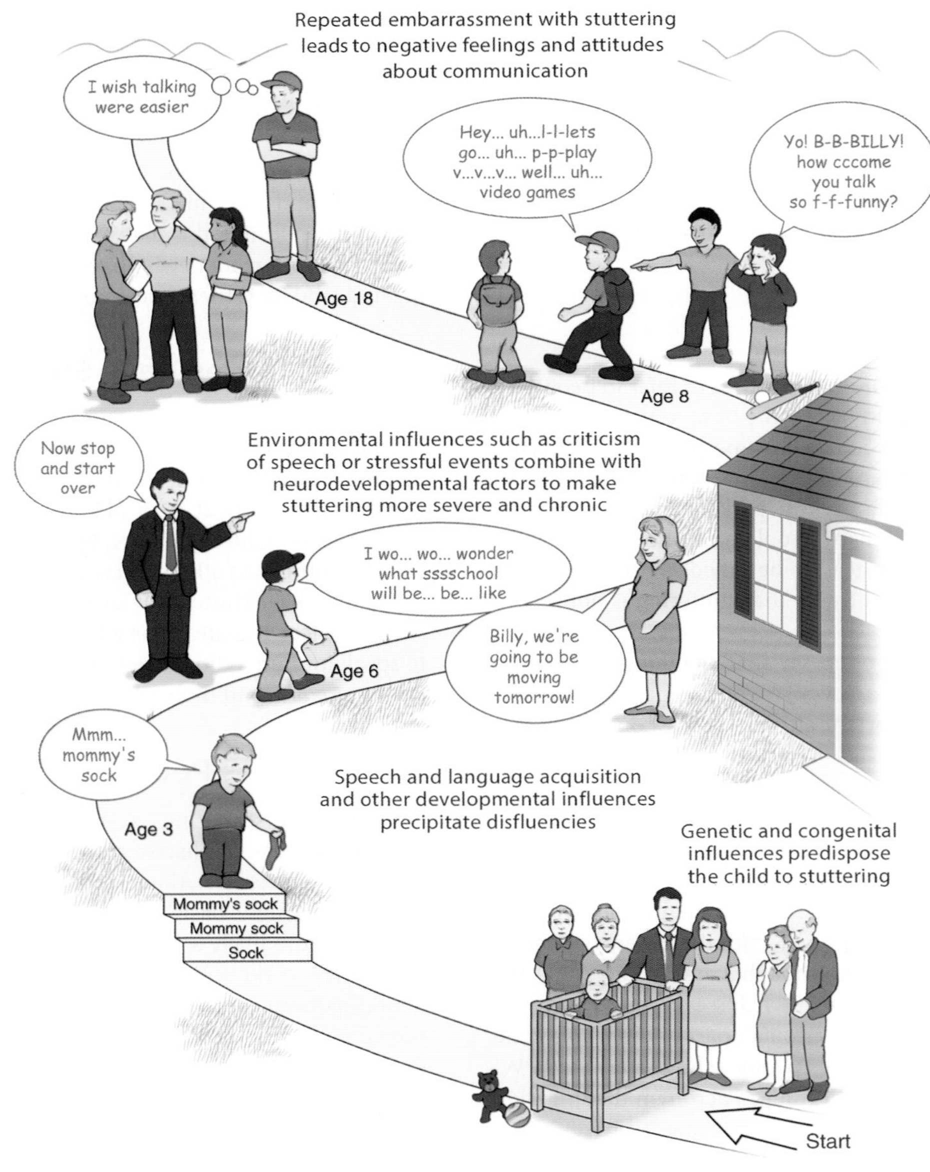

Figure 1.1 Factors contributing to the development of stuttering.

overview of many of the contributing factors in the evolution of stuttering. In this and the subsequent four chapters, I'll describe in detail our current understanding of these influences.

Can Stuttering Be Cured?

As implied above, it often cures itself. Many young children who begin to stutter recover without treatment. For others, early intervention may be needed to help the child develop typical fluency and prevent the development of a chronic problem. Once stuttering has become firmly established, however, and the child has developed many learned reactions, a concerted treatment effort is needed. Good treatment of mild and moderate stuttering in preschool and early elementary school children may leave them with little trace of stuttering, except perhaps when they are stressed, fatigued, or ill. Most of those who stutter severely for a long time or who are not treated until after puberty achieve only a partial recovery. Some of these people are able to learn to speak more slowly or stutter more easily and to be less bothered by their stuttering. Some, however, will not improve, despite our best efforts.

DEFINITIONS

Fluency

By beginning with a definition of fluency rather than stuttering, I am pointing out how many elements must be maintained in the flow of speech if a speaker is to be considered fluent. It is an impressive balancing act. Little wonder that everyone slips and stumbles from time to time when they talk.

Fluency is hard to define. In fact, most researchers have focused on its opposite, disfluency. (As I mentioned earlier in this chapter, I use the term disfluency to apply both to stuttering and to typical hesitations, making it easier to refer to hesitations that could be either typical or abnormal.) One of the early fluency researchers, Freida Goldman-Eisler (1968), showed that typical speech is filled with hesitations. Other researchers have acknowledged this and expanded the study of fluent speech by contrasting it with disfluent speech. Dalton and Hardcastle (1977), for example, distinguished fluent from disfluent speech by differences in the variables listed in Table 1.1. Inclusion of intonation and stress in this list may seem unusual. It could be said that speakers who reduce stuttering by using a monotone are not really fluent. We would argue that it is not their fluency but the "naturalness" of their speech that is affected. Nonetheless, both aspects will be of interest to the clinician working to help clients with all areas of their communication.

Starkweather (1980, 1987) suggested that many of the variables that determine fluency reflect temporal aspects of speech production. These include such variables as pauses, rhythm, intonation, stress, and rate that are controlled by when and how fast we move our speech structures. So, our temporal control of the movements of these structures determines our fluency. Starkweather also noted that the rate of information flow, not just sound flow, is an important aspect of fluency. Thus, a person who speaks without

TABLE 1.1 Variables Useful in Distinguishing between Fluent and Disfluent Speech*

Variable	Example of Disfluency
1. Presence of extra sounds, such as repetitions, prolongations, interjections, and revisions	If a speaker says "I-I-I nnnnneed to have uh my uh, well, I-I-I should get mmmmmy car fixed," he sounds disfluent.
2. Location and frequency of pauses	If a speaker says, "Whenever I remember to bring my umbrella (pause), it never rains," he sounds fluent. But if he says, "Whenever (pause) I remember to bring (pause) my (pause) umbrella, it never (pause) rains," he sounds disfluent.
3. Rhythmic patterning in speech	English is typically spoken with stressed syllables at relatively equal intervals; in general, stressed syllables are followed by several unstressed syllables. When marked deviations from this pattern occur, as when a speaker with cerebellar disease stresses all syllables equally, the speaker sounds disfluent.
4. Intonation and stress	If a speaker does not vary intonation and stress and is therefore monotonous, he may be considered disfluent. Abnormal intonation and stress patterns may also be considered disfluent.
5. Overall rate	If a speaker has a very slow rate of speech or has bursts of fast rates interspersed with slower rates, he may be considered disfluent.

*Suggested by Dalton and Hardcastle (1977).

hesitations but has difficulty conveying information in a timely and orderly fashion might not be considered a fluent speaker.

In his description of fluency, Starkweather (1987) also included the effort with which a person speaks. By effort, he means both the mental and physical work a speaker exerts when speaking. This is difficult to measure, but it may turn out that trained listeners can make such judgments reliably. Moreover, mental and physical effort may reflect important components of what it feels like to be a person who stutters.

In essence, fluency can be thought of simply as the effortless flow of speech. Thus, a speaker who is judged to be "fluent" appears to use little effort when speaking. However, the components of such apparently effortless speech flow are hard to pin down. As researchers analyze fluency more carefully, they may find that the appearance of excess effort may give rise to judgments that a person is stuttering. However, other elements, such as unusual rhythm or slow rate of information flow, may result in judgments that a person is not a fluent speaker, but is not a stutterer either. I will discuss aspects of fluency again when I relate some of the elements of fluency, such as rate and naturalness, to various therapy approaches.

Stuttering

General Description

At first, stuttering may appear to be complex and mysterious, but much of it is based on human nature and can be easily understood if you think about your own experiences. In some ways, it is like a problem you might have with a cell phone.

Imagine that you have a cell phone with intermittent problems, such as not holding a charge, dropping calls, and dropping words in the middle of a conversation. The listener may say, in an impatient voice, "What did you say? I can hardly hear you." Then momentarily the connection may clear up and you feel relief, only to be followed by exasperation when the call gets noisy again or is completely dropped (Fig. 1.2).

Compare this with the interruptions in communication caused by stuttering. The typical behaviors of stuttering—repetitions, prolongations, and blocks—often interfere with the smooth flow of information. It's not unusual, in my experience, for a listener to respond to my stuttering by asking, "What did you say?"

Returning to the cell phone analogy: When you realize the listener isn't hearing you, you might resort to talking louder or slower or just giving up and calling back later. Similarly, speakers who are stuttering usually react to their repetitions, prolongations, or blocks by trying to force words out or by using extra sounds, words, or movements in their efforts to become "unstuck" or to avoid getting stuck. Sometimes they just give up and say "Never mind."

If your cell phone calls were often hard to understand and calls were often dropped, you would probably develop some bad feelings about your phone. The first time it happened, you would be surprised. Then, as it happened more and more, surprise would give way to frustration. If you frequently had poor connections, dropped calls, and not holding a charge, you would begin to anticipate problems and become afraid they would happen whenever you tried to make an important call.

The person who stutters goes through many of the same feelings—surprise, frustration, dread. These feelings—in combination with the actual difficulty in speaking—may cause the stutterer to limit himself in school, in social situations, and at work. This might be similar to your responses to a troublesome cell phone. After months of problems, you would probably use a landline, e-mail, or other forms of communication.

Another aspect of any description of stuttering involves specifying what it is not. For example, an important distinction must be made between the stuttering behaviors just described and typical hesitations. Children whose speech and language are developing typically often display repetitions, revisions, and pauses—which are not stuttering. Neither are the brief repetitions, revisions, and pauses in the speech of most nonstuttering adults when they are in a hurry or uncertain. Chapter 7 describes the differences between typical disfluency and stuttering in more detail to prepare you for the task of differential diagnosis of stuttering in children.

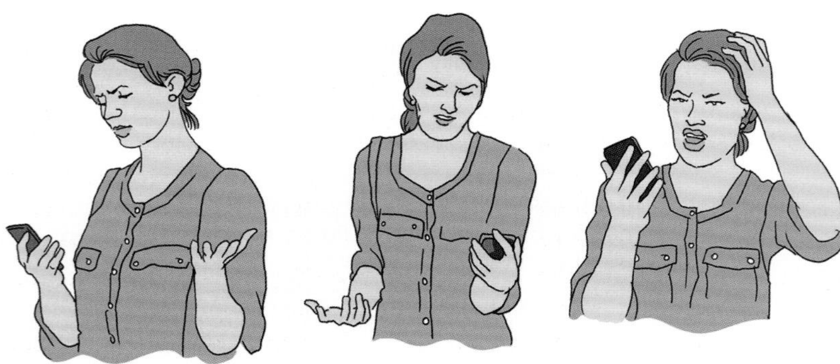

Figure 1.2 Stuttering can be like having a cell phone that doesn't always work.

A distinction should also be made between stuttering and certain other fluency disorders. Disfluency resulting from cerebral damage or disease or psychological trauma differs from stuttering that begins in childhood. In addition, stuttering differs from cluttering, another fluency disorder, which is characterized by rapid, sometimes unintelligible speech. These other fluency disorders may be treated somewhat differently than stuttering, although some of the same techniques that clinicians use with stuttering are also useful with these disorders. These other disorders are discussed in Chapter 15.

Core Behaviors

I have adopted the term "**core behaviors**" from Van Riper (1971, 1982), who used it to describe the basic speech behaviors of stuttering: repetitions, prolongations, and blocks. These behaviors seem involuntary to the person who stutters, as if they are out of her control. They differ from the "secondary behaviors" that a stutterer acquires as learned reactions to the basic core behaviors.

Repetitions are the core behaviors observed most frequently among children who are just beginning to stutter. Repetitions consist of a sound, syllable, or single-syllable word that is repeated several times. The speaker is apparently "stuck" on that sound and continues repeating it until the following sound can be produced. In children who have not been stuttering for long, single-syllable word repetitions and part-word repetitions are much more common than multisyllabic word repetitions. Moreover, children who stutter will frequently repeat a word or syllable more than twice per instance, li-li-li-li-like this (Yairi, 1983; Yairi & Lewis, 1984).

Prolongations of voiced or voiceless sounds also appear in the speech of children beginning to stutter. They usually appear somewhat later than repetitions (Van Riper, 1982), although both Johnson and associates (1959) and Yairi (1997a) reported that prolongations—as well as repetitions—may be present at onset. I use the term **prolongation** to denote those stutters in which sound or air flow continues but movement of the articulators is stopped. Prolongations as short as half a second may be perceived as abnormal, but in rare cases they may last as long as several minutes in adults who stutter severely (Van Riper, 1982). In contrast to my use of the term, earlier writers include stutters with no sound or airflow as well as stopped movement of the articulators in their definitions of prolongations (e.g., Van Riper, 1982; Wingate, 1964).

Repetitions and sound prolongations are usually part of the core behaviors of more advanced stutterers, as well as of children just beginning to stutter. Sheehan (1974) found that repetitive stutters occurred in every speech sample of 20 adults who stuttered. Indeed, 66 percent of their stutters were repetitions. Although many of their stutters were also prolongations, as defined above, how many is not clear, because Sheehan's definition of prolongations seems to differ from mine.

Blocks are typically the last core behavior to appear. However, as with prolongations, some investigators (Johnson and associates, 1959; Yairi, 1997a) have observed blocks in children's speech at or close to stuttering onset. Blocks occur when a person inappropriately stops the flow of air or voice and often the movement of her articulators as well. Blocks may involve any level of the speech production mechanism—respiratory, laryngeal, or articulatory. There is some evidence and much theorizing that inappropriate muscle activity at the laryngeal level characterizes most blocks (Conture, McCall, & Brewer, 1977; Freeman & Ushijima, 1978; Kenyon, 1942; Schwartz, 1974). Others disagree (Smith, Denny, Shaffer, Kelly, & Hirano, 1996).

As stuttering persists, blocks often grow longer and more tense, and tremors may become evident. These rapid oscillations, most easily observable in the lips or jaw, occur when someone has blocked on a word or sound. The individual closes off the airway, increases air pressure behind the closure, and squeezes her muscles particularly hard (Van Riper, 1982). You can duplicate these tremors by trying to say the word "by" while squeezing your lips together hard and building up air pressure behind the block. Imagine this happening to you unexpectedly when you were trying to talk.

People who stutter differ from one another in how frequently they stutter and how long their individual core behaviors last. Research indicates that a person who stutters does so on average on about 10 percent of the words while reading aloud, although individuals vary greatly (Bloodstein, 1944; Bloodstein & Ratner, 2008). Many people who stutter mildly do so on fewer than 5 percent of the words they speak or read aloud, and a few with severe stuttering stutter on more than 50 percent of the words. The durations of core behaviors vary much less, averaging around 1 second, and are rarely longer than 5 seconds (Bloodstein, 1944; Bloodstein & Ratner, 2008).

Secondary Behaviors

People who stutter dislike stuttering, to put it mildly. They react to their repetitions, prolongations, and blocks by trying to end them quickly if they can't avoid them altogether. Such reactions may begin as a random struggle to get the word out, but soon turn into well-learned patterns. I divide **secondary behaviors** into two broad classes: escape behaviors and avoidance behaviors. I make this division, rather than follow the traditional approach of dealing with secondary behaviors as "starters" or "postponements," for example, because my treatment procedures focus on the principles by which secondary behaviors are learned.

The terms "escape" and "avoidance" are borrowed from behavioral learning literature. Briefly, **escape behaviors** occur when a speaker is stuttering and attempts to terminate the stutter and finish the word. Common examples of escape behaviors are eye blinks, head nods, and interjections of extra sounds, such as "uh," which are often followed by the termination of a stutter and are therefore reinforced. **Avoidance behaviors**, on the other hand, are learned when a speaker anticipates stuttering and recalls (consciously or unconsciously) negative experiences he has had when stuttering. To avoid stuttering and the negative experience that it entails, he often resorts to behaviors he has used previously to escape from moments of stuttering—eye blinks or "uh"s, for example. But he employs these behaviors before attempting to say the word he expects to stutter on. Or, he may try something different, such as changing the word he was planning to say.

In many cases, especially at first, avoidance behaviors may prevent the stutter from occurring and provide highly rewarding emotional relief from the increasing fear that a stutter will occur. Soon these avoidance behaviors become strong habits that are resistant to change. The many subcategories of avoidances (e.g., postponements, starters, substitutions, and timing devices such as hand movements timed to saying the word) are described in Chapter 7.

When trying to decide if a secondary behavior is an escape or avoidance, just remember that an escape behavior occurs only after a moment of stuttering has begun, and an avoidance behavior occurs before the moment of stuttering begins.

Feelings and Attitudes

A person's feelings can be as much a part of the disorder of stuttering as his speech behaviors. Feelings may precipitate stutters, just as stutters may create feelings. In the beginning, a child's positive feelings of excitement or negative feelings of fear may result in repetitive stutters that he hardly notices. Then, as he stutters more frequently, he may become frustrated or ashamed because he can't say what he wants to say—even his own name—as smoothly and quickly as others. These feelings make speaking harder, as frustration and shame increase effort and tension and impede fluent speech. Feelings that result from stuttering may include not only frustration and shame but also fear of stuttering again, guilt about not being able to help oneself, and hostility toward listeners as well.

Attitudes are feelings that have become a pervasive part of a person's beliefs. As a person who stutters experiences more and more stuttering, he begins to believe that he is a person who generally has trouble speaking, just as you might believe that cell phone or your service is a lemon if you continue to have trouble calling. Adolescents and adults who stutter usually have many negative attitudes about themselves that are derived from years of stuttering experiences (Blood, Blood, Tellis, & Gabel, 2001; Daniels, Gabel, & Hughes, 2012; Gildston, 1967; Rahman, 1956; Wallen, 1960). A person who stutters often projects his attitudes on listeners, believing that they think he is stupid or nervous. Sometimes, however, listeners may contribute directly to the person's attitudes. Research has shown that most people, even classroom teachers and speech-language pathologists, stereotype people who stutter as tense, insecure, and fearful (e.g., MacKinnon, Hall, & MacIntyre, 2007; Turnbaugh, Guitar, & Hoffman, 1979; Woods & Williams, 1976). Such listener stereotypes can affect the way individuals who stutter see themselves, and changing a client's negative attitudes about himself can be a major focus of treatment.

The three components of stuttering—core behaviors, secondary behaviors, and feelings and attitudes—are depicted in Figure 1.3. The core behavior is the individual's block on the "N" in "New York." The secondary behaviors consist of postponement devices such as "uh," "well," and "you know" and substitution of "the Big Apple" for "New York." These secondary behaviors are avoidances. Feelings and attitudes are depicted as the individual's thoughts that he won't succeed in saying the word fluently and the individual's belief that listeners will think he is dumb because he stutters.

Functioning, Disability, and Health

Some time ago, the World Health Organization (WHO, 1980) adopted the International Classification of Impairment, Disabilities, and Handicaps to describe the consequences of various diseases and disorders. A number of authors have applied this framework to stuttering (Curlee, 1993; McClean, 1990; Prins, 1991, 1999; Yaruss, 1998, 1999). More than a decade ago, WHO changed its taxonomy to the International Classification of Functioning, Disability, and Health (ICF) (2001). Even more recently, they have devised a version that is specific to children and youth—the ICF-CY (WHO, 2007). In the following paragraphs, I will suggest ways in which this system may be applied to stuttering.

The taxonomy begins with "Functioning and Disability," wherein body structures and body functions are considered. Structures that are dysfunctional in stuttering, as brain imaging studies have shown, are cortical and subcortical structures, such as white matter tracts that may be critical for coordinating planning, execution, and sensory feedback for speech. Functions that differ in stuttering are the interruptions of speech flow that characterize the disorder. The ICF system becomes more useful when "Activity and Participation" are considered. Individuals who stutter may be affected to a greater or lesser extent in two of the ICF activity areas, "Speaking" and "Conversation." These are domains in which stuttering is noticeable. A third area, "Interpersonal Interactions," may also be affected if speaking and conversation are restricted by the stuttering to the extent that the person who stutters refrains from fully engaging with others thereby affecting his or her participation in different social roles (e.g., being a student or a family member).

A new and important section of the latest ICF system is titled "Contextual Factors." One component of this section is the "Environment." This is particularly relevant to individuals who stutter because people in the environment may range

Core Behavior
"I WENT TO N.... N.... NEW YORK"
Secondary Behavior
"I WENT TO.... UH.... WELL.... YOU KNOW.... UH.... UH.... THE BIG APPLE"
Feelings and Attitudes
"Where did you go last weekend?"
Oh no, I'll never get this word out. She'll think I'm really dumb.

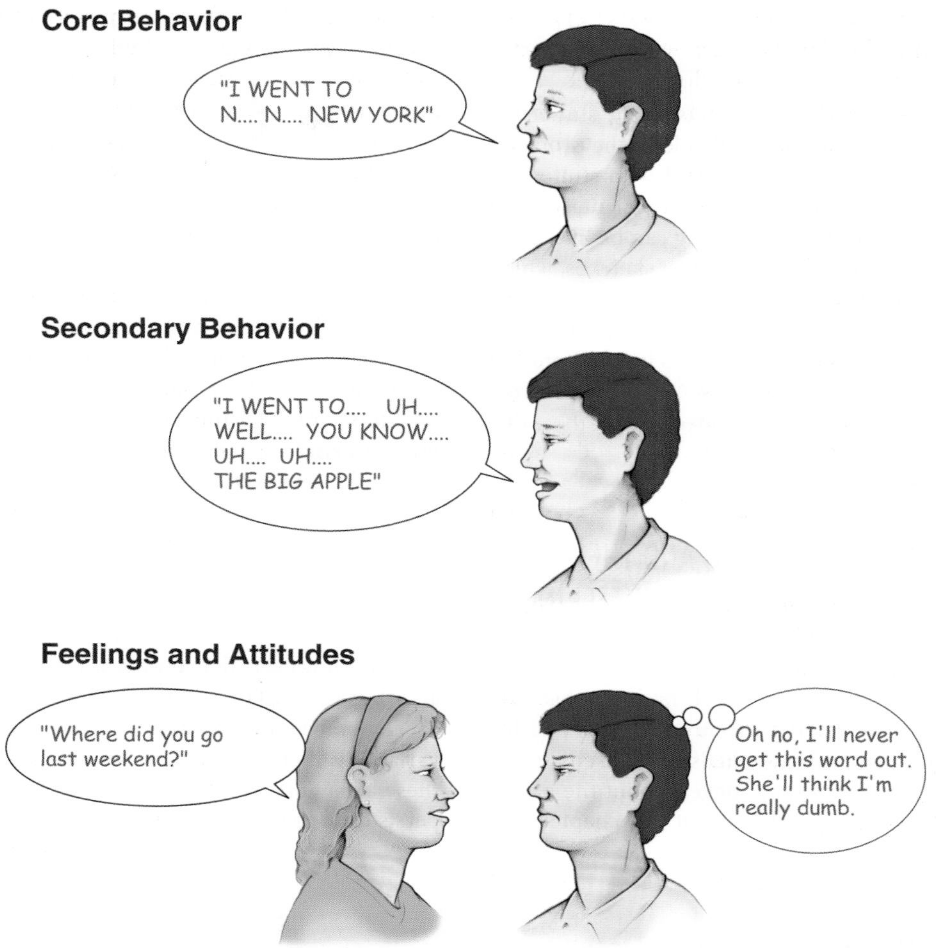

Figure 1.3 Components of stuttering: core behaviors, secondary behaviors, and feelings and attitudes.

from unsupportive (e.g., a home with great stress or classmates who tease a child) to highly supportive (e.g., a family that is accepting of the child and encouraging of her participation). Also under "Contextual Factors" is the category of "Personal Factors." These are the attributes of a person who stutters—her character and personality.

Consider the influence of environmental and personal factors on two individuals who stutter. The first is the successful former CEO of General Electric, Jack Welch, who authored *Jack: Straight from the Gut*. His assertive temperament and early acceptance of his stuttering by his family were no doubt important in helping him succeed in the high-pressure world of corporate boardrooms. From an early age, Welch refused to let stuttering stand in the way of his goals (Welch & Byrne, 2001). In contrast, actor James Earl Jones initially reacted to his stuttering in a vastly different way. When he was 6 years old, he was so traumatized by his stuttering that he pretended he was mute so he wouldn't have to speak. Only later, with the support of someone in his environment—a high school English teacher—did he begin to learn that he could overcome his stuttering by facing difficult situations and practicing reading aloud in front of an audience (Jones & Niven, 1993).

Other examples of men who had stuttered severely since childhood but obtained excellent college educations, were highly successful in business, and used their wealth to help others include Malcolm Fraser, who was a cofounder of the National Auto Parts Association and created the Stuttering Foundation of America, and Walter Annenberg, who established a media empire and later the Annenberg Foundation, a large philanthropic organization.

In all four cases, their functioning may have been impaired, but environmental and personal factors enabled them to overcome potential limitations in the domains of speaking and interpersonal interactions. You can see in this classification system why clinicians play a vital role in the lives of children and adults who stutter. They can influence environmental factors by helping families, teachers, and entire schools become supportive of the individuals who stutter and facilitative of increased fluency. And they can help build the personal attributes of each client through counseling, insightful listening, educating, and caring.

THE HUMAN FACE OF STUTTERING

Before I delve deeper into the basic facts about stuttering, I'd like to touch briefly on the personal side of the problem. Some of you may never have had a friend who stutters or may never have worked with a stutterer in treatment, so I will present several examples of what stuttering can be like. Even if you are familiar with stuttering, these brief sketches, which portray four individuals who differ in age and in their accommodations to stuttering, may expand your sense of what stuttering is like for the person who experiences it. I will present these case studies in the next few pages. You may also visit *thePoint* (thepoint.lww.com) to watch video clips of these different levels of stuttering.

BASIC FACTS ABOUT STUTTERING AND THEIR IMPLICATIONS FOR THE NATURE OF STUTTERING

This section relates some of the best-known "facts" about stuttering. These are established research findings that pertain to when and where stuttering occurs and how variable it is, in the population and in individuals. As I discuss these findings, I will point out what they suggest about the nature of stuttering. Thus, as you read the rest of this chapter, you will become increasingly aware of my perspective on the nature and treatment of stuttering.

Much has been made of the "**heterogeneity**" of stuttering; a number of authors have suggested that stuttering is not one disorder, but many. Researchers have proposed various divisions of the disorder, such as Van Riper's (1982) four "tracks" of stuttering development and St. Onge's (1963) triad of speech-phobic, psychogenic, and organic stutterers. There are also suggestions of different brain anomalies in some subtypes of individuals who stutter (Foundas et al., 2004). My approach is to focus on the majority of people who stutter—those whose stuttering begins during childhood without an apparent link to psychological or organic trauma. This most common type of stuttering has been called "**developmental stuttering**," because symptoms usually emerge gradually as a child develops, especially during the period of intense speech and language acquisition. I simply call it "stuttering." In denoting similar fluency problems that are associated with psychological problems, brain damage, cognitive impairment, and cluttering, I refer to their assumed etiology, such as "disfluencies associated with brain damage."

Note, however, that even within the group of individuals whose stuttering begins in early childhood during rapid speech and language development, there is a great deal of variability in the behaviors we call stuttering and in how these behaviors come and go as the child progresses toward persistence or recovery.

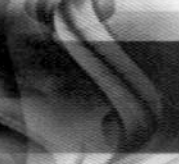

Case Examples

A Young Preschool Child: Borderline Stuttering

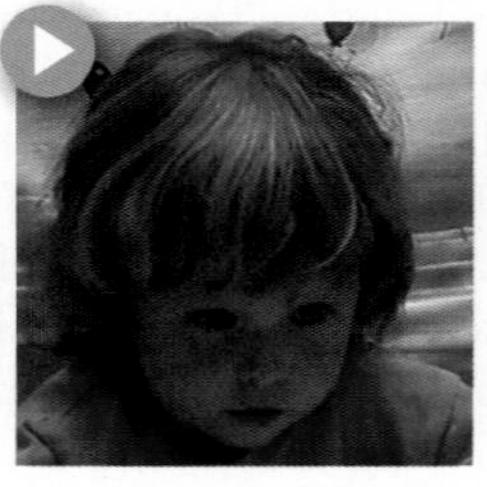

Ashley was a happy, outgoing child who was advanced in her language development; she spoke in well-formed sentences when she was 18 months old. Then suddenly, when she was 21 months old, she began to stutter. Her stuttering took the form of multiple repetitions, most often at the beginnings of sentences. For example she would say "I-I-I-I want some water" or "Ca-ca-ca-ca-can you lift me up?" Despite the fact that she would sometimes repeat a syllable 10 or more times before getting the word out, she didn't show obvious signs of frustration when she stuttered. She continued to develop language rapidly, talk copiously, and socialize easily.

About 6 months after she started stuttering, her parents contacted a speech-language pathologist who evaluated Ashley. The evaluation indicated that Ashley's language development was advanced for her age, that her phonological development was also advanced, and that she stuttered on 4 percent of the syllables she spoke. (This means that when a few minutes of her speech were analyzed and the number of syllables she spoke was counted, Ashley stuttered on 4 percent of those syllables.)

Ashley's parents told the clinician that they had no idea why Ashley started stuttering. She was happy, secure, and talkative; no big event occurred around the time of stuttering onset; and she didn't have any relatives who stuttered.

For a description of Ashley's treatment and its outcome, turn to Chapter 11.

continued

Discussion

The two segments in this video show Ashley talking about a picture (a cat named Cookie knocking a plant off a shelf) that the clinician has previously described to her. In the first segment, the clinician elicits Ashley's response by asking "What happened to Cookie, again?" Ashley's response is "Cat....nn...de-de-de .... Coo-Coo-[approximately 15 repetitions of this syllable]-Cookie knocked the plant down." In the second segment, the clinician says "Let's take another one. Tell me. Remember?" Ashley replies "Then Coo-Coo-Coo-Coo-Cookie knocked the plant down."

These segments are a pretty good illustration of what stuttering can be like when it first starts in a preschool child. What are the primary core behaviors that Ashley shows? Repetitions? Prolongations? Blocks?

When we are trying to determine whether a child needs immediate and direct treatment for stuttering, it is often helpful to assess the child's emotional reaction to her stuttering. Can you tell from the video whether Ashley is frustrated or embarrassed by her stuttering? What do you see in the video that gives you clues about this?

An Older Preschool Child: Beginning Stuttering

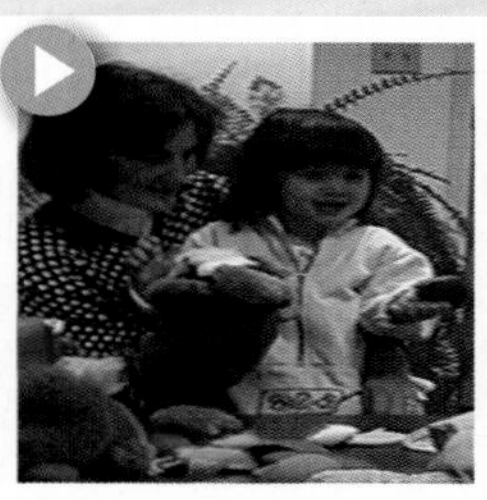

Katherine developed speech and language normally, speaking her first word at about 1 year and beginning to combine words at 15 months with complete fluency. When she was 3, after a particularly hectic Christmas holiday, she began to stutter. Her first disfluencies were easy part- and whole-word repetitions, but she soon began to tense her articulators, momentarily blocking the flow of speech until the word "popped out." Sometimes, when she was completely stuck for several seconds, she responded by hitting her parents or crying out. She also showed much less interest in talking and using new words and phrases.

Her parents soon brought her to a speech and language clinic for an evaluation. Katherine was found to be stuttering on 21 percent of the syllables she spoke—a very high percentage for any child. Her overall severity was assessed with the Stuttering Severity Instrument (Riley, 1994), which rated it as severe. Her receptive language was found to be far above average for her age. Her expressive language was found to be typical for her age, but it was likely that she was inhibited in expressing herself because of her stuttering. Her phonological development was found to be appropriate for her age.

For a description of Katherine's treatment, see Chapter 12.

Discussion

In Segment 1, Katherine responds to a question from her mother by saying "O-O-O-O...an...an...an...OK now...I think he is still hungry...[unintelligible]...a leaf." This may be an example of a child getting stuck on an attempt to say a word ("OK") and then, finding herself in a block, changing the word she tries to say (from "OK" to "and"). Then she is able to say the original word and go on.

In Segment 2, still with her mother, she is stuck on the first sound of the word "OK," then she seems to be able to move on to the "kay" but gets stuck there too, and so she doubles back to the "o" and finally finishes the word by pushing out of the stutter on "o" and then having a slight stutter on the first sound of "kay." Whew! You can see how much work this 3-year-old must do just to get a few words out. No wonder she doesn't seem as expressive as she did before her stuttering started.

In Segment 3, Katherine is playing with the clinician and says, "uh...nnnnn...ne...ne...nnnn...na...now, what is this?" The "uh" might be Katherine's way of getting ready for the stutter she anticipates on "now."

In Segment 4, Katherine is playing with both of her parents and says "Lo-look what I made. Oh... uh...bbbbb...buh...bbbbb...buh..." The first stutter is a part-word repetition ("lo-look") that is so mild it might be considered a **typical disfluency** in another context. But the second stutter (on a word beginning with "b") is quite a long stutter in which Katherine struggles heroically to produce the word but is interrupted by the door opening before she can finish. How would you describe this last stutter? Repetition? Prolongation? Block? What emotions do you think she's feeling? Why do you think so?

continued

A School-Age Child: Intermediate Stuttering

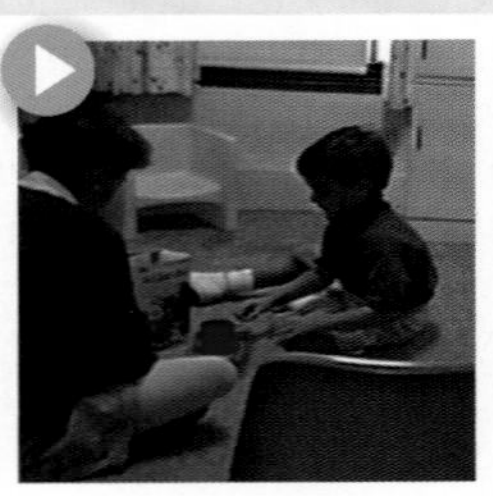

David was the second of three children in a family with no history of speech or language disorders. His speech was developing normally until age 4, when he began to show excessive part-word and whole-word repetitions. After several months, when David's stuttering had not decreased, his mother took him to his pediatrician who assured her it would resolve on its own.

When David was almost 6, his stuttering was growing steadily more severe, and he was avoiding talking in many situations. His mother then decided to consult a speech-language pathologist at a university clinic, who evaluated David. In the evaluation, David was stuttering on 8 percent of his syllables spoken; many stutters were tightly squeezed blocks with evident struggle behavior.

David's subsequent treatment and his current status as a 20-something-year-old are described in Chapter 13.

Discussion

In this video, you can see how stuttering may be more complicated as children grow older and become more self-conscious. In the video for the first child, Ashley's moments of stuttering seemed to pop up out of the blue and surprise her. In the video for the second child, Katherine's stuttering was a little more predictable to her, but it was mostly confined to those few words on which she got blocked. Now we will see that David's stuttering affects more of his entire speech pattern and is characterized by much avoidance and struggle.

In Segment 1, showing him talking with his mother, David's style of speaking is hesitant, with many stops, "ums," false starts, and changes in direction. He says something like "and then...it like that...and then...then put...um the same a-mount of...of...of...of ...um... [then some unintelligible words, after which he seems to give up on the sentence and begins counting]." As you can imagine, it's hard to assess what percentage of syllables are stuttered when David avoids saying the words on which he expects to stutter.

Segment 2 shows a block on the word "whoever," preceded by several words that seem to postpone David's attempt on this word. He says "and then ...uh ...whoever gets um ...um the four, four... an, an ... um ... um these [unintelligible word]." Do you think he expects to stutter on "whoever?" What are the cues that tell you so? What escape behaviors does David use as he struggles with this block?

In Segment 3, David has another block with a few avoidance behaviors before the stutter and escape behaviors during it. He says "He ... [unintelligible word] ... he goes home automatically because ... um ... because he-he has done the shortcut an-an he goes all the way home." Can you describe the avoidance and escape behaviors David shows in this clip?

An Adult: Advanced Stuttering

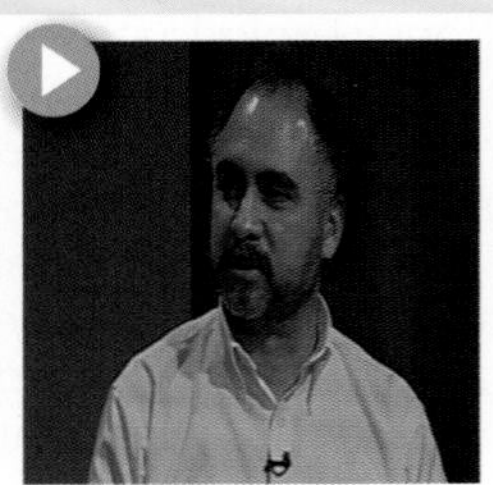

Sergio is a 44-year-old musician who has stuttered since he was 3 years old. Eight of his maternal aunts and uncles stuttered, suggesting a genetic origin to his problem. His stuttering began as multiple repetitions of one-syllable words and parts of words. Much of his speech was fluent, but whenever he was excited or hurried, Sergio's stuttering flared up, sending his parents into a state of alarm and concern for his future. At first, his father's solution for Sergio's stuttering was hitting him on the head with his knuckles when he blocked. When this failed and Sergio developed physically tense prolongations and blocks that occurred regularly in his speech, his parents took him to various therapists, including a hypnotist and a psychotherapist who prescribed tranquilizers. None of these seemed to have more than a temporary effect, and Sergio's stuttering grew steadily worse. During his elementary and junior high school years, he was frequently ridiculed for his stuttering, even by teachers, and Sergio found himself an outcast among his peers.

This changed, however, soon after "Beatlemania" swept through America. Sergio bought a guitar and taught himself to sing "I Want to Hold Your Hand" and other Beatles songs. As a result, his popularity with schoolmates shot up, even though his stuttering continued to worsen. He had so much difficulty speaking in class, and his teachers were so unsympathetic, that he finally dropped out of school and pursued a vagabond lifestyle as a singer and songwriter.

As he traveled, working various jobs by day and singing at night, Sergio continued to stutter severely, with one happy exception. When he was performing with his band, not only did he sing fluently, but

continued

he also spoke to the audience easily, announcing each number and making casual, funny comments between songs. As a result of his constant battle with stuttering, Sergio developed a wide variety of avoidances. He dodged making phone calls, and whenever he received calls, he used elaborate facial grimaces and starter sounds to fight his way through stutters.

Discussion

The telephone is a difficult situation for most people who stutter, and Sergio is no exception. Segment 1 shows Sergio talking about his past experiences on the phone when he had long silent blocks, and Segment 2 is a phone call Sergio made more recently. On both clips you'll see a mix of avoidance and escape behaviors that are now well entrenched in Sergio's speech pattern after years of stuttering. There are also some straightforward stutters without escape and avoidance behaviors that are witness to Sergio's attempts to stutter in a simpler way. See if you can identify the types of stutters that Sergio has on both segments, as well as his particular escape and avoidance behaviors, more of which are seen in Segment 2.

Onset

Imagine yourself in your doctor's office with an annoying cold that just won't go away—runny nose, sore throat, and cough. She asks you to describe when the first signs of your illness appeared and what they were like at onset. It is quite likely you won't remember exactly when your symptoms first occurred and exactly what they were like, especially if they came and went over the course of a week or two before they became persistent. This is the problem with determining the onset of stuttering. Parents are asked to recall exactly when the child's stuttering started and what it was like when they first noticed it; thus some of our information on onset—especially from older studies—may be inaccurate. The description of stuttering onset given here is relatively brief. More details are given in Chapter 7 when I describe the differences between typical disfluency and the beginning stages of stuttering.

Let's first consider the question of how old children are, on average, when they begin to stutter. In the earliest studies (e.g., Milisen & Johnson, 1936), researchers asked parents a year or more after the onset of stuttering had occurred to recall the age of stuttering onset in their children. The average age of onset, taken from nine pre-1990 studies summarized in Bloodstein and Ratner (2008), was roughly 4 years. After 1990, led by Ehud Yairi and his colleagues at the University of Illinois, researchers were careful to interview parents of children who began to stutter within the previous 12 months. In other words, they only included children whose stuttering had begun no more than a year before, so that parents' memories would be relatively fresh. Bloodstein and Ratner (2008) list six studies conducted after 1990 in which parents were interviewed closer to onset than in earlier studies. The average age of onset in these newer studies is about 33 months (2 years, 9 months). Thus, the newer studies are getting a more accurate picture of the age of onset, the age of onset is getting younger, or both.[1] The current consensus is that the onset of stuttering typically occurs just before age 3, and most onsets occur between ages 2 and 3.5 years (Yairi & Ambrose, 2005, 2013). Some older children—up to about age 12—may begin to stutter, but these are much rarer cases. Stuttering onset in adolescents and adults is likely to be a different form of disfluency—psychogenic or neurogenic—that I will discuss in Chapter 15, "Related Disorders of Fluency."

Next, let's look at the first signs of stuttering, as reported by parents. Most early reports of stuttering onset (e.g., Bluemel, 1932) indicated that simple, relaxed repetitions of syllables and words were the typical first signs of stuttering. However, some early studies (e.g., Taylor, 1937) and the carefully conducted interviews by Yairi (1983) found that, in many cases, parents described prolongations and blocks, along with signs of struggle, as the first stutters shown by their child. Yairi and Ambrose (2013) suggest that syllable and single-syllable word repetitions are by far the most common behavior that parents report as the first signs of stuttering. No matter what the first signs of stuttering are, excessive numbers of syllable repetitions seem to be a universal indicator of the presence of stuttering in a child (Yairi & Ambrose, 2005). This is an example of excessive syllable repetitions: "I-I-I-I-I-I-I don't want that." Repeating each syllable an excessive number of times (the number of "iterations") is a characteristic that

[1]Yairi and Ambrose (2005) ask whether the age at stuttering onset is getting younger and whether this reflects a general trend of earlier language acquisition. In this regard, Nan Ratner (personal communication, July 2009) has surveyed a number of language acquisition experts through the CHILDES discussion group, and their consensus seems to be that there is no clear evidence that the age of language acquisition (i.e., ages at which major language milestones are achieved) has changed over the last few decades. She points out, however, that there is some evidence from differing results achieved by older versus more recent studies of phonological development that children may be acquiring articulatory targets earlier. Whether this would affect the age of stuttering onset is not known.

clinicians use to distinguish children who are beginning to stutter from their peers who are developing typically.

Last, there is the question of whether onset is sudden, intermediate, or gradual. In other words, do parents notice very evident disfluencies seen in the course of a day or two, or do they realize only after several weeks of milder disfluencies that their child is having a problem? Remember our example of getting a cold and trying to remember the onset? No doubt some colds come on suddenly, with sore throat and runny nose appearing overnight and getting worse quickly. Other colds tiptoe into your life, with a sore throat that comes and goes and later turns into a runny nose and cough.

In contrast to the earliest reports on stuttering always having a gradual onset, Yairi and Ambrose (2005) found in their sample of 163 children many cases (41 percent) in which onset was reported to be sudden, with another group (32 percent) reported as intermediate, and a third group (27 percent) as gradual. Studies by Buck, Lees, and Cook (2002) and by Reilly et al. (2009) also found that about 50 percent of parents reported a sudden onset of their child's stuttering. These figures may be influenced by how attentive to their child's speech these parents were. No doubt, parents who had relatives who stuttered would have been more likely to recognize stuttering sooner.

Prevalence

The term "**prevalence**" is used to indicate how widespread a disorder is. Information about the prevalence of stuttering tells us how many people currently stutter. Accurate, up-to-date information on the prevalence of stuttering is difficult to obtain. The research literature contains studies having many methodological differences, which can result in wide differences in estimates of prevalence. For example, the prevalence of stuttering probably varies considerably with age, and not all studies measure stuttering in the same age groups. Moreover, definitions of stuttering may vary from study to study. Some studies may include typically disfluent individuals who are just passing through a short phase of excess repetitions; others may exclude them.

Beitchman, Nair, Clegg, and Patel (1986) assessed the prevalence of speech and language disorders in kindergarten children, using a representative sample. They retested children who failed the initial screening as well as a random sample of children who passed. The prevalence of stuttering in this sample of kindergarten children was 2.4 percent. Although this is only one study's finding, the care with which the data were collected increases its credibility.

Bloodstein and Ratner (2008) reviewed and summarized the results of 44 studies of school-age children in the United States, Europe, Africa, Australia, and the West Indies. These studies showed that the prevalence of stuttering throughout the school years is about 1 percent. Andrews et al. (1983) came to the same conclusion—about 1 percent of schoolchildren worldwide are likely to stutter at any given time. If the 2.4 percent prevalence among kindergartners noted above is valid, a considerable number of recoveries must take place between kindergarten and the upper grades.

Studies of prevalence over the entire life span are limited. Craig, Hancock, Tran, Craig, and Peters (2002) used telephone surveys to assess the life span prevalence of stuttering in Australia and found that the overall prevalence (from preschool to over 50 years) was a little less than 0.75 percent. Children from ages 2 to 10 showed a higher prevalence, about 1.5 percent. Prevalence dropped to near 0.50 percent in individuals older than that.

Incidence

The **incidence** of stuttering is an index of how many people have stuttered at some time in their lives. Like the data on prevalence, incidence figures are not clear-cut because different researchers have used different definitions of stuttering and methods for obtaining their data. Some researchers only report stuttering that lasted 6 months or more, not wanting to include shorter episodes of disfluency. Others report any speech behaviors that informants or parents considered to be stuttering. Estimates of incidence, when reports of informants and parents are considered, are as high as 15 percent, a figure that includes those children who stuttered for only a brief period (Bloodstein & Ratner, 2008). Many studies have considered only individuals who have stuttered at least 6 months and reported a figure of 5 percent for incidence (Andrews & Harris, 1964).

A review of more recent studies of incidence (since 2000) by Yairi and Ambrose (2013) considers the 5 percent figure to be low. For example, relatively recent studies by Dworzynski, Remington, Rijsdijk, Howell, and Plomin (2007) in the United Kingdom and by Reilly et al. (2009) in Australia suggest that the incidence figures for individuals who have stuttered at some time in their lives is likely to be at least 8 percent. This increase in lifetime incidence is probably caused not by more people stuttering but by improved procedures for gathering this information.

Recovery from Stuttering

Recovery from stuttering without treatment, also referred to as "spontaneous" or "natural" recovery, has long been a puzzling issue. Putting aside the important question about why children recover without treatment, there is debate about what percentage of children who start to stutter recover in this way.

Reviews of early research report findings that range from 20 to 80 percent natural recovery (Andrews et al., 1983; Bloodstein & Ratner, 2008). This wide range results from different methodologies used by different studies. Some asked large numbers of adults if they ever stuttered when they were children. This method, which is called "retrospective," may be affected by faulty memories, poor definitions of stuttering, and the inclusion of individuals who may have stuttered for only brief periods.

Recent research has proceeded more carefully, by first identifying a group of children close to the onset of their stuttering and then following them for several years without offering treatment and assessing how many recover and how many persist. Those who persist are then referred for therapy. Several studies using this methodology have been published. Yairi and Ambrose (1999) followed a group of 84 children for a minimum of 4 years after the onset of their stuttering and determined that over this span of time, 74 percent had recovered without treatment. Kloth, Kraaimaat, Janssen, and Brutten (1999) followed 23 children for 6 years and discovered that 70 percent had recovered. Mansson (2000) identified 51 children between the ages of 3 and 5 who started to stutter and found that 71 percent recovered within 2 years. When the follow-up continued for another few years until the children were 8 or 9 years old, recoveries were up to 85 percent. Mansson's data were closely approximated by a later study by Dworzynski et al. in 2007. These researchers studied 14,000 pairs of twins, some of whom were found to be stuttering between the ages 2 and 7. Repeated questionnaire assessments completed by parents indicated that by age 7, 87.55 percent of the children who had been stuttering earlier had recovered. Recent reviews, including Yairi and Ambrose (2013), estimate the percentage of children who recover from stuttering at 85 percent or higher. Whether these recoveries were completely "natural" is unclear. Some of the children may have received some form of treatment, direct or indirect.

Recovery versus Persistence of Stuttering

Several studies have compared children who recover and those who persist, to determine what might characterize children who recover. Research at the University of Illinois (Yairi & Ambrose, 2005) over the past 30 years indicates that there are several factors that are useful for indicating the likelihood that a child's stuttering will persist rather than disappear naturally. You may wish to follow up on this brief overview by reading the reference, given earlier, that describes these findings in detail. The following factors appear to be among the most important predictors reviewed by Yairi and Ambrose (2005):

Family history: When a child's family includes individuals whose stuttering persisted, there is increased risk of persistence.

Gender: Boys have a greater risk of persistence. However, girls typically recover more quickly; therefore, if a girl doesn't recover fairly soon after onset she may well persist in stuttering.

Age at onset: Children who begin to stutter "later" have a greater risk of persistence. Onsets occur most frequently between ages 2 and 3.5 years, so children with onset after 3.5 years are more at risk.

Trend of stuttering frequency and severity: Children whose stuttering (defined as part-word repetitions and single-syllable word repetitions, prolongations, and blocks) is not decreasing in frequency and severity over a period of a year after onset are at more risk of persistence.

Duration since onset: The longer the child continues to stutter beyond a year after onset, the greater the risk of persistence, especially for girls.

Duration of stuttering moments: Continued presence of more than one repetition unit, especially more than three (li-li-li-li-like this) is a sign of increased risk. Also, continued rapid repetitions are a sign of increased risk. Children who recover tend to have fewer repetition units (li-like this) and slower repetitions (li......like this).

Continued presence of sound prolongations and blocks: The percentage of prolongations and blocks at onset doesn't predict persistence, but if prolongations and blocks do not decrease as stuttering goes on, the child is more likely to persist.

Phonological skills: Children whose phonological skills are below the norms have a greater risk for continued stuttering.

Two other studies examined factors associated with recovery. A longitudinal study by Brosch, Haege, Kalehne, and Johannsen (1999) followed a group of 79 stuttering children for several years. The group that persisted in stuttering had a significantly larger proportion of left-handed children. Because this is a preliminary report from an ongoing study, caution should be exercised in considering this factor as critical to recovery. Nonetheless, the factor of laterality may be one of the additional genetic factors that influence recovery; replication of this work is critical. Brosch, Hage, and Johannsen (2002) also reported that acoustic measures of the children's fluent speech before stuttering onset and at several points after stuttering onset in the study were related to persistence of stuttering. For example, more variability in measures of voice onset time appeared to be related to persistence.

In the study by Kloth et al. (1999) described earlier, results indicated that children who recovered had a more mature speech motor system (as defined by less variability of articulatory rate), a slower speaking rate, and a mother whose interaction style was nondirective and whose language was less complex. Rommel, Hage, Kalehne, and Johannsen (2000) assessed the speaking environments of 71 children identified as stuttering soon after onset and followed them for 3 years. The mothers of those who recovered naturally compared to the mothers of those who persisted used less complex syntax and a smaller number of different words when talking to their children.

The findings of a recent neuroimaging study of white matter tracts throughout the brain in children who stutter by

Chang, Zhu, Choo, and Angstadt (2015) may shed new light on the persistence of stuttering. Younger children who stuttered showed many deficits (compared to control children) in white matter nerve tracts throughout the brain, suggesting a lack of efficient connectivity, including in the sensorimotor areas related to speech. Strikingly, older children who stuttered (children with persistent stuttering) continued to show less development of white matter tracts than their age-matched controls. However, the older control children's white matter tracts were more developed, compared to the younger control children. This developmental change was not as present in the older stuttering children, compared to their controls. This may indicate that persistence of stuttering (vs. recovery) is related to lack of maturation of the connective pathways among areas related to speech production.

If this finding about problems in the development of neural pathways is supported in future studies, we may find that there are many possible reasons for lack of maturation in the white matter tracts in children who persist in stuttering. Researchers looking at a number of related disorders have noted that the duration of breastfeeding in infancy correlates with presence or persistence of some disorders (Tanoue & Oda, 1989). Following this lead, Mahurin-Smith and Ambrose (2013) compared 17 children who persisted in stuttering with 30 children who recovered and found that the duration of breastfeeding in the persistent children was less than that in the recovered children (more so in boys). Their explanation of this finding was that the fatty acids in human milk have been shown to enhance neural development and influence the expression of certain genes.

In summary, early studies of recovery reported wide variations in results. Their findings depend on many factors—among them, the accuracy with which stuttering is differentiated from typical disfluency, whether the study is retrospective or longitudinal, and the size of the group studied. The most careful studies are longitudinal assessments of children who are identified soon after the onset of stuttering and are followed for several years (e.g., Mansson, 2005). In these studies, about 80 to 90 percent of the children who begin to stutter recover without formal treatment. Many factors have been suggested as associated with recovery. These include having relatives who recovered from stuttering or no relatives who stuttered; having an early onset of stuttering; showing a decrease in frequency and severity of stuttering in the year after onset; having a slower speech rate; having a more stable speech-motor system; having a mother who has a nondirective interaction style and uses less complex language when speaking to the child; being right-handed; having less severe stuttering (although some studies dispute this); having good phonological, language, and nonverbal skills; and being female. We now consider this last variable, the sex factor, in more detail. Recent research has focused on neurodevelopment, particularly of white matter tracts connecting areas of the brain that must coordinate to provide the timing and sequencing for fluent speech.

Sex Ratio

Studies of the sex ratio in stuttering were first published in the 1890s and have been published every decade since. With this steady stream of information, we ought to have reliable data on this phenomenon. In fact, we do. The results from studies of people who stutter at many ages and in many cultures put the ratio at about three male stutterers to every one female stutterer. There is strong evidence, however, that the ratio may increase as children get older. For example, Yairi (1983) reported that of 22 children who were 2 and 3 years of age and whose parents believed they were stuttering, 11 were boys, and 11 were girls. In a larger study of 87 children between 20 and 69 months, Yairi and Ambrose (1992b) found a male:female ratio of 2.1:1 overall, although the 20 youngest subjects, those under 27 months, showed a 1.2:1 ratio.

Bloodstein and Ratner's (2008) review indicated that the male-to-female sex ratio is about 3:1 in the first grade and 5:1 in the fifth grade, confirming the hypothesis that the sex ratio increases as children get older. Evidence of the increasing male-to-female ratio was provided by two other studies. Kloth and colleagues (1999) found a male-to-female ratio of 1.1:1 ratio near onset, which rose to 2.5:1 six years later. Mansson (2000) found a male-to-female ratio of 1.65:1 at the initial screening (age 3), which rose to a ratio of 2.8:1 two years later. The nearly even sex ratio among very young children who stutter and the gradually increasing proportion of boys who stutter may be a consequence of several factors. West (1931) presented data indicating that the change in sex ratio was the result of an increasing proportion of boys beginning to stutter in the late preschool and early school-age years. However, more recent data indicate that girls begin to stutter a little earlier than boys (Yairi, 1983; Yairi & Ambrose, 1992b) and recover earlier and more frequently (Andrews et al., 1983; Yairi & Ambrose, 1992b, 1999; Yairi, Ambrose, & Cox, 1996). A study in Australia (Reilly et al., 2013), however, is the lone finding that suggests boys recover more frequently than girls. This study only followed children between the ages 2 to 4, so that if many girls recovered after age 4, they were missed.

Females who stutter and don't recover by adulthood may be an interesting subpopulation to study. They may have inherited a stronger predisposition to stutter, may have been subjected to strong environmental pressures on their speech, or both (Andrews et al., 1983). Alternately, they may lack the "recovery factor" that most young female stutterers appear to have, or they may have inherited additional factors that interact with stuttering to inhibit recovery.

Variability and Predictability of Stuttering

Another important piece of background information about stuttering is how it varies in some ways, yet is surprisingly predictable in other ways. This predictability is an important clue to its nature. As we trace the research on stuttering's variability, we will see how this information reflects changing theoretical perspectives on the disorder.

Before the 1930s, stuttering had been commonly regarded as a medical disorder. Lee Edward Travis, the first person trained as a PhD to work with speech and hearing disorders, set up a laboratory at the University of Iowa in 1924 to study stuttering from a neurophysiological perspective. He hypothesized that stuttering was the result of an anomalous or inefficient organization of the brain's two cerebral hemispheres. To Travis and his fellow researchers, the variability of stuttering behaviors was seen as part of a larger, somewhat heterogeneous organic disorder, and an unimportant part at that. Far more relevant to their research were stutterers' brain waves, heart rates, and breathing patterns. But in the 1930s, psychologists at Iowa and elsewhere began taking a keen interest in behavioral approaches to the study of human disorders, which spilled over into research on stuttering. Scientists who had been trying to understand the neurophysiology of stuttering gradually began trying to examine the social, psychological, and linguistic factors that govern its occurrence and variability (Bloodstein & Ratner, 2008).

Anticipation, Consistency, and Adaptation

Before describing these interesting findings, I'll briefly explain these terms that are best understood in the context of someone who stutters reading a passage several times. "**Anticipation**" refers to an individual's ability to predict the words or sounds on which he or she will stutter (Johnson & Solomon, 1937; Knott, Johnson, & Webster, 1937; Milisen, 1938; Van Riper, 1936). "**Consistency**" is the tendency for people to stutter on the same words when they read a passage more than once (Johnson & Inness, 1939; Johnson & Knott, 1937). "**Adaptation**" is the finding that when speakers read a passage several times, they gradually stutter less and less over the course of five or six readings (Johnson & Knott, 1937; Van Riper & Hull, 1955).

These studies were usually carried out by the experimenter giving an individual who stutters a passage and asking him to read it aloud. Before reading it aloud, however, the individual is asked to read it to himself and mark the words he expects to stutter on. The experimenter then marks the words actually stuttered on and compares that with the individual's marked copy to see how much he has accurately anticipated which words he will stutter on. Then the experimenter has the individual read the passage again and, using a copy of the passage on which the previously stuttered words were marked, marks those words that were stuttered on in both readings. This assesses how consistent the individual is in his stuttering. And thirdly, the experimenter has the individual read the passage six consecutive times and observes whether the individual adapts to the reading task and stutters less and less with each reading.

These findings, called anticipation, consistency, and adaptation, respectively, changed some assumptions about the disorder. Stuttering, it seemed, was not simply a neurophysiological disorder. It showed characteristics of a learned behavior, as well.

These studies not only changed existing views of stuttering but also opened the door to new treatment possibilities. The reason was this: If much of stuttering is learned, it may be unlearned. The challenge was to determine how much is learned and how to help people who stutter develop new responses. Many of the treatment approaches we discuss later in the book use principles of learning to help clients acquire fluent speech, especially young children. Learning can also help older children and adults reduce the tension and avoidance of their old stuttering responses and speak with milder stuttering or none. Remember this. Learning principles will be critical to your clinical work.

Language Factors

One of the many stuttering researchers at the University of Iowa, Spencer Brown, pushed investigations of the predictability of stuttering into the realm of language. In seven studies completed over a stretch of 10 years, Brown found correlations between stuttering and seven grammatical factors during reading aloud. These findings were reported in a remarkable series of papers Brown published from 1935 to 1945 (Brown, 1937, 1938a, 1938b, 1938c, 1943, 1945; Brown & Moren, 1942; Johnson & Brown, 1935). Brown showed that most adults who stutter do so more frequently on:

- consonants
- sounds in word-initial position
- speech in a larger context (versus on isolated words)
- nouns, verbs, adjectives, and adverbs (vs. articles, prepositions, pronouns, and conjunctions)
- longer words
- words at the beginnings of sentences
- stressed syllables

These findings strongly suggest that stuttering is highly influenced by these linguistic factors.

Later investigators applied Brown's hypotheses to the speech of children who stutter. An advantage in studying language factors in children's stuttering is that the loci (places where stuttering occurs in speech) and frequency of stuttering might be less influenced by responses learned from years of stuttering and more by innate language processing characteristics. Indeed, researchers discovered that although stuttering in elementary school children follows the same linguistic patterns as adult stuttering, the loci and frequency of stuttering in preschool children are different. Stuttering in these very young children occurs most frequently on pronouns and conjunctions, not on nouns, verbs, adjectives, and adverbs. For these children, stuttering occurs not as repetitions, prolongations, or blocks of sounds in word-initial positions but as repetitions of parts of words and single-syllable words in sentence-initial positions (Bloodstein & Gantwerk, 1967; Bloodstein & Ratner, 2008). This led researchers to hypothesize that in its incipient stage, stuttering is located at the beginning of syntactic units (sentences, clauses, and phrases), as if the task of linguistic planning and preparation were a key ingredient in the recipe for stuttering (Bernstein Ratner, 1997; Bloodstein, 2001, 2002; Bloodstein & Ratner, 2008).

Conture (2001) and others (e.g., Byrd, Wolk, & Davis, 2007) have focused particular attention on the phoneme or sound selection component of linguistic planning in individuals who stutter. Findings that recovery from stuttering may be associated with good phonological skills, a slower speech production rate, and a stable speech-motor system suggest that some individuals who stutter may overcome a linguistic planning delay by relying on strengths in related language areas or by slowing their rates of speech production to compensate for such deficits. We will revisit these methods of dealing with stuttering when we discuss treatment approaches.

In summary, there are strong links between language and stuttering. As mentioned in the section describing onset, stuttering usually first appears when children are going through the most intense period of language acquisition (Bloodstein & Ratner, 2008). It is also clear that deficits in language (including phonology) often accompany stuttering and may predict its persistence (Yairi & Ambrose, 1999, 2005). Future studies may also confirm what several researchers have suggested, that even stutterers who show no clinically significant language disorders may have subtle subclinical language or phonological deficits that may contribute to their stuttering (e.g., Byrd et al., 2007). More information about the influence of language factors on stuttering will be found in the next two chapters.

Fluency-Inducing Conditions

One of the researchers at the University of Iowa, Oliver Bloodstein, wrote his PhD dissertation on "Conditions under Which Stuttering Is Reduced or Absent" (Bloodstein, 1948, 1950). In studying the speech of stutterers in 115 conditions, Bloodstein found that stuttering is markedly decreased in many of them. Some of these conditions are speaking when alone, when relaxed, in unison with another speaker, to an animal or an infant, in time to a rhythmic stimulus or when singing, in a different dialect, while simultaneously writing, and when swearing. In later studies, reviewed in Andrews, Howie, Dosza, and Guitar (1982), additional conditions were found to reduce stuttering. These conditions included speaking in a slow prolonged manner, speaking under loud masking noise, speaking while listening to delayed auditory feedback, shadowing another speaker (repeating what they say immediately afterward), and speaking when reinforced for fluent speech.

Various explanations have been proposed to account for the impact of these conditions. Most are compatible with the idea that stuttering has a substantial learned component and is affected by such external stimuli as communicative pressure. Recent brain imaging studies—reviewed in Chapters 2 and 3—indicate that cortical and subcortical networks for speech and language are impaired in people who stutter. This may make it difficult for a speaker to orchestrate rapid and coordinated production of phonological and lexical items, syntax, intonation, and other subcomponents of spoken language. Thus, many conditions may induce fluency by providing timing cues, reducing rate, lowering stress on vulnerable pathways, or marshalling attentional resources to overcome the limitations of the neurological system of a person who stutters.

An Integration

Modern research on stuttering has taken a long and complex journey from Travis's laboratory in Iowa in 1924. Yet, in many ways, those early findings are not irrelevant. Travis's theory of stuttering, which viewed it as a problem of coordinating the two sides of the brain for speech has reemerged as a view of stuttering as a problem of coordinating multiple brain networks for speech and integrating them with networks for language, cognition, and emotion. This juggling act breaks down in all speakers when the resources needed to process language, cognition, or emotion momentarily drain available central nervous system capacities, leaving too little capacity for the intricacies of rapid, smooth speech production. The result is typical disfluency. Those individuals who stutter appear to have even more than this typical trouble managing the needed multiple neural networks for speech production under conditions of high demand. They have inherited or acquired a more vulnerable speech production system—one that is less able to deal with the norm of rapid, smooth speech under a wide variety of conditions, perhaps because the neural pathways used to produce speech are not as efficient as they need to be.

In those children who recover naturally from stuttering, this vulnerable speech production system may heal itself and become more resistant to disruption. Because of the great neural plasticity of the very young, some children's brains will spontaneously develop new, more efficient pathways for speech, and these children will become entirely fluent. Others may recover because they learn to compensate by speaking more slowly or finding other ways to marshal their resources to overcome disfluency.

Children who persist in stuttering may have important neurodevelopmental differences from those who recover. The parts of their brains used in speech and language production—and the interconnections among these parts—may develop more slowly and less completely. Thus, they will have difficulty producing the lightening-fast sensorimotor coordinations needed for fluent speech. When their speech breaks down again and again, they are flooded with feelings of frustration and embarrassment. These emotions can cause children to tense their muscles during stutters and try to escape the moment of stuttering by squeezing and pushing out words, blinking their eyes and nodding their head. Anticipatory fears gradually develop as children stutter more frequently on certain words (e.g., their names) and in certain situations (e.g., meeting new people). These highly learned reactions—which are influenced by an individual's personality and the responses of people around the individual—become part of children's stuttering patterns and influence the way they think and feel about speaking.

This view is essentially the model of stuttering presented in this book. To state it more formally, stuttering is an inherited or congenital neurodevelopmental disorder of neural pathways in the brain that first appears when a child is learning the complex and rapid coordinations of speech and language production. Children who do not recover but persist in stuttering are those who may have more extensive deficits in these neural networks. They may also have more sensitive temperaments or other vulnerabilities. As stuttering persists, they learn maladaptive responses to their disfluencies. This learning is influenced by their biological temperament, developing social and cognitive awareness, and the response of people in their environment.

The next few chapters expand on this theme and prepare you to use this information in diagnosis and treatment.

SUMMARY

- Stuttering appears in all cultures and has been a problem for humankind for at least 40 centuries.
- It is characterized by a high frequency or severity of disruptions that impede the forward flow of speech.
- It begins in childhood and often becomes more severe as the child grows to adulthood unless he recovers with or without formal treatment.
- Core behaviors of stuttering are repetitions, prolongations, and blocks. Secondary behaviors are the result of attempts to escape or avoid core behaviors and include physical concomitants of stuttering, such as eye blinks, or verbal concomitants, such as word substitutions.
- Feelings and attitudes can also be important components of stuttering that reflect the individual's emotional reactions to the experience of being unable to speak fluently and to listener responses to her stuttering. Feelings are immediate emotional reactions and include fear, shame, and embarrassment. Attitudes crystallize more slowly from repeated negative experiences associated with stuttering. An example is the belief that listeners think you are stupid when they hear you stuttering.
- Stuttering begins between 18 months of age and puberty, but most often between ages 2 and 5 years, with a peak just before age 3. Its first appearance may be either a gradual increase in easy repetitions of words and sounds or a sudden onset of multiple repetitions, sometimes with prolongations or blocks as well.
- Prevalence of stuttering is about 1 percent. Incidence is about 5 percent. Recovery rate without professional treatment may be above 80 percent of children who ever stuttered. The male-to-female ratio in schoolchildren and adults is about 3:1 but may be lower, close to 1:1, in very young children who start to stutter. More girls recover during early childhood, increasing the proportion of males with the disorder after the preschool years.
- Many people who stutter are able to predict the words they will stutter on in a reading passage before reading it aloud (anticipation), and most tend to stutter on many of the same words each time in repeated readings of a passage (consistency). Stuttering frequency decreases for most stutterers when they read a passage many times (adaptation).
- Stuttering occurs more frequently in certain grammatical contexts. The nature of these grammatical contexts differs somewhat for adults and children.
- A variety of conditions reduces the frequency of stuttering. Their effects may be attributable to changes in speech pattern, reductions in communicative pressure, or both. Research on these fluency-inducing conditions suggests that stuttering may be decreased by conditions that reduce the demands on speech motor control and language formulation functions.
- Cortical and subcortical neural networks for speech and language may be slow to develop in children who stutter, particularly those whose stuttering becomes chronic. Many of these children who persist in stuttering develop cognitive, emotional, and behavioral responses to their stuttering. This can make the problem more difficult to treat and cause social, occupational, and academic difficulties for these individuals.

STUDY QUESTIONS

1. What might make some children's core behaviors progress from repetitions to prolongations to blocks?
2. What are the differences between core and secondary behaviors in stuttering?
3. From what other kinds of hesitation should stuttering be distinguished?
4. What are some feelings and attitudes people who stutter might have, and what is their origin? Are these feelings and attitudes ever experienced by people who don't stutter?
5. What is the age range for the onset of stuttering (the youngest and oldest ages at which onset is commonly reported)? Why might it occur at that time?
6. What is the difference between "incidence" and "prevalence?"
7. What problems do researchers encounter when they try to determine how many stutterers recover without treatment?
8. Why might the ratio of male-to-female stutterers change with age?
9. In what ways is stuttering predictable? In what ways does it vary?
10. Why is it difficult to answer the question, "What is the cause of stuttering?"
11. The International Classification of Functioning, Disability, and Health (ICF) indicates that with some conditions, interpersonal interactions may be affected. How might stuttering affect these interactions?
12. How can stuttering treatment help change factors affecting the individual in the ICF area called "Contextual Factors"?
13. How would you describe the etiology of stuttering to a parent who has had limited education and is not used to discussing abstract concepts?

SUGGESTED PROJECTS

1. Enlist the help of an adult who stutters, and have him teach you to stutter. Then ask him to go with you while you use some voluntary stuttering in public. Write a report (no more than a page) of what feelings you experienced and how people reacted to you.
2. Use an Internet search engine like Google to find an online discussion group of people who stutter and clinicians. Join the group and observe what issues they discuss.
3. Attend a support group for people who stutter.
4. Listen to some preschool children talking and note their typical disfluencies. Then listen to elementary school children talking, and compare their disfluencies to those of the preschool children.
5. If you are a fluent speaker, record your own speech and observe the types of disfluencies you hear. Do they differ from stuttering? In what ways?
6. Conduct a search on the Internet for resources that guide you to critically evaluate Web sites (e.g., https://www.library.georgetown.edu/tutorials/research-guides/evaluating-internet-content). Using that format, critically evaluate a Web site you find when searching for "stuttering" sites with your search engine.

SUGGESTED VIEWING

The King's Speech. This film depicts King George VI of England, who stuttered severely but found a great deal of help with his Australian speech therapist, Lionel Logue. The movie provides an excellent depiction of the emotions surrounding stuttering.
When I Stutter. This is a documentary film about stuttering made by John Gomez, SLP, of Keeneye Productions.

SUGGESTED READINGS

Bloodstein, O. (1993). *Stuttering: The search for a cause and cure.* Boston, MA: Allyn and Bacon.

This book is part history and part analysis, written with charm and clarity. Bloodstein covers early treatments for stuttering; the burgeoning of research in the 1930s, 1940s, and 1950s; and more recent findings in the realm of neurophysiology. His own orientation on the learning-environmental basis of stuttering comes through, but he gives good coverage of other possible factors as well. Bloodstein is particularly good at conveying the excitement that accompanies research.

Bobrick, B. (1995). *Knotted tongues: Stuttering in history and the quest for a cure.* New York, NY: Simon and Schuster.

A highly readable account of various treatments for stuttering throughout the ages and of famous people who stutter.

Carlisle, J. (1985). *Tangled tongue: Living with a stutter.* Toronto, ON: University of Toronto Press.

An eloquent autobiography by a man with a severe stutter and a great sense of humor.

Helliesen, G. (2002). *Forty years after therapy: One man's story.* Newport News, VA: Apollo Press.

An autobiography of someone who stuttered severely and was treated by Charles Van Riper, the world-renowned stuttering clinician. This book presents a unique view of stuttering therapy from the client's viewpoint.

Jezer, M. (1997). *Stuttering: A life bound up in words.* New York, NY: Basic Books.

A compelling, sensitive book about the frustrating and sometimes funny things that happen to someone growing up with a severe stuttering problem and learning to cope with it.

Murray, F. P. (n.d.). *A stutterer's story*. Memphis, TN: Stuttering Foundation of America (www.stutteringhelp.org).

An autobiography depicting the long struggle of someone who stuttered severely and spent his life searching for answers. The author describes his acquaintance with many of the pioneers of stuttering therapy.

Rabinowitz, A., & Chien, C. (2014). *A boy and a jaguar*. Boston, MA: Houghton Mifflin Harcourt.

A children's book that tells the true-life story of Alan Rabinowitz who stuttered severely and could only talk fluently to animals. Rabinowitz learned to manage his stuttering effectively and later was called the "Indiana Jones of wildlife conservation." This book received the American Library Association's Schneider Family Book Award.

Shields, D. (1989). *Dead languages*. New York, NY: Knopf.

This is a novel about a young boy who stutters. It conveys the feelings associated with being an individual who stutters in a world that prizes spoken language. It is recommended for students who would like to understand a child who stutters.

St. Louis, K. (Ed.) (2001). *Living with stuttering: Stories, basics, resources, and hope*. Morgantown, WV: Populore Publishing Company.

The life stories of 25 people who stutter and how they have coped with their stuttering.

2

Primary Etiological Factors in Stuttering

Chapter Objectives

After studying this chapter, readers should be able to:

- Describe the evidence supporting genetic inheritance of stuttering from (1) family studies, (2) twin studies, and (3) adoption studies
- Explain how genetic studies are done and what has been found about how chromosomes and genes are associated with stuttering
- Explain why congenital and early childhood factors are thought to contribute to a predisposition to develop stuttering and what some of these factors may be
- Describe the ways in which brain structures in stuttering individuals differ from those of nonstuttering individuals
- Describe the ways in which brain functions in stuttering individuals differ from those of nonstuttering individuals
- Describe changes in the brain that are associated with improvements in fluency as the result of treatment

Key Terms

Adoption studies: Investigations of stuttering in siblings who were adopted soon after birth and placed with different families. A higher incidence of stuttering among biological relatives than adoptive family members provides evidence of a genetic basis of stuttering rather than an environmental basis

Anomaly: A difference from the normal structure or function

Concordance (in twins): If one twin has a condition, such as stuttering, the other twin also has the condition

Congenital factor: A physical or psychological trauma that occurred at or near birth that may predispose an individual to develop stuttering

DNA: A double-stranded molecule passed on from a mother and a father to a child containing the "instruction book" for passing on traits

Family studies: Examination of family trees of individuals who stutter to determine the frequency and pattern of the occurrence of stuttering in relatives. These studies can answer questions such as whether males or females are more likely to have children who stutter and whether persistent stuttering (as opposed to natural recovery) is a trait that is inherited.

Gene: A segment of DNA that contributes to an individual's traits, such as height and weight

Genetic linkage studies: Because two or more genes connected with a disorder are physically close to each other on a chromosome, they are often inherited together in individuals who have that disorder. By comparing genes and chromosomes of family members who do have the disorder with those who don't, these disorder-related genes can be identified.

Natural recovery (from stuttering): Stuttering that disappears within a year or two after onset from natural causes rather than from treatment

Persistent stuttering: Stuttering that persists for several years after onset, beyond the time at which natural recovery is likely to occur

Predisposition: A susceptibility to developing a condition

Twin studies: Research on the co-occurrence of stuttering of both members of a twin pair if one twin stutters; questions such as whether identical twins show more concordance than fraternal twins can be answered, shedding light on the extent of a genetic basis of stuttering

Whole brain intrinsic network connectivity: Networks throughout the brain can be compared between those who stutter and those who don't. Looking for networks is in contrast with looking only at specific areas of the brain—a localizationist approach.

WHAT DO WE KNOW ABOUT CONSTITUTIONAL FACTORS IN STUTTERING?

We know a lot. There is much more to be learned, of course, and you may be able to contribute to our knowledge yourself. But let's start with what we do know about factors inherent in the person—aspects of their constitutional makeup—that influence their stuttering. This knowledge may help you counsel people who stutter and parents of children who stutter to help them understand that stuttering is not their fault. You will also be able to explain that, despite the biological basis of stuttering, much of the handicap of stuttering can be overcome. Think of the many famous and successful people, like Emily Blunt, James Earl Jones, Bruce Willis, Carly Simon, and former Vice President Joe Biden, who have stuttered and have largely conquered their problem.

In addition to putting this knowledge to clinical use, you may be interested in contributing to the science of stuttering. Information in this chapter can be helpful to future researchers who may find new and more effective interventions based on what they will discover. As you read about the information that I present here, keep your creative portals open; that way, you may come up with new ideas that could solve a remaining riddle related to the causes of stuttering.

In this chapter, I give you an overview of the heredity of stuttering and the possible influence of childhood brain injury on the disorder. Then I describe how differences and deficits in specific areas of the brain may be associated with stuttering. Figure 2.1 gives a quick impression of the areas we will cover. The chapters that follow will help you understand how all these details about heredity and brain structure and function may result in the speech production difficulties that result in stuttering.

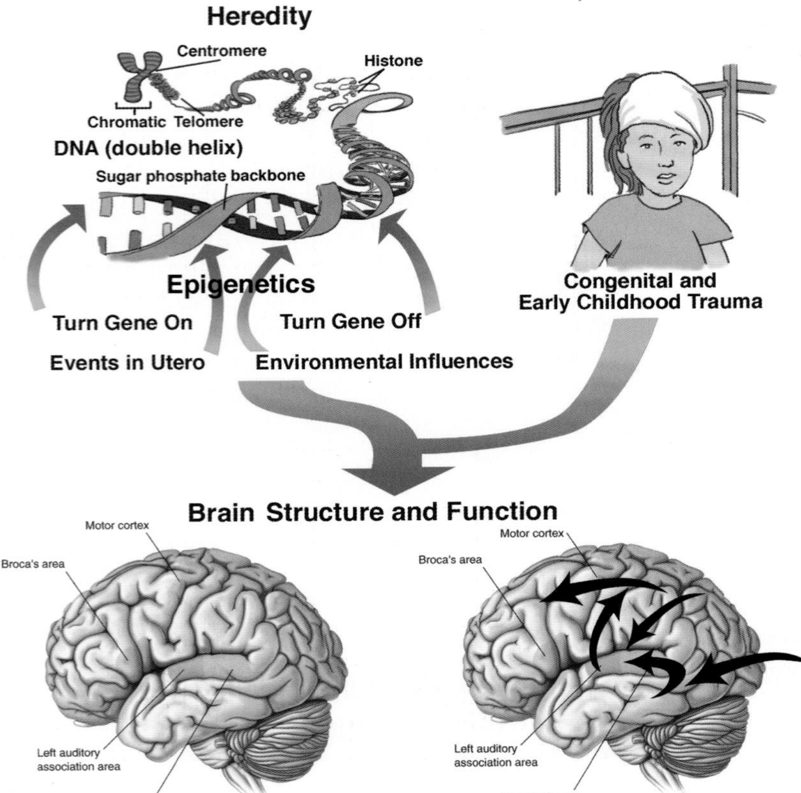

Figure 2.1 Constitutional factors in stuttering.

HEREDITARY FACTORS

Remember when you realized you were beginning to resemble your parents in some ways? Or that you look like your sister or brother? Obviously, many traits that make parents and children so similar are inherited. It wasn't until the mid-eighteen hundreds that we began to understand how this works. Two individuals contributed a vast amount to our understanding of heredity. One was the Augustinian monk, Gregor Mendel, whose experiments in breeding varieties of peas gave rise to his insights about genetic inheritance in people. He established the principle that each parent in a breeding pair contributes equally to the genetic makeup of the offspring, and he developed the understanding of dominant and recessive traits (see Fig. 2.2 and related text for more on genes). Another major contributor to the science of genetics was Charles Darwin. Darwin is quite relevant to the topic of this book because he is thought to have inherited stuttering from his famous grandfather, Erasmus Darwin (Thomson, 2009).[1] Charles Darwin's theory of evolution (natural selection) suggested that while specific characteristics (such as height and skin color) could be inherited by one generation from another, variations in how those characteristics expressed themselves produced slight differences in members of a species. These differences favored some individuals more than others, depending on the environment. The most useful traits for surviving in the species' environment will be passed on to future generations because those individuals possessing them would thrive and reproduce most successfully. For example, deer who can run at astonishing speeds can escape predators and thereby survive to produce more offspring. Thus, deer have evolved to be fast runners.

Let's go back to stuttering. The idea that stuttering is inherited because it often runs in families is a fact long recognized by researchers (e.g., Bryngelson, 1935). For many years, researchers debated about what this meant. Some suggested that the appearance of stuttering in several generations of a family must mean that it is caused by an inherited neurological difference or **anomaly**. Others disagreed, countering that religious beliefs often run in families too but aren't inherited. Some researchers argued that stuttering develops in response to a critical attitude toward normal disfluency that has been handed down from one generation to the next (Johnson & associates, 1959). A child whose parents were critical of her normal disfluencies would grow afraid of speaking because of their critical remarks and would "hesitate to hesitate." This would start a spiral of more hesitations leading to greater criticism, greater fear, more disfluencies, and so on.

[1]Erasmus Darwin was a famous British physician, natural philosopher, physiologist, slave-trade abolitionist, inventor, and poet. He was known to have had a severe stutter, but obviously it didn't hold him back.

For many years, researchers aligned themselves with one side of the argument or the other: Is stuttering inherited or are critical attitudes just passed down? Currently, however, there is broad agreement that stuttering is frequently inherited (Bloodstein & Ratner, 2008; Kraft & Yairi, 2012; Yairi & Ambrose, 2005, 2013). In other words, for many people who stutter, one or both of their parents had some **predisposition** to stuttering that was transmitted in their genes. Current thinking may be due to new strong evidence about heredity in stuttering but is probably also due to the rise of less deterministic views of heredity. Research has shown, for a number of inherited disorders, that genes do not work alone. Stuttering, asthma, migraine headaches, and many other disorders are seen as the result of heredity and environment acting together, with elements of chance thrown in (Kidd, 1984). The interaction between heredity and environment is something we commonly encounter.

For example, a few summers ago, I grew all my tomato plants from the same seed packet, giving them an identical heredity. But I planted some near Burlington, in a relatively warm environment (for Vermont), and I planted others in the Northeast Kingdom of Vermont, a colder, cloudier summer environment. As you might guess, by mid-August, the tomatoes near warmer, sunnier Burlington were plump and red, while those in the Northeast Kingdom were smaller with many shriveled blossoms, showing that environment had a strong differential effect on heredity. And so it is with stuttering.

A child in one family may inherit genes predisposing him to stutter, but his environment may be so low-key that stuttering never develops. A different child, inheriting similar genes, may grow up in a culture that favors rapid speech and a fast-paced lifestyle and begin to stutter at age 3.

In this chapter, I review four approaches to the study of heredity and stuttering: family studies, twin studies, adoption studies, and genetic studies. These different ways of gathering evidence all suggest that for many individuals, stuttering is partly attributable to heredity. These methods complement each other because no single method can provide all the information we want and because they can provide converging insights into what is really going on when we think about how genetics is involved in stuttering. The insights we gain from these studies are vital in counseling individuals and families about the nature of their child's stuttering.

The studies that I review are a good example of the increasing rigor of science as it progresses. Investigations of heredity in family studies were often casual in the 1930's, using only parents' reports to determine if a child was stuttering and not using control groups in their studies. Twin studies and adoption studies had tighter methodology and strongly suggested what portion of stuttering was the result of heredity and what portion was from environmental factors. Genetic studies that actually examined participants' DNA were more rigorous still and were often able to pinpoint exact genes and chromosomes that were related to stuttering. We'll begin with the most casual studies.

Family Studies

Table 2.1 summarizes the studies that I discuss here. I begin by summarizing research from early studies. These provide the first clear scientific evidence that stuttering has a strong genetic component. However, as you'll see, these studies had several weaknesses (these weakness are detailed in Felsenfeld, 1997; Yairi, Ambrose, & Cox, 1996). First, researchers only studied families with stuttering and did not use closely matched control families. Second, their subjects were adults who stuttered. This excluded subjects (children) who had begun to stutter and then recovered while still young. Another weakness in several early studies is that parent reports of children's speech—rather than observation by the experimenters—were used to determine whether a child stuttered or not. Relying solely on parent reports might introduce some errors. Let's look at some of those pioneering studies, which are interesting despite their flaws.

The first among those early reports on the genetics of stuttering were published by a group of researchers in Newcastle, England (Andrews & Harris, 1964; Kay, 1964). They compared the family histories of older children who stuttered with those of children who didn't. They found good evidence for inheritance of stuttering: Children who stuttered had far more relatives who stuttered. They also found that stuttering was different in males and females. Males were more likely to stutter, but females who stuttered were more likely to have relatives who stuttered. This means that something about boys makes them more vulnerable to stuttering. And something about girls makes them more resistant to stuttering so that in order to develop stuttering, girls need to inherit more genetic material (i.e., more stuttering relatives passing on a tendency to stutter).

Ten years after the Newcastle studies, researchers at Yale University confirmed these early findings that males are more vulnerable to stuttering and females are more resistant (Kidd, 1977; Kidd, Kidd, & Records, 1978; Kidd, Reich, & Kessler, 1973). Kidd (1984) concluded that these patterns were best explained by an interaction between the environment and a combination of several genes.

A decade later, researchers at the University of Illinois (Ambrose, Yairi, & Cox, 1993) studied the family histories of children who had just been diagnosed with stuttering. These younger children were a mix of children who would later recover from their stuttering and children who would persist. They found, like the earlier studies, that the children who stuttered had far more stuttering relatives than control children and more stuttering relatives were male. Unlike past studies, however, these researchers found that male and female children who stuttered had similar chances of having relatives who stuttered. Thus, the inheritance of stuttering was supported. But unlike Kay (1964), they found no evidence that females needed more "stuttering genes" to account for their stuttering.

TABLE 2.1 Summary of Family Studies of Stuttering

Authors, Date	Major Findings	Implications
Andrews and Harris, 1964; Kay, 1964	Children who stuttered had more relatives who stuttered than children who didn't. More males than females stuttered. Females who stuttered were more likely to have relatives who stuttered.	Stuttering seems to be inherited. Males are more susceptible to stuttering. Females who stutter are likely to have more genetic "loading" in order to overcome female resistance to stuttering.
Kidd, 1977; Kidd et al., 1978; Kidd et al., 1973	More males stuttered than females; females who stuttered had more relatives who stuttered. This team developed statistical polygenetic model of stuttering.	Confirmed findings by Andrews and colleagues that stuttering is often inherited. They suggested that stuttering is best explained by interaction of several genes and environment.
Ambrose et al., 1993, 1997	Used very young children just after onset, thus a mix of persistent and those who may recover. Found that male and female children had equal chance of having relatives who stutter. Found females more likely to recover. Persistence runs in families.	Confirmed earlier studies indicating stuttering is often inherited. Children who stutter from families with persistent stuttering are more likely to persist.
Viswanath et al., 2004	These researchers suggest that persistent stuttering and recovered stuttering may be two different disorders.	It may be possible someday to predict if a child will recover from stuttering.

Four years later, the Illinois group published another study of children who were assessed soon after the onset of their stuttering (Ambrose, Cox, & Yairi, 1997). They followed the children for 36 months and categorized them into those who completely recovered from stuttering and those whose stuttering persisted for more than 36 months after initial evaluation. The researchers found that the sex ratios of the two groups were quite different. In the persistent group, the male-to-female ratio was 7:1, but it was about 2:1 in the recovered group, indicating a much higher percentage of boys in the persistent group. This provides more evidence that girls are more likely to recover than boys.

A second finding was that persistence tended to run in families. In other words, children who did not outgrow their stuttering were likely to come from families in which relatives who had stuttered also persisted in their stuttering. Conversely, children who recovered were likely to come from families in which relatives who initially stuttered became fluent when they grew older. Further analysis of their data led the authors to propose that persistent and recovered stuttering are transmitted by the same major gene or genes but that those individuals whose stuttering persisted had additional genetic factors that affected recovery. A contrasting view is given by Viswanath, Lee, and Chakraborty (2004). Their studies of family members of persistent stutterers led them to hypothesize that persistent and recovered stuttering are two genetically different disorders, meaning that two or more different genes are involved. Other aspects of their work confirmed that stuttering is inherited through a dominant gene (a gene related to stuttering can come from just one parent rather than requiring one from each parent). They also found, like other studies, that males are more susceptible and that if a parent (rather than a more distant relative) stutters, inheritance is more likely.

Family studies have clinical relevance as well as giving us a window into the nature of stuttering. As a clinician, you can ask families whether they have relatives who stutter and then find out if these relatives recovered. If they did, the preschool child you are evaluating has a good chance of recovering himself. If the child had relatives who stuttered, you can inform the parents about the likelihood that their child's stuttering was inherited. This may relieve their guilt that they may have caused the stuttering by something they did or didn't do. As an example of this, I have a friend whose parents both stuttered. They originally met at a stuttering therapy center in New York City and made improvements to their speech, but they continued to stutter noticeably throughout their lives. Their first child, my friend, began to stutter at age 4, but neither parent was willing to talk with him about their stuttering or his. His stuttering persisted and he grew up thinking it was unmentionable. But when he had children and one of them began to stutter, he did some reading and talked to professionals. This led him to conclude that he was not to blame. His son hadn't imitated him nor had he caused his son's stuttering by something he did. Thus, unlike his parents, he felt comfortable talking openly about his own stuttering to his son and reassuring his son that stuttering was okay. His son has grown up with only a mild stutter and no self-consciousness about it.

Let's go back to the researchers in Illinois for a moment. They examined a number of genetic and seemingly non-genetic factors that might predict recovery or persistence and thereby might be useful in deciding which children are in immediate need of treatment. In an early study, Yairi, Ambrose, Paden, and Throneburg (1996) found that predictors of recovery include (1) good phonology, language, and nonverbal skills; (2) family members who had recovered from stuttering; and (3) early age of onset of stuttering. Some of the factors that impede recovery, such as problems in phonology or language, might be determined by other genes accompanying a gene related to the initial onset of stuttering. In a study a few years later (Yairi & Ambrose, 1999), the Illinois group expanded this list of factors; this larger list, which includes eight factors, was presented in Chapter 1 in the section titled "Recovery versus Persistence of Stuttering" (page 17). In addition to the three factors just mentioned, attributes that predict recovery include (4) being female, (5) decreasing severity and frequency of stuttering during the period after onset, (6) currently having stuttered less than a year, (7) having fewer repetition units (li-like this) and slower repetitions (more time between iterations, li......like this), and (8) decreasing number of prolongations and blocks (if they occur at all).

Before we leave the topic of family studies, Yairi et al. (1996) suggested that future studies (1) look for subgroups of stutterers that may have different genetic etiologies, (2) examine family members who don't stutter to find factors that may resist stuttering, and (3) search for environmental factors that may interact with genetic factors to precipitate or maintain stuttering.

Twin Studies

The twin studies I discuss are summarized in Table 2.2. **Twin studies** of stuttering have shown that the disorder occurs much more often in both members of identical (monozygotic) twin pairs than in both members of fraternal (dizygotic), same-sex twin pairs (Andrews, Morris-Yates, Howie, & Martin, 1991; Felsenfeld et al. 2000; Howie, 1981; Luchsinger, 1944; Seeman, 1937). To use the vocabulary of genetics, there is higher **concordance** of stuttering in identical than in fraternal twins. This supports the hypothesis that stuttering is inherited, but it doesn't reveal exactly what is inherited.

In addition to providing evidence of genetic factors in stuttering, twin studies demonstrate that heredity does not work alone. In one of the twin studies, although there was higher concordance for stuttering among identical twins, some identical twin pairs were discordant (Howie, 1981). Specifically, Howie found that in 6 of the 16 identical twin pairs, 1 twin stuttered but the other didn't. This means that even though both members of the twin pair had the same genetic inheritance, something else must have been operating. This may not be surprising when one learns that genes must interact with the environment to produce their effects (e.g., LeDoux, 2002). A gene might not express itself in stuttering unless, for example, there is some kind of prenatal or postnatal stress on the child. In the case of stuttering, where there may be several genes working together to produce a chronic disorder, the situation is even more complex because several genetic tendencies may need to interact with different aspects of the child's internal and external environment to create stuttering. No wonder more than a third of the pairs were discordant (6/16 or 37.5 percent) in the Howie study.

An estimate of the relative proportions of genetic and environmental influences was suggested in a later study involving 3,810 unselected (from Australian Twin Registry) twin pairs (Andrews et al., 1991). Analyses of stuttering in these 3,810 unselected twin pairs estimated that 71 percent of the variance (the probability of whether or not one would stutter) was accounted for by genetic factors, and 29 percent was accounted for by the individual's environment (including factors influencing the fetus, such as maternal stress), as well as factors after birth (such as family conversational style or serious childhood illness). Felsenfeld and colleagues (2000) followed this with a study of a new sample of 1,567 twin pairs and 634 individuals from the same Australian Twin Registry. They found 17 monozygotic and 8 dizygotic twin pairs who were concordant for stuttering and 21 monozygotic and 45 dizygotic twins who were discordant for stuttering. Statistical analyses estimated that "additive genetic effects" (the effects of different genes working together) accounted for 70 percent of the variance and that an individual's unique environment accounted for 30 percent of the variance. These proportions are essentially the same as those found by Andrews and colleagues (1991) and support the now-common assumption that genes and environment interact to set the stage for stuttering.

Five years after the study by Felsenfeld et al., Ooki (2005) studied 1,896 twin pairs, also comparing concordance in identical and fraternal twins. Using sophisticated statistical techniques, Ooki determined that the proportion of genetic influence on stuttering in males was 80 percent and 85 percent in females. It is interesting that the females' rate of stuttering showed slightly more genetic influence than the males'. Perhaps this echoes the evidence that females have some resistance to stuttering. For a female to develop stuttering, more genetic influence is needed.

Dworzynski, Remington, Rijsdijk, Howell, and Plomin (2007) discovered interesting differences between a group of twins who recovered from stuttering ($n = 950$) and a group who persisted ($n = 150$). In the recovered group, concordance for stuttering was 40 percent for identical twins and 20 percent for fraternal twins. However, in the persistent stuttering group of twins, the concordance was 19 percent for identical twins and 0 percent for fraternal twins. This suggests

TABLE 2.2 Summary of Twin Studies of Stuttering

Authors, Date	Participants	Major Findings	Implications
Howie, 1981	30 pairs of same-sex twins, in each of which at least one twin stuttered	62.5 percent concordance in identical twin pairs; 23 percent in fraternal twin pairs In 6 of 16 identical twin pairs, one twin stuttered and the other didn't, implicating nongenetic factors	Evidence for inheritance of stuttering but also evidence for nongenetic factors
Andrews et al., 1991	3,810 unselected twin pairs	71 percent of variance attributed to genetic factors; 29 percent attributed to individual's fetal and postpartum environment	Evidence for inheritance
Felsenfeld et al., 2000	1,567 pairs and 634 individuals from Australian Twin Registry	70 percent of variance attributed to "additive genetic effects"; 30 percent attributed to environment	Evidence for inheritance Similar findings as in previous studies
Ooki, 2005	1,896 twin pairs	80 percent variance attributed to genetic factors in males; 85 percent in females	Slightly more genetic effect in females may be related to their natural resistance to stuttering
Dworzynski et al., 2007	950 twins who recovered from stuttering; 150 twins who persisted	40 percent concordance for identical twins vs. 20 percent for fraternal twins among recovered twins 19 percent concordance for identical twins vs. 0 percent for fraternal in persistent twins	Suggests that persistent stuttering may be the result of multiple genes being inherited; that is, concordance may be less likely in persistently stuttering fraternal twins if more than one gene must be inherited
van Beijsterveldt et al., 2010	105,000 total twin pairs For categorization, parents described speech characteristics	Concordance higher in identical vs. fraternal twins categorized as "probably stuttering" and as "high nonfluency"	
Rautakoski et al., 2012	1,728 total twins	2.3 percent of total twins said they had stuttered at one time; 28 percent of those individuals said they continued to stutter Concordance rates indicated that 82 percent of variance due to additive genetic effects; 18 percent due to nonshared environmental factors	Provides further evidence of the major influence of genes on stuttering and a minor influence of twins' nonshared environment

that the genetics of **persistent stuttering** are complex. As we noted previously, the family studies of Ambrose et al. (1997) indicated the possibility that while recovered and persistent stuttering are transmitted by the same major gene(s), persistent stuttering itself may have additional genetic factors that make recovery more difficult (or genetic factors that facilitate recovery). The findings of Dworzynski and colleagues (2007) may support this supposition because there is so little concordance in the persistent fraternal twin group—meaning that to get concordance, the same array of multiple genes (the "additional genetic factors") must be transmitted. This is far less likely in fraternal twins.

van Beijsterveldt, Felsenfeld, and Boomsma (2010) conducted a twin study using a very large participant pool: 105,000 twin pairs at age 5. They reduced the usual problem of parent identification of their children as stuttering by asking parents merely to estimate the frequency of repetitions, prolongations, and blocks they observed in their children's speech. Children were categorized by the experimenters as "probably stuttering" or "high nonfluency," or as having typical speech. Concordance for probable stuttering was higher in identical twins, supporting the genetic/heritability hypotheses. It was notable that high nonfluency also appeared to be genetically based (see Barasch, Guitar, McCauley, & Absher, 2000 for more on a commonality between stuttering and high levels of typical disfluency).

Fagnani, Fibiger, Skytthe, and Hjelmborg (2011) used a large participant pool (33,317) of adults from the Danish Twin Registry, employing questionnaires to ascertain whether they had ever stuttered. They found that 9 percent of the males and 5 percent of the females reported stuttering at some point in their past. There was significantly greater concordance in monozygotic twins and estimated that 70 percent of the variance in stuttering probability was due to heredity and the other 30 percent was due to environment or environment-gene interaction. This matches the findings of Andrews et al. (1991) and Felsenfeld et al. (2000) but with a much larger sample. Similar findings were reported by Rautakoski, Hannus, Simberg, Sandnabba, and Santtila (2012), using self-report from adults in a study of 1,728 twins in Finland. They indicated that 82 percent of the variance could be attributed to additive genetic effects and 18 percent to nonshared environmental influences.

In an interesting aside, Bloodstein and Ratner (2008) questioned the assumption that influence on stuttering that was not accounted for by genetic factors must be attributed to environmental factors. Research using animal models suggests that identical twins sometimes have discordance for certain traits not because of environmental influences but because of variations in the way two identical embryos develop. Some of these variations may be related to "epigenetics," which are non-DNA factors that are inherited and influence the expression of genes as effects on specific behaviors or phenotypes. Readers wishing to understand developments circa 2005 in genetics, epigenetics, and other principles of gene variability may want to view "Ghost in Your Genes," a Public Broadcasting System NOVA program on genetics (http://www.pbs.org/wgbh/nova/genes/). An online search for "epigenetics Ghost in Your Genes" provides brief summaries of the content.

Adoption Studies

Adoption studies are summarized in Table 2.3. Because the birth records of adopted children are often difficult to obtain, studies of adopted stutterers are rare. Nonetheless, they can be helpful because they offer larger contrasts in environmental factors than seem to be available in twin studies, where family environments are somewhat shared. Bloodstein (1961a) and Bloodstein and Ratner (2008) presented information

TABLE 2.3 Summary of Adoption Studies

Authors, Date	Participants	Major Findings	Implications
Bloodstein, 1961a; Bloodstein and Ratner, 2008	13 adopted individuals who stuttered	Four of the 13 individuals reported having relatives who stuttered in adoptive families	Four is a larger number than would happen by chance. May imply these four individuals may have been influenced by adoptive family members who stuttered
Felsenfeld, 1997	No information on number of individuals	Preliminary data only summarized as from both biological and adoptive families Stuttering in biological families was a better predictor	Data suggested stuttering in biological families was more predictive of stuttering in subject than stuttering in adoptive families

obtained from 13 adopted individuals who stuttered whom Bloodstein interviewed about stuttering in their adoptive families (information on their biological families was not available). Four of the 13 reported having relatives who stuttered in their adoptive families, which is higher than would be expected by chance. This small sample, without data from biological families, supports the possibility that environmental factors may have an effect. If the relatives in the adoptive family were key figures, such as a parent or older sibling who was close to the child, this would be stronger evidence for the influence of the environment on stuttering. Unfortunately, this information is not available.

Felsenfeld (1997) reported some preliminary data on a small sample of adopted children who had speech disorders (primarily stuttering) and for whom data were available from both adoptive and biological families. These data indicated that a history of stuttering in the biological families was slightly more predictive of disorders in these children than was stuttering in the adoptive family.

Again, the evidence from family and twin studies suggests that both genetic and environmental factors influence whether or not a child will stutter and that genetic inheritance appears to contribute more strongly. Methods developed relatively recently allow more direct examination of the genetics of families with and without members who stutter; these will be discussed in the next section.

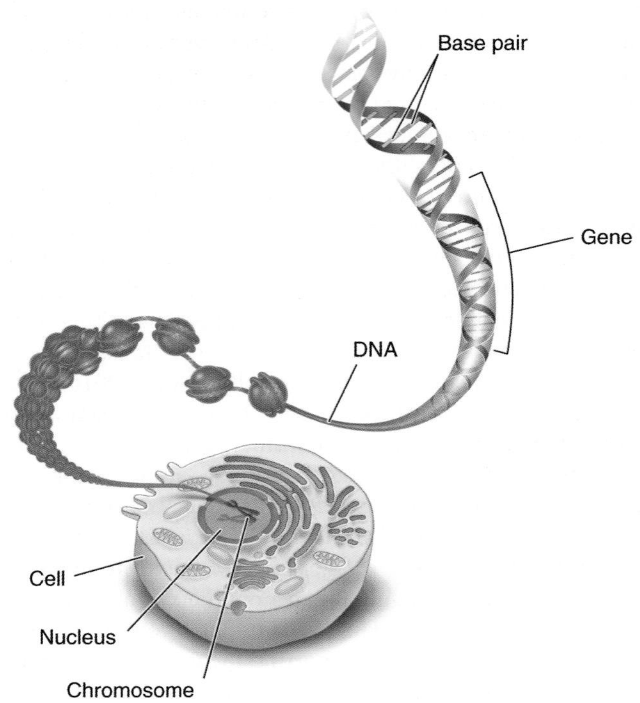

Figure 2.2 Chromosomes and gene.

Genes

Genes are the basis of inheritance. They are sequences of **DNA** that determine traits—like your hair color and the shape of your ears. Genes ride on chromosomes that are worm-like strings of DNA contained in the nucleus of every cell. Figure 2.2 will give you a visual impression of these dynamos of heredity.

Genetic Linkage Studies

Genetic linkage studies can be difficult to understand. The Stuttering Foundation produced a video in 2013 in which one of the scientists, Dennis Drayna, explains his work in this area (https://www.youtube.com/watch?v=HK-TyKKW-ok; or Google "YouTube Dennis Drayna genes and stuttering").

Drayna and his colleagues at the National Institutes of Health have carried out genetic linkage studies using large numbers of families to try to isolate genes for stuttering (for an early overview, see Drayna, 1997). The term "genetic linkage" refers to the fact that the genes related to a disorder may be physically close together (linked) on the chromosome when they are inherited. Genetic linkage analysis compares the chromosomes of family members who have a trait with those of family members who do not. In this way, the approximate chromosomal location of the stuttering gene or genes can be identified. Genetic linkage analysis is in accord with the view that stuttering, like most inherited disorders, is the result of more than one gene. To use the proper term, stuttering is thought to be "polygenic."

To begin their hunt for a stuttering gene, Drayna and his colleagues studied families in which there is more than one individual who stutters. They studied 68 families in North America and Europe and found evidence that genes on chromosome 18 may be related to stuttering in this family (Shugart et al., 2004). Because these are a set of genes that control intercellular communication, this finding suggests that such intercellular communication may be important among neurons involved in speech production and that when such communication goes wrong, the flow of information for speech production may be discoordinated.

Several years later, Drayna, his students, and his colleagues joined with geneticists in Lahore, Pakistan, to continue the hunt for stuttering genes. They chose Pakistan because tradition encourages marriage within families (cousins marrying cousins), and this produces a smaller degree of genetic variation that results in a greater concentration of genetic disorders. Kang et al. (2010) published a study in the prestigious New England Journal of Medicine that reported on 123 Pakistani individuals who stuttered as well as 270 individuals in the United States and England who stuttered. They also used a control group of 372 individuals in these three countries who didn't stutter. Mutations of three genes (the genes were called *GNPTAB*, *GNPTG*, and *NAGPA*) on chromosome 12 were found to be associated with stuttering. Some individuals showed mutations of gene *GNPTAB*, others had mutations on *GNPTG*, and still others had mutations on *NAGPA*. The work of all three genes is related to controlling enzymes in a cell's lysosome structure—the part of a cell involved in recycling cell waste products. It is important to note that there are known genetic disorders (e.g., mucolipidoses) of this waste recycling process that affect joint, skeletal, and other body components. These disorders affect brain development, resulting in delays in movement coordination, and some forms of mucolipidoses are accompanied by speech problems (National Institute of Neurological Disorders and Stroke, 2011). Additionally important is the fact that one of the genes, *GNPTG*, is associated with motor control and emotional regulation by way of the gene's expression in (i.e., their effects on) the cerebellum and the hippocampus. It is noteworthy that the hippocampus is affected because it helps regulate emotions, and emotion-related responses are important in stuttering.

Further exploring the findings described above, Lee, Kang, Drayna, and Kornfield (2011) provided stronger evidence that mutations in one of these genes—*NAGPA*—may cause stuttering. The effect of the mutations is to diminish enzyme activity in cells. The authors caution that not enough is known about exactly how neuronal deficits affect speech to be able to explain how these mutations result specifically in stuttering. Nonetheless, one hypothesis about the underlying mechanism relating diminished enzyme activity in cells' lysosome structure was proposed by Budde, Barron, and Fox (2014). Through a meta-analysis of many studies of differences in individuals who stutter, they concluded that the diminished activity related to lysosomal processing may underlie incomplete myelination of white matter tracts important in speech motor control. The incomplete myelination hypothesis will be discussed again when I present findings on white matter tracts later in the chapter. Interestingly, for more than 50 years (Karlin, 1947), there have been hypotheses that incomplete myelination of nerve tracts, a factor that could lead to less efficient transmission of electrical impulses, helps cause stuttering.

There have been many genetic linkage studies in the last 15 years and more are being published every year. Rather than describe each study, I have created a table of these studies (Table 2.4) that summarizes this research. In addition, a review article appearing a few years ago (Yairi & Ambrose, 2013) gives an overview of genetic research up to that date. If you wish to know the very latest on the genetics of stuttering, conduct a search using a research database such as Ovid MEDLINE or PubMed, using the two terms "stuttering" and "genetics." Another approach—not using families with many individuals who stutter—to studying genes is described in the next section.

A Genome-Wide Association Study

Kraft (2010) took a different approach to the study of genetics and stuttering. Rather than a genetic linkage study in which DNA is compared among family members, she carried out a genome-wide association analysis of the genes of 84 persistent stutterers and 107 controls in which the DNA of a population of unrelated individuals is examined. Kraft was interested not in the chromosomes that were associated with stuttering but in the genes themselves. She scanned the DNA of all of her participants, looking for "markers" that distinguished the DNA of stuttering participants. She didn't find a clear, single gene that characterized stuttering but instead identified 10 "candidate genes" that were statistically more likely to appear in the DNA of those who stuttered. These genes could be subdivided into the three ways in which they may lead to stuttering—through effects on (1) neural development, (2) neural function, and (3) behavior. Some genes (e.g., one labeled *FADS2*[2]) were associated both with neural development and neural function. In the behavior category were some genes that happened to have been identified with such disorders as autism, alcoholism, and Alzheimer's. As Kraft points out, much future work needs to be done to understand the mechanisms that would allow some combination of these genes to pave the way for a child's stuttering.

The next section moves from heredity as a causal factor in stuttering to congenital and early childhood trauma as alternative etiological explanations of stuttering. These factors can also be considered "constitutional" and may account for the many individuals who stutter who have no family history of stuttering or related disorders.

CONGENITAL AND EARLY CHILDHOOD TRAUMA STUDIES

One of the first studies to look closely at stutterers who had no family history of stuttering—West, Nelson, and Berry (1939)—examined a sample of 204 people who stuttered and found that 100 of them reported no family history of stuttering. Of these 100, 85 reported **congenital factors** or early childhood factors that may have been related to the onset of stuttering. These factors included infectious diseases, diseases of the nervous system, and injuries—all reported to have occurred just prior to stuttering onset, although the exact proximity to onset was not reported. Thus, these factors may have created a constitutional predisposition for the development of stuttering. (Of course, a stronger design would have looked at a second sample of people who did not stutter in order to be sure that 85 out of 204 people don't tend to report those levels of suspicious factors.)

A later study by Poulos and Webster (1991) found that 57 of the clients in a clinic sample of 169 adults and adolescents who stuttered reported no family history of stuttering. Of these without family histories, 37 percent reported

[2]This gene is a fatty acid that may be related to findings discussed in Chapter 1 that suggest breastfeeding may help prevent persistent stuttering (Mahurin-Smith & Ambrose, 2009).

TABLE 2.4 Summary of Genetic Studies of Stuttering

Authors, Date	Participants	Major Findings	Implications
Cox and Yairi, 2000	Community of Hutterites in North Dakota	Chromosomes 1, 13, and 16 identified as possibly being the locus of genes related to stuttering	Early evidence that specific chromosomes related to some individuals' stuttering may have been found
Shugart et al., 2004	68 families in North America and Europe	Evidence for stuttering related to genes on chromosome 18	These genes may be related to intercellular communication in speech production areas of the brain
Riaz et al., 2005	44 Pakistani families	A locus on chromosome 12q may contain a gene related to stuttering in these families No evidence found for linkage on chromosome 18 (see above)	Stuttering is probably a complex trait transmitted by non-Mendelian inheritance and can be caused by genes on different chromosomes, as seen in different studies
Kang et al., 2010	123 individuals who stuttered in Pakistan	Mutations found in 3 genes on chromosome 12: *GNPTAB*, *GNPTG*, and *NAGPA*	These mutations affect recycling cell waste products, sometimes producing known genetic disorders Possible source of motor control and emotion effects in stuttering individuals
Raza, Riazuddin, and Drayna, 2010	Large, consanguineous Pakistani family with many individuals with persistent stuttering	Significant linkage found on chromosome 3Q13.2-3q13.33	One individual with this genetic linkage did not stutter but may have outgrown childhood stuttering Provides more evidence of inheritance of stuttering
Raza, Amjad, Riazuddin, and Drayna, 2012	Family in Lahore, Pakistan, with 14 members who stuttered	Linkage found for several genes on chromosome 16q	Evidence for new locus for stuttering gene
Raza et al., 2012	Family of 71 individuals in Cameroon, of whom 33 have persistent stuttering	No single locus for stuttering was found; instead, evidence found for linkage to loci on previously reported 3q and 15q and new finding of loci on 2p, 3p, 14q and new region of 15q	Strong evidence for linkage at several loci
Han et al., 2014	602 unrelated cases of persistent stuttering	*FOXP2* and *CNTNAP2* genes seen in verbal dyspraxia and SLI not found in stuttering individuals	Genetic neuropathological origins of stuttering differ from those in dyspraxia and SLI
Raza et al., 2015			Findings suggest problems in intercellular communication (cf., Shugart et al., 2004)
Chen et al., 2015	502 Chinese families with dyslexia and 502 without	Stuttering risk genes *GNPTAB* and *NAGPA* shown to be associated with dyslexia	Common genes associated with stuttering found in dyslexic families
Raza et al., 2016	1,013 unrelated individuals who stutter from around the world	Mutations in genes *GNPTAB*, *GNPTG*, and *NAGPA* were shown to be related to stuttering but also to serious mucolipidosis disorders Stuttering individuals did not show any mucolipidosis disorders	Mutations of these genes in stuttering are different from those is mucolipidosis These mutations are estimated to occur in 16 percent of stuttering individuals worldwide

congenital or early childhood factors that may have been associated with the onset of stuttering, whereas only 2.4 percent of the clients having a positive family history of stuttering reported such factors. The factors reported included anoxia at birth, premature birth, childhood surgery, head injury, mild cerebral palsy, mild retardation, and experiencing intense fear.

A study by Alm and Risberg (2007) examined a group of 32 individuals who stuttered to look for etiological subgroups. Twenty-three of the 32 (72 percent) who stuttered had family histories of stuttering. Seventeen of the 32 (53 percent) had sustained neurological lesions prior to onset of stuttering. Of note is the finding that seven of the nine individuals with no family history of stuttering (78 percent) reported preonset neurological lesions. This is further support for the hypothesis that two different predispositions may contribute to stuttering—genetic inheritance and brain injury.

Two studies looked at a brain-injured population and assessed whether it comprised more individuals who stuttered than in the general population. In the first, Böhme (1968) examined a sample of 313 individuals who had sustained brain damage at birth or in early childhood; 24 percent of those 313 developed stuttering (compared to 5 percent in the general population). Unfortunately, no information is given about family history of stuttering in those who developed it, but the implication drawn was that congenital or early childhood brain injury can often result in stuttering. In a similar study, Segalowitz and Brown (1991) surveyed more than 600 high school students to ascertain how many had experienced head injury during their childhoods. Of the students, 92 reported head injury, and, of those, nine (about 10 percent) reported having been diagnosed with stuttering. However, it was not clear if the stuttering appeared after the head injury. The authors found that there was a significant relationship between having a head injury and being diagnosed with stuttering, particularly for those children who were unconscious for a period of time after the head injury. Again, there is no information as to whether some of the children who stuttered and had head injuries also had family histories of stuttering.

The fact that neurological or psychological traumas may be associated with childhood stuttering in those without family histories of stuttering is not surprising. Adult onset of stuttering is often associated with head injury, neurological disease, stress, or psychological trauma as I will describe in Chapter 15, "Related Disorders of Fluency." Thus, mechanisms similar to those precipitating adult onset may be involved in childhood stuttering in the absence of family history of stuttering, but this possibility raises as many questions as answers. Why would some children (and adults), but not others, begin to stutter as a result of intense fear or brain injury? Which brain structures and functions affected by head injury and neurological disease result in stuttering? How are they similar to and how do they differ from the effects of inheriting a predisposition to stutter?

In relation to the last question, a number of investigators have looked at whether individuals who stutter who have family histories of stuttering showed any differences in their stuttering behavior, such as severity, compared with those without family histories. Andrews and Harris (1964) and Kidd, Heimbuch, Records, Oehlert, and Webster (1980) found no differences in the stuttering of those with and without family histories of stuttering. However, Janssen, Kraaimaat, and Brutten (1990) looked at a wider variety of speech and language-related variables in several different age groups. They found several significant differences (as well as similarities) between the group with family histories of stuttering and the group without such histories. In terms of similarities, the groups did not differ significantly in responsiveness to treatment, reading ability, or speech-related anxiety. However, when stuttering behaviors were examined closely, those with family histories of stuttering showed more prolongations and blocks than those with no family history of stuttering, although the frequency of repetitions was the same for both groups. Another difference between the groups was that those with positive family histories for stuttering showed significantly longer durations of voiced segments of speech and significantly greater variability in length of unvoiced segments during fluent speech than those with no family history of stuttering. The authors interpreted this finding by suggesting that the stutterers with positive family histories were slower and more variable in their fluent speech. What might this mean?

From these studies, we can conclude that individuals with family histories of stuttering have inherited greater neuromotor instability than those without family histories of stuttering—an instability that produces more prolongations and blocks and that may require the individual to speak more slowly to maintain fluency. This is not to say that those without family history of stuttering did not inherit the predisposition to stutter. Their family histories may contain other speech-related deficits (e.g., articulation problems), and their underlying neuromotor anomalies may result in stuttering. Future research can try to answer this question: Do individuals who stutter but have no family history of stuttering have more family history of other speech and language disorders than the general population?

Table 2.5 summarizes the important findings regarding congenital and early childhood factors as possible etiologies of stuttering.

BRAIN STRUCTURE AND FUNCTION

Brain functions and structures act as link between what you've just been reading about—genetic predisposition or neurological trauma as a possible distal cause of stuttering—and the behaviors of stuttering that we see and hear. If studies show evidence of delays or disruptions of the brain's processing of speech, then we can look for the effect in mistimed or discoordinated movements in speech structures. Because

TABLE 2.5 Summary of Congenital and Early Childhood Factors in Stuttering

Authors, Date	Participants	Major Findings	Implications
West et al., 1939	204 individuals who stuttered	100 of the 204 participants reported no family history of stutter, and 85 reported congenital or early childhood factors, such as nervous system diseases and injuries	Early indication that congenital or early childhood factors may create predisposition for stuttering
Poulos and Webster, 1991	169 individuals who stuttered	57 individuals reported no family history of stuttering. Of these, 37 percent reported congenital or early childhood events that might be related to stuttering predisposition. These included anoxia at birth, premature birth, head injury, experiencing intense fear. Only 2.4 of those with family history reported such events.	Further evidence that congenital and early childhood factors may predispose a child to stuttering
Alm and Risberg, 2007	32 individuals who stuttered	78 percent of those with no family history of stuttering reported "neurological lesions" prior to the onset of stuttering	Genetic factors may explain only some of the causal factors in the onset of stuttering

of neurological processing problems, the brain's instructions to the articulators may be in the wrong sequence, or feedback from movements in progress may erroneously inform the speech production part of the brain that a movement is wrong and must be redone or stopped. You can imagine how this could result in the repetitions, prolongations, and blocks that characterize stuttering.

In the following sections, I review studies of brain function and brain structure in separate sections even though they obviously influence each other. The influence goes both ways. Not only does an anomalous structure (such as less dense nerve fibers) result in slow or discoordinated transmission of information, but the converse may be true as well: repeated dysfunction may cause changes in structures.

As you read about specific anatomical areas, consult Figure 2.3 to orient yourself to landmarks related to speech and language production.

Brain Function Differences in People Who Stutter Compared with People Who Do Not Stutter

Some of the earliest research on the brain and stuttering was conducted in the 1920s, as I described in Chapter 1. Because of the limited technology available at that time, brain function rather than brain structure was the target of researchers' questions. They could see the brain not working quite right, but they couldn't yet see into brain nerves and networks. At that time, researchers had a new tool—electroencephalography (EEG)—they could use to measure brain waves, which are the "signatures" of the electrical activity in the brain as it works. EEG had been developed by Hans Berger, in part because of his interest in mental telepathy (see his biography on Wikipedia). By the late 1920s, Lee Edward Travis at the University of Iowa used it to study the brains of people who stutter, as you will see in the following sections.

Cerebral Dominance for Speech

Both old and new studies have shown that individuals who stutter have greater activity in their right hemispheres than in their left hemispheres, during both fluent and stuttered speech. Just to remind you, this is the reverse of the pattern shown by fluent typical subjects who show considerable left-hemisphere activity and little right-hemisphere activity during speech. Figure 2.4 shows this difference between adults who stuttered and those who didn't. The activity seen in the right hemispheres in adults who stuttered was often in those very areas that are in the same place in the other hemisphere as the left-hemisphere areas most active in fluent speakers. These are usually referred to as "homologous" areas.

These findings about greater right hemisphere activity (compared with left-hemisphere activity) suggest that left-hemisphere structures for speech and language in individuals who stutter may have deficits or delays in development. This may prompt these individuals' use of homologous right-hemisphere structures, which themselves may not be as suited for rapid speech production as left-hemisphere structures (Geschwind & Galaburda, 1985; Kent, 1984). This may result in stuttering, especially under the stress of increasing language demands as well as interference from nearby right-hemisphere centers for emotion.

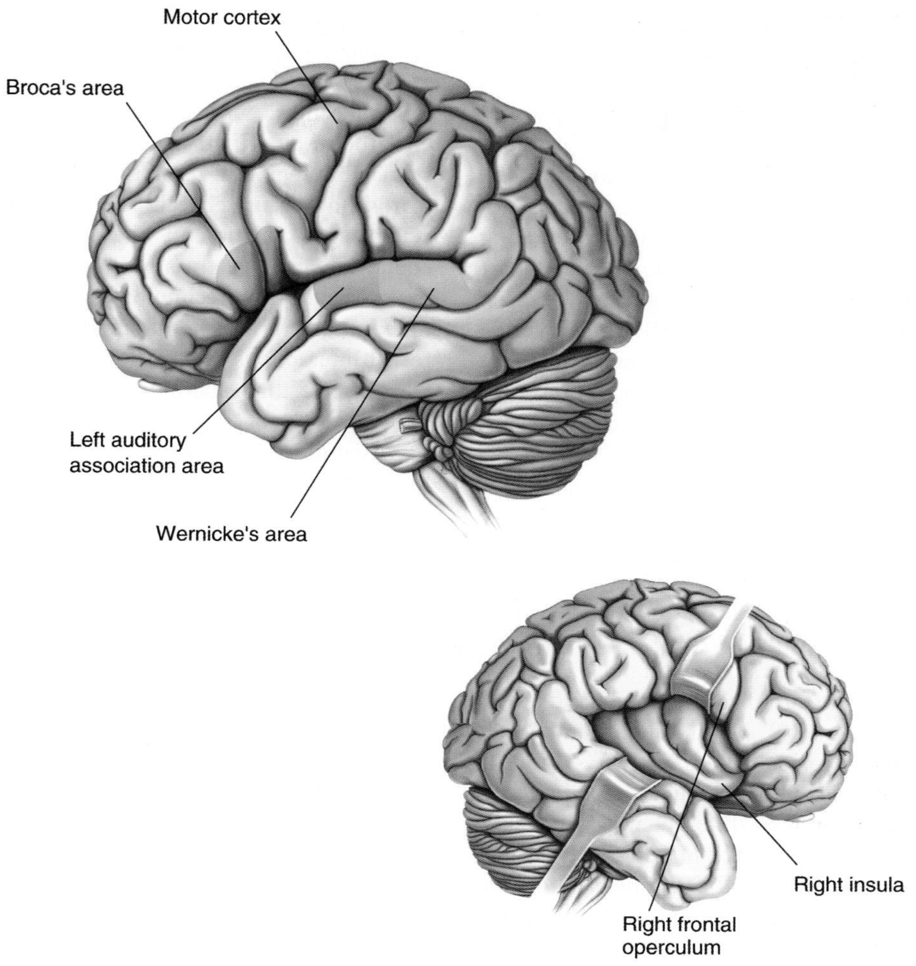

Figure 2.3 Areas in the left and right sides of the brain that may be involved in speech and language processing in stutterers and nonstutterers.

Electroencephalographic Studies

Samuel Orton and Lee Edward Travis (Orton, 1927; Orton & Travis, 1929; Travis, 1931) used EEG to measure brain waves in stuttering and nonstuttering subjects. Their hope was to find proof that the brains of stutterers didn't show the normal left-hemisphere dominance during speech and that this difference might account for the mistiming of signals sent from the brain to muscles of the speech production system. EEG studies are carried out by pasting electrodes to the surface of

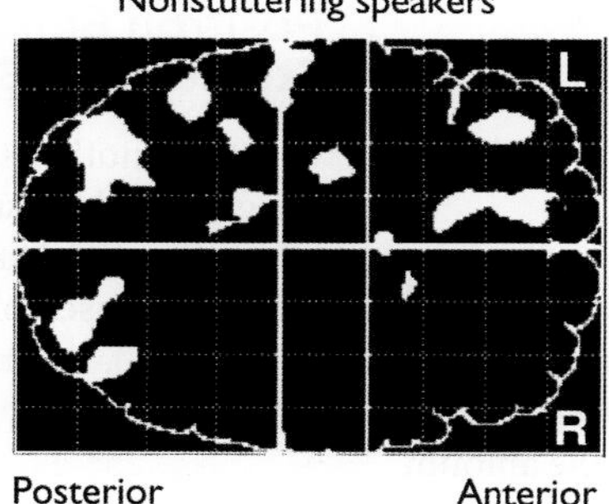

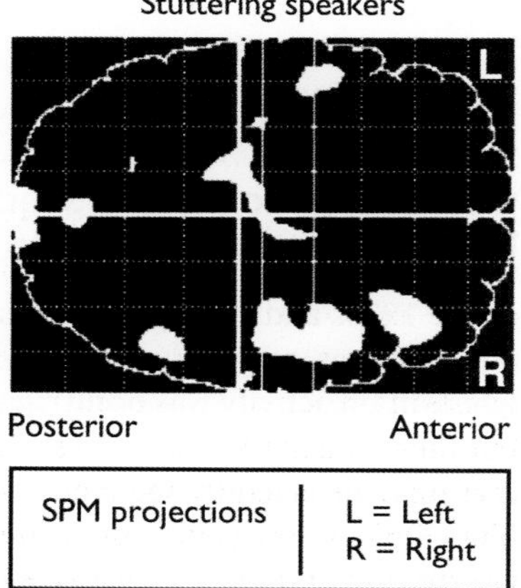

Figure 2.4 PET scans of brains of nonstuttering **(left)** and stuttering **(right)** adults while reading aloud. SPM, statistical parametric mapping. (From De Nil, L. F., Kroll, R. M., Kapur, S., & Houle, S. (1995, December). *Silent and oral reading in stuttering and nonstuttering adults: A positron emission tomography study*. Paper presented at the Annual Convention of the American Speech-Language-Hearing Association, Orlando, FL, with permission.)

the scalp to measure the electrical activity of the brain lying several millimeters below. This procedure, like any assessment of the brain, was fraught with methodological quandaries (Bloodstein, 1995). For example, how faithfully would electrical activity on the scalp mirror the activity of brain cells several millimeters below? How do we know that the electrical activity recorded isn't created by muscle contractions during speech or even the result of the subject blinking her eyes or wiggling her nose? How do we know which part of the brain is active when we see the squiggles on the chart paper that represent electrical impulses? These sources of variability made it likely that the EEG studies by different scientists in different laboratories would produce widely different findings due to different methodologies and different interpretations of the data.

Despite these problems, many EEG studies of people who stutter and those who don't have been conducted. Some interesting findings have turned up. However, as with other experimental results, you should be cautious about accepting the results as final proof. Several EEG studies supported the notion that the brains of people who stuttered functioned differently, although other studies did not. EEG studies by Douglass (1943), Ponsford, Brown, Marsh, and Travis (1975), Travis and Knott (1937), Zimmermann and Knott (1974), many by Moore and his colleagues (e.g., Moore & Haynes, 1980), and a study by Boberg, Yeudall, Schopflocher, and Bo-Lassen (1983) showed in different ways that individuals who stuttered tended to have more activity on the right side of the brain during speech and especially during stuttering than did those who didn't. This activity seemed to involve structures in the right hemisphere that were in locations similar to those in the left hemisphere that control speech and language. One of those areas is called the right frontal operculum (see Fig. 2.3) and is in the same location in the right hemisphere that Broca's area is in the left hemisphere (Fox, 2003). Although this was not exactly what Orton and Travis had predicted in their theory, it was close. Whereas the Orton-Travis theory hypothesized that individuals who stuttered lacked hemispheric dominance, findings from these EEG studies suggested that rather than lacking dominance, individuals who stutter may be more likely to have a right-hemisphere dominance for speech and language (whereas nonstutterers generally have left-hemisphere dominance).

Cerebral Blood Flow Studies: A More Detailed Look at Different Areas of the Brain

In the 1970s and 1980s, researchers developed new technology that was more precise than EEG in detecting exactly where brain activity was occurring by measuring the amount of blood flowing to those areas. Cerebral blood flow (CBF) is usually detected by injecting a radioactive tracer into the bloodstream and taking the equivalent of x-ray pictures of the amount of radioactivity given off. The greater the amount of neural activity in an area, the greater the blood flow in that area and the greater the amount of radioactivity given off.

Interpretation of CBF and other brain imaging studies must take into account many different variables that can influence the results (Ingham, 2001). Two such variables are the spatial and temporal resolution of each technology. In other words, how accurately can CBF determine exactly where the activity is occurring and when it's occurring? Early studies could only observe areas of the brain in a relatively general way, but improved technologies have allowed researchers to differentiate the activity of different areas in more detail and reveal interactions among brain areas. Besides the problem of how good the resolution is, other variables that can influence outcomes of brain imaging studies are the gender of the participants, the severity of their stuttering, whether or not they've had speech therapy, what tasks the participants perform in the study, and techniques used to analyze the data (Lauter, 1995, 1997). Keep these factors in mind as you read about the research in this area.

Wood, Stump, McKeehan, Sheldon, and Proctor (1980) published the first study of CBF in stuttering, using only two participants. They found greater activity in the right-hemisphere region corresponding to Broca's area (the right frontal operculum, remember?) than in Broca's area (left hemisphere) itself during stuttering before treatment with the drug haloperidol.[3] After 2 weeks of treatment with haloperidol, both participants showed that the greater activity had shifted from right- to left-hemisphere speech areas. The second CBF study of stuttering was not published until 11 years later. Pool, Devous, Freeman, Watson, and Finitzo (1991) studied the brains of 20 adults who stuttered using single photon emission computed tomography, an improved technology that enabled scientists to view the brain from multiple angles and obtain better images of what was going on. The principal finding from this study was that the stuttering group showed less left-hemispheric dominance compared to controls in areas that are believed to be associated with language processing (middle temporal lobe), speech motor control (inferior frontal lobe), and motor initiation (anterior cingulate).

Positron Emission Tomography Studies and Beyond

In 1995, another CBF study took advantage of a new brain imaging tool, positron emission tomography (PET), which allowed researchers to make more accurate inferences about where increased blood flow was occurring in the brain (Wu et al., 1995). A large team of researchers studied the brains of four adults who stuttered and a matched group of control

[3]Early experiments with haloperidol had shown success with Tourette syndrome. It was then tried with children who stuttered and found to be helpful. Most later studies had mixed results. Because haloperidol often has adverse effects, it is no longer used for stuttering.

participants in two conditions: reading aloud alone and reading in unison with someone else, which is called "choral reading." As you may remember from Chapter 1, when individuals who stutter read aloud along with someone else, they become more fluent. This research revealed that two important speech and language areas of the brain—Broca's area and Wernicke's area, both in the left hemisphere (see Fig. 2.3)—showed decreased activity (compared to their normal-speaking controls) when participants were stuttering under typical speaking conditions compared to when they were fluent during choral reading. Why might this be? Broca's area is responsible for organizing and executing speech motor output. Wernicke's area is the storehouse for the sounds that form words—the phonological representations that are called upon before the motor commands are given (see Sussman, 2016). These functions may have been shifted away from Broca's and Wernicke's areas to right-hemisphere homologous areas. Right-hemisphere areas are not designed for typical rapid speech and may have been unable to function well enough to produce fluency. In this experiment, choral reading, for some reason, may have "turned on" left-hemisphere speech areas, which are designed for typical rapid reading.

In November 1995, three different research groups using PET brain imaging tools presented their findings at the annual convention of the American Speech-Language-Hearing Association in Orlando, Florida (De Nil et al., 1995; Ingham, Fox, & Ingham, 1995; Wu et al., 1995). As the presentations were given, the excitement in the room was palpable because so many of their findings were similar, although the groups were working entirely independently. Here at last was clear evidence that the brains of people who stutter worked differently than those of people who don't. Years of previous speculation and studies suggesting anomalous cerebral dominance, inadequate laterality, auditory processing problems, and language dysfunction in stuttering seemed to be confirmed. These findings and others are reviewed below, organized by the types of anomalies they suggest. I have chosen to describe the anomalies by whether they are overactivations or underactivations in various areas of the brain. Then, I have described two other sets of findings: those on brain changes after stuttering therapy, and anomalies in the structure and functions of white matter nerve tracts that convey information.

Brain Overactivation during Stuttering

Many studies have shown that certain areas of the brain show higher levels of activation in those who stutter than in controls. Sometimes this is present during stuttering, but it has also been shown in fluent speech. Researchers have suggested that some of the overactivations may be important etiological factors (causing stuttering), while others may be compensatory (attempts by the brain to compensate for low activity in key areas by activating areas not usually used for speech).

Overactivation of Right-Hemisphere Cortical Areas during Stuttering

A common finding by several of the brain research teams in 1995 and afterward is that individuals who stutter demonstrate high levels of activity in the right hemisphere when they are speaking, especially when they are stuttering, as illustrated in Figure 2.4.

The focus of this activity is greatest in right-hemisphere structures that are homologous to those in the left hemisphere used by normal speakers (Braun et al., 1997a, 1997b; De Nil, Kroll, Kapur, & Houle, 2000; Fox et al., 1996, 2000). One active right-hemisphere area (right frontal operculum) may be compensating for an underactive Broca's area that is thought to be usually used in planning the phonetic structure of an utterance to be spoken (Kent, 1997). Another area in the right hemisphere commonly found to be active during stuttering is the right insula (Fox, 2003). In the left hemisphere, the insula may function as a connection between Wernicke's area (which may be important for phonological representations of words and auditory monitoring of one's own speech) and Broca's area (Ingham, Ingham, Finn, & Fox, 2003).

A meta-analysis of many brain studies that compared people who stuttered and controls (Brown, Ingham, Ingham, Laird, & Fox, 2005) confirmed that a major anomaly in those who stutter was a general overactivation of right-sided areas that are homologous to left-sided areas active for speech production: the right frontal operculum, rolandic operculum, and right anterior insula. These findings of overactivity in right-hemisphere areas were confirmed in a more recent meta-analysis (Budde et al., 2014). It should be noted that these more recent researchers also observed that a common finding was overactivation in left-hemisphere areas related to motor control of speech compared to nonstuttering peers, perhaps as a result of the extra effort required to speak.

Researchers have considered two possible explanations for the overactivation of right-hemisphere structures during stuttering. One is that during embryonic development, the right side of the brain, instead of the left, becomes "wired" to be the primary speech and language area (e.g., Geschwind & Galaburda, 1985). This may result in some difficulty speaking because right-hemisphere structures are not generally suited for the rapid processing of signals required for speech (such as the quick transitions in many consonant-vowel combinations). When a child with this right-hemisphere "wiring" for speech develops language beyond the single-word stage, stuttering may emerge as he tries to produce multiword utterances at the typically fast speech rates used for longer sentences (Kent, 1984; Malecot, Johnston, & Kizziar, 1972). A second hypothesis is that the child who stutters initially tries to use left-hemisphere regions for speech and language, but the neural networks for speech and language fail to function adequately and result in stuttering. Only then does the child's brain begin to use right-hemisphere structures in a compensatory way to try to achieve more normal speech, similar to the way in which some individuals with aphasia use right-hemisphere structures to compensate for damaged areas in the left hemisphere (e.g., Sommer, Koch, Paulus, Weiller, & Buchel, 2002; Weiller et al., 1995).

Several researchers have provided evidence in favor of the second (compensation) hypothesis. Braun and colleagues (1997a, 1997b) found that activations of right-hemisphere sensory areas were negatively correlated with stuttering; that is, these regions became more active as speech became more fluent. Moreover, researchers in Germany (Neumann et al., 2003) found that right-hemisphere activations were greater in participants who stuttered moderately compared to those who stuttered severely, suggesting that right-hemisphere activity may indeed be a way in which individuals could partially overcome dysfunctions in the left-hemisphere areas. In other words, the moderate stutterers used more compensatory right-hemisphere activity to reduce the severity of their stuttering.

It is possible, of course, that both hypotheses are correct—that some individuals develop right-hemisphere processing for speech and language before they begin to stutter, and others develop right-hemisphere processing after they begin to stutter, as a compensatory response. Still others may in fact process speech and language in both hemispheres simultaneously. Each of these options is probably inefficient and may create the dyssynchrony in processing assumed to result in stuttering. Future research examining changes in the processing of individuals who stutter as they develop from early childhood would be very helpful in sorting this out.

Overactivation in Midbrain Areas

A number of researchers have reported unusually high levels of activity in midbrain structures that, via pathways to the cerebral cortex, may influence speech movements. Specifically, some structures of the basal ganglia have been shown to be overactive in those who stutter (e.g., substantia nigra, subthalamic nucleus, red nucleus, globus pallidus) (Fox et al., 1996; Watkins, Smith, Davis, & Howell, 2008). This midbrain area is important in speech motor activity, via loops that send signals from the cortex to the basal ganglia, which then send "go" or "no go" signals to the supplementary motor area (SMA), which itself is responsible for initiating the respiratory, phonatory, and articulatory movements needed for speech. Excess activity in the basal ganglia associated with stuttering could possibly result in inhibitory signals sent to SMA that would prevent the initiation of speech movements. Another perspective, given by Alm (2004), is that the excess right-hemisphere SMA activity during stuttering reported by Fox and colleagues (1996) may be the result of inadequate left-hemisphere SMA activity due to basal ganglia dysfunction in stutterers. Excess right-hemisphere pre-SMA activity in individuals who stutter was also found in the meta-analysis conducted by Budde et al. (2014).

Underactive Brain Areas during Stuttering

Several areas of the brain, including both motor and sensory centers, have been found to be underactive in stuttering. Because speech motor control involves the integration of motor and sensory information, it is not surprising that this is sometimes reported in these studies.

Underactivity in Speech Motor Areas

Watkins and colleagues (2008) found that during speech production, individuals who stutter showed decreased activity compared to controls in areas related to using sensory and motor information and planning sequential movements: ventral premotor, rolandic opercula, and sensorimotor cortex on both sides of the brain. This underactivity was in the same area of the brain as the structural differences found by Chang, Erickson, Ambrose, Hasegawa-Johnson, and Ludlow (2008)—less dense white matter tracts connecting articulatory planning and sensory feedback areas. Thus, structural differences seem to result in functional deficits that presumably interfere with the smooth flow of speech. The researchers point out that the fact that the decreased activity is present on both sides of the brain and is widespread may account for the findings that, unlike in cases of unilateral and limited brain lesions, these individuals' brains were unable to develop "work-arounds" to compensate for the problem allowing them to speak at all, even if disfluently.

Underactivity in Auditory Areas

Many brain imaging studies of stuttering have shown a lack of activity in the superior temporal lobe, including auditory association areas and Wernicke's area (Braun et al., 1997a, 1997b; De Nil, Kroll, Lafaille, & Houle, 2003; Fox et al., 1996, 2000). The meta-analysis by Brown and colleagues (2005) mentioned earlier indicated that a common finding among several of these studies was that auditory areas in both hemispheres were underactivated, suggesting that in individuals who stutter mechanisms for guiding their speech by self-hearing were not functioning properly. Budde et al. (2014) followed up the meta-analysis by Brown et al. and found that the 17 studies they analyzed showed that during speech, individuals who stuttered showed less activity in left auditory cortex than did controls. They also found that activity was reduced in both the auditory cortices when the stuttering individuals were stuttering compared to when they were fluent. Watkins et al. (2008) found in their study of adolescent and young adult stutterers that underactivity was notable in Heschl's gyrus, a part of the auditory cortex that is important for processing speech sounds. Evidence of dysfunction in auditory areas during stuttering is especially pertinent in light of the many studies that have shown that stutterers may have difficulty performing auditory processing tasks (e.g., Barasch et al., 2000; Kent, 1984; Molt, 1997) and that fluency can be induced by changing the way stutterers hear their own speech (e.g., Brayton & Conture, 1978; Howell, El-Yaniv, & Powell, 1987).

How does auditory self-monitoring affect fluency? It may provide a stimulus to synchronize or integrate the sequence of activities that run in parallel when a speaker decides what she will say, selects the linguistic elements for it, and executes the utterance. Thus, the asynchrony or timing disturbance that many researchers see as the basis of stuttering (e.g., Kent, 1984; Perkins, Kent, & Curlee, 1991; Van Riper, 1982) may be caused by a paucity of signals that can help synchronize the sequence for speech output. Therapies (e.g., Van Riper, 1973) that emphasize proprioception may be increasing the amount of information to use for synchronizing speech the client has by focusing their attention on another feedback modality. Specifically, therapies that focus on the use of slow speech, gentle onsets, and light articulatory contacts may help clients more easily use feedback to guide and synchronize their speech motor commands.

Other functions besides monitoring one's own speech may also reside in the underactivated regions of the auditory cortex. For example, Wernicke's area may be important for storing the phonological representations of words (Caplan, 1987; Paulesu, Frith, & Frackowiak, 1993; Sussman, 2016). Activation of this region of the brain, therefore, may be a key stage in phonological planning for speech production. Lack of adequate activation during stuttering may reflect a deficit in the sequence of phonological selection, phonetic planning, and motor execution.

Connectivity Deficits in White Matter Tracts

In a study of adults who stutter, Chang, Horowitz, Ostuni, Reynolds, and Ludlow (2011) discovered structural connectivity deficits in white matter tracts in the left hemisphere that linked inferior frontal areas (these areas may be involved in programming speech movements) and premotor cortex (these areas may be involved in sensory guidance of speech movements). Moreover, deficits in functional connectivity in these tracts were found both for speech and nonspeech movements, which would help explain findings that show poorer performance among stutters for tasks like repeating sentences (Walsh, Mettel, & Smith, 2015) and finger-tapping (Subramanian & Yairi, 2006). In addition, Chang et al. found heightened functional connectivity for stutterers compared to nonstutterers in the right hemisphere, which may have been a compensation for left-hemisphere deficits.

In one of the first multimodal neuroimaging studies of young children, Chang and Zhu (2013) compared both structural and functional connectivity in white matter tracts of 56 children 3 to 9 years old who stuttered versus their fluent peers. They found deficiencies in the networks connecting auditory-motor and basal ganglia-thalamocortical areas in the children who stuttered. These deficiencies were hypothesized to create problems in planning and carrying out speech movements. Findings of this study included evidence that girls who stutter showed higher connectivity in auditory-motor tracts than boys who stutter. In a later publication, Chang (2014) expanded on the sex differences in neuroimaging studies of boys and girls that may be important in our understanding of why girls are more likely to recover from stuttering than boys. Chang's review of research in this area makes it clear that girls' brains show earlier development in many areas, including those areas that underlie speech and language development. Therefore, they may be able to move out of a period of disfluency more rapidly and therefore be less prone to the reinforcements that may underlie persistent stuttering.

Table 2.6 presents two meta-analyses of brain imaging studies of stuttering that include many of the best publications on brain function differences. Meta-analysis is a way of statistically analyzing a large number of studies on the same topic and summarizing what findings are common among them.

Brain Structure Differences in People Who Stutter Compared with People Who Do Not Stutter

Research on structural differences in brains of people who stutter (compared to research on functional differences) has begun relatively recently. Several studies between 2000 and 2007[4] examined the brain anatomy of adults who stuttered by measuring the shape, size, and density of speech and language areas. The findings suggested that sensory, planning, and motor areas in the left hemisphere of these individuals developed differently from those in matched nonstuttering individuals. For example, white matter tracts, which convey information from sensory centers in the left hemisphere (which, e.g., store phonological representations of sounds) to motor execution areas of the left hemisphere, have been shown to be less dense than those in typical speakers. However, the same tracts were found to be denser in the right hemisphere of those who stuttered. It is perhaps a consequence of the right hemisphere takeover of some typical left-hemisphere functions, mentioned earlier.

By 2008, neuroimaging researchers had developed techniques that were safe enough to use with children for the purposes of examining brain structures. In that year, two groups of investigators published studies of school-age children who had stuttered in their preschool years. One study of children who recovered from stuttering compared them both to those who hadn't and to a control group (Chang et al., 2008) and showed that, compared to the control group, both recovered and persistent stutterers had reduced volumes of gray matter around Broca's area, the part of the brain you probably remember by now is associated with motor control for speech. They also found reduced volume in bilateral temporal lobe areas that may be related to auditory perception of speech. The subgroup of children who persisted in stuttering (but not the subgroup who recovered) also showed less dense

[4]These include Beal, Gracco, Lafaille, and De Nil (2007), Fondas, Bollich, Corey, Hurley, and Heilman (2001), Foundas and colleagues (2004); Jäncke, Hänggi, and Steinmetz (2004), and Sommer, Koch, Paulus, Weiller, and Büchel (2002).

TABLE 2.6 Summary of Recent Meta-Analyses of Studies of Brain Function Differences in People Who Stutter

Authors, Date	Participants	Major Findings	Implications
Brown et al., 2005	Meta-analysis of eight studies focusing on both stuttering and control participants	"Neural signatures" of stuttering were described as overactivity in right-hemisphere areas homologous to speech areas in the left hemisphere; absence of activity in auditory areas used to monitor one's own speech; high level of activity in an area of the cerebellum not activated in controls	Suggests that findings support an "efference copy" dysfunction in stuttering; in other words, the predicted sensory outcome of the motor plan for speech is typically compared with what the speech output actually is, and thus, errors can be detected and the motor plan can be corrected See Chapter 6 for a description of efference copy dysfunction (the "Reduced Capacity for Internal Modeling" theory)
Budde et al., 2014	Meta-analysis of 17 studies, following up on Brown et al. (2005), using many more studies and participants and a more rigorous statistical meta-analysis	Confirms the "neural signatures" found in Brown et al. meta-analysis The SMA, implicated in other studies, was found to be more active in individuals who stutter than in controls, especially during stuttered speech	Suggests that continued meta-analyses of brain imaging studies of stuttering may lead to better models of stuttering and eventually to treatments that can be personalized to fit an individual's particular deficits

white matter tracts connecting areas associated with phonological representations of sounds to speech motor execution areas, the same deficit as discovered in adult stutterers, described earlier. This finding was reported again in a second 2008 study of slightly older children in that same year, indicating that this structural abnormality in the left hemisphere may well be a major factor in stuttering (Watkins et al., 2008).

The 2008 findings of the two groups cited above were replicated by Cykowski, Fox, Ingham, Ingham, and Robin (2010), using more extensive brain imaging technology. They found that the most robust difference between adults who stutter and those who don't is in left-hemisphere white matter fiber tracts that communicate between the inferior parietal cortex (sensory integration) and the ventral frontal cortex (motor planning). As in earlier studies, the authors found that in individuals who stutter compared to individuals who don't, certain nerve fibers aren't structured as effectively to conduct impulses along the directional flow of the nerve bundle. Thus, conduction is not as fast as it might be. The fiber tract implicated in Cykowski et al. is called the superior longitudinal fasciculus (SLF III). It is illustrated in Figure 2.5. This tract connects speech output planning areas of the ventral frontal cortex with sensorimotor integration areas of the inferior parietal lobe. Cykowski and his colleagues speculated that the etiology of the less efficient transport structure of the white matter tracts in individuals who stutter may be a result of reduced myelination of nerves in these pathways.

As mentioned earlier, this explanation is essentially a reprise of Karlin's (1947) hypothesis that "the basic cause for stuttering is a delay in the myelination of the cortical areas in the brain concerned with speech" (p. 319). Karlin pointed out that the myelin sheath surrounding nerves functions to

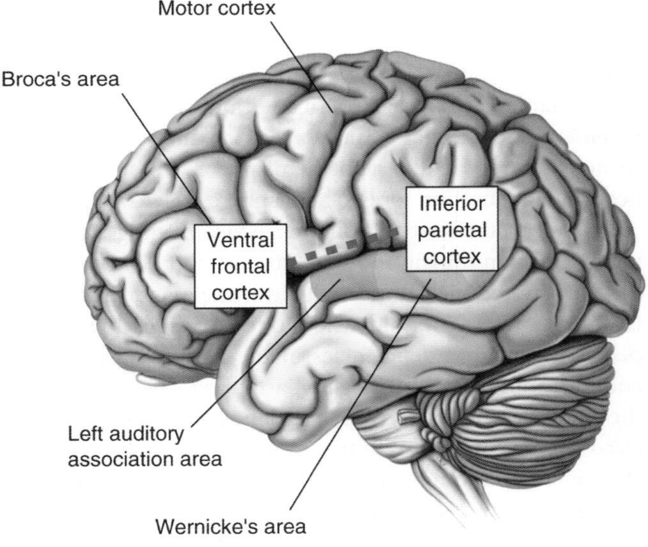

Figure 2.5 The superior longitudinal fasciculus III is a bidirectional pathway between the inferior parietal cortex (sensory integration) and the ventral frontal cortex (motor planning).

insulate them. This insulation speeds the flow of electricity, just as it does in the electric transmission lines outside your house. Incomplete myelination of some nerves results in slower transmission in those nerves, and thus, where many different nerves are working together in a network, the slow transmission in some nerves could result in actions that are less well coordinated. Karlin further pointed out that myelination occurs earlier in girls than in boys (Flechsig, 1927), which may help explain the greater persistence of stuttering in boys.

An important effect of reduced myelination in these bidirectional nerve pathways may be that, in addition to slowing transmissions, without adequate insulation provided by the myelin sheath, these pathways may also be vulnerable to "cross talk" from high levels of activity in emotion and language processes. By cross talk, I mean the disruption of some pathways by activity in others. The term itself comes from discussions of electric transmission lines but seems relevant here. Vulnerability of poorly myelinated fibers to interference by emotional activity seems possible given the evidence that the left frontal cortex is active for positive emotional arousal (e.g., Davidson, 1995) and the evidence reported by Johnson, Walden, Conture, and Karrass (2010) that stuttering may increase during positive emotional arousal, not just negative emotional arousal. Furthermore, emotion-related disorders (e.g., pediatric bipolar disorder) are reported to be associated with decreased myelination in the SLF (Pavuluri & Passaroti, 2008). Taking these finding together, increased stuttering during high levels of emotion may be the result of disruptions in neural transmission in poorly myelinated white matter tracts in speech areas of the brain. These disruptions then may cause mistiming of the signals that, in turn, result in discoordinated movements.

In addition to the effects of emotion on stuttering, the effects of language processing may sometimes overwhelm neural "transmission lines" because so much information must be passed back and forth at such high speeds (e.g., longer sentences are spoken more quickly; Malecot et al., 1972). Karlin (1947) pointed out that stuttering first appears when "sentence formation and flow of language has become more fully developed" (p. 319), implying that this increased demand of more developed language is too much for the pathways that are not fully myelinated, with stuttering as a result. Cykowski and colleagues (2010) also suggest that speech-language demands (such as the production of low-frequency or more complex words that require more careful monitoring) can put enough stress on the less myelinated fiber tracts to provoke stuttering.

Later studies have continued to support earlier findings about deficits in white matter nerve tracts in children who stutter. For example, Chang, Zhu, Choo, and Angstadt (2015) used a technique called fractional anisotropy to analyze white matter fiber integrity throughout the brain in 37 children who stutter comparing them with 40 matched control children, all between ages 3 and 10. Fractional anisotropy involves looking at the alignment of water molecules in the white matter tracts. Well-aligned water molecules in these tracts promote rapid and efficient transmission of information back and forth between areas of the brain. Chang and her colleagues' findings suggested widespread white matter connectivity deficits in children who stutter, not only in left-hemisphere cortical areas linking premotor, motor, and auditory systems but also in areas outside the left hemisphere, affecting interhemispheric communication and cortical-subcortical pathways. These deficits would obviously hinder speech-motor coordination in children who stutter.

Because Chang et al. (2015) studied so many children in such a wide age range, they could effectively compare the brains of younger children with those of older children in both the stuttering and nonstuttering groups. They found that white matter integrity increased with age in both groups. However, the children in the stuttering group showed less increase with age compared to the nonstuttering group. In addition, increases in white matter integrity were uneven and inconsistent in the stuttering group, compared to the nonstuttering group. White matter deficits shown by the analysis were significantly correlated with the age of the children in the stuttering group. This led the authors to surmise that there are continuing white matter deficits with persistent stuttering, because the older children had not recovered. In other words, "It is likely that [white matter] differences become more exaggerated with age as stuttering persists" (p. 705).

In this same study, Chang and her associates (2015) also investigated whether children with more severe stuttering showed white matter integrity differences (from nonstuttering children) compared to children with less severe stuttering. They found that differences in white matter deficits did indeed differentiate the more severely stuttering children from the less severe children. Some of the areas that were deficient in the severe stutterers were connections with the laryngeal motor cortex. The authors note that these poorer connections would involve white matter tracts linking the laryngeal motor cortex with surrounding cortical areas involved in the "integration of proprioceptive and tactile feedback from the orofacial, respiratory, and laryngeal regions during voice production" (quoted by Chang et al. from Simonyan & Horowitz, 2011, p. 203). Therefore, it would not be surprising if problems in integrating feedback during speech would result in severe stuttering.

The study by Chang et al. (2015) is clearly an important one because it was the first to show white matter deficits in many areas of the brain in young children who stutter, to suggest what might distinguish recovery from persistence, and to find connectivity differences that distinguish mild and moderate stuttering from severe stuttering.

Whole Brain Intrinsic Network Connectivity

The imposing title of this section signals a new perspective on how brain differences in people who stutter are investigated. Much of the previous research described in this chapter has used a "localizationist" approach. In other words, researchers have looked at differences in structure and function in specific areas of the brain, such as speech-motor and auditory processing areas in the left hemisphere. Whole brain studies examine activity in the entire cortex. Chang et al. (2017) reported on the study of 42 children who stutter and 42 controls who were given repeated brain scans over a period of several years. Some of the children who stuttered were persistent in their stuttering, and others recovered over the span of the study. The brain scans used were termed "rsfMRI" because they were done while the children were in a resting state, rather than speaking. Resting brain scans allow the natural interconnectivity (or lack thereof) of different networks to be viewed. This resting interconnectivity is termed "default mode network" or DMN. Without going into too much detail about the particular networks involved, the results can be summarized as follows:

> *One of the aberrant connections found was between the DMN and the posterior cingulate cortex, which is involved in attention. Because of the influence that dopamine can have on this connection, this finding was cited as some support for the hypothesis that stuttering is characterized by excess dopamine.*

Some of the anomalous connections in the DMN—including those related to speech motor control—were found in children who stutter, whether they recovered or not.

Children who persisted in stuttering also tended to show abnormal connectivity in networks associated with attention and executive function.

Overall, stuttering was associated with abnormal connectivity in networks associated with attention, motor performance, perception, and emotion. This finding may help explain why there is such variability in stuttering (connectivity changes over time) and why stuttering may co-occur with other disorders such as attention deficit disorder and anxiety. This study is probably the first of many that will follow, exploring abnormal connectivity in networks of individuals who stutter (Table 2.7).

Changes in Brain Activity after Treatment

Both short-term and long-term treatment outcome studies using brain imaging suggest that areas of the left hemisphere that were previously underactivated were reactivated after effective treatment and that right-hemisphere sites became more normally activated (i.e., less overactivated) (Boberg et al., 1983; De Nil et al., 2003; De Nil & Kroll, 1995; Kroll, de Nil, & Houle, 1999; Kroll, De Nil, Kapur, & Houle, 1997; Moore, 1984; Neumann et al., 2003, 2005; Neumann & Euler, 2010; Wood et al., 1980). A chapter by Neumann and Euler (2010) has additional details about brain changes following treatment using the Kassel Stuttering Therapy (KST) program. This approach changes the client's speech pattern, using prolonged speech, easy onsets, and smooth transitions, all using computer-guided feedback. Neumann and Euler (2010) suggest that successful treatment activates left-hemisphere areas near those that were deficit before treatment.

Figure 2.6—from Neumann et al. (2003)—depicts the differences in brain activity in people who stutter (1) before treatment, (2) immediately after treatment, and (3) 2 years after treatment. It is evident that activity levels shift from greater in the right hemisphere to greater in the left hemisphere following treatment.

An fMRI study by Kell et al. (2009) compared the recovery processes of 13 male adults who stuttered and were given treatment with those of a fluent control group and a matched group of adult males who recovered on their own as adults, without treatment. These findings were reviewed in Neumann and Euler (2010) as noted above, but some of the details are of interest here. Those subjects who were still stuttering at the time of the fMRI scans showed right-hemisphere "compensation" (use of right-hemisphere structures for speaking), which was not very effective in generating fluency. However, after treatment, the same subjects showed generally increased left-hemisphere activation for speech. But the adults who had recovered unassisted from their stuttering had specific left-hemisphere activation very near to areas of white matter that are found to be dysfunctional in persistent stuttering. The gray matter area associated with unassisted recovery was Brodmann's area 47/12—an area in the inferior frontal cortex thought to be important in linguistic processing and timing structure in music (e.g., Levitin & Menon, 2003). In these individuals who recovered on their own, the white matter areas were functioning well. The authors suggest that this reflects plasticity in the adult brain, wherein the white matter anomalies repaired themselves as a part of the recovery process. Some of the authors who have studied stuttering therapy (e.g., Kell et al., 2009) suggest that the effect of treatment may be to re-establish in the left hemisphere mechanisms that integrate auditory feedback with proper timing for speech production, leading to increased fluency.

A recent publication by Ingham, Ingham, Euler, and Neumann (2017) reviewed a large number of studies of neural changes associated with recovery—both natural and after treatment. Among the treatments this paper reviewed was the Modified Phonation Interval (MPI) approach that had been reported by Ingham, Wang, Ingham, Bothe, and Grafton (2013) and Ingham, Ingham, Bothe, Wang, and Kilgo (2015). This approach teaches clients to change the length of the phonated portion of their utterances, inducing fluency. In the first of these papers, the authors reported that the brain change most related to successful treatment was increased activity in the left putamen, a structure critical for the regulation of movement. The left putamen has been identified in other research as one of the brain structures than normalizes after stuttering treatment (e.g., Neumann and Euler, 2010).

The publication by Ingham et al. (2017) also reviews the effects of various types of brain stimulation on stuttering. Readers are encouraged to read this paper to learn more about new approaches to treatment (see Suggested Readings for the full citation).

TABLE 2.7 Summary of Relatively Recent Studies of Brain Structure Differences in People Who Stutter

Authors, Date	Participants	Major Findings	Implications
Chang et al., 2008	School-age children	Reduced volume of gray matter around Broca's area Reduced volume in bilateral temporal lobe areas related to auditory perception Persistent stuttering was associated with less dense white matter tracts connecting areas for phonological representation of sounds to motor execution areas (replicated by Watkins et al., 2008)	Clear indications that children who stutter show structural deficits in key areas related to speech production (not just adults who have been stuttering for years)
Cykowski et al., 2010	Adults	Deficits in myelination of white matter tracts connecting sensory integration areas with motor planning areas	Possible deficits in effective connectivity in areas related to speech production, which may lead to discoordination among many interconnecting pathways critical for smooth speech production Possible potential for interference with speech production by language overload and emotional arousal
Chang et al., 2015	37 children who stuttered and 40 matched controls	Widespread white matter connectivity deficits in children who stutter. These deficits were found not only in left-hemisphere areas linking premotor, motor, and auditory systems but also affecting interhemispheric and cortical-subcortical communication	Children with persistent stuttering and children with more severe stuttering were more likely to show these white matter deficits
Chang et al., 2017	42 children who stuttered and 42 controls Brain scans repeated over a period of years as children developed	Resting brain scans showed widespread anomalies in the connections between the resting networks and those associated with speech motor control, attention, executive function, perception, and emotion	Helps to explain why stuttering can be so variable because connections varied over the course of development Suggests why stuttering may co-occur with many other disorders such as those affecting attention and anxiety

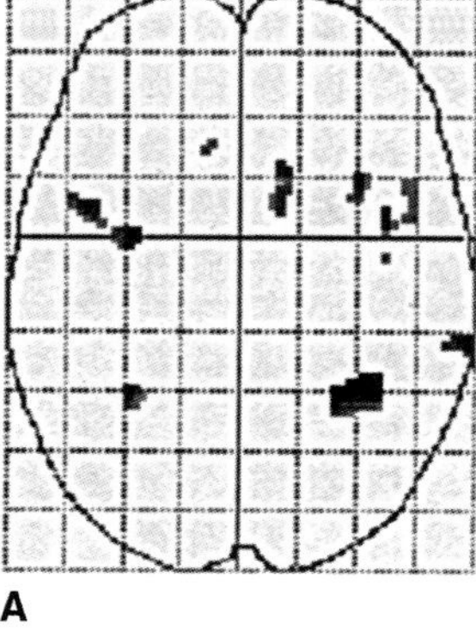

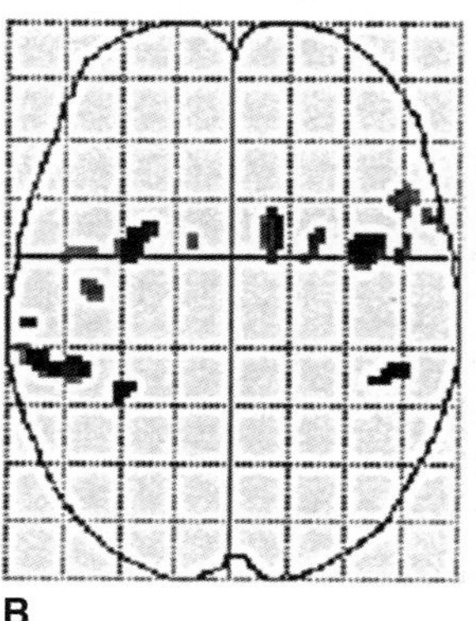

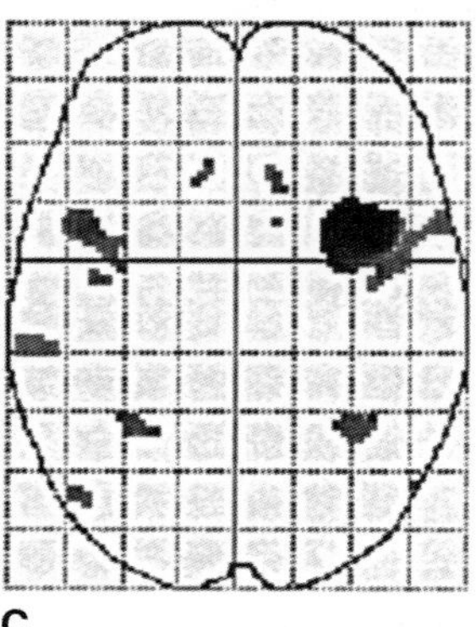

Figure 2.6 Overt reading: statistical parametrical maps of between-group comparisons (people who stutter vs. people who do not stutter) **(A)** before therapy, **(B)** immediately after therapy, **(C)** 2 years after therapy. (Reprinted from Neumann, K., Euler, H. A., von Gudenberg, A. W., Giraud, A. L., Lanfermann, H., Gall, V., et al. (2003). The nature and treatment of stuttering as revealed by fMRI: A within- and between-group comparison. *Journal of Fluency Disorders, 28*(4), 381–410, with permission from Elsevier.)

SUMMARY

- Stuttering appears to have a genetic basis in many individuals. However, twin studies and adoption studies confirm that genes must interact with environmental factors for stuttering to appear.
- Recent research identifies some genes associated with stuttering in some individuals.
- Stuttering may have its etiology in congenital factors for some stutterers. These may include physical trauma at birth or in utero, cerebral palsy, retardation, and emotionally stressful situations.
- Slightly more boys begin to stutter than girls, but girls are more likely to recover, so by school age and beyond, there are many more boys who stutter than girls.
- Early childhood stuttering may be either transitory, in which the child recovers naturally within 18 months, with no or minimal treatment, or persistent, in which the child, if not treated, stutters 3 years or more.
- Persistent and transitory stuttering appear to be the result of a common genetic factor (either a single gene or several), but the persistent form of stuttering probably has additional genetic factors that impede recovery.
- Natural recovery from stuttering seems to be associated with the following factors: (1) good scores on tests of phonology, language, and nonverbal skills; (2) either no family history of stuttering or family members who had natural recovery from stuttering; (3) early age of onset of stuttering; and (4) being a girl.
- Brain imaging studies of adults who stutter have shown various anomalies during speaking and especially during stuttering. One anomaly is overactivation in right-brain areas homologous to left-hemisphere speech and language structures typically used by nonstutterers. Another anomaly is deactivation in the left auditory cortex.
- Neuroanatomical differences seen via brain imaging include (1) anomalies in the planum temporale (related to auditory processing) and in gyri (raised areas on the brain's surface) in speech and language areas and (2) less dense and less myelinated white matter fiber tracts connecting speech perception, planning, and execution areas.
- Inducement of short-term or long-term fluency in stutterers is accompanied by decreases in right-hemisphere activations and increases in activation of left-hemisphere speech, language, and auditory areas.

STUDY QUESTIONS

1. How does each of the areas—family studies, twin studies, and adoption studies—provide evidence that stuttering is inherited?
2. A couple comes to you for advice. They tell you they are thinking of having children but are worried because each has a relative who stutters. What more information would you like to get from them? What would you tell them about the likelihood that they would have a child who stutters and whether they should be concerned?
3. How do studies provide evidence that stuttering is a product of both heredity and environment?
4. How would you summarize the brain imaging studies to someone who is not a professional in our field?
5. Why do most of the brain imaging studies use right-handed males as participants?
6. Researchers have found many differences between groups of stutterers and nonstutterers. Why can't we always say that these differences cause stuttering?
7. What research finding in this chapter do you think has the most relevance for the treatment of stuttering? Defend your answer.

SUGGESTED PROJECTS

1. Talk to someone who stutters and plot out his or her family tree, noting relatives who stutter and relatives who have other speech, language, or learning problems.
2. Make a family tree of your own relatives indicating which, if any, currently have or have had speech, language, hearing, or learning disabilities. Describe how you got the information and what the disabilities are.
3. On which side of your brain do you process speech and language? Find out how you could ascertain this information by asking speech-language pathology researchers or audiologists you know if they have tests you could take to find out. If this doesn't lead to a test for this kind of laterality, search the Internet for self-administered tests, which tell you whether you are more "left-brained" or more "right-brained." Does the answer make sense to you? (I came out more right-brained).

SUGGESTED READINGS

Doidge, N. (2007). *The brain that changes itself.* New York, NY: Penguin Books.

This is an inspiring book by a psychiatrist interested in neuroplasticity. It describes research suggesting that the brain is more changeable that previously believed.

Doidge, N. (2016). *The brain's way of healing.* New York, NY: Penguin Books.

A follow-up to Doidge's 2007 book. This one has many stories of individuals who overcame serious brain injuries and diseases by helping their brains change and thereby modify their disorders.

Etchell, A., Civier, O., Ballard, K., & Sowman, P. (2017). A systematic literature review of neuroimaging research on developmental stuttering between 1995 and 2016. *Journal of Fluency Disorders, 55*, 6–45. doi:10.1016/j.jfludis.2017.03.007

This is a relatively recent review of both brain structure and function differences in people who stutter.

Ingham, R., Ingham, J., Euler, H., & Neumann, K. (2017). Stuttering treatment and brain research in adults: A still unfolding relationship. *Journal of Fluency Disorders, 55*, 106–119. doi:10.1016/j.jfludis.2017.02.003

A good review of the effects of treatment on the brain and explorations of potential new approaches to treatment.

Neumann, K., & Euler, H. (2010). Neuroimaging and stuttering. In B. Guitar, & R. McCauley (Eds.), *Stuttering treatment: Established and emerging approaches* (pp. 355–377). Baltimore, MD: Lippincott Williams & Wilkins.

This chapter begins with a history of brain imaging and stuttering and then describes the most important findings in structural and functional brain imaging related to stuttering. This is followed by a section on neuroimaging findings before and after treatment, a specialty of the authors.

3

Sensorimotor, Emotional, and Language Factors in Stuttering

Chapter Objectives

After studying this chapter, readers should be able to:

- Describe differences in these areas found between groups of individuals who stutter and groups of individuals who don't: (1) sensory processing, (2) central auditory processing, (3) dichotic listening, (4) auditory feedback, (5) sensorimotor control, (6) reaction time, (7) fluent speech, and (8) nonspeech motor control
- Suggest why differences in each of these areas could be related to stuttering
- Describe how language development and performance in individuals who stutter have been found to differ from individuals who don't
- Describe the ways in which stuttering and emotion may be related

Key Terms

Anomaly: A difference from the normal structure or function

Proprioception: Sensory information from the body that conveys position of structures and movement of structures

Sensorimotor control: The way all movement is carried out with sensory information used before, during, and after to improve the precision of movement

Sensory processing: Activity of the brain as it interprets information coming from the senses, such as sounds arriving via the ears and auditory nerves

Temperament: Aspects of an individual's personality, such as sensitive versus thick skinned, that are thought to be innate rather than learned

The organization of this chapter reflects the flow of causality I offered in previous editions. Starting with the most distant factors, genetics and epigenetics result in brain structure and function **anomalies**. These, in turn, result in deficits in sensorimotor control of speech that give rise to the occurrence of stuttering. Language and emotion also have a strong influence on sensorimotor control of speech, affecting whether or not stuttering occurs, when it occurs, and how severe it is.

Other authors have expressed similar views. Conture and Walden (2012) and Walden et al. (2012), who propose a "dual diathesis-stressor" model of stuttering, suggested that stuttering is influenced by both emotion and speech-language factors, with many individual differences. Smith and Weber (2017) presented a theoretical perspective on stuttering ("Multifactor Dynamic Pathways Theory") suggesting that stuttering onset and development are best explained by complex and changing interactions among speech motor, language, and emotional factors. They emphasize that no single factor can explain stuttering, but it is best seen as emerging from the interplay of the many attributes and anomalies that underlie speech production. As with the Conture and Walden model, Smith and Weber emphasize that different children will have different combinations of factors (changing over development) that determine whether stuttering will occur or not.

SENSORIMOTOR FACTORS

As you can see in Figure 3.1, sensory and motor factors that influence stuttering emerge from an individual's brain structure and function. For example, brain areas that are underactivated or overactivated and white matter tracts that are less dense are likely to disrupt the precisely timed sequences of motor movements that produce speech. Thus, the genetics and epigenetics that influence brain structure and function ultimately affect the onset and development of rapid and fluent speech or stuttering.

Researchers have investigated deficits underlying the ability to produce rapid and fluent speech by studying sensory and motor abilities of people who stutter compared to those who don't. Both sensory and motor abilities are important because precisely timed articulator movements require sensory feedback to hit their targets. This section reviews the findings from studies over many years that have led theorists and experimenters to conclude that a "cause" of stuttering is poorly timed, discoordinated movements of the muscles and structures involved in speech. Both sensory and motor deficits are thought to contribute to this discoordination. Van Riper (1990) surmised long ago "that stuttering is essentially a neuromuscular disorder whose core consists of tiny lags and disruptions in the timing of the complicated movements required for speech."

Sensory Processing

There are at least two arguments to support the position that fluency may be affected by sensory processes. First, patients with various injuries and diseases have taught us that normal speech depends on intact auditory as well as proprioceptive (feeling of position and movement) and tactile (feeling of touch) feedback. Therefore, researchers have been curious to determine whether, in people who stutter, abnormal speech might be the result of some disturbance of sensory feedback. Second, experiments that have altered **sensory processing**, such as delayed auditory feedback (Black, 1951; Lee, 1951), have created repetitions, prolongations, and blocks in normal speakers, prompting scientists to ask whether this disturbance of feedback might be the cause of stuttering.

Central Auditory Processing

As you will remember from the brain imaging studies reviewed in Chapter 2, several researchers have suggested that areas of the auditory cortex are underactivated during stuttering (Beal, Gracco, Lafaille, & De Nil, 2007; Brown, Ingham, Ingham, Laird, & Fox, 2005; Budde, Barron, & Fox, 2014); others have found structural anomalies in the auditory cortex (Foundas, Bollich, Corey, Hurley, & Heilman, 2001). Still others have discovered reduced density in the white matter fibers that support sensorimotor integration in speech production of individuals who stutter (Chang, 2014; Chang 2010; Chang & Zhu, 2013; Chang, Zhu, Choo, & Angstadt, 2015; Sommer, Koch, Paulus, Willer, & Bücher, 2002). It would not be surprising, then, if these brain anomalies affect both the fluency of speech production and the accuracy of speech perception.

Speech and Sound Perception

Researchers have demonstrated that individuals who stutter (compared to control subjects) have deficits in perceiving speech and other sounds under conditions that stress auditory perceptual processing[1] (Hall & Jerger, 1978; Herndon, 1967; Kramer, Green, & Guitar, 1987; Liebetrau & Daly, 1981; Molt & Guilford, 1979; Toscher & Rupp, 1978). Interestingly, one study, which did not find these differences, used individuals who stuttered after they had received treatment (Hannley & Dorman, 1982). This finding may be explained by evidence that treatment for stuttering repairs

[1]For example, the Synthetic Sentence Identification/Ipsilateral Competing Message test and the Masking Level Difference test

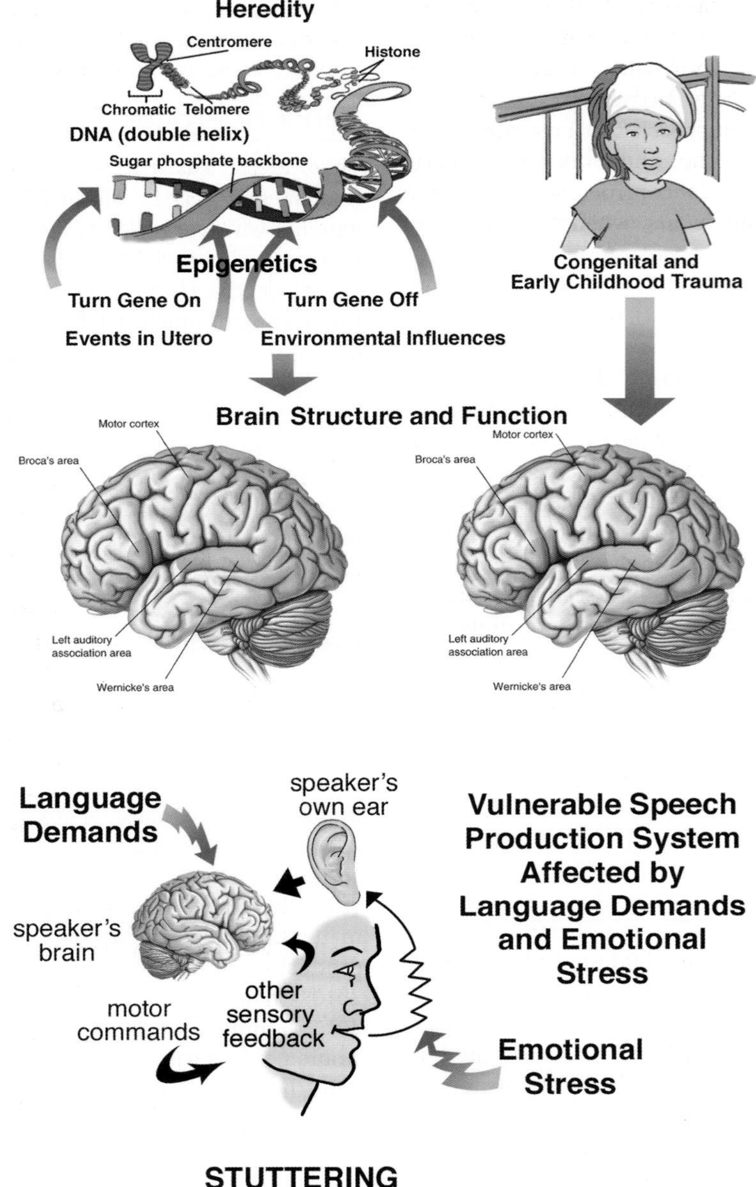

Figure 3.1 Constitutional factors in stuttering.

deficits in auditory processing (De Nil, Kroll, Lafaille, & Houle, 2003; Ingham, 2003; Kell et al., 2009; Neumann et al., 2003; Stager, Jeffries, & Braun, 2003).

Another unexpected finding about speech and sound perception is that when more fluent and less fluent nonstuttering speakers are compared on tests of auditory perception, the more fluent speakers perform significantly better than the less fluent speakers even when they are not speakers who stutter (Barasch, Guitar, McCauley, & Absher, 2000; Wynne & Boehmler, 1982). This might reflect some commonality in the neurophysiological functioning between people who stutter and typical speakers who are highly disfluent. It suggests that intact central auditory processing is required for complete fluency.

Brain Electrical Potentials Reflecting Auditory Processing

Studies of electrical brain activity in response to auditory stimuli have provided further evidence that auditory processing is abnormal in individuals who stutter. A variety of studies have shown that some or all of groups of individuals who stutter have abnormalities in neural electrical activity when responding to a variety of auditory stimuli (Dietrich, Barry, & Parker, 1995; Hampton & Weber-Fox, 2008; Hood, 1987; Molt, 1997). While most found significant group differences, Hampton and Weber-Fox only found a subgroup of individuals who stuttered who showed differences from controls. This finding is reminiscent of the subgroup of individuals who stuttered described in the Foundas et al. (2004) study with an anomalous rightward asymmetry in the planum temporale (PT) who showed a greater improvement in fluency while speaking under delayed auditory feedback than did those individuals who stuttered with more typical PT asymmetry. In other words, not all individuals who stutter may have auditory processing anomalies. A subgroup may have both structural and functional deviations from the norm, and this group may benefit from therapeutic approaches that help them compensate for these deviations.

Dichotic Listening Tests

More support for the notion that individuals who stutter have abnormal auditory processing comes from dichotic listening studies. These experiments deliver simultaneous auditory stimuli to right and left ears (and thus to the opposite hemisphere because the neural pathways from the ear to the brain are more efficient going to the opposite hemisphere) and look for evidence that one hemisphere or the other is dominant in being able to more accurately perceive the stimuli. Most (but not all) of these studies indicate that individuals who stutter do not show the right-ear (left hemisphere) advantage that typical speakers show (Blood, 1985; Blood & Blood, 1989; Brady & Berson, 1975; Curry & Gregory, 1969; Davenport, 1977; Liebetrau & Daly, 1981; Quinn, 1972; Rosenfield & Goodglass, 1980; Sommers, Brady, & Moore, 1975; Strong, 1977).

Sensory Processing Other Than Auditory

The few studies that have been conducted of other sensory systems besides auditory also show some deficits, but the results are mixed. Baker (1967) found that people who stutter performed more poorly than typical speakers on tests of oral sensation. However, this finding was not replicated by Jensen, Sheehan, Williams, and LaPointe (1975). In fact, a review article by Namasivayam and van Lieshout (2011) suggests that the literature does not support the hypothesis of deficits in orosensory function in stuttering. However, on a test that required subjects to match spatially ordered visual patterns with temporally ordered auditory patterns, Cohen and Hanson (1975) found that individuals who stuttered performed more poorly than those who didn't. Chuang, Fromm, Ewanowski, and Abbs (1980) evaluated abilities of individuals who stuttered to make the smallest movements possible with their jaws and tongues. The stuttering group had significantly larger "difference limens" (smallest detectable difference) with or without the assistance of visual feedback for such movements. This means that they did not have the degree of fine sensorimotor control of the jaw and tongue that the nonstuttering group did. De Nil and Abbs (1991) followed up this study and demonstrated that individuals who stuttered had less **sensorimotor control** for minimal movements with their jaws, lips, and tongues (but not finger movements) compared to individuals who did not stutter, when using only kinesthetic feedback. There were no differences between the groups when using visual feedback. The review by Namasivayam and van Lieshout (2011), mentioned previously, did suggest that individuals who stuttered appeared to benefit from increased kinesthetic feedback by using larger articulatory movements or by using a slower speech rate. This temporary increase in fluency via increased kinesthetic feedback is advocated as a therapeutic strategy called "**proprioception**" that is described in the chapters on treatment of school-age children and treatment of adults.

Summary of Findings on Sensory Processing

Together with the findings about the auditory system, these studies of other sensory modalities may indicate that as a group, individuals who stutter have some difficulty using auditory, touch, and movement information to control speech. But Namasivayam, van Lieshout, McIlroy, and De Nil (2009) provided evidence that individuals who stutter are as capable as those who don't in using sensory feedback to stabilize speech motor control in the face of experimental perturbations (masking noise and tendon vibration). If they are as good as individuals who don't stutter at using sensory feedback to nullify the effects of external interference with speech movements, individuals who stutter may be using sensory feedback to also nullify the effects of internal interference with speech (i.e., their innately poorer speech motor skills). In other words, when individuals who stutter are fluent, as they naturally are some of the time, they may be achieving this fluency by making extra use of sensory feedback (van Lieshout, Hulstijn, & Peters, 2004). In summary, this literature is full of conflicting findings, and it is not clear whether all individuals who stutter have deficits in sensory feedback or only a subgroup. It is possible that deficits in sensory processing may be quite widespread in individuals who stutter, but that it varies in people tested in these experiments depending on the task and on the day. After all, stuttering itself varies from day to day in each of us who have the disorder. Table 3.1 summarizes sensory processing factors in stuttering.

Sensorimotor Control

Reaction Time

Reaction time studies are used to examine sensorimotor control in speech production because in stuttering, it is thought that timing may be particularly compromised. Figure 3.2 depicts an example of a reaction time experiment. The participant is told to watch the computer screen for a picture of an object and to say the name of the object the instant it appears. The time between the appearance of the object on the screen and the first sound or movement made by the participant is her reaction time. As indicated, reaction time involves sensory analysis, response planning, and response execution. It is therefore a potentially useful measure in stuttering research if it is thought that the core deficit is a delay in some aspect of sensory processing, planning, or motor execution.

TABLE 3.1 Sensory Processing Factors in Stuttering

Important Findings	Major Implications
Individuals who stutter show the following differences from their fluent peers: Poorer central auditory processing, especially with regard to temporal information. Poorer perception of speech and nonspeech sounds, under difficult listening conditions. Brain waves of people who stutter may have longer latencies and lower amplitudes when listening to linguistically complex stimuli. May be true of only a subgroup of individuals who stutter. Some dichotic listening studies have found that people who stutter have less right-ear/left-hemisphere advantage. More evident in more severe stutterers and more likely when stimuli are linguistically complex. A small number of studies suggest people who stutter may be poorer at processing tactile, kinesthetic, and visual information. Masking and other changes in the way that people who stutter hear themselves speaking can decrease the frequency and severity of stuttering.	Dysfunction of auditory system implicated as a contributing factor in the etiology of stuttering. May also be true of other sensory systems. Nonfluent typical speakers may also show some of these deficits, suggesting a link between these two groups. Treatment may improve deficits in sensory processing. Temporary fluency can be obtained by masking or distorting auditory feedback. Possible use in treatment.

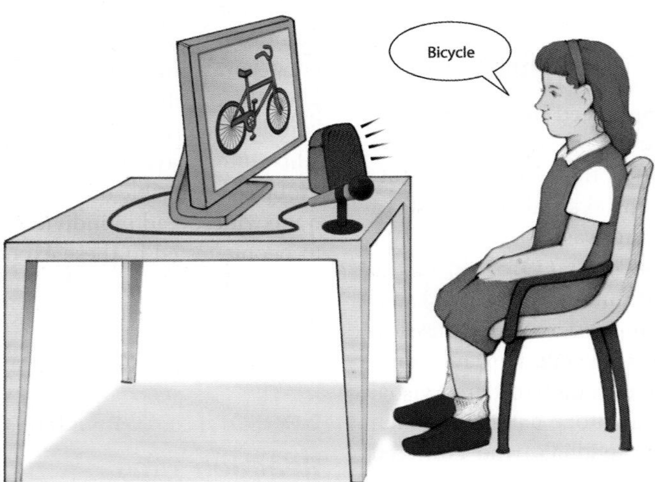

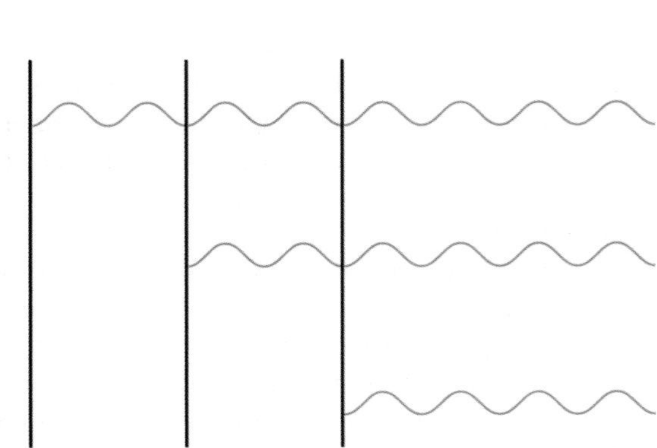

Figure 3.2 Processing stages in a reaction time task.

Among the early experiments demonstrating sensorimotor control difficulties related to stuttering were those that found that people who stutter were slower than nonstutterers in initiating and terminating a vowel sound in response to a buzzer (Adams & Hayden, 1976; Starkweather, Hirschman, & Tannenbaum, 1976). Later experiments showed that people who stutter were slower than people who don't in reacting with respiratory (exhalation) and articulatory movements (lip closing) (McFarlane & Prins, 1978; Watson & Alfonso, 1987). They were also slower whether they were responding to auditory or visual signals (e.g., Cross & Cooke, 1979). Children who stutter were also found to have slower reaction times in studies by Cross and Luper (1979, 1983), Cullinan and Springer (1980), Maske-Cash and Curlee (1995), and Till, Reich, Dickey, and Sieber (1983).

Although not all studies showed clear-cut significant group differences, De Nil (1995) pointed out that about 75 percent of the 44 voice reaction time studies that he reviewed found that people who stutter were significantly slower than people who don't stutter and that most of the other studies showed trends in that direction. He further noted that when investigators used linguistically meaningful stimuli to test reaction times (words or sentences, rather than isolated sounds), 80 percent of the studies found significant differences between people who stutter and people who don't. These findings are likely to be related to the evidence from brain imaging studies indicating that individuals who stutter have anomalies in areas used for sensorimotor processing of speech and language. Not surprisingly, these anomalies may affect sensorimotor reaction times on nonspeech tasks, but are most evident in tasks requiring linguistic processing.

Studies of Fluent Speech

The fluent speech of individuals who stutter has been a focus of numerous studies because clues to the nature of stuttered speech may be hidden in these individuals' fluent utterances. That is, the deficits that create moments of perceptible stuttering may sometimes be present, but so subtle that stuttering itself does not appear. However, fine-grained analysis of this apparently fluent speech may show tiny differences in coordination and timing. Here are some findings related to that idea: Acoustic studies have demonstrated that, on average, people who stutter have longer vowel durations, slower transitions between consonants and vowels, and delayed onsets of voicing after voiceless consonants even when speaking fluently (Colcord & Adams, 1979; DiSimoni, 1974; Hillman & Gilbert, 1977; Starkweather & Myers, 1979). The results of these acoustic studies have been supported by "kinematic" research, which has measured the movements of speakers' speech structures (e.g., Alfonso, Story, & Watson, 1987; Zimmermann, 1980). As a group, people who stutter tend to move their lips and jaws more slowly, even during fluent speech, than do people who don't stutter (e.g., Zimmermann, 1980). Kinematic research has also shown that some individuals who stutter demonstrate abnormal sequencing of articulator movement onsets and velocities (Caruso, Abbs, & Gracco, 1988). Walsh, Mettel, and Smith (2015) demonstrated that boys who stutter showed less stability in motor speech control, compared to girls who stutter and less stability compared to fluent children. Other kinematic studies, however, have not found group differences or have found them only in individuals who had recently undergone therapy (e.g., McClean, Kroll, & Loftus, 1990), which may have taught them to speak more slowly. Smith and Weber (2017) provide an excellent review of many studies from their research group at Purdue University that have shown that both children and adults who stutter have less stable articulatory coordination than their peers.

Three different explanations have been put forth by researchers for why many individuals who stutter speak more slowly or use different sequences of articulatory movements than nonstuttering speakers even when they are fluent. First, some researchers think that these findings reflect delays or other dysfunctions in processing incoming and outgoing signals. Individuals who stutter may be unable to process neural signals fast enough to make the rapid, precise movements of normal conversational speech, especially when they are under the stress of planning a complex sentence or competing with other talkers. Their delays in voicing onset, slower transitions, and abnormal sequencing during fluent speech may just reflect a slower mechanism working at its limited rate. Second, other researchers, perhaps more skeptical ones, have suggested that such differences simply reflect the way individuals who stutter have learned to talk to avoid stuttering, either on their own or as a result of therapy, and this way of speaking keeps them fluent even with an inefficient speech motor system. In their review of the evidence supporting a "speech motor skills" approach to stuttering, Namasivayam and van Lieshout (2011) suggest that a slower speech rate in the fluent speech of individuals who stutter is a compensatory strategy that gives the speaker more time to use sensory feedback to guide articulator movement. This increased sensory feedback is thought to stabilize the speech motor system and prevent stuttering.

Yet a third interpretation of slower movements on the part of people who stutter in fluent speech is that these slow movements are the result of heightened tension in muscles having antagonistic functions for speech production (Starkweather, 1987). For example, increased tension in both muscles that move a structure forward (agonists) and muscles that hold it back (antagonists) would make movement of that structure considerably slower. Imagine two people pulling a rope in opposite directions. Even if one were stronger, that person would make slow progress in her direction because the other, weaker person would create a drag. These slowed movements of speech structures in those who stutter would account for not only slower reaction times but also the longer movement durations in their fluent speech.

Findings from a number of studies support this third view. They have shown that people who stutter co-contract agonist and antagonist muscles of both the laryngeal (Freeman & Ushijima, 1975; Shapiro, 1980) and articulatory (Guitar, Guitar, Neilson, O'Dwyer, & Andrews, 1988) muscle groups during stuttering. These studies, like Starkweather's (1987) review, have noted that such co-contraction of agonist and antagonist muscles appears even in some of the apparently fluent speech of stutterers. This finding has led many researchers to posit that stuttering is not an "all-or-nothing" event (Adams & Runyan, 1981; Bloodstein, 1987; Smith & Kelly, 1997). Sometimes, people who stutter may speak freely, without a trace of excess tension. At other times, they may have excess tension that isn't heard by listeners as stuttering. At still other times, muscle tension may be great enough that both listeners and the person who stutters are acutely aware of stuttering. This continuum of fluency reflects the subjective impression of many individuals who stutter, including me.

It should be noted that not all researchers believe that excess muscle tension is an important component of stuttering. Walsh and Smith (2013), for example, did not find evidence of perioral muscle tension in preschoolers who stutter. As you will see, in Chapters 5 and 6, I make the argument that tension is a response to stuttering that may appear as children experience excessive disfluencies that feel "out of control." It may be that the preschoolers that Walsh and Smith studied were not reacting to their disfluencies with tension (their stuttering was not threatening to them yet) or that the researchers' measurements—limited to perioral muscles—did not reflect tension in other musculature.

Nonspeech Motor Control

Researchers have been curious about whether stuttering is the result of a general motor timing/coordination problem rather than a problem limited to speech production. In a study of both sequential finger movements and sequential counting aloud fluently, Borden (1983) found that individuals who stuttered severely, but not those who stuttered mildly, were slower than their fluent peers in executing both finger movement and speech tasks. Thus, severely stuttering individuals may have substantial deficits in certain sensorimotor tasks, but those who stutter mildly may only have slight deficits, and these may require special task conditions to be revealed.

Webster (1993a) developed a finger movement task—10 years after Borden's study—in which participants tapped four numbered keys in a predetermined sequence. To make the task somewhat like speech, participants were assigned a novel sequence of keys at the beginning of each trial (3-2-4-1 or 4-1-2-3, etc.). In both timed and untimed tests, subjects who stuttered made more errors sequencing and were slower initiating the task but were comparable to their fluent peers in execution time (once the movement was started). Unlike Borden's study, no effort was made to analyze the results by subjects' stuttering severity. Webster thought that these results suggested that individuals who stutter may have difficulty in "response planning, organization, and initiation" (Webster, 1993b, p. 84) of novel sequences of movements.

To answer the question of why this difficulty may be present only intermittently in individuals who stutter (after all, they have a great deal of fluent speech), Webster (1993b) postulated what others (Cross, Sweet, & Bates, 1985; Curlee, 1993; Peters & Guitar, 1991) have also considered that at times, such as under emotional stress, there is "cross talk" or interference with speech motor control. Specifically, activity in the right hemisphere interferes with sequential movement control in the left hemisphere.

To test this, Webster used a task in which participants performed sequential finger tapping with the right hand while turning a knob with the left hand, in response to an auditory signal. If his hypothesis were true, the stuttering group's left-hemisphere–controlled finger tapping would be vulnerable to interference by the right-hemisphere–controlled knob turning. Indeed, the stuttering group's performance was significantly poorer than that of the nonstuttering group on both tasks.

Webster (1997) then wondered whether interference of left-hemisphere sequential movement control mechanisms might be the result of an inability to focus attention on the left-hemisphere task and ignore interference from a competing source, whether from the right or left hemisphere. To test this, Webster used a procedure developed to investigate attention focus in right- and left-handed people. Participants were required to tap twice with one hand for every tap they made with the other hand. They were tested with the right-hand double tapping and the left-hand single tapping, as well as vice versa. The individuals who didn't stutter were able to perform the task significantly better when they tapped twice with the right hand and once with the left; however, people who stuttered and nonstuttering left-handers performed the task equally well with either hand doing the double tapping. Webster interpreted this outcome as suggesting that individuals who stutter and left-handed individuals who didn't stutter did not have the ability to focus predominantly on the left hemisphere, but had equal focus on both, making their left hemispheres vulnerable to interference from other activities. Webster's model of stuttering, derived from these experiments, postulates that individuals who stutter are unable to protect the integrity of speech production centers from interference or "cross talk" from emotions or other ongoing processes. It is not clear why all left-handers don't stutter. I would presume that this model proposes that individuals who stutter have both a deficit in the sequencing of processing underlying speech production (unlike fluent left-handers) as well as an inability to focus on the left hemisphere.

Following up on Webster's studies, Subramanian and Yairi (2006) experimented with a version of the finger-tapping task, using not only individuals who stuttered and controls but a third group of "high-risk" participants. The high-risk individuals were parents or siblings of the subjects who stuttered—of special interest because they were thought to be carriers of genetic material that could create stuttering except for the absence of some critical factor that would presumably cause them to stutter, too. All participants were right-handed. They all tapped in several conditions, including tapping at a comfortable rate and at a fast rate. Among the findings of this study was evidence that in the comfortable rate condition, the stuttering group and the high-risk group were slower than the control groups. However, in the fast rate condition, the stuttering group tapped faster than either of the other groups, both with their right hand and with their left hand. Along with their high rate, the stuttering group also had higher variability in tapping rate than either group.

Of great interest was the finding that in this fast rate condition, the high-risk group had slower tapping rates than either the stuttering group or the control group but had relatively low variability. The authors speculated that these findings may reflect that those in the stuttering and high-risk groups have motor systems that operate best at slow rates. When there is pressure to operate at a faster rate, the high-risk group is able to control their rate and maintain stability (low variability). But under this pressure, the stuttering group taps very rapidly, pushing their motor systems beyond their optimal operating speed, causing them to become unstable (high variability).

It is not too great a leap to imagine that individuals who stutter speak more rapidly than is optimal for their speech planning and execution systems, thus becoming disfluent. It is also possible that close relatives of individuals who stutter who may have inherited a predisposition for stuttering don't develop stuttering because they are able speak at slower speech rates, more appropriate for the limitations of the speech motor production system. When I read this finding, I was reminded of meeting a young man at a social gathering who said the he had a first cousin who stuttered, but he himself didn't. As I talked with the young man, I realized that he talked quite slowly (but fluently). This seemed to confirm the hypothesis that some relatives of individuals who stutter may have some genetic material for stuttering but are able to control their speech rates and thereby remain fluent. But several weeks afterward, I realized this was an example of "confirmatory bias"—confirming your hypotheses on the bases of selected observations. I was ignoring the many fluent and fast-talking relatives of people who stuttered whom I had met over many years.

But back to the idea that those who stutter may be talking more rapidly than their speech production systems allow: This perspective was supported by research of Kloth, Janssen, Kraaimaat, and Brutten (1995, 1998) who found that in a high-risk-for-stuttering population (one or more parents stuttered) of 93 children studied prior to onset of stuttering, the 26 children who did develop stuttering spoke more rapidly than the 67 children who didn't. However, both groups' speech rates were within the normal range.

Subramanian and Yairi (2006) also found evidence that could support Webster's (1997) hypothesis that individuals who stutter suffer from an inability to focus entirely on the left hemisphere when performing motor tasks. Instead, people who stutter may activate both hemispheres for speech, as brain imaging studies have shown (e.g., Brown et al., 2005; Budde et al., 2014). Subramanian and Yairi's (2006) data showed that when participants were asked to tap simultaneously with both hands, but tap twice as fast with one hand than with the other, the stuttering and high-risk participants (parents and siblings of the subjects who stuttered) performed equally well with either the right or left hand tapping twice as fast. The control group participants were better when they tapped twice as fast with their dominant (right) hand as with their left hand. This finding supports the speculation that the stuttering and high-risk groups did not suppress the right hemisphere and focus entirely on the left hemisphere. Another similarity to Webster's (1997) findings was that Subramanian and Yairi's (2006) stuttering group required more trials to learn to tap twice as fast with one hand than the other. Webster's similar finding that stuttering subjects took longer to initiate a pattern of tapping led him to speculate that it reflects a difficulty initiating speech movement at the beginning of an utterance, thus stuttering more at the beginnings of phrases.

Subramanian and Yairi's (2006) finding that adults who stutter manifest greater variability in a nonspeech motor task was also found in children who stutter. Olander, Smith, and Zelaznik (2010) studied 17 children who stuttered and controls, ages 4 to 6, using a task that required children to clap their hands in time to a metronome and then continue to clap at that rate after the metronome was turned off. Their results indicated that although 40 percent of the children performed like the control group, 60 percent showed variability outside the range of the controls. They speculated that nonspeech motor variability may be related to speech motor control deficits and that these deficits might be predictive of recovery or persistence of stuttering. However, Hilger, Zelaznik, and Smith (2016) found in a larger study (70 children who stuttered) that there were no differences—between children who stuttered and those who didn't—in the timing of hand clapping in preschool children. The authors suggest that the use of a large sample is vital to assessment of differences between those who stutter and those who don't.

The last studies of nonspeech motor control I will review concern the use of auditory input to control motor output. A common paradigm in these studies is to have participants track or follow the changing frequency (pitch) of a target sound with a second sound, called a "cursor." A computer controls the pitch changes in the target's sound, and participants follow these changes by using their hand or their jaw to move a lever that changes the pitch of the cursor. Using this paradigm, Sussman and MacNeilage (1975) found that normal speakers made fewer errors tracking the target sound when the cursor tone was presented to the right ear and the target tone to the left ear. Those who stuttered, on the other hand, made equal numbers of errors whether the cursor tone was in the right ear and the target tone in the left or vice versa, suggesting that they did not have a left-hemisphere advantage for integrating auditory information with motor output as the nonstutterers did.

Researchers in Australia replicated and extended this work on tracking (Neilson, 1980; Neilson & Neilson, 1987, 1988) using both visual and auditory targets and cursors.

They demonstrated that participants who stuttered were significantly poorer using auditory targets and cursors than when using visual ones. They also showed that when both stuttering and nonstuttering participants practiced the tasks beforehand, the differences between the groups were even larger than when they had not practiced. The Neilsons proposed that those who stuttered were slow in developing a mental auditory-motor model of the relationship between their movement of the cursor control and the resulting sound change. They further hypothesized that the basic deficit in stuttering is difficulty in forming or accessing auditory-motor models of what speech movements are needed to produce the sounds they want to make. The Neilsons' perspective on stuttering is given in detail in Chapter 6. I suspect that the Neilsons would agree that individuals who stutter can use their auditory-motor models better in situations where the demands on their neural resources are low but have more trouble when the demands are high.

Brain imaging studies have provided evidence of possible neural substrates underlying the difficulty that individuals may have in accessing auditory-motor models of speech sounds. Chang et al. (2015) reported that the biggest differences in white matter tracts, between individuals who stutter and those who don't, are in "areas supporting auditory-motor and somatosensorimotor integration for speech motor production" (p. 706). These areas are apparently crucial for using stored auditory-motor models of sounds to plan and execute the articulatory gestures needed for speech.

As the Neilsons were working on their experiments in Australia, researchers at Baylor University College of Medicine in Texas were also studying the auditory-motor tracking abilities of individuals who stutter. In a series of publications (Nudelman, Herbrich, Hess, Hoyt, & Rosenfield, 1992; Nudelman, Herbrich, Hoyt, & Rosenfield, 1987, 1989), these researchers described experiments that required participants to hum along with a tone that suddenly changed pitch. The pitch of the target tones was sometimes changed rapidly, sometimes slowly, while researchers measured how quickly participants could change their humming to match the changing pitch of the auditory target tone. The researchers found that the subjects who stuttered were significantly slower than those who didn't in responding to changes in the target's frequency, suggesting that subjects who stutter need more time to process auditory signals and make motor responses. Once again, we find that research has produced evidence that, as a group, people who stutter have difficulty performing sensorimotor tasks. This may be related to the findings of Chang (2010), Change et al. (2015), Cykowski, Fox, Ingham, Ingham, & Robin (2010), and Sommer et al. (2002) that brain areas used for sensory integration are not efficiently connected to motor planning/motor execution areas. Chang, Horowitz, Ostuni, Reynolds, & Ludlow (2011) found this lack of connectivity between programming and premotor areas for nonspeech as well as speech movements in adults.

Table 3.2 summarizes sensorimotor control factors in stuttering.

TABLE 3.2 Sensorimotor Control Factors in Stuttering

Important Findings	Major Implications
Compared to nonstutterers, individuals who stutter appear to have these differences:	There is a possibility that training in auditory speech motor control could improve fluency.
Reaction times in people who stutter are slower, especially when linguistically meaningful stimuli are used.	Evidence that individuals who stutter are slower at a variety of tasks suggests that slower speech rate may facilitate fluency.
Fluent speech in individuals who stutter is slower, with longer vowels, slower transitions, and delayed onset of voicing. They are also slower and make more errors on nonspeech tasks of sequencing. This may be truer for more severely stuttering individuals.	If people who stutter try to speak at fast rates, they may be more likely to stutter because of unstable speech motor control.
Although individuals who stutter are slower tapping at a comfortable rate, they are faster than controls during fast-tapping conditions but more variable. Close relatives of stutterers have slower tapping rates than stutterers and controls but less variability.	It is possible that some close relatives of people who stutter may be predisposed to stutter but may prevent stuttering by speaking more slowly. Modeling slow speech by parents of young children at risk may prevent stuttering by inducing a slower speech rate in children.
Results of hand-tapping task experiment suggested that individuals who stutter are not as able to focus on left-hemisphere motor control and may be vulnerable to interference from the right hemisphere or other areas of the left hemisphere.	Brain imaging studies support findings of poorer auditory-motor control in people who stutter because of anomalies in auditory-motor areas of the brain.
Individuals who stutter are poorer at auditory-motor tracking; they may not have left-hemisphere advantage for auditory-motor tracking, and they may be slower at developing a mental model of auditory-motor relationships.	

LANGUAGE FACTORS

Language factors may play an important role in the onset and development of stuttering because language processing can place extra demands on speech production. In the previous chapter on constitutional factors, I described several possible determinants of stuttering. These include heredity, congenital and childhood brain injuries, and the resulting neurological structure and function deficits in people who stutter. These neurological deficits may, in turn, result in a "vulnerable" sensorimotor system for producing speech. That is, the system may be compromised because a smaller volume of gray matter and less myelinated white matter tracts in speech-related areas may require extra neuronal resources to compensate for these deficits in order to produce speech at normal rates. Here, the word "vulnerable" means that the sensorimotor system may break down under stress. Language—the topic of this section—appears to be one of those stresses.

The very onset of stuttering itself—which occurs in most children between the ages of 2 and 5 years—has been linked to rapid pace of language acquisition at this same time (Bloodstein & Ratner, 2008; Smith & Weber, 2017; Yairi & Ambrose, 2005). You can imagine that if a child has a vulnerable speech production system and needs extra neural resources to maintain fluency, the competition for those resources is intense as language is being acquired, resulting in the breakdown of the child's speech. Even when these children have grown older and have mastered language production, their use of long, complex sentences at rapid rates while planning the next parts of a narrative may make them momentarily more vulnerable to stuttering, as the literature shows.

Studies of language effects on fluency in children began with demonstrations that children who stutter are more likely to have language deficits or "dissociations" among language components than their fluent peers (e.g., Anderson & Conture, 2000; Anderson, Pellowski, & Conture, 2005; Ntourou, Conture, & Lipsey, 2011; Zackheim & Conture, 2003). Several studies have used event-related potentials (an electroencephalographic or EEG measure) to assess neural correlates of language processing in children who stutter. They have shown that young children who stutter (compared to their fluent peers) have anomalies in brain activity related to language processing (e.g., Mohan & Weber, 2015; Usler & Weber-Fox, 2015). Some of these studies have also shown that a few of these anomalies predict whether the children will recover from stuttering or not. In their review of many studies of stuttering children compared to their peers, Smith and Weber (2017) remind us that (1) there are many individual differences in language ability and performance in children who stutter, with some children having above-average abilities and others below; (2) complex interactions among language skills and between language and speech skills will be different for different children; and (3) these interactions involve many subsystems that are developing rapidly during childhood; thus stuttering in individual children will emerge at different times from different combinations of factors.

Research on the effect of language on stuttering in adults may be somewhat easier to conduct than in children because adults can be trained to do complex tasks that challenge their speech and language processing. The trick is to develop these complex tasks. One example of such research is the work of Hans-Georg Bosshardt (e.g., 1999, 2002, 2006), who found that in many cases, adults who stutter are poorer at tasks requiring linguistic processing while engaging in other cognitive activities. Bosshardt's interpretation of his results describes the connection between language and stuttering by hypothesizing that individuals who stutter have speech production systems that are less protected (than typical speakers) from the heavy demand of complex language. Remember that linguistically complex sentences are spoken faster, so that yet another demand (faster rate) is added when language becomes more complex.

Another approach to examining language processing in adults who stutter was developed by Anne Smith's research group at Purdue University. Rather than adding on cognitive processing tasks, as Bosshardt did, Kleinow and Smith (2000) studied the stability of articulator coordination (using a measure of stability called "spatiotemporal index") during fluent speech as their subjects were asked to produce more linguistically complex utterances. The underlying assumption was that adults who stutter have vulnerable speech production systems that would show "breakdown" in articulatory coordination even before any stuttering surfaced. Kleinow and Smith demonstrated that longer and more syntactically complex sentences produced significantly more instability in the speech production of individuals who stutter, compared to their simpler and shorter sentences. The same was not true for individuals who don't stutter. Kleinow and Smith interpreted these findings as suggesting that in individuals who stutter, speech production systems are more vulnerable to breakdown when language complexity is great. Ten years later, Smith, Sadagopan, Walsh, and Weber-Fox (2010) found increasing interarticulatory coordination breakdown as phonological complexity increased for adults who stutter but not controls. Similarly, findings about syntactic complexity have been reported by Smith, Goffman, Sasiekaran, and Weber-Fox (2012) and by MacPhereson and Smith (2013). Table 3.3 summarizes language factors in stuttering.

EMOTIONAL FACTORS

Emotions have many components—physiological arousal, expressive behaviors, and conscious experience. I will touch upon these as I review the research on stuttering and emotions.

TABLE 3.3 Language Factors

Important Findings	Major Implications
Stuttering onset is often associated with language development. Children who stutter appear to have slightly less robust language processing abilities. More stuttering occurs in more complex sentences; stuttering is influenced by linguistic factors such as lexical class of word, length, and location in a sentence. More linguistically complex stimuli result in poorer performances by individuals who stutter on many speaking tasks.	Findings of deficits in language processing and more stuttering under greater linguistic demands support a model of stuttering wherein a vulnerable speech production mechanism breaks down under the demands of language learning and using more complex language. To help develop an idea of possible causal roots when evaluating a child who has recently begun to stutter, it is important to determine if the child is/was in a period of intense language development when stuttering started. A complete evaluation of a child who stutters should include assessment of receptive and expressive language. Decreasing linguistic load on children who are beginning to stutter may reduce their stuttering. In addition, the use of pauses and slower speech rate in older children and adults who stutter may increase fluency by decreasing linguistic demands on the speech production system.

Stuttering as a Result of Emotional Arousal

Relatively few studies have investigated whether momentary increases in emotional arousal are associated with occurrences of stuttering. A direct connection between emotional arousal and stuttering-like behavior in people who didn't stutter was suggested by an important, but almost forgotten, study conducted many years ago by Harris Hill (1954). Subjects were trained to produce a sentence describing a picture in response to a red light flashing on. After several trials, when the red light came on, they were then given a mild electric shock while speaking the sentence. Subsequently, no shock was given during sentence production, but the red light was assumed to be associated with electric shock. When speaking under the anticipation of shock when the red light flashed on, subjects produced "compulsive and preservative" repetitions, prolongations, and blocks. Hill reported that many responses appeared to be "indistinguishable from what is generally termed stuttering. [Moreover, the responses of several subjects] would have been classed as severe [stuttering] in any speech clinic" (p. 302). Electromyographic sensors on the sternocleidomastoid muscle detected increased muscle tension during these stutter-like responses. The sternocleidomastoid is a neck muscle that is easily accessible and may show generalized physical tension. Thus, it appears that even individuals who don't stutter will show stuttering-like behaviors under threat of penalty, and some people who don't stutter show severe instances of this. This study demonstrates that emotion (probably negative arousal, in this case) can result in disfluencies, as well as increase muscle tension in anticipation of stuttering.

Several researchers have examined how stuttering frequency and severity, in people who stutter, are affected by emotional arousal. Three studies in the 1990s found that when people who stutter are more emotionally aroused—assessed by various physiological measures like heart rate, skin conductance, and level of cortisol—they stutter more (Caruso, Chodzko-Zajko, & McClowry, 1995; Miller, 1993; Weber & Smith, 1990). The study by Weber and Smith examined the period just preceding moments of stuttering as well as during stuttering and found that for both conditions, higher levels of autonomic arousal were associated with instances of stuttering. Additionally, severity of moments of stuttering was associated with higher levels of autonomic arousal.

Other studies have used a more indirect approach, using emotionally laden words to examine the effect of emotional arousal (low vs. high arousal) on the speech production system. Hennessey, Dourado, and Beilby (2014) found that people who stutter had longer speech reaction times (i.e., took longer to begin to say the word) in response to emotionally loaded words compared to neutral words. These longer reaction times correlated significantly with the amount of stuttering that subjects showed in conversational speech recorded in the same session. This suggests that the speech production system of those who stutter is vulnerable to emotion and more so for those who stutter more frequently. Similar results were found by van Lieshout, Ben-David, Lipski, and Namasivayam (2014) who showed that aspects of the speech production system of people who stutter were affected by saying emotionally loaded words. While stuttering didn't occur, reaction time to begin to speak and articulator movement coordination were affected by the threatening words (e.g., "rape" and "loser"). These five studies are indirect support for the hypothesis that emotional arousal has an effect on the speech of those who stutter more than those who do not.

Anxiety and Sensitive Temperament in People Who Stutter

This section reviews research on whether people who stutter are more anxious than people who don't. Do they carry around more worry and dread about events in the future? Also, do they have a **temperament** that is more easily emotionally aroused?

Anxiety

Just to make sure that we're on the same page about anxiety, I'm not referring to the immediate effect of encountering something threatening, like a coiled snake or a strange creature under your bed. That immediate emotion we usually call fear. Anxiety, on the other hand, is a more ongoing emotion that usually involves worries about something bad that might happen in the future. Like many questions about stuttering, questions about anxiety and stuttering wrestle with the issue of cause and effect. Does anxiety cause stuttering or does stuttering result in anxiety—or do effects occur in both directions?

An early study of anxiety and stuttering is of interest because of what it might tell us about emotion, speech physiology, and stuttering. Horovitz, Johnson, Pearlman, Schaffer, and Hedin (1978) looked at a phenomenon called the stapedial reflex, which had been previously shown to increase during anxiety in normal speakers. The stapedial reflex is muscle contraction in the middle ear, triggered by activation of the internal branch of the superior laryngeal nerve just prior to speaking, decreasing the loudness with which a speaker hears her own voice. The researchers found that individuals who stutter demonstrated an increased stapedial reflex when they became more anxious (as measured by a physiological assessment of anxiety—the amount of sweat on the subject's palm), compared to a low-anxiety condition. A group of matched fluent speakers showed no increase in stapedial reflex when their anxiety increased. Participants in both groups increased their anxiety (sweated more) by imagining themselves in stressful speaking situations. Although the results of this study are hard to interpret, it appears to show that an increase in anxiety in stutterers may result in changes in speech-related physiology even when only imagining some difficulty speaking. It may be relevant that the increase in stapedial reflex may have been brought about by an increase in laryngeal nerve activity (McCall & Rabuzzi, 1973). This connection between autonomic arousal and heightened laryngeal muscle activity may reflect a conditioned response that becomes part of the learning, which many believe maintains stuttering in some individuals. I will revisit this connection between laryngeal tension and autonomic arousal when I discuss temperament and stuttering in Chapter 6.

Researchers have asked whether people who stutter are generally more anxious than people who don't. Some of the authors I cited earlier, who showed that physiological evidence of greater anxiety was associated with more stuttering (Caruso, Chodzko-Zajko, Bidinger, & Sommers, 1994; Miller, 1993; Peters & Hulstijn, 1984; Weber & Smith, 1990), also compared anxiety (autonomic arousal) between a group of people who stuttered and a control group in a situation that involved speaking. They found no differences between the groups.

Because anxiety and stuttering have long been a controversial topic, Ashley Craig edited a special issue of *Journal of Fluency Disorders* (volume 40, 2014) devoted to this subject. Nine studies—some of them analyzing the literature and others presenting new experimental results—comprised the special issue. I recommend reading this issue of the journal to get an in-depth view of stuttering and anxiety. My "take" on the findings is that the authors generally agreed that the anxiety relevant to stuttering is the social anxiety that derives from a speaker's repeated experiences stuttering in social situations. Sometimes, the listener's reaction to the stuttering is clearly negative; at other times, the speaker interprets a relatively neutral reaction as negative. Both experiences create a general dread of speaking and expectations of negative listener reactions, but this varies greatly among individuals. Social anxiety, of this type, contributes to the problem of stuttering in several ways. It causes people who stutter to develop avoidance behaviors related to the moment of stuttering as well as to speaking situations. The anxiety is also part of the suffering experienced by people who stutter, making it imperative that, to the extent a specific client does have anxiety, this part of the problem is treated along with the speech itself.

Sensitive Temperament

Many of us who work with children who stutter have often heard parents describe their children as particularly sensitive. Upon questioning, these parents frequently say that even before stuttering began, the child was more easily upset by changes in routine or was shyer with strangers than her siblings. These emotional and behavioral characteristics may be a part of the child's inherited temperament. The idea of different people having different temperaments goes back at least as far as the ancient Greek physician Hippocrates who suggested that personalities could be categorized as sanguine, choleric, melancholic, or phlegmatic. These different temperaments were thought to be determined by different bodily fluids or "humors." Today, we think of temperament as determined by genes and epigenetics, interacting with the environment.

Jerome Kagan's (e.g., Kagan, 1994b; Kagan, Reznick, & Snidman, 1987) work on temperament has influenced my thinking about the relationship between temperament and stuttering. His view of temperament places children on a continuum from cautious and shy (inhibited) to fearless and outgoing (uninhibited). Much of his research has studied children on the extreme ends of this continuum; he has used behavioral observation and acoustic/physiological measurements to compare the two groups. Among his many observations, he and his colleagues have found that more inhibited children (children who are typically fluent; he has never studied children who stutter) show an increase in laryngeal muscle tension under more stressful conditions (Kagan et al., 1987). This finding may be related to changes in the topography of stuttering as it progresses, as I suggest in Chapter 5.

Mary Rothbart (e.g., 2011) has also done extensive research on temperament in typical children. She and her coworkers conceptualize temperament as based in the child's biology and observed as difference in children's reactivity[2] and self-regulation. Reactivity refers to how arousable the child's motor, cognitive, and emotional systems are to various stimuli. Self-regulation refers to how the child deals with those stimuli, for example, avoiding negatively arousing situations. A number of studies have used Rothbart's model of temperament to compare children who stutter and those who don't using the Children's Behavior Questionnaire (CBQ) (Rothbart, Ahadi, Hershey, & Fisher, 2001). I summarize these results and other relevant studies after a brief historical account of how various authors have speculated that temperament may play an important part in the development of stuttering.

Theoretical Considerations about Stuttering and Sensitive Temperament

An important early conceptualization of stuttering, temperament, and anxiety can be found in Brutten and Shoemaker's (1967) landmark book *The Modification of Stuttering.* Rather than using the term "temperament," they referred to "individual differences in conditionability and autonomic reactivity." They suggested that some individuals have predispositions to stutter because they are constitutionally more likely to have an anxiety-based speech breakdown under stressful conditions. Moreover, these individuals are also thought to be more conditionable because of their autonomic reactivity, making it more likely that initial breakdowns under stress will develop into highly learned stuttering behaviors.

Following Brutten and Shoemaker (1967), a number of authors have speculated about the possible importance of considering this kind of reactive temperament in gaining a better understanding of the nature of stuttering (e.g., Bloodstein, 1987, 1995; Bloodstein & Ratner, 2008; Conture, 1990; Guitar, 1997, 1998, 2000; Peters & Guitar, 1991; Walden et al., 2012). Many of us have suspected that a reactive temperament, for example, might trigger increased struggle, physical tension, and avoidance in children when they are initially disfluent and thus create a learned cycle of mild stuttering begetting more severe stuttering, leading to chronic stuttering. On the other hand, a placid temperament in equally disfluent children might allow them to stay relaxed, ignore the disfluencies, and thereby outgrow early stuttering. Questionnaire studies have found indications that both adults and children who stutter are more sensitive than nonstutterers. This has been corroborated by studies of physiological measures of sensitivity, to be discussed (Anderson, Pellowski, Conture, & Kelly, 2003; Karrass et al., 2006; Zengin-Bolatkale, 2016).

With evidence in hand that at least some individuals who stutter have more sensitive temperaments, we need to ask how this may shed light on the disruption of fluency by emotion. Psychologists who study temperament have looked carefully at the regulation and expression of emotion in persons with sensitive temperaments. Studies of both normal and brain-damaged patients provide good evidence that the regulation of emotion is a lateralized function (Kinsbourne, 1989; Kinsbourne & Bemporad, 1984). In other words, some emotion-based behaviors are more regulated by one cerebral hemisphere or another. Emotions regulated by the left hemisphere seem to motivate such behaviors as approach, exploration, and action, whereas emotions regulated by the right hemisphere motivate behaviors such as avoidance, withdrawal, and the arrest of action. Studies of electrical activity in the brain indicate that individuals with sensitive temperaments are right hemisphere dominant for emotionally based behaviors (Ahern & Schwartz, 1985; Calkins & Fox, 1994). This means that if individuals who stutter are temperamentally reactive as a group, they may have an inborn proclivity toward behaviors motivated by right-hemisphere emotions—avoidance, withdrawal, and the arrest of action.

How this may affect speech is not yet clear, but Webster (1993b) speculates that when individuals who stutter are emotionally aroused, then right-hemisphere proclivities, such as avoidance and withdrawal, could affect their left-hemisphere supplementary motor areas (SMAs), interfering with planning and initiation of speech. My own speculation about the relationship between emotion and stuttering is that one important aspect of right hemisphere–dominant, emotionally based behaviors is the arrest of ongoing behavior. This phenomenon is especially well described by Jeffrey Gray (1987), a psychologist who has studied the central nervous system's response to stress. He proposes that when an individual experiences fear or frustration, a behavioral inhibition system in the brain increases three distinct forms of behavior: (1) freezing, which involves widespread muscular contractions that produce tense and silent immobility; (2) flight; or (3) avoidance. It is possible that such behaviors may be manifested in speech by both core behaviors (repetitions, prolongations, and blocks) and secondary behaviors (escape and avoidance).

Indirect support for this possibility can be found in the unpublished dissertation by Wendy Coster (1986) (cited in Kagan et al., 1987). Coster found that more sensitive children manifest their reactivity by generating higher levels of physical tension, particularly in laryngeal muscles, when they are speaking in unfamiliar or threatening situations. I suspect that some children who are both sensitive and have motor speech systems vulnerable to breakdown under stress may respond to these breakdowns (disfluencies) by increasing physical tension, especially in laryngeal muscles. As Van Riper (1971) has observed, "When the child becomes aware of his basic stuttering behaviors as frustrating or unacceptable to others, tension appears in the speech musculatures involved in the repetitions and fixations" (p. 123). This physical tightening

[2]Kagan also used the phrase "highly reactive" to describe children whom he labeled as inhibited.

of muscles may further interfere with speech, producing the abruptly terminated repetitions, as well as prolongations, pitch rises, and blocks that develop in many children when stuttering persists. Other children who are highly sensitive and predisposed to have motor speech breakdowns may begin their disfluencies with tense prolongations and blocks in response to emotionally difficult situations. The heterogeneity of individuals who stutter and their unique patterns of stuttering will be discussed further in upcoming chapters on developmental factors and on learning.

More speculation about the effect of emotion on stuttering is prompted by brain imaging studies that have shown extensive activity during stuttering in an area called the right insula, shown in Figure 2.3 in the last chapter (Fox, 2003), and the anterior cingulate cortex (Braun et al., 1997a, 1997b; De Nil, Kroll, Kapur, & Houle, 2000). Both of these areas have strong connections with the amygdala (Allman, Hakeem, Erwin, Nimchinsky, & Hof, 2001; Habib et al., 1995), which is a major structure in fear conditioning (LeDoux, 2002, 2015). It is possible that some of the right-hemisphere activity that is heightened during stuttering and reduced during induced fluency may reflect negative emotional arousal. My reasoning is as follows. First, many of the studies reviewed in the previous chapter suggest that in individuals who stutter, speech planning and production are localized in right-hemisphere regions homologous to Broca's, Wernicke's, and interconnecting areas. Second, emotions lateralized to the right hemisphere in the human brain are those associated with fear—avoidance, escape, and arrest of ongoing behavior (Gray, 1987; Kinsbourne, 1989). Third, because strong emotions tend to dominate the neural processes in surrounding areas (LeDoux, 2002), these emotions may disrupt ongoing speech processing in ways analogous to how they affect all behavior, including avoidance behaviors, escape behaviors, and blocks.

The section you have just read—on emotions and stuttering—suggests that emotions play a major role in the development of stuttering. In some cases, emotions may also play a role in the cause. An interesting theoretical perspective on stuttering and emotions has been proposed by Conture and Walden (2012) and Walden et al. (2012). Although their view ("dual diathesis-stressor model of stuttering") incorporates both emotional variables and speech-language variables, I will only describe what they hypothesize about emotions. They suggest that children who stutter may have constitutional predispositions (diatheses) that make them highly emotionally reactive to novel stimuli. This predisposition will be greater or lesser in different children. For the predisposition to be "activated," the child must encounter some environmental stress. Thus, the child may stutter more or less in any given situation, depending on the stress he experiences and the degree of predisposition he has. The stimulus the child is reacting to in this case is the experience of having some difficulty speaking (disfluencies or other speech disturbances). The child's emotional reaction to the difficulty will increase the difficulty in a cyclical fashion, with early emotional reactions to milder disfluencies causing them to become more severe, which in turn would cause stronger emotional reactions, resulting in even more struggle and avoidance behaviors. Of course, any given child will have other predispositions, such as language or speech deficits that will interact with the emotional diathesis.

Complete theoretical models of stuttering must, of course, incorporate all of the constitutional factors described in this and the previous chapter—genetics, epigenetics, brain structure and function, sensory processing, sensorimotor control, language, and emotion (see Smith & Weber, 2017). In addition, developmental and environmental factors must be included as well. An unexpected connection between genetics, emotion, and stuttering comes from a study mentioned earlier, by Kang et al. (2010). This work has identified a gene associated with stuttering (GNPTG) that is associated with both motor control and emotional regulation. Exploration of how individuals with this gene respond to treatment and how treatment may be adjusted to modify the effect of this gene would be a vital step forward.

Empirical Evidence about Stuttering and Sensitive Temperament

Greater sensitivity in children who stutter has been reported by several studies. Fowlie and Cooper (1978) reported that mothers of children who stutter viewed them as more sensitive than did mothers describing children who do not stutter. In a questionnaire study, Oyler (1992) found that adults who stutter were more emotionally sensitive than were adults who don't stutter; however, this hypersensitivity could be the result of many years of stuttering. Oyler and Ramig (1995) found that parents of children who stutter rated them as more sensitive than did control parents rated nonstuttering children.

Using the concept of "difficult" temperament, which includes some aspects of sensitivity as well as restlessness and impulsiveness, both Wakaba (1998) and Embrechts and Ebben (1999) found that parents of children who stuttered rated their children as having this type of temperament to a greater degree than did parents of nonstuttering children. LaSalle (1999) presented a paper indicating that, in contrast to parents of young children who don't stutter, parents of young children who do stutter rated their children as having high frustration reactions and lack of persistence. Both of these traits have been associated with sensitive temperament (Thomas & Chess, 1977). Anderson et al. (2003), using the Behavioral Style Questionnaire (McDevitt & Carey, 1978), found that parents of children who stutter rated their children as slower to adapt to novelty compared with how parents of nonstuttering children rated their children. They related this to Kagan's (1989, 1994b) description of this personality trait as also being more shy and fearful when encountering unfamiliar events and people. More evidence of children who stutter having a more reactive temperament comes from an important study by Karrass et al. (2006). Their findings, using a scale of children's reactions to everyday stressful situations completed by parents, suggested that when compared to nonstuttering children, children who stutter are more emotionally reactive and are less able to regulate their emotional responses. The authors speculated that these traits may make it more likely that children who stutter will react emotionally to their disfluencies, producing more disfluencies in a cycle of reactivity and increasing stuttering, which the authors call "reverberant interaction."

Kurt Eggers conducted several studies on children who stuttered compared with those who did not (Eggers, 2012). His initial study included 69 children who stuttered and 149 children who did not; all children were between 3 and 8 years old. Using the CBQ (Rothbart et al., 2001), Eggers found that children who stuttered scored higher in negative reactivity (Kagan's category of "inhibited") and lower in self-regulation. Relating this to Rothbart's interpretation of these factors, this study suggests that children who stutter tend to have greater motor, cognitive, and emotional responses to stimuli. They also may show more inhibition and avoidance (see Fig. 1.1 in Eggers, 2012).

Compared to the research on temperament in children who stutter, only a small amount of research has been done on adults. Some researchers (e.g., Kagan, 1994a, 1994b) have advocated for physiological or behavioral studies, rather than parent rating of children's temperament. In this spirit, using a physiological measure of sensitivity, Guitar (2003) found that the acoustic startle responses of adults who stutter were significantly greater than those of adults who do not. The startle paradigm, which measures the magnitude of the eye blink in response to a burst of white noise, is believed to differentiate individuals whose nervous systems have low thresholds of arousal from those whose nervous systems require larger stimuli to react (Vrana, Spence, & Lang, 1988). Moreover, that paradigm has been used to demonstrate differences between children who have been categorized as temperamentally inhibited and those categorized as temperamentally uninhibited (Snidman & Kagan, 1994). Guitar (2003) also found substantial correlations between startle responses and scores on the nervous subscale of the Taylor-Johnson Temperament Analysis (Taylor & Morrison, 1996). That subscale assesses the individual's tendency to be tense and excitable.

It should be noted that two later studies, Alm and Risberg (2007) and Ellis, Finan, and Ramig (2008), failed to replicate Guitar's (2003) findings. This suggests that a sensitive temperament may not be a characteristic of all adults who stutter, and it is certainly not a trait limited to those who stutter. To the extent it is a component of stuttering for many individuals, it probably interacts with a basic predisposition for difficulty with speech motor control.

Some studies of sensitive temperament in children who stutter have used electrophysiological measures of brain activity as well as parent questionnaires to compare children who stutter with those who don't. Zengin-Bolatkale (2016, 2017) used late positive potential (LPP)—a measure of EEG activity in response to stimuli—to assess both groups' response to pleasant and unpleasant pictures. Higher levels of LPP are thought to reflect emotional reactivity, and this study was able to show that children who stutter had significantly more emotional reactivity to unpleasant pictures, and this reactivity was significantly correlated with parent report of the child's sensitive temperament. Zengin-Bolakale (personal communication, November 27, 2017) also showed that this emotional reactivity was significantly and positively correlated with the children's severity of stuttering.

The findings that children who stutter are more temperamentally reactive are important because they point toward why some children who have vulnerable speech production systems may begin to stutter under relatively normal stress. They also help us understand why some of these children are susceptible to conditioning that can turn mild intermittent stuttering into more severe and persistent stuttering. This will be explored more fully in Chapter 5, on learning. Table 3.4 summarizes emotional factors in stuttering.

TABLE 3.4 Emotional Factors in Stuttering

Area of Interest	Important Findings	Major Clinical Implications
Anxiety	Many, but not all, studies find that individuals who stutter are not more anxious than individuals who don't stutter, but a few do indicate they are more anxious.	For many individuals with persistent stuttering, their treatment programs may benefit from components that facilitate the unlearning of fear-based stuttering behaviors.
Autonomic Arousal	Anxiety or autonomic arousal in individuals who stutter is associated with stuttering. Emotion caused by threat of electric shock can cause disfluencies even in individuals who don't stutter.	Treatment should consider addressing anxiety and fear in clients who manifest them.
Temperament	There is some evidence that children and adults who stutter tend to have a more sensitive or inhibited temperament; there is speculation that this may be related to right-hemisphere activity associated with stuttering. Sensitivity may influence physical tension.	There may be a subgroup of particularly reactive/sensitive individuals who need more focus on emotions during treatment.

SUMMARY

- Strong evidence indicates that individuals who stutter have deficits in sensory processing, such as auditory perception, cortical speech processing, dichotic listening, and control of movement using kinesthetic feedback. These deficits may signal some weakness in use of sensory information to make movements used in speech production.
- Many studies have found that sensorimotor responses, like reaction times, in individuals who stutter are slower than in typical speakers. Movements in fluent speech are also slower, reflected by acoustic and kinematic measures.
- Individuals who stutter appear to have deficits not only in speech motor control but also in nonspeech motor tasks, such as sequential finger tapping and using auditory input to control motor output.
- Many researchers have theorized that stuttering occurs because some individuals—through heredity or cerebral injury—have a vulnerable speech production system that may break down under stress of various kinds.
- One type of stress that may produce stuttering in such a vulnerable system is from demands of language. It is hypothesized that the demands of language learning during, especially during ages 2 to 5, may overwhelm the speech system and result in the onset of stuttering. In adults, it has been shown that those who stutter show problems in motor speech coordination as the components of language (e.g., syntax or phonology) become more complex.
- Another stress that may cause breakdown in a vulnerable speech motor system may come from emotional arousal. Heightened emotion has been shown to affect those who stutter more than those who don't. In addition, there is evidence that a sensitive temperament may characterize both adults and children who stutter, making them more prone to emotional reactivity and less ability to regulate responses to emotion. Emotion may interfere with smooth motor coordination, lead to more muscle tension, and make classical conditioning (learned emotion-based responses) more likely.

STUDY QUESTIONS

1. There were many findings about sensory deficits in people who stutter. How would sensory deficits result in stuttering, which is a motor disorder?
2. What are some reasons why individuals who stutter might be slower in their reaction times and in speech movements during fluent speech?
3. Why would people who stutter have problems with motor movements that have nothing to do with speech?
4. Explain how language demands might cause the onset of stuttering between ages 2 and 5.
5. Given that adults have already learned their languages, why would adults who stutter have more stuttering with utterances that are more complex?
6. Do you think stuttering causes people to be more sensitive or do you think more sensitive people tend to stutter?
7. Why would an easily emotionally reactive person be more likely to be affected by classical conditioning? (You may need to find out more about classical conditioning to answer this. See Chapter 5.)
8. Researchers have found many differences between groups of people who stutter and their fluent peers. Why can't we say that these differences cause stuttering?
9. What research finding in this chapter do you think has the most relevance for the treatment of stuttering? Defend your answer.

SUGGESTED PROJECTS

1. Assess your own reaction time under different conditions. Use a stopwatch (how fast can you turn it on and off?) or similar instrument to determine your reaction time. Try this under many different conditions, such as at several times during the day and when sick or tired versus when feeling alert. Determine what variables affect your reaction times, and determine whether it is true for other people. Using this information, suggest why different studies of reaction times in individuals who stutter get different outcomes.
2. Find a temperament test (many are available online at no cost), and take it yourself. Do you think the results accurately describe you? Here's one to start with: www.TemperamentQuiz.com/.

SUGGESTED READINGS

Bloodstein, O., & Ratner, N. (2008). *A handbook on stuttering.* (6th ed.). Clifton Park, NY: Delmar Learning.

This is the most recent edition of a classic reference book on stuttering. It provides a thorough update of "the most important research in stuttering." Moreover, it is quite easy to read.

Craig, A. (Ed.). (2014). Anxiety and stuttering [Special issue]. *Journal of Fluency Disorders*, 40.

This issue of the journal contains review articles as well as empirical research on the relationship between anxiety and stuttering. It gives a good overview of this topic as of 2014.

Maassen, B., Kent, R., Peters, H., van Lieshout, P., & Hulstijn, W. (Eds.). (2004). *Speech motor control in normal and disordered speech*. Oxford, UK: Oxford University Press.

This book contains updated chapters by many scientists who presented their findings at a conference on speech motor control in 2001. Although not all of the contents are directly related to stuttering, there is much of great interest to clinicians and researchers interested in the neurophysiological bases of speech and stuttering.

Smith, A., & Weber, C. (2017). How stuttering develops: The multifactorial dynamic pathways theory. *Journal of Speech, Language, and Hearing Research*, *60*, 2483–2505.

This article is an excellent review of research—much of it from Smith and Weber's own research group—supporting a view that motor, linguistic, and emotional factors combine and interact to precipitate and maintain childhood stuttering.

StutterTalk: Changing how you think about stuttering…one podcast at a time (www.stuttertalk.com).

This Web site is a gold mine of information about stuttering research and treatment. Founder Peter Reitzes and other hosts interview scientists, clinicians, and people who stutter about stuttering—its nature and treatment. At present, there are more than 500 recorded interviews you can listen to on your computer or mobile device. Episodes 571, 568, 564, 561, and 558 are interviews on topics covered in this chapter on constitutional factors in stuttering.

Van Riper, C. (1982). *The nature of stuttering* (2nd ed.). Englewood Cliffs, NJ: Prentice-Hall.

Although somewhat dated, this book reviews an impressive amount of world literature on stuttering, from as long ago as the 20th century BC *In a synthesis of the research, Van Riper presents his venerable hypothesis that stuttering is a disorder of timing.*

Yairi, E. & Ambrose, N. G. (2005). *Early childhood stuttering*. Austin, TX: Pro-Ed.

The authors give an in-depth description of the results of 14 years of research on the development of stuttering conducted at the University of Illinois. Chapters are devoted to the onset and development of stuttering, characteristics of children's disfluency, genetics, and cognitive, psychosocial, and motor factors in stuttering. Elaine Paden and Ruth Watkins contributed chapters on phonological and language abilities of children who stutter, respectively. Like Wendell Johnson's magnum opus The Onset of Stuttering, this book reflects a monumental effort focused on childhood stuttering.

4

Developmental and Environmental Factors in Stuttering

Chapter Objectives

After studying this chapter, readers should be able to:

- Explain how factors related to physical development can interfere with fluent speech
- Explain how factors related to speech and language development can interfere with fluent speech
- Explain how, in some cases, increasing language development may decrease disfluencies

- Explain how factors related to cognitive development can interfere with fluent speech
- Explain how factors related to social-emotional development can interfere with fluent speech
- Describe the evidence for the role of parents, the speech-language environment, and life events in the onset and development of stuttering

Key Terms

Competition for neural resources: This is the concept that the brain has a limited amount of resources that can be applied to tasks such as learning to speak and learning to walk. If some task requires a great deal of attention or involves extensive neural activity, other tasks performed at the same time will have fewer resources and may thus be less well performed.

Life events: Happenings in a child's life that may stress the child, such as parents' divorce or being hospitalized

Speech and language environment: The communication style that characterizes people in a child's environment—usually his or her home. For example, some parents, siblings, and other relatives of a child may speak very rapidly, use advanced forms of language, or interrupt the child frequently. These aspects of the speech and language environment are thought to stress the child.

The two preceding chapters described the constitutional factors that put a child at risk for stuttering. These factors usually lie dormant until the child's language reaches the two-word stage or even later. At that time, motor and cognitive abilities are also developing rapidly, and the child's environment is often a busy household with competing demands and distractions. These are the conditions under which stuttering first appears, then disappears, continues, or grows worse.

Developmental and environmental influences can be pressures that bring on stuttering, but they can also ameliorate or protect. A child's rapidly developing language abilities may enable her to keep up with a desire to produce long and complex sentences, thus bridging a gap that might otherwise have resulted in stuttering. Parents may be able to change a child's environment, so that demands from a garrulous, fast-talking family can be tempered by more one-on-one time when a parent talks slowly to a child and lets him speak when he wants on a topic of his choosing, while she listens.

Figure 4.1 depicts the influence of developmental and environmental factors on the onset and development of stuttering.

The developmental and environmental factors that interact with constitutional factors to give rise to stuttering often work quietly. The ordinariness of the child's life when stuttering first appears is reflected in this observation by Van Riper (1973, p. 81):

> *In the great majority of children we have carefully studied soon after onset, we were unable to state with any certainty ... what precipitated the stuttering. In most instances there simply were no apparent conflicts, no illnesses, no opportunity to imitate, no shocks or frightening experiences. Stuttering seemed to begin under quite normal conditions of living and communicating.*

Because children's lives often seem so normal when stuttering first emerges, research to determine critical developmental and environmental factors affecting its onset and progression has not produced conclusive results. This is a domain of educated guesses and tentative hypotheses. Evidence for developmental factors is inferred from the fact that almost all onsets of stuttering occur when children are developing most rapidly during their preschool years (Andrews et al., 1983; Bloodstein & Ratner, 2008; Wingate, 1983; Yairi & Ambrose, 2005, 2013). Evidence of environmental influences comes in part from clinical reports of particular stresses sometimes associated with the onset of stuttering and its remission when these stresses are lessened (e.g., Jones, Choi, Conture, & Walden, 2014; Van Riper, 1973, 1982). Environmental factors are also implicated by higher incidences of stuttering in those cultures that appear to be more competitive, with high standards and less tolerance of differences, like the United States and Japan. By contrast, in New Guinea, among Polar Eskimos, and in the aborigines of Australia, where cultural pressures to conform may be less, there is apparently a lower incidence (Bloodstein & Ratner, 2008). Finally, some sources of evidence for genetic factors in stuttering are also evidence for environmental factors. Genetic studies—described in Chapter 2—show that genes alone cannot account for the occurrence of stuttering in all children, but rather some other factors—probably environmental—must also play a part (e.g., Andrews, Morris-Yates, Howie, & Martin, 1991; Fagnani, Fibiger, Skytthe, & Hjelmborg, 2011; Felsenfeld et al., 2000; Ooki, 2005; Van Beijsterveldt, Felsenfeld, & Boomsma, 2010). However, this research has not been able to identify with certainty which environmental factors might be involved.

In this chapter, I have divided developmental and environmental factors into separate sections, although they do not operate independently. For example, if a child is in the early

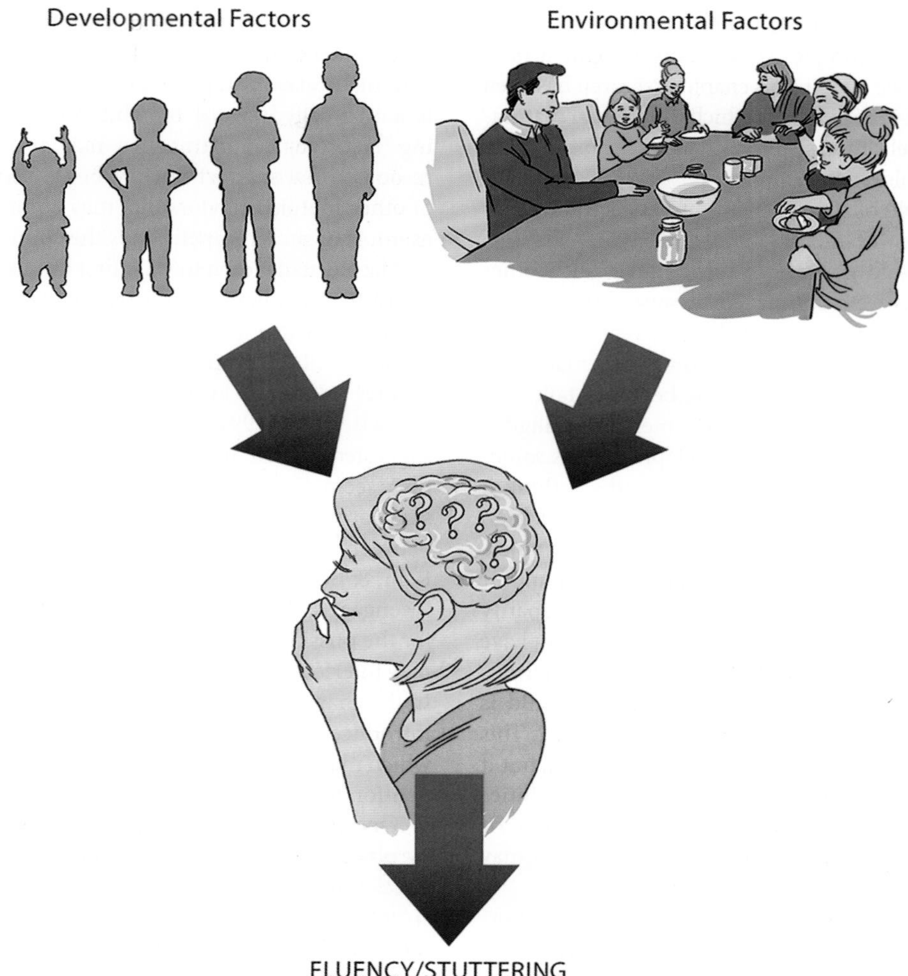

Figure 4.1 Predisposing constitutional factors interact with developmental, environmental, and learning factors to precipitate or worsen stuttering.

stages of speech and language learning, it may be hard for her to keep up with a chattering, interrupting, and raucous household. Excess disfluencies and then perhaps stuttering may appear because of this interaction pattern. Every child and every family are different, of course. Thus, an evaluation needs to explore recent changes in each child's developmental level and the challenges of her environment.

DEVELOPMENTAL FACTORS

My view of how developmental factors affect children's fluency assumes that there is in the growing child **a competition for neural resources**. That is, the brain must share its resources in coping with the "great blooming, buzzing confusion" (James, 1890) of the sounds, sights, and feelings of childhood. Like a computer, the brain can work on several things at once—but as the brain nears its maximum capacity, the more tasks it performs simultaneously, the more slowly and less efficiently it does each one. For humans, there are some ways in which multiple things can be done simultaneously. If the tasks are dissimilar, such as driving a car and talking about the weather, there is less interference between them. On the other hand, if the tasks are similar, such as rubbing your stomach while patting your head, there is more interference between them (Kinsbourne & Hicks, 1978). The problem of shared resources is more acute in children because their immature nervous systems have less processing capacity to draw on (Hiscock & Kinsbourne, 1977, 1980). Some children are especially at risk for straining their developing resources. Their speech and language skills may be delayed, yet they have to compete in a highly verbal environment. Or, their language development may surge ahead of their speech motor control skills, giving them much to say, but limited capacity to say it rapidly and fluently. It is as though they were trying to herd a dozen cats through a small door, in a hurry, resulting in a slight catastrophe. Children with some unevenness in their development of different skills may become excessively disfluent as other developmental demands—for example, physical and cognitive growth—compete with their ability to coordinate the complex movements of rapid, articulate speech. As you'll see later in this chapter, research has been carried out to quantify the extent to which differential maturation of components related to speech and language production is characteristic of children who stutter.

Here is an example of the competition between burgeoning language and slower motor abilities. Several years ago, I evaluated a 4-year-old girl whose uncle and grandmother stuttered. Her parents were concerned because she had been repeating words and sounds excessively for a year and a half, sometimes up to 20 times per instance. However, her language development was well above average; she began to talk with single words at 9 months and to produce sentences intelligibly at 12 months. In contrast, her motor development was somewhat slower; she had not walked until 18 months. I think it is possible that her disfluencies emerged as a result of a high proportion of her cerebral resources being used to formulate and express language with less mature capacities for motor activities, including fluent speech. In other words, a disparity between language facility and motor speech ability may have been an important contributor to the emergence of stuttering.

To appreciate how many skills and abilities the child is developing at the same time, look carefully at Figure 4.2. This chart covers only social, motor, and language domains, but it is clear that children have to master many different abilities simultaneously. If a child's development is slower in one or more areas (i.e., dyssynchronous), her road to maturity may be steep at times.

The question of dyssynchronous development is an important one, because if it involves domains relevant to producing fluent speech, dyssynchrony may be a contributing factor in stuttering. To understand dyssynchrony, imagine trying to prepare a huge dinner, but having trouble getting all the parts of the meal ready at the same time. The roast beef may be done, but the string beans are not fully cooked. Another example is a tricycle factory (Fig. 4.3) that sometimes malfunctions because some parts of the tricycle are ready to be assembled when other parts are delayed. If the team preparing the wheels is much slower than the team making the frames, delays will result. Extra resources will be suddenly needed by the wheel team to resolve the problem, taking away resources from other teams, making the factory go into momentary disarray (i.e., stuttering).

So, let us look at some of the domains of development and how they might contribute to the onset of stuttering.

Physical and Motor Development

Demands of Physical and Motor Development

The mother of a 3-year-old child who recently began to stutter told me "Whenever he has a spurt of physical growth, his stuttering seems to increase." Why would this be? Between ages 1 and 6 years, children grow by leaps and bounds. Their bodies get bigger. Their nervous systems form new pathways and new connections. Their perceptual and motor skills improve with maturation and practice. This intensive period of growth is a two-edged sword for children predisposed to stuttering. Neurological maturation may provide more neuronal resources that support fluency, but it also spurs development of other motor behaviors that may compete with fluency. An example of such competition is the common observation that children usually learn to walk first or talk first, but not both at the same time. For example, Netsell (1981, p. 25) said of this trade-off, "The practice of walking or talking seems sufficient to 'tie up' all the available sensorimotor circuitry because the toddler seldom, if ever, undertakes both activities at once." Likewise, Berk (1991, p. 194), in his text on child development, suggested "when infants forge ahead in spoken language, they seem to temporarily postpone mastery of new motor skills or vice versa." Other possible evidence for competition between cognition and motor control (Beurskens, Helmich, Rein, & Bock, 2014) also suggests that if one domain is heavily engaged, the other domain may suffer deficits. This argues for the possibility that rapid physical and motor development may interfere with the cognitive resources needed for fluency. In the chapter on theoretical perspectives on stuttering, I will introduce the "capacities and demands" view of stuttering, which may be a useful framework for understanding the competition for resources that I have been discussing.

One particular challenge to speech motor control posed by physical development in children is rapid change in the vocal tract between ages 2 and 5 years. During this time, structures in a child's head, neck, and torso undergo their most accelerated growth; moreover, different structures grow at different rates (Kent & Vorperian, 1995, 2007). As children's speaking mechanisms change—the shape, size, and biomechanical properties of muscles and bones are different one day from the way they were the previous day—children continue to produce intelligible speech. Callan, Kent, Guenther, and Vorperian (2000) hypothesize that children maintain a stable speech output in the face of daily changes in their speech structures by using feedback to continuously update the motor commands they send to their muscles to produce specific sounds. What their brains told their muscles to do yesterday must be adapted to the new size, shape, and biomechanical properties of the vocal tract today. Auditory feedback, integrated with proprioceptive and other muscle feedback, helps children discover errors in their motor commands and adjust the commands to the new dimensions.

You can see from these demands of speech motor development just described that the preschool child's brain is occupied with a multitude of tasks to keep up with his or her developing speech mechanism. No wonder that children with a fragile speech motor system—children predisposed to stutter—will develop repetitions and prolongations as they juggle the demands of growing, changing sensorimotor mechanisms, the need to speak ever faster, and the ability to employ increasingly more complex language.

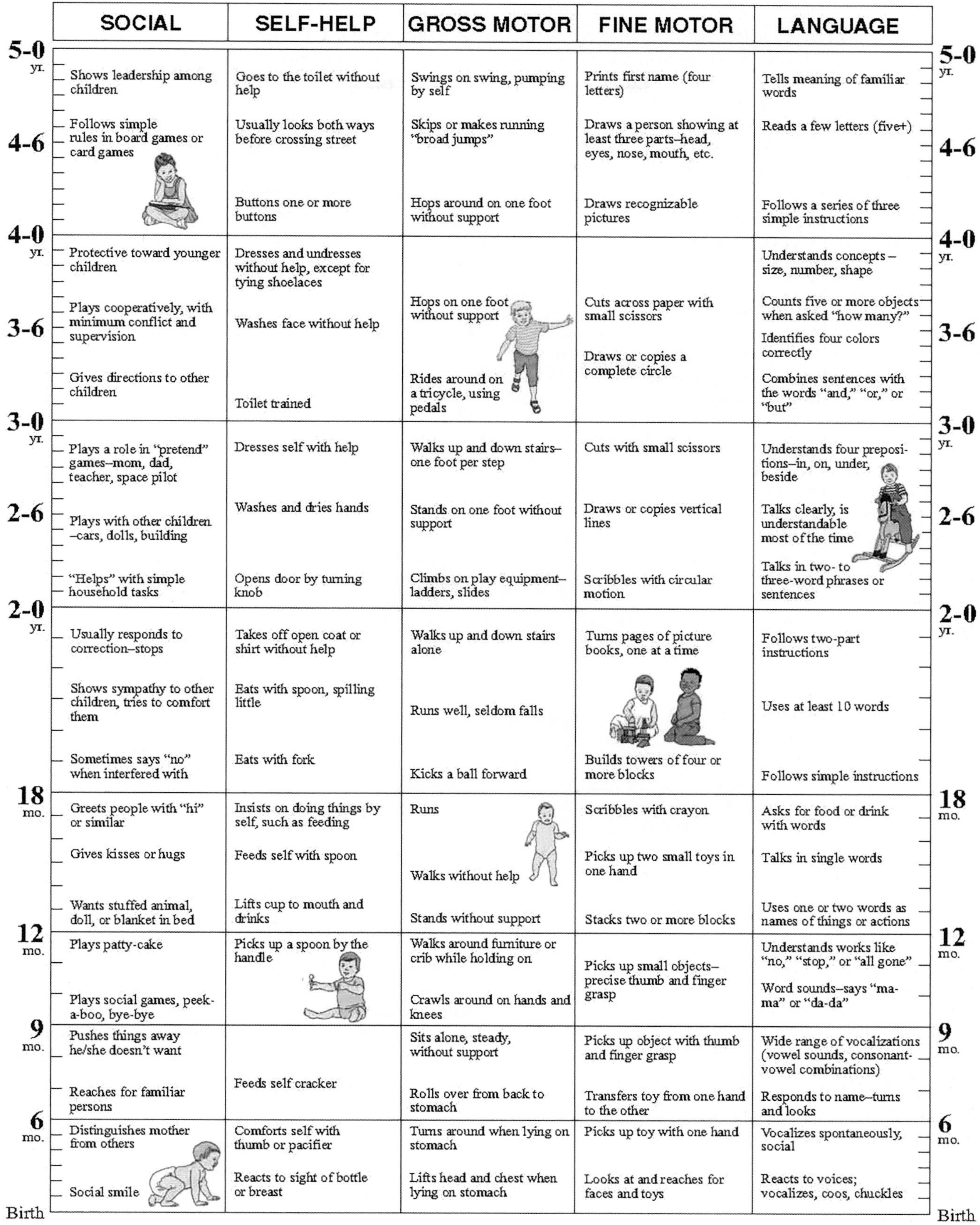

Age	SOCIAL	SELF-HELP	GROSS MOTOR	FINE MOTOR	LANGUAGE
5-0 yr. – 4-0 yr. (4-6)	Shows leadership among children Follows simple rules in board games or card games	Goes to the toilet without help Usually looks both ways before crossing street Buttons one or more buttons	Swings on swing, pumping by self Skips or makes running "broad jumps" Hops around on one foot without support	Prints first name (four letters) Draws a person showing at least three parts–head, eyes, nose, mouth, etc. Draws recognizable pictures	Tells meaning of familiar words Reads a few letters (five+) Follows a series of three simple instructions
4-0 yr. – 3-0 yr. (3-6)	Protective toward younger children Plays cooperatively, with minimum conflict and supervision Gives directions to other children	Dresses and undresses without help, except for tying shoelaces Washes face without help Toilet trained	Hops on one foot without support Rides around on a tricycle, using pedals	Cuts across paper with small scissors Draws or copies a complete circle	Understands concepts – size, number, shape Counts five or more objects when asked "how many?" Identifies four colors correctly Combines sentences with the words "and," "or," or "but"
3-0 yr. – 2-0 yr. (2-6)	Plays a role in "pretend" games–mom, dad, teacher, space pilot Plays with other children –cars, dolls, building "Helps" with simple household tasks	Dresses self with help Washes and dries hands Opens door by turning knob	Walks up and down stairs– one foot per step Stands on one foot without support Climbs on play equipment– ladders, slides	Cuts with small scissors Draws or copies vertical lines Scribbles with circular motion	Understands four prepositions–in, on, under, beside Talks clearly, is understandable most of the time Talks in two- to three-word phrases or sentences
2-0 yr. – 18 mo.	Usually responds to correction–stops Shows sympathy to other children, tries to comfort them Sometimes says "no" when interfered with	Takes off open coat or shirt without help Eats with spoon, spilling little Eats with fork	Walks up and down stairs alone Runs well, seldom falls Kicks a ball forward	Turns pages of picture books, one at a time Builds towers of four or more blocks	Follows two-part instructions Uses at least 10 words Follows simple instructions
18 mo. – 12 mo.	Greets people with "hi" or similar Gives kisses or hugs Wants stuffed animal, doll, or blanket in bed	Insists on doing things by self, such as feeding Feeds self with spoon Lifts cup to mouth and drinks	Runs Walks without help Stands without support	Scribbles with crayon Picks up two small toys in one hand Stacks two or more blocks	Asks for food or drink with words Talks in single words Uses one or two words as names of things or actions
12 mo. – 9 mo.	Plays patty-cake Plays social games, peek-a-boo, bye-bye	Picks up a spoon by the handle	Walks around furniture or crib while holding on Crawls around on hands and knees	Picks up small objects– precise thumb and finger grasp	Understands works like "no," "stop," or "all gone" Word sounds–says "ma-ma" or "da-da"
9 mo. – 6 mo.	Pushes things away he/she doesn't want Reaches for familiar persons	Feeds self cracker	Sits alone, steady, without support Rolls over from back to stomach	Picks up object with thumb and finger grasp Transfers toy from one hand to the other	Wide range of vocalizations (vowel sounds, consonant-vowel combinations) Responds to name–turns and looks
6 mo. – Birth	Distinguishes mother from others Social smile	Comforts self with thumb or pacifier Reacts to sight of bottle or breast	Turns around when lying on stomach Lifts head and chest when lying on stomach	Picks up toy with one hand Looks at and reaches for faces and toys	Vocalizes spontaneously, social Reacts to voices; vocalizes, coos, chuckles

Figure 4.2 Child development in the first 5 years. (Courtesy Harold Ireton, Ph.D.)

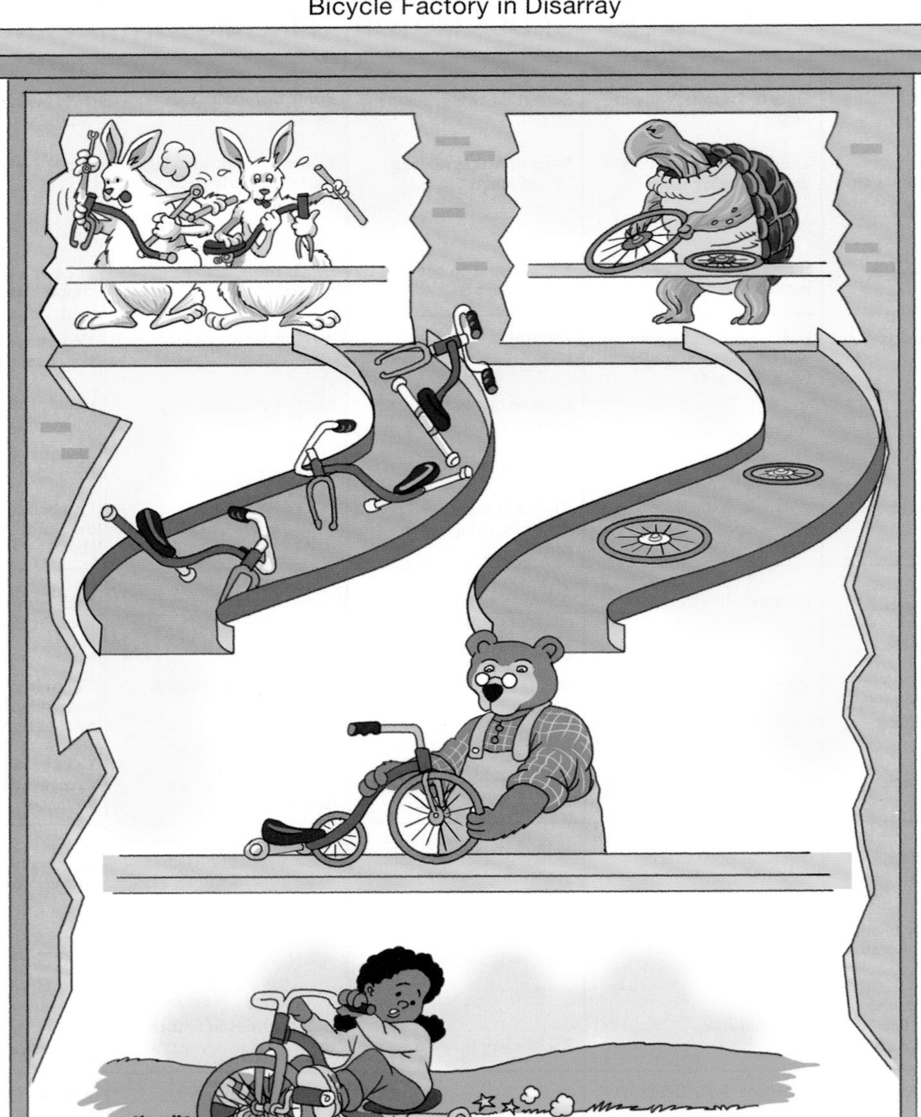

Figure 4.3 A tricycle factory in disarray and using extra resources.

Delays in Motor Development

Evidence from brain imaging studies presented in Chapter 2 (e.g., Chang et al., 2015; Choo et al., 2016; Cykowski, Fox, Ingham, Ingham, & Robin, 2010; Sommer, Koch, Paulus, Weiller, & Buchel, 2002) suggests that the neurological structures, pathways, and networks used to produce sounds and words may be inefficient (less well myelinated, where myelin provides a form of insulation that carries signals more efficiently) in children who stutter. These neural pathways and networks are crucial in helping the child speak accurately as his or her system changes in development. When children with compromised neural pathways are ready to speak and need quick access to the stored plans for production, this access may be slow in coming, and stuttering may result.

Problems in neural networks related to speech production may be detected using various measures of motor coordination or movement stability. A review of earlier studies of motor coordination in people who stutter can be found in Bloodstein and Ratner (2008). Some studies suggested deficits in speech motor control and some did not. More recent studies have provided stronger evidence that children who stutter have a delay in development of motor control. Many of these studies have been conducted by experimenters at Purdue University. As mentioned in the section on nonspeech motor control in the previous chapter, Olander et al. (2010) demonstrated a deficit in motor timing during a rhythmic clapping task in a large subgroup of preschool children who stutter. When tested on nonsense words produced fluently in a later study (Smith, Goffman, Sasisekaran, & Weber-Fox, 2012), preschool children who stuttered showed more variability (more like younger children) in articulator movement than did the control children. MacPherson and Smith (2013) assessed speech motor variability when children who stutter speak fluently. They found that many, but not all, of the stuttering children had greater variability (less stability) than their nonstuttering peers in articulator movements even during fluent speech. The Purdue group then followed these children to see if there were differences in measures of speech-motor abilities during the time that some of them recovered and some didn't. For example, Spencer and Weber-Fox (2014) found that tests of accuracy of phonological production and nonword production showed a greater deficit in those children who persisted in stuttering than those who did not. A year later, similar conclusions about persistent stuttering were published. Researchers at the University of Illinois (Ambrose, Yairi, Loucks, Seery, & Throneburg, 2015) followed a large cohort of 58 children who stuttered. They observed the children from near the onset of their stuttering to several years later when many had recovered. Their findings in language and temperament measures will be discussed later, but their findings in motor development support the conclusions of Spencer and Weber-Fox described above. Specifically, the Illinois researchers demonstrated that children who persisted in stuttering tended to show more immature speech motor development for their age compared to both the children who recovered and those who had never stuttered when motor performance was measured acoustically.

Absolute delays in development may not be as important in stuttering as differences in the rate of development among components. Building on previous research (Anderson, Pillowski, & Conture, 2005) that compared the relative maturation of different components of the speech-motor-language system, Choo, Burnham, Hicks, and Chang (2016) compared children who stuttered with children who didn't on many aspects of performance and also compared white matter tract density of the two groups using diffusion tensor imaging. These researchers found more dissociations (uneven abilities) in the development of motor performance in children who stuttered compared to typical children. In fact, they found delays and uneven development in speech and language areas as well as motor performance. This was more pronounced in boys and all left-handed children who stuttered. These delays and dissociations in motor development were also reflected in brain imaging data suggesting less dense white matter tracts (in the children who stuttered compared with those who didn't) in areas supporting speech motor and auditory-motor development.

Summary of the Effect of Physical and Motor Development on Fluency

The demands of motor development on neural resources will affect even typically developing children. Typical children may have to postpone learning complex levels of phonology morphology, syntax, and semantics as they master walking, climbing, hopping, and kicking a ball. Children with compromised speech motor development (including children who stutter) may be affected even more.

Evidence for delayed motor development in children who stutter has been accumulating in recent years. These delays appear to be greater in children who persist in stuttering rather than those who recover.

Research suggests greater dissociations (uneven abilities) in the relative development of motor abilities and language abilities in children who stutter compared to those who don't. Such dissociations may contribute to the onset or persistence of stuttering because of the strain this may put on neural resources (Anderson et al., 2005; Coulter et al., 2009).

Speech and Language Development

Language Learning and the Onset of Stuttering

In Chapter 3, I said that language growth may affect fluency because individuals who stutter may have a fragile speech production system that would be stressed by the demands of producing more and more complex language. I also suggested that children in the process of learning language may be particularly prone to disfluencies—both normal disfluencies and stuttering—because of the heavy load that learning a new and complex skill intimately associated with speaking puts on neural resources for speech production as it is becoming more automatic. In this section, I want to expand on this idea that early language learning can be the stress most frequently associated with the onset of stuttering.

Here's a quick review of what the child is learning at this time: Between the ages of 2 and 3, a child's vocabulary jumps from 50 to well over 500 words; in fact, toward the end of this year, five to seven new words may be learned each day (Studdert-Kennedy, 1987). At the same time, the child's single-word utterances develop into successive single-word pairs with sentence-like intonations and durations and then to multiword sentences (Branigan, 1979; Veneziano, 2013). Thus, the child's speech graduates from a simple "syllable-timed" prosody for single words to complex prosodic rhythms that span multiple words (Allen & Hawkins, 1980). As the child expands sentences, he also overhauls his language storage system. At first, his shelves are stocked with whole words in the form of articulatory routines or gestural patterns; then, he must change strategies and begin to stock, not whole words, but segments that can be combined in various ways to form a multitude of words (Kent, 1985; Nittrouer, Studdert-Kennedy, & McGowan, 1989; Sternberger, 1982, Tilsen, 2016). During these same preschool years, the child also progressively learns active, negative, and passive constructions as well as present, future, and past tenses. Further, he increases the length and linguistic complexity of his sentences together with the rate of his utterances as he increasingly tries to synchronize the rates and rhythms of his speech with those of his family, with whom he has a growing urge to communicate (Prelock & Hutchins, 2019; Velleman, 2015).

This huge array of language and speech production tasks is a challenge even to the fluency of nonstuttering children. Normal disfluencies of children also increase from ages 2 to 4, peaking when they tackle the task of producing long, complex sentences (Ito, 1986). It is not surprising, then, that children begin stuttering during this same period.

Many clinician-researchers have speculated on the connection between language learning and stuttering. Dalton and Hardcastle (1977) commented that "it is tempting to see the ever-increasing demands on linguistic competence and articulatory proficiency as major factors in the onset of some disfluency" (p. 69). Sheehan (1975) said, "The age of onset of stuttering is consistently related to certain stages in the developmental sequence. Most notably, the 'period of resonance,' or high readiness in language learning…is also the period during which stuttering develops and flourishes" (p. 142). Andrews and colleagues (1983) pointed to the demands placed on speech by rapidly developing language, noting that "stuttering [has] a maximal frequency of onset at a time when an explosive growth in language ability outstrips a still-immature speech-motor apparatus" (p. 239).

Many studies of children have found that greater length and complexity of language are associated with more stuttering. This is a developmental factor because stuttering may first appear when children use longer and more complex utterances. For example, research on natural conversational speech of children who stutter has shown that more complex utterances contain more stuttering (Brundage & Bernstein Ratner, 1989; Gaines, Runyan, & Meyers, 1991; Logan & Conture, 1995; Yaruss, 1999; but see Hollister, Van Horne, & Zebrowski, 2017 for a different view). Some research suggests that utterance length may have a greater effect on stuttering than does complexity (Hollister et al., 2017; Logan & Conture, 1995; Wilkenfeld & Curlee, 1997; Yaruss, 1999). Experimental studies, in which children were asked to produce both more and less complex utterances, show that children who stutter (Bernstein Ratner & Sih, 1987; Stocker & Usprich, 1976) and fluent children (Gordon, Luper, & Peterson, 1986; Haynes & Hood, 1978; Pearl & Bernthal, 1980; Yaruss, Newman, & Flora, 1999) increase their disfluencies as language complexity is increased. Unfortunately, there is little longitudinal research that directly bears on the question of how and when emerging language is associated with normal disfluency or stuttering. However, a study of articulatory coordination variability in both typically developing children and children who stuttered indicated that both groups demonstrated more variability for longer sentences (McPherson & Smith, 2013). This suggest that as both typically developing and stuttering children use longer utterance as they mature, articulatory coordination may become less stable, giving rise to increased normal disfluency as well as stuttering.

One of the few studies of the appearance of disfluencies in individual children over time was Norma Colburn's analysis of the disfluencies of four nonstuttering children using data originally gathered by Lois Bloom for her work on normal language development. Published reports of Colburn's analysis (Colburn & Mysak, 1982a, 1982b) suggested that these children's normal disfluencies did not emerge when they first learned a new language construction but appeared as they began to master a new construction and started using it regularly. Explanations suggested for this result include the possibility that a child who has learned, but not completely automatized, the use of a new construction allocates fewer resources than are necessary for its production (Kent & Perkins, 1984) or the possibility that as a child masters the new construction he produces it at an increased rate, thereby straining capacity (Starkweather, 1987).

A single-case study by Frank Wijnen (1990) was used to explore the relationship between syntax acquisition and normal disfluencies. Weekly speech samples were obtained from a boy from age 2 years, 4 months to 2 years, 11 months. The number of repetitions, revisions, and incomplete phrases was assessed in relation to the length and complexity of utterances. It was reported that disfluencies were randomly distributed initially, but eventually clustered on function words and sentence-initial words and then declined. Although speech rate was not measured (increased rate might have accounted for some of the increase in the child's disfluencies), the number of disfluencies was not highly correlated with length of utterance. Instead, Wijnen concluded that the eventual decline in the child's disfluencies was associated with his mastery of a routine type of sentence (pronoun + verb + some other word) and that the early stages of learning this routine involved so much of his processing capacity that speech production was short-changed and disfluencies resulted. This preliminary study needs to be followed up with many more cases to test the hypothesis that the process of first learning to make sentence productions more automatic through routinization of several sentence types is related to increased normal disfluency.

What is happening in the brain to precipitate stuttering during this speech and language growth spurt? You will remember from Chapter 2 that brain imaging studies of children who stutter have shown some anomalous patterns of activity during speech. For example, there are abnormally high levels of activity in some regions of the right hemisphere and abnormally low levels in some areas of the left. In addition, recent findings with children who stutter suggest that white matter tracts connecting areas of the brain used for integration of articulator planning, sensory feedback, and motor execution are compromised (e.g., Chang et al., 2008, 2015). Thus, planning and production of speech and language may have to rely on weak neural pathways and compromised gray matter areas that may be slow or inefficient. But the demands grow ever greater as a child produces longer, faster, and more complex sentences. Tasks using different neural networks for segment selection, grammatical formulation, and prosodic planning must be orchestrated precisely so that each element is in place at the proper time as utterances are produced. If some components are ready but others are delayed, initial sounds or syllables may be repeated, prolonged, or even blocked, waiting for all the elements of each sentence to be put together in the brain. We will revisit this scenario in the next section.

Before we leave the topic of language development and the onset of stuttering, I would like to bring up the view that language development may, in some cases, decrease stuttering. A longitudinal study by Hollister et al. (2017) examined the language development and disfluencies of three groups of children: typically developing children, stuttering children who would recover, and stuttering children who would persist in stuttering. Their findings indicated that of the three groups, only the children who would recover had fewer disfluencies as their mastery of grammar and syntax increased (independent of age). This suggests that as the recovering children could more easily manage the demands of producing longer sentences, their speech production systems would not be stressed.

Delayed and Deviant Language Development

For an example of a child whose language was delayed and then developed stuttering, watch the video of David Wilkins' mother in which she describes the onset of her son's stuttering. Go to *thePoint* and watch Video 4-1 "A Mother's Experience with Her Child's Stuttering."

Because available evidence suggests that stuttering arises from constitutional differences (e.g., inheritance or congenital injury), it is natural to wonder whether the brain anomalies that give rise to stuttering also delay overall language development as well. Delays in language development could co-occur with stuttering, but not cause it. On the other hand, language delays could cause children to become frustrated with their difficulty expressing themselves and consequently develop fears about speaking, which could lead to stuttering (c.f., the anticipatory avoidance response theory of stuttering; Bloodstein & Ratner, 2008) described in the chapter on Theories of Stuttering. A study many years ago indicated that language-delayed children have a significant amount stuttering-like disfluencies when they are given therapy—significantly more disfluencies than matched language-delayed children not in therapy and matched typically developing children (Merits-Patterson & Reed, 1981). This suggests that the combination of language delay and pressure to produce language may generate signs of stuttering.

What is the evidence for language delays in children who stutter? Some published studies have found that language delays or difficulties are more common among children who stutter than those who don't, but the findings are neither simple nor clear-cut, and their implications are unclear. After surveying many studies of language abilities in children who stutter, Nippold (2012) concluded that there are no differences in language capability in children who stutter compared to those who don't and that language deficits are not associated with stuttering onset, nor its persistence. Supporting this position, Watts, Eadie, Block, Mensah, and Reilly (2014) examined language abilities in a large community sample of children ages 2 to 5 (181 children stuttered; 1,438 did not). They found that the children who stuttered scored higher on all the language measures. It should be noted that many of the younger children who stuttered may have later grown out of stuttering, so the sample is probably a mix of recovered and persistent children who stuttered. In contrast to these and Nippold's findings, research groups in Illinois and Wisconsin (Ambrose et al., 2015) compared 58 children who stuttered (ages 2–4) with 40 who did not over a period of several years. By the end of the study, the children who stuttered at the first visit could be classified as Persistent (n = 19) or Recovered (n = 39). Analysis of standardized language testing indicated that the Persistent group did significantly poorer than either the Recovered or the Control group on the first tests of language, even though their language was within the normal range. The Recovered group was similar to the Controls on all language tests. In summary, as a single group, children who stutter appear to have similar language skills compared to fluent children. However, when the stuttering children are subdivided into those who persist in stuttering and those who recover, the persistent stuttering children score slightly lower in measures of language. This finding could be affected by the possibility that the persistent stuttering children could have been more severe at the first assessment and thus may have been more reluctant to speak or not as experienced in speaking and thus appear to have slightly less developed language.

A number of researchers have approached the language question in a slightly different way. A possible reason for the conflicting findings about language delay in children who stutter may be that absolute levels of language skills may vary considerably in children who stutter. Some may have above-average ability in one area of language while they have average ability in another area. Some may have below-average ability in one area and average in another. This may result in group averages that are within the typical range but many individual cases where there is a disparity in the child's abilities in subcomponents of language, as it is usually assessed. Research has suggested that this very phenomenon—unequal rates of maturation of subcomponents of speech and language production—may be an important contributor to stuttering. Neuropsychologists studying neurological patients developed a statistical procedure to identify when "dissociations" (unequal abilities in subcomponents) were truly occurring (Bates, Appelbaum, Salcedo, Saygin, & Pizzamiglio, 2003). Anderson, Pellowski, and Conture (2005) used this statistical procedure to test for dissociations among speech and language skills in 45 children who stuttered and 45 who did not. They found that the group of children who stuttered had generally poorer speech and language skills but were still within the normal range. However, three times as many children who stuttered had dissociations among speech and language skills than those who did not stutter. The authors hypothesized that these dissociations may lead to stuttering because neural resources may be suddenly taken away from fluent speech production to resolve the mismatch between the readiness of some components to be produced compared to others.

The work of Choo, Burnham, et al. (2016), mentioned earlier in regard to motor development, revealed more dissociations among language areas in children who stuttered compared to typically developing children and less white matter coherence in "left dorsal language pathways" that support these language areas. This disparity in dissociations was particularly pronounced among boys who stuttered compared to girls and in left- compared to right-handed children who stuttered.

Summary of the Effect of Speech and Language Development on Fluency

The onset of stuttering, commonly between ages 2 and 5, is the period when children are most intensively learning to understand and produce language. It has been suggested that the heavy load on neural resources during language learning puts an extra strain on the child's speech production system and stuttering may come and go during this period, particularly if the child's speech production system is less robust, or even fragile, compared to that of children who do not stutter.

Research studies are conflicted about whether children who stutter have language delays compared to children who do not. There may be a subgroup of children whose language, while within the normal range, is somewhat delayed. These children may be those whose stuttering persists.

Some components of speech and language may be developing more slowly than other components in some children who stutter. This dyssynchrony in development may put an extra strain on the speech production system and result in stuttering. In these children, the white matter nerve tracts supporting language also appear to be developing more slowly or abnormally.

Cognitive Development

I use the phrase "cognitive development" to refer to the growth of perception, attention, working memory, and executive functions that play roles in spoken language but that can be considered separate from it, although intertwined with it as well.

Cognitive development may affect stuttering in two ways. First, growth spurts in cognitive development may trigger the onset of stuttering or may exacerbate it. Second, as a child who stutters develops more advanced cognitive abilities, he is more likely to become aware of and even self-conscious about his stuttering.

Cognitive Development Related to the Onset and Fluctuation of Stuttering

Parents frequently report that the onset of their child's stuttering occurs under the most normal of circumstances—no extra stresses in the household and no apparent increases in the child's anxiety. The same "normal circumstances" are also frequently true for sudden changes in the ongoing stuttering of a preschool child—suddenly, his stuttering is worse, and just as suddenly, it's better. One factor that may not be obvious to the parent but nonetheless may be an influence on stuttering is the child's cognitive growth. Earlier in this chapter, I suggested that aspects of physical development may affect stuttering; for example, learning to walk may make great demands on sensorimotor abilities, making fewer resources available for fluency. Now, I am proposing that learning to think, remember, problem-solve, and plan may make great demands on neural resources, leaving fewer resources available for rapid production of fluently spoken language.

This argument has been made before. Lindsay (1989) pointed out that during Jean Piaget's "preoperational period" of childhood development from 2 to 6 years, a child goes through a series of transitions in which new cognitive learning must be assimilated and consolidated with current knowledge. These transitions are times when a child's linguistic and cognitive systems are temporarily unstable before new concepts are mastered. As a consequence, children's speech and language production during this period of adjustment may be vulnerable to disfluencies.

Even in children with stable, age-appropriate cognitive function, high cognitive demands in their communicative environments may make stuttering temporarily worse (Starkweather, 1987). Consider, for example, how "on the spot" a 4-year-old child feels when asked to play "telephone" with a group of people. In this parlor game, participants sit in a circle, and one person starts by whispering a complex message to the person next to him or her. The last person to receive the message has to say aloud what they heard. The fun comes from the fact that the whispered message gets hilariously distorted in its journey around the circle. The agony comes from the fact a child who stutters has to remember what he heard and say it to the next person and sometimes say it aloud to the whole circle. Even decades later, this experience still haunts me.

A number of studies suggest that the incidence of stuttering is unusually high in individuals who have cognitive impairments, such as those with a developmental disability, especially Down syndrome (Kent & Vorperian, 2013; Van Borsel, Moeyaert, Rosseel, van Loo, & van Renterghem, 2006; Van Riper, 1982). An explanation has been suggested by Starkweather (1987) who noted that developmentally delayed individuals are slower in their overall acquisition of speech and language. Their extended period of acquisition may make them more vulnerable to speech breakdown because competition between language acquisition and motor speech production for limited neurological resources occurs over a relatively long period of time.

Individuals who have had traumatic brain injury, which usually affects cognitive functions such as memory and attention, also have an increased risk for fluency disorders (Jokel, De Nil, & Sharpe, 2007; Stasberg, Johnson, & Perry, 2016; Theys, van Wieringen, & De Nil, 2008). This may be because typically rapid and complex speech and language production depend on fully functioning perception, attention, working memory, and executive functions. When these processes are compromised, breakdowns in spoken language are likely to result. As an example, consider the effect of a faulty working memory on rapid retrieval of vocabulary or syntax. If some components of language are mistimed in relation to others, repetitions of words or syllables may result, just as an engine with an unsteady fuel supply will stop and start, stutteringly.

Yet another link between cognition and stuttering was found in a study by Yairi and colleagues (1996) indicating that poorer cognitive skills are associated with lack of ability to recover from stuttering. Of the study's 32 children who began to stutter, 12 continued to stutter for 36 months and perhaps longer. The two groups of stutterers, those who recovered and those who did not, were compared with a control group of nonstuttering children on an intelligence test—the Arthur Adaptation of the Leiter International Performance Test (Arthur, 1952). The group of children who continued to stutter scored significantly lower than the nonstuttering control group, although their mean score was not below the norm for the test. However, the children in the recovered group performed just like the control group. Thus, some abilities associated with cognition may be related to a neural resilience allowing recovery from stuttering. In other words, children with slightly higher cognitive functioning may have the extra resources needed to reorganize their speech and language processing, allowing them to develop a work-around for the problem causing them to stutter.

The research by Choo et al. (2016) that I cited earlier assessed cognitive functioning in the group of children who stuttered and the group who did not. As with speech, language, and motor measures, the children who stuttered scored below the nonstuttering children on cognitive measures and exhibited dissociations among these areas. They also showed less dense white matter tracts in areas underlying all these skills and abilities.

Cognitive Development and Reactions to Stuttering

In the preceding section, I have suggested that children's cognitive development may influence the onset of stuttering—or momentary increases in stuttering—through competition for resources in the child's brain. Now, I would like to suggest that the role of cognitive development is also important in explaining how and when a child begins to form negative attitudes and beliefs about herself and her speech. Between ages 3 and 4, children's cognitions mature enough so that they internalize the standards of behavior of those around them, including peers (Fagan, 2000). It is only at this point, according to Lewis (2000), that children can evaluate how they are performing in comparison to others and will experience the "self-conscious" emotions of embarrassment, pride, shame, and guilt.

In regard to stuttering, once children who stutter compare their speech with others, they are likely to conclude that they are doing something wrong. Because some of the conclusions that children who stutter draw about their speech may come from other children's reactions to their speech, a study by Ezrati-Vanacour, Platzky, and Yairi (2001) is of importance. These researchers looked at awareness of stuttering in typically developing children and found that some children were aware of stuttering in puppets at age 3, but most were not aware until age 5. Notably, most children at age 4 showed a preference for fluent speech, suggesting a negative evaluation of disfluent speech. Thus, peers of children who stutter may respond negatively to the speech of stuttering children at this age.

A study by Boey et al. (2009) found that children as young as 2 years old appear to have some awareness of their own stuttering, although it is not clear that they are comparing their speech to other children. The signs of awareness of the youngest of these children were more in terms of being frustrated or angry, and it was not until they were older that they were showing some sadness about their speech, which may reflect comparison with other children.

The authors of a meta-analysis of 18 studies on the attitudes of children who stutter (Guttormsen, Kefalianos, & Naess, 2015) concluded that negative communication attitudes increase with age, in both preschoolers and in school-age children. It was suggested that this increase in negative attitudes may arise from more negative experiences with speech, including bullying, as children get older. This meta-analysis is a rich source of information for readers who want to delve deeper into communication attitudes, as well as emotional and behavioral reactions to stuttering.

Emotions such as embarrassment and shame that arise from the increasing cognitive maturity of children who stutter and their peers may play an important role in the discomfort children feel when they stutter, and thus, it may affect the persistence of the stuttering. The emotions that some children feel about their stuttering may be an important factor that gives rise to increases in tension, escape, and avoidance responses that may make stuttering a self-sustaining disorder and increasingly difficult to overcome. In my experience, most children who recover completely from stuttering with or without treatment are younger than 5, perhaps a significant age, given the evidence cited above about self- and peer awareness of stuttering. Emotional, as well as social, factors will be considered in the next section.

Summary of the Effect of Cognitive Development on Fluency

The stresses of going through each new stage of cognitive development may deplete the extra neural resources some children need to compensate for a vulnerable speech motor system. Stuttering may appear or worsen during this stress. Children who have cognitive limitations (or even slightly less than typical cognitive abilities in some areas) may be more stressed during cognitive development as they try to compensate for these limitations. This also may precipitate or worsen stuttering. As children who stutter advance in cognitive development, they become more likely to be aware of their stuttering and may develop negative attitudes toward communication as a result.

Social and Emotional Development

In this section, I discuss how children's development in the preschool years may involve social challenges and emotional stresses that may trigger or worsen stuttering. It may be helpful to start with evidence and speculation about exactly how these kinds of stresses affect fluency.

Interference of Speech by Emotion

At some time in your life, you have probably experienced the effects of strong emotion on your speech. If you've been nervous when talking in front of an audience, your voice may have quavered or you may have been talking faster than you meant to but couldn't help it. When you get really worked up, like when you have to make a phone call in an emergency, rapid breathing and tension in your larynx can make it difficult to talk. The same sort of interference by emotion may be even more prevalent in early childhood, because a child's speech neural networks are immature, are not fully myelinated, and may not be buffered from "cross talk," or interference by the limbic (emotional) system structures and pathways involved in the regulation and expression of emotion (e.g., Dolcos & MacCarthy, 2006). Such interference may be even more likely among many children predisposed to stutter. Their slower maturing speech production system may not be optimally localized or adequately insulated from interference and may be closer to centers of emotion in the right hemisphere, a hypothesis I discussed in Chapter 3. Thus, when such children are emotionally aroused, fluency may suffer because neural signals for properly timed and sequenced muscle contractions may be interrupted in some way. I see evidence of this when I ask parents when their child first began to stutter. They frequently tell me that they noticed stuttering for the first time when their child was highly excited about something.

Excitement is commonly mentioned in the literature as a stimulus that elicits disfluency. Starkweather (1987) noted "all children speak more disfluently during periods of excitement." Dorothy Davis (1940), who conducted one of the first studies of normal disfluency, reported that of the 10 situations in which children showed repetitions in their speech, "excitement over own activity" was when they most frequently repeated sounds and words. In a later study, Johnson and associates (1959) asked parents of children identified as stuttering to describe the situation in which they first observed their child's stuttering. They most often reported that the first appearance of stuttering occurred when the child was in a hurry to tell something or was in an excited state. Thus, both stuttering and normal disfluency seem to occur most often or noticeably during states of transitory emotional arousal.

Further evidence of the relationship between heightened emotion and stuttering comes from a study by Ntourou et al. (2013) that examined emotional reactivity and emotional regulation in children who stutter. Among other things, they found that children who stuttered showed more negative emotion in an experimental task designed to disappoint them than children who didn't. There was also a tendency for children who stutter to show more stuttering while speaking when they were trying to regulate their negative emotions. In discussing their results, the authors concluded that "...present findings support the notion that emotional processes are associated with childhood stuttering and may possibly contribute to the difficulties that at least some CWS have establishing normally fluent speech" (p. 271). As to how emotions exert that influence, they suggest that "...children's emotional arousal may divert limited attentional resources from an already, for some CWS, vulnerable speech-language planning and production system (e.g., Ntourou, Conture, & Lipsey, 2011) and in turn contribute to disruptions in their speech fluency" (p. 270).

Having explored the connection between emotions and the occurrence of stuttering, let us now turn to children's progress through stages of social-emotional development and their influences on fluency.

Stages of Social and Emotional Development

As children grow, they pass through several stages of social and emotional development, some of which may provoke more stress than others. Rothbart (2011) describes the development of many personality features during childhood that result from the interaction between the child's inborn attributes such as temperament and the child's environment, including parents and peers. For example, the attachment between an infant and her mother can be a critical foundation for the growing child's sense of security and her ability to learn to cope with stress and to regulate her own emotions. If the child experiences a mother who is able to meet her needs, to sooth her when she is distressed, she develops better coping skills and her ability to attach to others. If attachment to the mother is not secure, stresses will have a greater negative effect on the child. All this, of course, is greatly affected by the child's biological inheritance, including temperament. These interactions are described in detail by Rothbart (2011).

Emotional Security

As a young child grows older, other members of the family besides the mother play a role in social and emotional changes. Although a child's father and siblings comprise a wider support system, a child's resentment at having to share his mother's attention may elicit feelings of anger, aggression, and guilt. It seems possible that if such feelings are punished or ignored, transient disfluency or more severe stuttering may result in some children.

One of the more common provocations for feeling resentment is the birth of a sibling. I discuss the effect of a sibling's birth on fluency later in the section on environmental factors, but it warrants mentioning here too because a child's strong emotions may often reflect his developmental level as well as the environmental event that triggered the emotions. Theodore Lidz (1968, p. 246), a developmental psychiatrist with interests in speech and language, provided this example:

Psychoanalytically oriented play therapy with children also indicates that many of their forbidden wishes and ideas have relatively simple access to consciousness. A 6-year-old boy who started to stammer severely after a baby sister was born was watched playing with a family of dolls. He placed a baby doll in a crib next to the parent dolls' bed and then had a boy doll come and throw the baby to the floor, beat it, and throw it into a corner. He then put the boy doll into the crib. In a subsequent session, he had the father doll pummel the mother doll's abdomen, saying, "No, no!" At this point of childhood, even though certain unacceptable ideas cannot be talked about, they are still not definitely repressed.

Many threats to feelings of security can create emotional stress that may disrupt the speech of children who are predisposed to stutter. As we will see in the section on treatment, we have found that therapy strategies that increase a child's sense of security and help him learn to speak more fluently will suffice for many children who begin stuttering under these emotional stresses.

Development of Self-Consciousness and Sensitivity

As we noted earlier in the section on cognitive development, the emergence of self-consciousness, which begins during the child's second year and gradually increases, may be another source of social and emotional stress. This reflects the child's growing awareness of how he is performing relative to adult expectations. Although this process is not thoroughly understood, Jerome Kagan presents an interesting description of it in his book, *The Second Year* (1981). In a relevant example, Kagan proposes that the self-corrections a child makes in his speech are evidence of this self-awareness. Taking this further, we can surmise that increasing self-awareness in a child who is excessively disfluent might lead to self-corrections and stoppages that only worsen the problem.

In Chapter 3, in a section on temperament, we discussed the hypothesis that people who stutter, as a group, may have unusually sensitive temperaments. Research on temperament in nonstuttering children, especially the longitudinal studies of Calkins and Fox (1994) and Kagan and Snidman (1991), indicates that the social-emotional traits of fearfulness and withdrawal that accompany more sensitive temperaments can change over the course of a child's preschool years. Some children become better able to regulate their temperamental tendencies, but others remain hostage to their temperaments. Such individual adaptations may be crucial in determining which children who begin to stutter will continue to do so and which will stop.

Reports on sensitive temperament have included the positive as well as negative aspects of this personality type. In an overview article, Ellis and Boyce (2008) suggest that a reactive temperament in a child may produce very different outcomes, depending on whether a child encounters a stressful environment or a nurturing one. For example, Boyce et al. (1995) found that, compared to relatively unreactive children, sensitive children in stressful environments had more respiratory illnesses than typical children, whereas sensitive children in nurturing environments had fewer. In other words, a sensitive temperament can give a child protection against illness if the environment is favorable. What are the implications for stuttering? We will revisit this in Chapter 6, "Theories About Stuttering," but it is pretty clear that a nurturing environment would help a sensitive child predisposed to stuttering be less reactive to his disfluencies.

I previously cited several studies that support the hypothesis that many children who stutter are born with a sensitive temperament. However, a strong case has been made for the opposite view—that children who stutter, as a group, do not have an inherently sensitive temperament, but that developmental and environmental factors have given rise to the anxiety and sensitivity often seen in children who stutter. Smith, Iverach, O'Brian, Kefalianos, and Reilly (2014) reviewed many studies related to anxiety and sensitive temperament in stuttering and concluded that there is no clear evidence for an inherited anxiety or hypersensitivity. They suggest that repeated negative social consequences of stuttering, in later childhood and adolescence (and beyond), give rise to increased anxiety in many people who stutter. Others disagree (e.g., researchers at Vanderbilt University, including Jones et al., 2014; Ntourou et al., 2013; Walden et al., 2012). A strong and data-based answer to this question has been made by Eggers (2012). He found that children who stutter have higher "negative reactivity" and lower "self-regulation" than children who do not stutter. My impression of his findings and those of the researchers at Vanderbilt is that they strongly suggest that these temperamental differences are inherent, rather than a consequence of stuttering.

Summary of the Effect of Social and Emotional Development on Fluency

Many of the normal social and emotional stresses that children experience as they grow up may result in disfluent speech, although the evidence is mostly anecdotal.

Children who are neurophysiologically predisposed to stutter may be especially prone to disfluency when social conflicts and emotions create extra "noise" in their neural circuitry for speech. This would be particularly true for those children who are both predisposed to stuttering and who have emotionally reactive temperaments. This combination of constitutional traits could be associated with the onset and development of stuttering. They may also be related to the persistence of stuttering in some children.

Some researchers believe that emotional reactivity and anxiety are not one of the causes of stuttering but the result of social encounters in which negative listener reactions create the anxiety and sensitivity. Others think that emotional reactivity or sensitivity is innate.

Important findings, key speculations, and clinical implications about developmental factors are summarized in Table 4.1.

TABLE 4.1 Developmental Factors in Stuttering

Area of Interest	Important Findings and Key Speculations	Clinical Implications
Development in General	Competition for neural resources may diminish resources available for speech-motor control	When a child is going through a period of intense developmental growth in any domain, stuttering may increase.
Physical and Speech Motor Skill Development	Physical growth can compete with neural resources for speech. Developmental changes in the speech motor system require neural resources to continually update sensorimotor "maps" for fluent speech. Evidence that children who stutter—especially those who persist—have less mature speech motor control than typical children. Some studies suggest that uneven development of speech motor abilities in children who stutter may be as detrimental to fluency as delayed development.	Possibility that adult modeling of slower speech rate could promote fluency. Predicting which children will persist in stuttering rather than recover may be possible using measures of speech motor control.
Speech and Language Development	Evidence that as children learn to use longer and more complex sentences, both typical disfluencies and stuttering increase. Conflicting studies about whether children who stutter are more delayed than those who don't. However, several studies found that children with persistent stuttering are more delayed (than typical or those who recover) in language when tested when they first begin to stutter. Even this research, however, found that children who stutter have language within the normal range. Some researchers have found among stuttering children "dissociation" or uneven development of subcomponents of language, even though overall language scores of children who stutter are not different from those of typical children. As with uneven development of motor abilities (see above), these disparities in development of language subcomponents may drain neural resources as stuttering children try to cope with them.	Adult models of shorter and less complex sentences may promote fluency in children beginning to stutter.
Cognitive Development	In the preschool years, children pass through several stages of cognitive development. At each new stage, neural resources may be taxed, stressing the fragile speech motor system of children at risk for stuttering. This competition for resources may precipitate or worsen stuttering. Individuals with cognitive limitations—such as those with Down's syndrome—appear to be at greater risk for stuttering (or excess disfluencies) because of competition for neural resources during development (and thereafter). Some evidence shows that children who stutter have slightly lower scores on cognitive assessments. There is also evidence that children who persist in stuttering may have slightly lower (but in normal range) scores on cognitive assessments. Although a few younger children who stutter may be unaware of their stuttering, most children do develop awareness and negative attitudes toward their stuttering. These negative attitudes increase with age—perhaps because of more negative experiences—and may contribute to the persistence of stuttering.	Information about fluctuations of stuttering with cognitive development may help parents understand why stuttering can be better at some times and more severe at others. They may be reassured they aren't causing the changes. Parents with children who have cognitive limitations may find this information helpful to understand their child's speech. Evidence of slightly lower than average cognitive scores may predict persistence and warrant immediate treatment. Treatment of stuttering should take into consideration negative communication attitudes in children who stutter. Children with little awareness of their stuttering may benefit from indirect treatment. Children who are negatively aware of their stuttering may need treatment components that change attitudes as well as behaviors.

TABLE 4.1 Developmental Factors in Stuttering (*Continued*)

Area of Interest	Important Findings and Key Speculations	Clinical Implications
Social and Emotional Development	Increases in emotion tend to be associated with increases in stuttering. As children grow, they pass through various stages of social and emotional development, some of which may be stressful and precipitate more stuttering. Threats to a child's sense of security, for example, may increase stuttering. The development of self-consciousness, especially in sensitive children, may cause them to feel more negatively about their stuttering.	Heightened emotion—whether positive or negative—may temporarily increase stuttering. This may explain otherwise puzzling changes in stuttering. Increasing a child's sense of security may help increase fluency. Children who are negatively aware of their stuttering may be helped by treatment procedures that decrease this negative emotion, such as playing with stuttering.

ENVIRONMENTAL FACTORS

Environmental factors that influence the onset and progression of stuttering are stresses and pressures in the child's home, playground, and daycare or school. One example is a conversational style in the child's home that is characterized by lots of interruptions and rapid, complex speech that is beyond the child's level. As you can imagine, there are many things in a child's environment—some subtle and some not so subtle—that can add enough stress to a child with a predisposition to stutter to trigger the onset and promote the growth of stuttering. Environmental stresses interact with genetic factors as well as developmental pressures to have their effect on the child. Table 4.2 summarizes environmental factors that may influence children's stuttering.

I begin the discussion of environmental factors by reviewing research on the most important factor in family environments—the parents.

Parents

In the 1930s and 1940s at the University of Iowa, Wendell Johnson developed the "diagnosogenic" theory of stuttering (Johnson et al., 1942). This theory proposed that a child's parents were the cause of stuttering because they misdiagnosed normal disfluencies as stuttering. Parents' reactions to the "stuttering" then caused the child to try to avoid these normal disfluencies and, in avoiding them, the child hesitated and struggled in a way that eventually became real stuttering. Johnson's diagnosogenic theory generated a great deal of research on parents of stutterers. Were they different from the parents of nonstutterers? Were they unusually critical? Did they have unreasonably high standards of speech?

Studies by Johnson and his colleagues trying to answer these questions suggested that parents of children who stuttered appeared to be more critical and perfectionistic and had higher standards of behavior than parents of children who did not. These findings, as well as details about the types of disfluencies reported by parents, were collected and published in a book titled *The Onset of Stuttering: Research Findings and Implications* (Johnson & Associates, 1959). Johnson interpreted these data as showing a great deal of similarity between the disfluencies of stuttering and nonstuttering children. He suggested that the same disfluency types that parents of nonstuttering children considered normal were reported by parents of stuttering children as the earliest signs of stuttering. Johnson used this as evidence to support the diagnosogenic hypothesis that the problem was parents' interpretation of their child's disfluencies, or as some often put it, "the problem was not in the child's mouth but in the parent's ear."

Later researchers disagreed. McDearmon (1968), for example, argued that Johnson's findings actually showed that the disfluencies of normal children were notably different from those in the stuttering children. Syllable repetitions, sound prolongations, and complete blocks were reported to have occurred much more frequently in the stuttering children, whereas phrase repetitions, pauses, and interjections were reported more frequently in the nonstuttering control group. This reinterpretation of Johnson's data and new findings about genetic and constitutional factors in stuttering have caused the diagnosogenic view of stuttering to be largely abandoned.

More recent studies of parents of children who stutter and parents of typically speaking children focused on parent characteristics rather than disfluency types. In a summary of these studies, Yairi (1997b) found mixed results. Some indicated that parents of stutterers were more anxious or more rejecting, while others found no differences. On balance, Yairi suggests, it seems likely that some children who stutter grew up with parents who were a little more demanding or anxious than average, and this may have made a difference. Assuming they already had a constitutional predisposition to

TABLE 4.2 Environmental Factors in Stuttering

Area of Interest	Important Findings and Key Speculations	Clinical Implications
Parents	Theory that parents caused stuttering by misdiagnosing normal disfluencies has been disproven. Some evidence shows that parents of children who stutter may be a little more anxious and demanding than parents of typical children, but other research refutes this idea. Parents may be more hypervigilant about disfluencies if they have family members who stutter, but there are no data confirming this.	Families should be reassured that there is no evidence that parents or families cause stuttering. In a diagnostic evaluation, parent-child interactions should be evaluated to assess whether there may be demands on the child that could be reduced to see if this improves fluency. Parents will benefit from learning what aspects of their child's speech is typical disfluency, compared to actual stutters.
Speech and Language Environment	There is evidence that some parents of children who stutter speak to their children with a higher speech rate, interrupt more, ask more questions, and use more complex language, compared to parents of typical parents. But because there are conflicting data, it is probably best to assume that parents of children who stutter may be using speech and language at nearly normal levels but their children would benefit from less conversational pressure.	For younger children, treatment may focus on helping parents and families use slower speech rates, allow their children plenty of time to talk without interruptions, ask fewer questions (but use comments instead), and use language at the child's level.
Life Events	Stuttering may first appear or worsen after stressful life events, such as emotional trauma. This cause of stuttering may be more likely in cases where there is no family history of stuttering.	If onset or worsening of stuttering is associated with an emotional life event, child should receive psychological counseling as well as stuttering therapy. When the clinician is qualified, these may be carried out by the same individual.

stutter, these children's early speech may have been peppered with disfluencies, which would have alarmed their parents. The children then, picking up on their parents' dismay, may have become self-conscious about their minor disfluencies and thus have unwittingly added tension and struggle, which blossomed into more noticeable stuttering. However, the strong conclusion is that parents do not cause their children to stutter, although they may have passed along genes that increased the risk for stuttering.

It is interesting to speculate that in some cases, a child's hypersensitivity to parents' concern and the child's increased tension as a response to his disfluencies are a component of an overall vulnerable temperament found in some children who stutter (Anderson, Pellowski, Conture, & Kelly, 2003; Choi, Conture, Walden, Jones, & Kim, 2016; Eggers, 2012; Karrass et al., 2006; Oyler & Ramig, 1995; Walden et al., 2012), which may be inherited. The parents, the genetic source of these temperaments, may be the anxious, overprotective mothers or fathers that have been described in the literature on parents of stutterers. Such children are, therefore, in double jeopardy for persistent stuttering because of the children's own temperaments and because one or both parents, having a sensitive temperament themselves, may be overly concerned about their children's stuttering. On the other hand, some parents may have a beneficial and calming effect on their child's vulnerable temperament, making it possible for a child who begins to stutter and who is emotionally reactive to recover from stuttering. In a discussion of environmental influences on biological predispositions of children who do not stutter, Calkins and Fox (1994, p. 209) said that "the child's interactions with a parent provide the context for learning skills and strategies for managing emotional reactivity."

Once again, we see that influences on stuttering are numerous and complex, coming from both the child and the environment. Some of these influences may precipitate stuttering, others may interact to make remission difficult, and still others may provide the kinds of support that make remission possible.

Summary of the Effect of Parents on Fluency

The "diagnosogenic" theory of stuttering onset—that parents cause stuttering because they misdiagnose normal disfluencies as stuttering—has been largely refuted.

Some research suggests that parents of children who stutter may be a little more demanding or perfectionistic than parents of typical children. The results, however, are mixed and some studies find no differences between these two groups of parents.

It is possible that any stress that comes from parents may be the result of the fact that stuttering is often inherited and parents may have relatives who stutter, making them hypervigilant about stuttering in their children. Or, these parents may have a hypersensitive temperament (which they may have passed on to their children), making them (and their children) more anxious and reactive to an excess of disfluencies.

Speech and Language Environment

Because every preschool-age child is tuned into the speech and language around him, especially that of his parents, the communication style surrounding him may be an important influence on the child who stutters. Van Riper (1973) expressed the situation this way: "Stuttering usually begins at the very time that great advances in sentence construction occur, and it seems tenable that, when the speech models provided by the parents or siblings of the child are too difficult for him to follow, some faltering will ensue" (p. 381).

Many other clinical researchers have also speculated that **speech and language environments** are a potential source of stress for children who stutter (e.g., Gottwald, 2010; Richels & Conture, 2007; Shapiro, 1999; Starkweather, Gottwald, & Halfond, 1990; Zebrowski & Kelly, 2002). Several of them have also developed treatment programs based on this potential stress. Table 4.3 lists a variety of sources of possible stress from the speech and language environment.

In addition to treatments, theoretical models have emerged to explain how the speech and language environment influences children's stuttering. Crystal (1987) proposed an "interactive" view of many speech and language disorders, which suggested that demands at one level of language production (e.g., syntax) may deplete resources for other levels (e.g., prosody or phonology) and result in breakdown. His supporting data nicely illustrate how stuttering may be exacerbated by a child's use of advanced language. He presented evidence that the more complex the syntax and semantics that a child used, the more he stuttered. Starkweather (1987), describing a demands-and-capacities view of stuttering, commented "the production of speech and the formulation of language place a simultaneous demand on the young person. If the demands in either of these two dimensions are excessive, performance in the other dimension may be reduced." These two views imply that stuttering may increase when an individual uses longer words, less frequently occurring words, more information-bearing words, and longer sentences. Stuttering may also increase when the individual is uttering a more linguistically complex sentence. By implication, the child's speech and language environment—usually conversation by adults talking to the child—may be responsible for influencing a child to use more advanced language.

What do we know about the speech and language of parents of children who stutter and its influence on stuttering? Research has concentrated on four major characteristics of parent speech: (1) rate of speech, (2) interruptions of children's speaking, (3) frequency of questions that parents ask children, and (4) the linguistic complexity of parent speech. I'll summarize the research in each area.

TABLE 4.3 Possible Speech and Language Stressors

Stressful Adult Speech Models	
Rapid speech rate	Complex syntax
Polysyllabic vocabulary	Use of two languages in home
Stressful Speaking Situations for Children	
Competition for speaking	Hurried when speaking
Frequent interruptions	Frequent questions
Demand for display speech	Excited when speaking
Loss of listener attention	Many things to say

Rate of Speech

Susan Meyers and Frances Freeman (1985a, 1985b) compared the speech of mothers of stuttering children with that of mothers of nonstutterers. They found that mothers of children who stuttered spoke more rapidly than did the mothers of nonstutterers. This may be critical, since a mother's high speech rate may encourage a child to try to speak faster than his optimal speed (e.g., Jaffe & Anderson, 1979). The possibility that rapid speech rates may lead to stuttering is consistent with Johnson and Rosen's (1937) finding that adults who stutter were more likely to stutter when they spoke more rapidly than their habitual rates. Children who stutter may be even more vulnerable to fluency breakdowns during rapid speech than adults who stutter by virtue of the fact that children's natural rates of speech are slower and their temporal coordination less than those of adults (e.g., Kent, 1981).

However, Kelly and Conture (1992) found no differences in the speaking rates of mothers of these two groups of children. In a subsequent study, Kelly (1994) found no differences in the rates of fathers of the two groups. Using another method to compare rates, Yaruss and Conture (1995) found no differences in the articulatory rates (the rate at which each individual phrase is spoken, in contrast to "speaking rate," which includes pauses between phrases) between mothers of stuttering children and mothers of nonstuttering children.

However, the latter researchers did find a significant correlation between children's severity of stuttering and parent-child differences in speaking rate; greater differences in parent-child speech rates were associated with more severe stuttering in the children. These results could have been obtained if more severely stuttering children talk more slowly than other children and their parents have speech rates similar to other parents in the study. It is also possible that greater parent-child differences in rate make a child who already stutters more severe.

A study by Dehqan, Bakhtiar, Panahi, and Ashayeri (2008) found results that appear to confirm the findings of Yaruss and Conture (1995). They assessed mothers' speaking rates, their children's rates, and the severity of their children's stuttering and found that faster rates by mothers were associated with more severe stuttering in their child. As expected, the more severe the child's stuttering, the slower was his speaking rate. This study suggests many follow-up questions: (1) Did these mothers' speech rates increase from the time of their child's stuttering onset to when it was measured? (2) If the mothers were taught to slow their speech rates, would the frequency of their children's stuttering decrease? (3) If the parents were taught to use a response-contingent intervention such as Lidcombe Program, would the mothers' speech rates decrease as their children's stuttering severity decreased?

Interruptions

Another suspected stress, in addition to rapid speech rates, is the frequency with which parents (or other listeners) interrupt their children. One of Meyers and Freeman's reports (1985a) presented some unexpected evidence about interruptions. The mothers of both stuttering and nonstuttering children interrupted most frequently when a child was disfluent. It seems possible that such parental interruptions, some of which may have been elicited by the child's disfluencies, may in turn elicit changes in the child's speech. Some children might increase tension and rate, thereby developing the struggled behaviors of stuttering. Others might suppress disfluencies to avoid interruptions and eventually be "taught" by parents not to be disfluent.

In a later study, Kelly and Conture (1992) found no significant differences in the interruptions of mothers of stuttering children and those of mothers of nonstuttering children. However, a closer inspection of their data revealed a correlation between the duration of "simultalk" (one person talking at the same time another is talking) of the mothers of children who stutter and the severity of their stuttering. Thus, mothers of more severe stutterers did more simultalk when their children were talking than did mothers whose children stuttered less severely. In a later study of fathers, Kelly (1994) found no differences in the interruptions of fathers of children who stutter and those of fathers whose children don't stutter. Moreover, the correlation between these fathers' simultalk and severity of stuttering was not significant.

In an unusual study, Livingston, Flowers, Hodor, and Ryan (2000) deliberately interrupted the speech of several children who stuttered (ages 5–6) and found that stuttering did not increase very much. They were reluctant to emphasize reducing parental interruptions of children who stutter, especially for this age group.

Asking Questions

Another variable of children's speech and language environments that has been studied is the extent to which parents ask questions. Meyers and Freeman (1985a) found no significant difference in the number of questions asked by mothers of children who stutter compared to mothers of children who do not. Langlois, Hanrahan, and Inouye (1986), however, did find significant differences when making a similar comparison. Langlois and Long (1988) then conducted an experimental treatment of a 4-year-old who stuttered, in which the mother was taught to reduce the number of questions she asked, among other changes. After 16 treatment sessions in which the mother had markedly reduced her number of questions and given her child more speaking turns, the child no longer stuttered. This finding is especially interesting because it is tempting to assume that asking questions results in more stuttering. However, subsequent studies tested this assumption and failed to support it. In a study of eight stuttering children in conversations with their parents, Weiss and Zebrowski (1992) found that the children stuttered less when they answered questions than when they made assertions. This appeared to be related to the fact that questions were often answered with brief responses, but assertions by children were often longer utterances. A more direct test of the effect of parents asking questions was carried out by Wilkenfeld and Curlee (1997), who used a single-subject ABAB design to vary an adult's verbal behavior (questions vs. comments) in conversations with a child who stuttered. Their results with three children who stuttered demonstrated that stuttering did not appear to be related to whether the adult asked questions or commented but was more likely to occur in either condition when the child's utterances were longer.

Complexity of Language

Most studies of parents' speech have focused on comparing parents of children who stutter with parents of children who do not. Kloth et al. (1999) took a different approach, with a longitudinal study of speech and language of parents whose children were at risk for stuttering. They assessed the complexity of the mothers' language, measured in terms of mean length of utterances in words in conversations with their child, both before and immediately after the onset of stuttering. They found that the language of the mothers of children who persisted in stuttering was significantly more complex than that of the mothers of children who recovered, when measured both before their children began to stutter and again after stuttering began. In a later study of persistent and recovered stutterers, Rommel, Hage, Kalehne, and Johannsen (2000) assessed the complexity of the language of 71 mothers soon after their children had begun to stutter, rather than before stuttering began. They followed these children for 3 years and found that one of the more powerful predictors of whether or not a child would recover was "the linguistic demands to which the child is exposed" (p. 181). More specifically, these researchers found that the more complex the mother's syntax (mean length of utterance or MLU) and the greater number of different words she used in talking to her child, the more likely that her child would not recover over the following 3 years. The language abilities of the children themselves had no predictive value (Rommel et al., 2000).

Using a more traditional approach rather than looking at persistence and recovery, Miles and Ratner (2001) assessed the complexity of the language of parents of children who stuttered, gathering samples of conversations from 12 mother-child pairs involving stuttering children and 12 involving fluent children. All children were between 27 and 48 months of age, and the stuttering children were within 3 months of the onset of their stuttering. Mothers' utterances were assessed for syntactic complexity, lexical diversity and rarity, and mean number of utterances per turn. No significant differences between the mothers of the stuttering children and the mothers of the fluent children were found. These studies suggest that parents of children who stutter may not use more complex language than parents of typically speaking children, but for at-risk or stuttering children, less complex language is associated with better likelihood of recovery.

Summary of the Effects of Speech and Language Environment on Fluency

Speech models by parents, siblings, and others may precipitate or worsen stuttering if they are too far above the child's level. This may occur because of the demand on already stressed neural resources.

Although the evidence is equivocal, four characteristics of parents' (or other speakers') speech and language have been shown to be associated with children's stuttering: speech rate, interruptions, frequency and type of questions, and language complexity.

Life Events

Certain **life events** can deliver a blow to a child's stability and security. When this happens, stuttering may suddenly appear out of nowhere, or previously easy repetitions may be transformed into hard, struggled blocks. To move to a new home, to be hospitalized for an operation, or to have parents divorce is difficult for any of us, but it is especially difficult for children. Although there are not many published studies supporting this idea, Van Riper (1982) discusses reports of emotional stress triggering the onset of stuttering but is cautious about accepting all the clinical anecdotes in the literature. In my own case, a move from Connecticut to South Carolina was associated with a worsening of my stuttering,[1] and the move back to Connecticut a few years later was associated with it becoming noticeably worse. In an odd coincidence, as I was writing this section, I got an e-mail from an SLP asking advice about a child who had experienced just such a life event. This child was from a family of migrant workers and had begun to stutter after he and his family became homeless for several months. I am hoping that after some help with the emotional trauma, accompanied by therapy for his stuttering, he will improve his fluency and become a happy, mostly fluent boy again. As you might imagine, many children go through stressful experiences and adapt to them without apparent major problems. But children who are more sensitive often show the effects of such events in their speech. Kagan (1994a) noted that some children who begin life with relaxed temperaments might even become shy and fearful under the onslaught of stressful events. This may well set the stage for stuttering if other constitutional factors predispose the child for it. You may wonder what the mechanism is by which stress can precipitate or worsen stuttering. I don't know the answer, but it seems likely that if a child's brain pathways for speech and language are compromised, extra resources are needed to maintain fluency. When stress increases negative emotions such as anxiety, it seems possible that the negative emotions would consume the extra resources. However, it still leaves us with an incomplete picture. How exactly do extra resources compensate for deficits? How does anxiety consume extra resources?

There is little research on the relationship between stressful life events and stuttering, but many authors have observed the connection. Starkweather (1987), for example, wrote, "All children speak more disfluently during periods of tension—when moving or changing schools, when their parents divorce, or after the death of a family member" (pp. 146–147). These increases in disfluency could easily result in the onset of stuttering or in increased stuttering in children who are vulnerable to such stresses. Johnson and associates (1959) noted that the following events were among the 16 situations in which parents first noticed their child's stuttering: (1) child's physical environment changed (e.g., moving to a new house); (2) child became ill; (3) child realized his mother was pregnant; and (4) a new baby arrived. In discussing the onset of stuttering, Van Riper (1982) acknowledged that various studies have found no differences in the amount of emotional conflict in the homes of children who developed stuttering versus those who didn't. However, he went on to note, "Nevertheless, we have studied individual cases in which

[1]Before my family moved to South Carolina, I had few recollections of stuttering, but on the day of our arrival, our new neighbors asked me my brother's name. I got so jammed up on "Lenny" that in despair I just told them "I don't know." Ever after, I have had trouble with the sound /l/.

stuttering did seem [to be] triggered by such conflicts, and it is difficult for us to ignore these experiences" (p. 79).

My own clinical experience is similar. In the past several years, for example, during which I've evaluated dozens of children who stutter, I've encountered four children in four different families who began to stutter when their parents were in the early stages of divorce. However, this turmoil was not the only factor in their stuttering. Three of the children had relatives who stuttered, and the father of the fourth child stuttered himself. Moreover, all four were preschoolers and were probably experiencing various growth and development pressures. But for all of them, their parents' divorce appeared to be a factor that pushed them from normal speech to stuttering.

In another case of a life event precipitating stuttering, I evaluated a 9-year-old girl who began to stutter when her classroom teacher had an emotional breakdown that was apparent in the classroom. The teacher's outbursts of anger and crying, interspersed with high demands for rapid performance on frequent examinations, were apparently extremely stressful for this student. Under this stress, she developed tight blocks, with physical tension at the level of the larynx and abdomen. Even though I was convinced through extensive interviews with the family that the child had no prior stuttering, I noted several predisposing factors for stuttering. First, her younger sister had significant learning disabilities, including auditory processing problems. Second, her mother described herself and her daughter who stuttered as shy and emotionally reactive. These two factors—a family history of learning disability and a vulnerable temperament—may have provided a fertile matrix for the sudden germination of stuttering when a stressful life event occurred. Happily, after a year of treatment, this child became fluent. This child, now a young woman, discusses this stressful time with her mother in Video 4-2 "Onset of Stuttering Related to a Stressful Life Event" on *thePoint*.

In a few cases, traumatic life events appear to precipitate stuttering in children who appear to have no genetic predisposition to stuttering. As cited in Chapter 2 on constitutional factors, Poulos and Webster (1991) examined 57 clients with no family history of stuttering and found that 37 percent reported childhood events or illnesses that were associated with stuttering onset. For example, three individuals reported experiencing intense fear associated with the onset of stuttering. These fears arose from being attacked by an animal, being bombed during a war, or being alone in a thunderstorm. When this sort of life event triggers stuttering, a predisposition for stuttering may or may not have existed prior to the event, rather than a genetic inheritance specifically of stuttering. Other neurologically predisposing conditions such as ADHD (Alm & Risberg, 2007) or sensitive temperament (Karass et al., 2006) may have existed in these children. Other life events, such as head injury or diseases of the nervous system, may precipitate stuttering without a predisposing condition because the event may damage the speech motor control system.

TABLE 4.4 Stressful Life Events That May Increase a Child's Disfluency

The child's family moves to a new house, a new neighborhood, or a new city.
The child's parents separate or divorce.
A family member dies.
A family member is hospitalized.
The child is hospitalized.
A parent loses his or her job.
A baby is born, or a child is adopted.
An additional person comes to live in the house.
One or both parents go away frequently or for a long period of time.
Holidays or visits occur, which cause a change in routine, excitement, or anxiety.
There is a discipline problem involving the child.

Table 4.4 lists some of the life events that I have found to be stressful to children's fluency.

Summary of the Effects of Life Events on Fluency

Many clinicians have suggested that stressful life events may precipitate stuttering or increase its severity. Some research suggests that among individuals who stutter without family history of stuttering, there is more evidence of emotional trauma, sickness, or injury associated with the onset of stuttering than in those with family history of stuttering. This suggests that in some cases, stressful life events, rather than a genetic inheritance of stuttering, can cause stuttering.

In the preceding section, I described the environmental factors that can interact with developmental factors and with a child's constitutional predisposition to produce and worsen stuttering. Fortunately, some of these environmental factors can be modified or compensated for to improve fluency.

SUMMARY

- Physical and motor development uses a great deal of neuronal resources in the brain, perhaps leaving fewer resources available for speech fluency. This may be potentially crucial in children with compromised or delayed neural systems for speech production.
- Children's learning of phonology, morphology, syntax, and semantics may strain resources for the establishment of fluent speech. In addition, *differences in the rate of development* of different components of speech and language may result in more disfluency.

- The demands of cognitive development (memory, attention, executive function) may stress the development of fluency, resulting in the onset or increase in stuttering.
- Normal social and emotional conflicts in children predisposed to stutter may trigger onset or worsening of stuttering.
- Communication stress in the home (rapid speech rates, interruptions, constant questions, and overly complex language) may precipitate or worsen stuttering.
- Traumatic or stressful life events may trigger or worsen stuttering in children who have a family history of stuttering and/or have a vulnerable temperament.

STUDY QUESTIONS

1. The effect of a child's development on fluency has been likened to the effect of multiple tasks for a computer. Explain this analogy.
2. It has been said that children usually do not learn to walk and talk at the same time. What does this suggest about how motor development might affect fluency?
3. There is a high incidence of stuttering among individuals with cognitive impairment. What might this suggest about the relationship between cognition and fluency?
4. What aspects of social and emotional development might threaten fluency?
5. What evidence is there that emotional arousal might increase disfluency?
6. What is the possible connection between atypical hemispheric localization and the effects of emotion on fluency?
7. Why would children's speech and language development be likely to put greater pressure on fluency than would their physical or cognitive development?
8. What aspects of parents' behavior might put pressure on a child who is disfluent?
9. Identify several characteristics of parents' speech that may create difficult models for a disfluent child to emulate.
10. Name several life events that have been suggested to increase a child's disfluency.
11. The communicative failure and anticipatory struggle view proposes that experiencing a communication failure may cause a child to anticipate difficulty speaking and begin to stutter as a result. What characteristic of the child may be another important factor?
12. Johnson and associates' (1959) revised view of stuttering suggested that it results from an interaction among the following three factors: (1) the extent of the child's disfluency, (2) the listener's sensitivity to that disfluency, and (3) the child's sensitivity to his own disfluency and to the listener's reaction. Relate these factors to constitutional, developmental, and environmental factors in stuttering.

SUGGESTED PROJECTS

1. Record a natural speech sample from someone who stutters, and analyze the relationship between the occurrences of stuttering and the linguistic level of the utterances in which they occur.
2. Develop an experimental protocol to assess the relationship between linguistic variables and stuttering. For example, compare the variables of length of utterance, syntactic level of utterance, and phonological complexity of utterance on the likelihood of the utterance being stuttered.
3. Interview several people with typical speech and ask them if they had major life events in their childhood that impacted their lives. Compare these events with the life events mentioned in this chapter that may affect stuttering.
4. Study the effect of your speech rate on other people by designing and carrying out an experiment in which you vary the speed at which you talk. Record conversations in which you talk slowly for several minutes and then talk rapidly for several minutes. Measure the effect on your conversational partner's speed of talking. You will need to practice varying your rate beforehand.
5. In the section called Speech and Language Development, research on language abilities of children who stutter is reviewed. Some studies found that children who stutter have poorer language abilities, and other studies did not. Review these studies and suggest what might be causing this disagreement in the literature.

SUGGESTED READINGS

Andrews, G., & Harris, M. (1964). *The syndrome of stuttering.* London: W. Heinemann Medical Books.

These authors present data from longitudinal studies of 1,000 families in Newcastle, England. The interpretation of results presents evidence that both genetic and environmental influences are at work to create stuttering. This book gives an early version of the "capacities and demands" view that stuttering is due to a lack of capacity for some aspect of speech and language processing.

Bernstein Ratner, N. (1997). Stuttering: A psycholinguistic perspective. In R. Curlee, & G. Siegel (Eds.), *Nature and treatment of stuttering: New directions* (2nd ed., pp. 99–127). Boston, MA: Allyn & Bacon.

This is an insightful review of the many connections between language and stuttering. The author's background allows her to use linguistic theories and evidence from child language studies to discuss how language influences the loci of stuttering in speech, how parent-child interactions may affect stuttering, how language development may be important in stuttering onset, and the role of feedback on speech, language, and stuttering development.

Bloodstein, O., & Ratner, N. (2008). Inferences and conclusions. In O. Bloodstein, & N. Ratner (Eds.), *A handbook on stuttering* (pp. 332–336). Clifton Park, NY: Thompson-Delmar Learning.

This chapter presents the communicative failure and anticipatory struggle view of stuttering onset. Bloodstein and Ratner muster evidence summarized in earlier chapters of this handbook to argue convincingly that stuttering develops from an interaction between the child and his environment.

Choo, A., Burnham, E., Hicks, K., & Chang, S. E. (2016). Dissociations among linguistic, cognitive, and auditory-motor neuroanatomical domains in children who stutter. *Journal of Communication Disorders, 61*, 29–47.

This article examines dissociated (uneven) development across speech, language, cognitive, and motor domains and relates those findings to density of white matter nerve tracts. Important implications for persistent versus recovered stuttering are provided.

Crystal, D. (1987). Towards a "bucket" theory of language disability: Taking account of interaction between linguistic levels. *Clinical Linguistics and Phonetics, 1*, 7–22.

This is a theoretical discussion of interaction among levels of speech and language, with an illustrative case of a child whose stuttering increases when language demands are greater. The article makes a clear argument for the influence of speech and language development on stuttering.

Guttormsen, L., Kefalianos, E., & Naess, K. A. (2015). Communication attitudes in children who stutter: A meta-analytic review. *Journal of Fluency Disorders, 46*, 1–14.

This is an excellent overview of the many studies that have been conducted on the attitudes of children who stutter toward speaking. Their findings include evidence that children who stutter have much more negative attitudes about speaking than their fluent peers and that these negative attitude increase with age. The authors discuss the bidirectional nature of these attitudes: more negative attitudes can create more severe stuttering and more severe stuttering can result in experiences that make attitudes more negative.

Hollister, J., Van Horne, A., & Zebrowski, P. (2017). The relationship between grammatical development and disfluencies in preschool children who stutter and those who recover. *American Journal of Speech-Language Pathology, 26*(1), 1–13.

In its introductory review of the literature, this article presents a good description of how language demands may interact with language abilities to produce disfluencies. One important finding presented is that for children who recover, as their mastery of syntax and grammar increases, their disfluencies decrease. Relationships between frequency of disfluencies and sentence length and sentence complexity were also explored.

Johnson, W. (1959). *The onset of stuttering*. Minneapolis, MN: University of Minnesota Press.

This book presents extensive data on parents' perceptions of the onset of their child's stuttering, compared with other parents' perceptions of their child's normal disfluency. Johnson eloquently lays out his view of stuttering as the product of an interaction between the child's disfluency, his sensitivity, and the listener's reactions.

Paden, E. P. (2005). Development of phonological ability. In E. Yairi, & N. Ambrose (Eds.), *Early childhood stuttering* (pp. 197–234). Austin, TX: Pro-Ed.

This chapter focuses on the phonological development of children who stutter with particular emphasis on comparisons between children who recover without intervention and those who persist in stuttering. The author brings to light several aspects of her research that are intriguing puzzles for future researchers to solve.

Watkins, R. V. (2005). Language abilities of young children who stutter. In E. Yairi, & N. Ambrose (Eds.), *Early childhood stuttering* (pp. 235–251). Austin, TX: Pro-Ed.

Although current evidence reviewed in this chapter suggests that language abilities of children who stutter and those who don't are similar, language factors appear to play an important role in stuttering. The author discusses several interesting relationships between language and stuttering, including the role of language factors in the occurrence of stuttering in an utterance and the finding that early onset of stuttering is often associated with advanced language skills.

5

Learning and Unlearning

Chapter Objectives

After studying this chapter, readers should be able to:

- Explain classical conditioning, operant conditioning, and avoidance conditioning
- Describe how each of these types of conditioning plays a role in the development of stuttering
- Describe what the tension response is, what it is a response to, and how it affects the development of stuttering
- Describe the role of learning new behaviors and unlearning old ones in the treatment of stuttering

Key Terms

Avoidance conditioning: A learning process that teaches an individual to engage in behavior that prevents an unpleasant consequence. It is thought to combine classical and operant conditioning in the following way. If the daily paper or the television news frequently upsets you, you associate that medium with unpleasant feelings (classical conditioning). You then discover that if you stop reading the paper or watching TV news, you don't become nauseous, and you engage more and more in this avoidance behavior because it is rewarded (operant conditioning).

Classical conditioning: Learning caused by the association of a neutral stimulus with a stimulus that strongly provokes a response. The conditioning process will cause the formerly neutral stimulus to eventually provoke the response. If you have encountered an angry bear in a familiar forest that was neutral before, that forest will now be likely to provoke fear or at least caution the next time you enter it.

Conditioned response (CR): A response that is triggered by a CS (conditioned stimulus). In the example below of a CS, you're feeling hungry and salivating when a bell is rung if you haven't eaten.

Conditioned stimulus (CS): A neutral cue that becomes associated with the UCS and then triggers the response that was produced by the UCS. In our food example, a bell might be rung repeatedly when you haven't eaten and food is presented. Eventually—through classical conditioning—you would salivate when the bell is rung if you are hungry even though no food is presented.

Operant conditioning: Learning caused when a behavior is immediately followed by a reward or punishment or the relief from punishment. If you experience delight when you eat a Dove Bar™, then you are likely to eat more Dove Bars. If you get sick after eating your first Dove Bar, you are not likely to eat more.

Unconditioned response (UCR): A response that occurs naturally and automatically (without learning) when an unconditioned stimulus (UCS) is present. An unexpected loud noise makes you blink. The blink is the UCR (unconditioned response).

Unconditioned stimulus (UCS): This is a sight, sound, smell, or other cue that automatically (unconditionally) brings on a response. For example, the smell of food (UCS) when you haven't eaten makes you salivate and feel hungry.

To help you understand the last four key terms related to unconditioned and conditioned stimuli and responses, imagine that you fell in love with someone (UCS) and were excited by their presence (UCR), and they had a particular smell from perfume, shampoo, or lotion (CS), the repeated pairing of the CS (smell) with the UCS (someone you love) would condition you. Eventually, the smell (CS) would make you excited (now CR) even if the person you love is absent.

"I-I-I-I didn't d-d-d-do it!" a two-and-a-half-year-old child says after she dumps her glass of milk on the table. With this first stutter, the stage is set for learning. Depending on the child's genetic risk factors, developmental age, sensitivity, and listeners' reactions, the learning can be quick and the stuttering can soon be on its way to persistence. Alternatively, if developmental and environmental factors are in her favor, the child may completely recover. If natural recovery doesn't occur, early treatment can be the antidote, preventing persistent stuttering. And finally, if stuttering perseveres, the learned behaviors that constitute the real handicap can be unlearned.

Before I begin to discuss learning and unlearning, I'd like to warn you that these topics are complex and involve some fancy terminology. I hope that by presenting concepts and terminology in several different ways, the underlying ideas will become second nature to you. Ideally, then, you can use them to create effective evaluation and therapy strategies.

LEARNING

In this section, you will find out about how learning works in the development of stuttering, so that you will understand your client's stuttering behaviors and then be able to help him change them. Specific types of learning are often referred to as different kinds of conditioning. These include classical conditioning, operant conditioning, and avoidance conditioning. As I describe the ways in which stuttering behaviors are learned, I will be drawing on many sources, but two books have been particularly helpful: *Learning and Behavior: A Contemporary Synthesis* by Mark Bouton (2016) and *Anxious: Using the Brain to Understand and Treat Fear and Anxiety* by Joseph LeDoux (2015). For more details on them, see the Suggested Readings at the end of the chapter.

Classical Conditioning

Classical conditioning was first described by the Russian physiologist Ivan Pavlov. As with many discoveries, it was a surprise. Pavlov and his colleagues were studying how dogs digested their food, which they assessed by measuring the dogs' saliva when they were fed. One morning when Pavlov first walked into his laboratory in his white coat and bushy beard, he noticed that the dogs salivated just in response to seeing him, even though he hadn't fed them. Pavlov realized that the dogs associated his coming into his lab with their food. Just his appearance triggered their salivation. Experimenting with different cues, he tried ringing a bell just before they were fed. After many pairings (the conditioning), he saw results—the bell alone elicited salivation without the food.

Note that the bell is the stimulus used in the rarefied atmosphere of a laboratory. Everyday classical conditioning happens in a more complex context. For example, if you are a graduate student and you get an e-mail every time you are assigned a new task, you may be conditioned to feel panic if your schedule is already full and your phone or laptop "pings" to tell you you've got another e-mail. The incoming e-mail ping is your Pavlov's bell.

Pavlov's observation provided the first scientific understanding of classical conditioning. Since then, classical conditioning has been studied extensively, and scientists have been able to describe how it takes place. Figure 5.1 depicts the "paradigm" (a model or diagram of how a process takes place) for classical conditioning.

For classical conditioning to take place, several things must occur:

- A stimulus that reliably elicits a response must be present. This stimulus is called the **unconditioned stimulus (UCS)**. The response it elicits—often a reflexive or hardwired response—is called an **unconditioned response (UCR)**. For humans, encountering a snake when walking is often a UCS for a threat response such as freezing in your tracks.
- Then, a neutral stimulus that doesn't elicit any particular response is paired with the UCS. The neutral stimulus is called the conditioned stimulus (CS) because it will be conditioned to elicit a response. In the example of the snake, a neutral stimulus might be a pile of rocks.
- After repeated pairing of the CS (the pile of rocks) with the UCS (the snake, which reliably elicits the UCR of freezing), the CS is then presented without the UCS, and voila! The CS elicits the freezing (which then becomes a CR). If you have encountered snakes around a pile of rocks many times, the next time you suddenly stumble upon a pile of rocks while hiking, you will then momentarily freeze in your tracks (and probably look around for snakes).

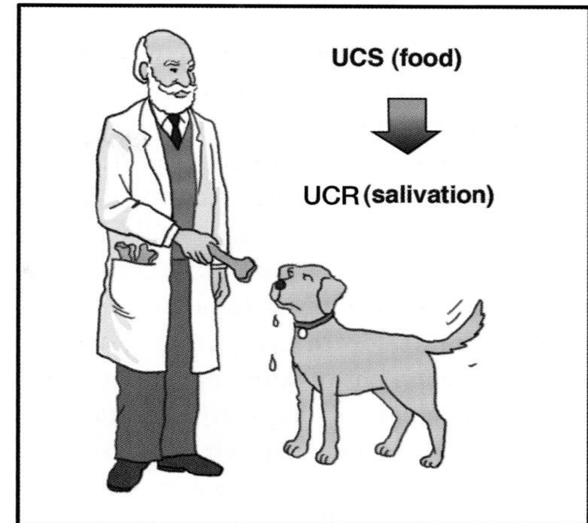

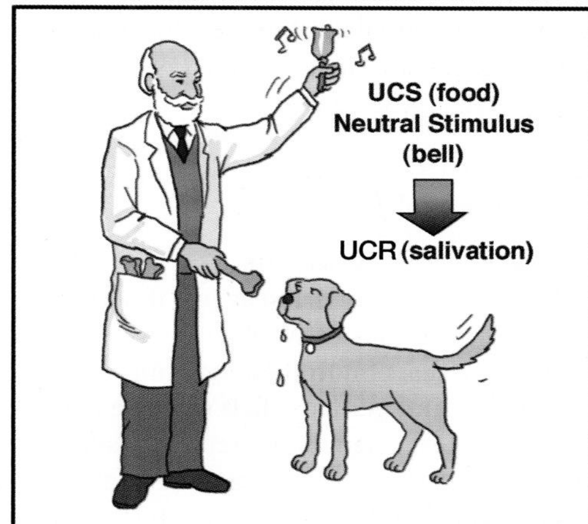

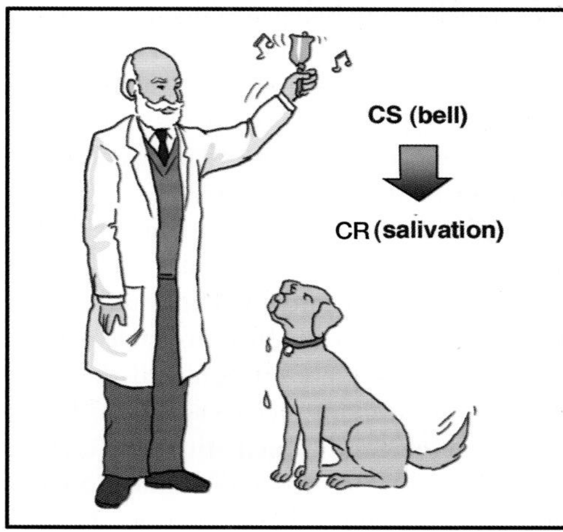

Figure 5.1 Classical conditioning paradigm. Dog salivates naturally when given food. Food is paired frequently with sound of bell. Bell without food eventually elicits salivation without the food. CR, conditioned response; CS, conditioned stimulus; UCR, unconditioned response; UCS, unconditioned stimulus.

Classical Conditioning and Stuttering

An excellent theoretical account of classical conditioning and stuttering was provided by Eugene Brutten, a speech-language pathologist, and Donald Shoemaker, a psychologist, who worked together at the University of Southern Illinois (Brutten & Shoemaker, 1967). They hypothesized that the earliest stuttering symptoms (often repetitions) result from the cognitive and motor disorganization that occurs when a child's anxiety or negative emotion is associated with speech.

Although the description of classical conditioning and stuttering I give here owes much to Brutten and Shoemaker's (1967) pioneering work, I believe classical conditioning is seldom responsible for the earliest signs of stuttering. Instead, I believe, along with Van Riper (1982), that "the real contribution of classical conditioning theory as it is applied to stuttering lies in its ability to explain the *development* of the disorder (italics mine)." I also agree with a similar assessment by Starkweather (1987, p. 372) that "it seems likely that [neuro-]physiological sources play more of a role in stuttering onset, whereas conditioning processes play more of a role in stuttering development."

If you follow the arc of most children's stuttering development, you will see that in most cases, the earliest signs of stuttering are multiple part- and single-syllable whole-word repetitions without tension or hurry. The child often doesn't notice them at first. These appear to be the result of dyssynchronies in the child's speech production system caused by delays in the development of some neural circuits and systems. Some components of the word or phrase to be produced are ready to be articulated while others are not. The part that is ready for production is spoken, but it is repeated, awaiting the next part. In the following section, I describe how those relatively simple disfluencies become transformed into more complex stuttering.

Classically Conditioned Components of Stuttering

Initial Conditioned Stimulus

The initial stuttering disfluencies, as just described, are most often excessive repetitions of syllables or words. At first, the child may have no reaction to these repetitions. Gradually, as they go on and on and perhaps elicit negative reactions from listeners, the child experiences the repetitions (on a nonconscious level) as threatening. This may be because the child, who has been speaking fluently up to this point, suddenly experiences something in his speech that is out of his control. The threat or alarm caused by these out-of-control repetitions triggers a response to stop them. This response, in my opinion, is increased physical tension of the muscles of speech and perhaps other muscles as well. This is a co-contraction of agonist-antagonist muscle pairs to increase stiffness (and thus control) of muscle groups in response to the "perturbations" of out-of-control repetitions (Guitar, Guitar, Neilson, O'Dwyer, & Andrews, 1988). Such a hardwired, instantaneous response to threat may be related to the uncontrollable nature of these perturbations when they are encountered during speaking (Fig. 5.2). When this response occurs again and again, the disfluencies become the **conditioned stimulus (CS)** that elicits the tension response, which becomes a **conditioned response (CR)**. Once this conditioning has taken place, the individual's experience of threat doesn't have to be present all the time for the repetitions to elicit the tension response.

Like other threat responses, the tension response in stuttering is probably processed through the amygdala.[1] It is nonconscious and may be the specific increased muscular tension[2] described by Bloodstein in his theory of stuttering (Bloodstein, 1975).

Spread of Conditioning

Classical conditioning is an active and continuing process. When a child is disfluent and experiences the tension response, a host of other stimuli are present in that context. When the child stutters, he or she is talking to someone, uttering a particular word or sound, speaking in a particular room, and talking about a particular topic. Because of the power of classical conditioning, the pairing of these other stimuli with the CS (conditioned stimulus) of the out-of-control repetitions gives the other stimuli the potency to elicit the tension response when the child is disfluent but also even before any disfluencies occur. The particular sound on which he stutters, for example, may become conditioned to elicit the tension response, so in the future he is more likely to produce that sound with tension. As conditioning takes place again and again, the stimulus becomes a complex of many things, including words and sounds, listeners, and physical surroundings or situations. This chaining of stimuli is called "higher-order conditioning" or "second-order conditioning." Gradually, past experiences of the threat stored in the medial temporal lobe memory systems (LeDoux, 2015) create conscious fear in the child, and this adds to the dynamics of the spread of conditioning.

It is important to note that to maintain the effects of the repetitions causing the tension response, negative emotion must occur periodically (cf, discussion by Bouton, 2016, of remembering, forgetting, and extinction in learning). Stuttering must occasionally be experienced as a threat for it to continue to elicit the tension response. It seems likely to me that listener responses of alarm or dismay may contribute to the threatening nature of the runaway repetitions. In children who are cognitively advanced enough, the threat that is a nonconscious perception is gradually conceptualized by the child as fear. Another thing that may happen is that the individual begins to imagine that the listener has a negative response even though the listener response may be actually neutral. In other words, as the child develops cognitively, he develops beliefs that his stuttering is bad and listeners will always be impatient with him when he stutters.

The spread of conditioning to other conditioned stimuli results in changes in stuttering as well. Initially, a child might emit several repetitive disfluencies or a long prolongation before the tension response occurs. Soon, however,

[1]LeDoux (2015) devoted his recent book to the argument that "fear conditioning" is really "threat conditioning." Humans and other animals, he suggests, respond reflexively to danger with rapid, nonconscious behaviors that try to cope with the danger. The explicit labeling of the experience as fear comes later with conscious processing of the threat.

[2]Many others have suggested that increased tension is a common reaction to the feeling that one is unable to control one's actions. For example, Oliver Bloodstein has suggested that "Whenever we are faced with the threat of failure in the performance of a complex activity demanding accuracy or skill, we are likely to make use of abnormal muscular tension" (Bloodstein & Ratner, 2008, p. 46). Reacting to walking on a slippery surface illustrates this nicely.

Classical Conditioning in the Development of Stuttering
Lo-lo-look at the cat
Child has a few loose and easy repetitions
Parent has calm, acceptable demeanor
Whe-whe-whe-whe-whe-whe-where is the mou-mou-mou-mou-mou-mou-mouse?
Child has more frequent and longer repetitions that seem out of control.
Parent shows alarm and concern
Lllllllllook. The caaaaaaaaaat has the mmmmmmouse.
Child has tension response to stutters that seem out of control. Repetitions turn to prolongations and blocks.
Child notices parent's alarm and concern

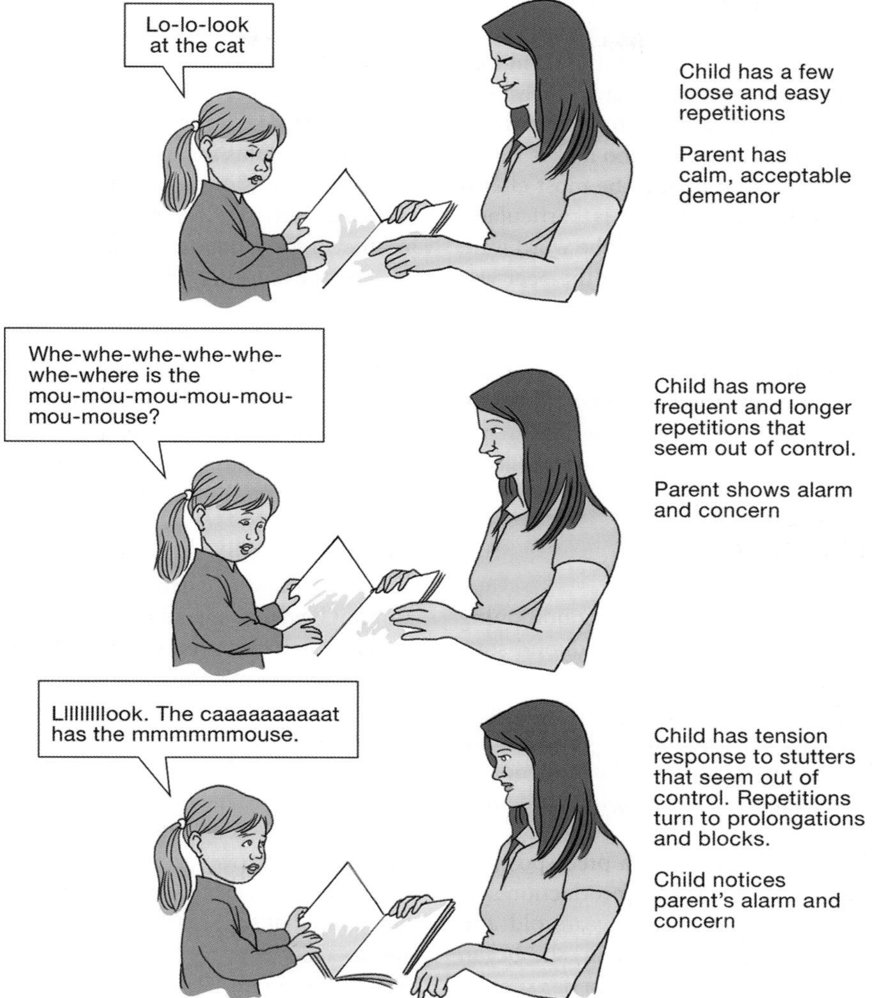

Figure 5.2 Classical conditioning in the development of stuttering.

muscle tension occurs earlier and earlier in the stutters. When other conditioned stimuli, such as words, elicit the tension response, the easy repetitive disfluencies may not occur at all. Instead, a child may increase muscle tension on the very first sound he or she tries to utter, resulting in the "fixed articulatory postures" that are a sign of advancing stuttering.

As a child's stuttering frequency increases as a result of the spread of conditioning to more and more stimuli, the duration of the child's stuttering may also increase. This can be explained by the fact that the tension response soon becomes a stimulus that itself elicits more tension. After all, the tension response (co-contracted muscles) makes it harder to utter a word, and the experience of "squeezing hard" without being able to speak for a second or two elicits greater perception of threat, leading to a longer tension response.

Individual Differences in Conditioning

Before we leave our discussion of classical conditioning, I would like to touch on the topic of individual differences and conditioning. The rapid learning and widespread generalization that is apparent in most stuttering may parallel the "prepared classical conditioning" of some animals that are rapidly and deeply conditioned to such naturally dangerous objects as snakes (Mineka, 1985). Preparedness in animals—humans included—refers to sensitivity to various objects that could have caused harm to our ancestors (e.g., snakes and spiders). Evolution favored humans, and other animals who were more sensitized to them would have had a greater chance for survival. Thousands of years later, rapid conditioning can occur in individuals with temperaments that are more alert to threatening stimuli. For example, individuals with an anxious temperament are more prone to acquire fears and phobias (Biederman, Rosenbaum, Chaloff, & Kagan,

1995; Mineka & Oehlberg, 2008), and animals that have been exposed to stressful situations—especially those that are unpredictable and uncontrollable—are more easily classically conditioned (Mineka & Oehlberg, 2008; Shors, Weiss, & Thompson, 1992). Thus, it seems likely that those children who stutter and who are especially sensitive may rapidly condition to such threatening stimuli as being unable to say a word, a critical listener response, or a peer who makes fun of the child's stuttering. This conditioning may be most etched into memory if that word, listener, or peer is particularly important to the child, as might be the case if the word were the child's name, the listener was his parent, or the peer was a close friend or sibling. Brutten and Shoemaker (1969) and Brutten (1986) have made a similar point: that individual differences in emotional reactivity and conditionability are important factors in the developmental patterns of stuttering. These differences may also relate to stuttering persistence versus recovery.

Illustration of Classical Conditioning and Stuttering

Let me give you a description of how classical conditioning might actually work in the development of childhood stuttering. I would like to use a girl named Ashley (Fig. 5.3) as an example because, with her kind permission, I have been able to provide a video clip of her early stuttering. You can find the video clip on *thePoint* under "Chapter 1: Introduction to Stuttering. Video 1-1 A Young Preschool Child: Borderline Stuttering."

Let's assume that Ashley was born with a predisposition to stutter in the form of a vulnerable speech production system. When Ashley was just two-and-a-half years old and her language development was galloping along, she began to have easy whole- and part-word repetitions in her speech, like "I-I-I" and "whe-whe-whe-when." She didn't even notice them at first.

But, as Ashley's repetitions occurred more and more often, she began (I believe nonconsciously) to try to stop them. She put her hand over her mouth at first and then started squeezing her speech muscles, much as you would tense up your body if your car started sliding around on an icy road and headed for a tree. In Ashley's case, her repetitions were typically most frequent (and she tensed up to stop them) when her mother asked her questions about a picture book they had read together. This context eventually became a conditioned stimulus for Ashley's tension response.

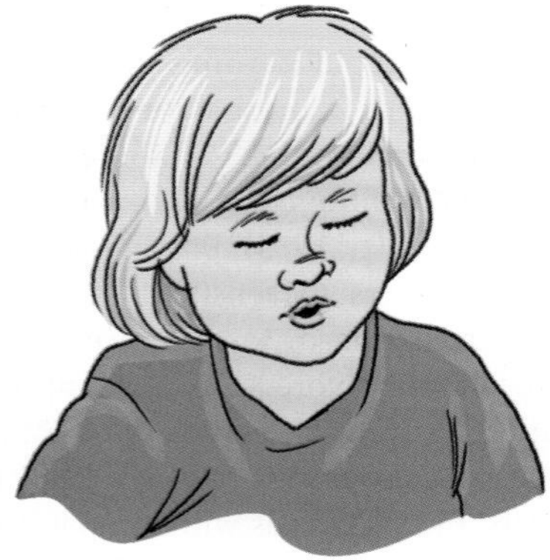

Figure 5.3 Ashley: a young preschool child with borderline stuttering (see Video 1-1 on *thePoint*).

Ashley's tension response was at first a UCR: automatic, nonconscious. However, day after day, the context of her mother asking questions and the repetitions that followed elicited the tension response. Then, the context of her mother asking questions elicited the tension response whenever Ashley tried to answer. That is, because Ashley had often experienced repetitions in answering her mother's questions about the picture book, and she had responded with increased tension, the context of her mother asking questions (previously a neutral stimulus) became a conditioned stimulus for the tension response (previously a UCR) and that became a CR.

Although Ashley's increasing tension in response to her repetitions first occurred with her mother asking her questions, it began to spread or generalize to more and more situations. After many repeated pairings, Ashley began to stutter and do so more tensely to other people and in other places. Several things were responsible for this development of her stuttering. First, the stimulus or cue of her mother became associated with other listeners who asked questions, and then to when Ashley herself initiated the conversation, such as when she asked "Whe-whe-whe-whe-when are we going home?" Then, over time, she may have been subliminally aware of "proprioceptive" (sensation in the articulators) cues signaling that she was tensing her muscles before even starting to talk. This, in turn, triggered tension that made her repetitions more tense and gradually changed some of the stutters into prolongations and blocks.

Operant Conditioning

Here, I will describe another aspect of learning that is key in the development of stuttering: operant conditioning. It differs from classical conditioning in that classical conditioning focuses on the pairing of two stimuli (food and a bell), whereas **operant conditioning** deals with a behavior and its consequences (a rat pushing a lever and receiving a food pellet). In the 1930s and 1940s, a psychologist named B.F. Skinner conducted a series of experiments that involved putting a rat in a box that had a lever mechanism for delivering a food pellet. Whenever the rat accidentally hit the lever in the box, a food pellet would roll out of a storage container, and, of course, the rat would gobble it up. The rat soon learned to hit the lever deliberately rather than accidentally to receive a food pellet reward. This approach to learning is called operant conditioning, and it happens when an animal (or person) is free to make a response whenever it wants and the response is followed by some consequence. For example, you are free to push an elevator button whenever you feel like it to get the elevator to stop on your floor. You quickly learn to push the button when you want the elevator (your positive reinforcement). You've probably learned it so well that you push the button multiple times if the elevator doesn't come quickly enough.

Operant conditioning is simply the occurrence of a consequence after a behavior is performed that change in the frequency of the behavior. Consequences can be one of three things:

- A positive reinforcer (such as a food pellet), which increases the behavior that preceded it (lever pressing)
- A negative reinforcer (such as experiencing an electric shock and then having it stop). This may be a little harder to grasp, but it works because it is a reinforcer because it terminates an unpleasant experience. If a rat is placed on electric grid and given a continuous shock, the rat will make random movements. One of the random movements may include jumping off the electric grid onto the floor of the cage. This jump will stop the animal from feeling the shock and will increase (reinforce) the behavior (jumping off an electrified grid).
- A punishment (a sudden loud noise) during a behavior, which decreases the behavior (a dog's barking)

Operant Conditioning and Stuttering

Many clinicians and researchers have suggested that the complicated stuttering behaviors we see in most adults who stutter result from a combination of classical and operant learning (Brutten & Shoemaker, 1967; Van Riper, 1971, 1982). Their views are that whereas classical conditioning is probably responsible for the child's learning to respond to certain stimuli with tension injected into repetitions, prolongations, and blocks, operant conditioning teaches the child to use a variety of secondary behaviors in response to the unpleasantness of being stuck. A common secondary behavior is pushing with the articulators to finish a word that is stuck because of the tension that is meant to stop the stutters. If simple pushing doesn't work, then the individual may add a sudden movement of the face or eyes or even of the arms or legs to escape from feeling "jammed up" by having muscle groups that are so tense that movement is impossible. A typical facial movement to release a word is squeezing the eyes shut. The first time this occurs, it might be the result of random struggle behavior. When the squeezing is followed by release of the word, this relieves the emotional pain of being stuck in a stutter and feeling frustrated and embarrassed. The negative reinforcement—escaping a painful experience—makes it more likely the speaker will use the same eye squeezing when stuttering happens again. Thus is born part of an individual's own pattern of stuttering. However, the squeezing of the eyes may not always work to release the stutter, and when it doesn't, the speaker needs to add something else like making a sound such as "uh." Then, the several "escape behaviors"—pushing with the articulators, squeezing the eyes shut, and saying "uh," one right after the other—become part of the speakers' habitual way of responding to being stuck in a stutter. Sometimes one is used and not the others, but in most cases the child develops a repertoire of escape behaviors.

Illustrations of Operant Conditioning and Stuttering

Ashley, the child we described earlier as being classically conditioned to respond to various speaking-related cues with tension, soon began to show escape behaviors as part of her pattern of stuttering. For example, when she was stuck in a repetitive stutter, she would often just stop trying to say the word and continue talking, omitting the stuttered word. This was an escape behavior that was negatively reinforced because she used it when she was stuck in a stutter to escape the uncomfortable feeling and thus it was rewarded by relief from that feeling. The video of Ashley shows that escape behavior.

Another child, Katherine, who was a year older than Ashley, developed much tenser blocks than Ashley. After a few months of increasingly tense repetitions and prolongations, Katherine's stuttering had become complete blocks. These blocks created even greater negative emotion, which elicited even greater tension, in a worsening spiral. Katherine's escape behaviors—developed initially from a panicky flailing of her arms when she was jammed up—became swinging her arm to hit her mother until the block was released. See Video 1-2 "An Older Preschool Child: Beginning Stuttering" for an example of this.

Avoidance Conditioning

Avoidance conditioning has been something of a puzzle to learning theorists because it could be considered a type of operant conditioning, but psychologists have been hard-pressed to identify what the reinforcement is (Bouton, 2016). That is, if a child who has previously enjoyed going to his friend's house suddenly starts avoiding his friend's house, why is that rewarding? Probably the best explanation of the dynamics of avoidance learning was given by the psychologist O.H. Mowrer in his "two-factor theory" (Mowrer, 1939; Mowrer & Lamoreaux, 1942). Bouton (2016) suggests that Mowrer's description of avoidance learning is generally accepted today by psychological scientists. Mowrer suggested that the first factor in avoidance learning is pavlovian or classical fear conditioning, in which the organism (typically a rat in Mowrer's lab) was given a warning signal such as a buzzer that was followed by an electric shock. In this way, the buzzer became a conditioned stimulus for fear that was aroused because of the impending shock. The rat would be then taught that if it leapt to another part of its "shuttle box" when the buzzer sounded and the shock was given, the shock stopped. Soon, the rat learned to jump to another part of the box when the buzzer sounded, before the shock was given. The rat could thus avoid the shock by jumping to the safe part of the box when the buzzer sounded. Mowrer postulated that the buzzer elicited fear. This was a key element in the classical conditioning component. But then the avoidance was reinforced by the reduction of fear. This reinforcement was the operant conditioning component. This explanation was confirmed in many later experiments by a legion of psychologists (e.g., Brown & Jacobs, 1949; Miller, 1948). According to Bouton (2016), Mower's two-factor theory has been the basis for the analysis and treatment of many human behaviors such as the "agoraphobia" that often accompanies panic disorder and obsessive-compulsive disorder such as compulsive hand washing. In agoraphobia, the individual stays home and avoids public places because of a learned fear of crowds that might result in a panic attack. In compulsive hand washing, the person washes his hands frequently because of a learned fear of germs. Treatment often consists of systematically extinguishing the fear by helping the patient accept the fear and gradually become calm in a threatening situation, with the help of the therapist. LeDoux (2015) supports Mowrer's model as a basis for treatment but suggests that it is not fear that is extinguished but the nonconscious defensive state that is triggered by the conditioned stimulus. If components of the defensive state in stuttering are nonconscious, extinguishing it in people who stutter will require creativity.

In the example I gave earlier, in which a child suddenly starts avoiding his friend's house, we would probably find that classical conditioning has caused the friend's house to trigger a defensive state in the child. This could happen if the friend had a birthday party in his house and his parents had invited a clown to perform at the party. The child who developed the avoidance behavior may have been terrified by the clown, and thus the friend's house became a conditioned stimulus associated with the defensive state triggered by the scary clown. Once that association has been made, the child's avoidance of his friend's house is rewarded by easing the defensive state ("fear," if it is conscious) when they meet somewhere else—not the friend's house, but the child's own house.

Avoidance Conditioning and Stuttering

The history of stuttering theory and speculation is brimming with ideas about the cause of stuttering itself being avoidance behavior. Many figures in the stuttering hall of fame have formulated a view of stuttering as essentially an avoidance reaction to being punished for normal nonfluency: "stuttering is an anticipatory, apprehensive, hypertonic avoidance reaction" (Johnson, 1938); "the stutterer has originally established an avoidance reaction" (Wischner, 1950); stuttering is a result of "anticipatory struggle" (Bloodstein, 1958). I think it's more accurate to put avoidance behaviors among the secondary symptoms that appear after stuttering has started and learning has taken place, rather than an explanation of its onset. As you now know, stuttering's onset is probably the result of a vulnerable speech production system breaking down under stress. However, I think avoidance is a key concept in the development of stuttering and therefore an important aspect of treatment. Avoidance behaviors in stuttering are probably triggered both by nonconscious and conscious cues. These are cues signaling that the person is about to be trapped in a stutter. The avoidance behaviors—such as putting in extra sounds before starting a feared word, substituting easy words for ones that may be stuttered, or not volunteering in a class discussion—are learned because they reduce the threat and fear and are thus negatively reinforced. They become part of the individual's stuttering pattern, they maintain the emotional response to stuttering, and they may need to be identified and confronted in treatment.

Illustration of Avoidance Conditioning and Stuttering

David began stuttering when he was 3 years old; the onset of his stuttering occurred after his parents were away for a weekend and he and his sister were taken care of by a babysitter. David's mother recalled that she first noticed David's stuttering right after that weekend, while driving him somewhere in the family car with David in a car seat behind her. He started to say something and he got stuck in a tense repetitive stutter, something like "I-I-I-I-I" and immediately put his hand over his mouth. In the months following, when he got stuck in a stutter, he would roll his eyes and tense his jaw. It wasn't long before he began to use avoidance behaviors such as putting in extra sounds before saying a feared word and changing how he pronounced words (see how he says "amount" in the video described below) to keep from stuttering on them.

Some examples of David's avoidance behaviors are in the video clip of him on *thePoint*: Video 1-3 "An Elementary School Child: Intermediate Stuttering." In Segment 1, notice how he puts in extra words like "and then" and extra sounds like "um" to reduce the fear he feels as he tries to say what he wants to say but can't. In Segment 2, he uses "and then" and another sound like "um" to postpone his attempt on "whoever." In Segment 3, talking to the clinician, he again uses repetitions of "he" to reduce fear as he gets up his courage to say "automatically"—on which he blocks and pushes back in his chair to escape from the block and finish the word. David's avoidance behaviors were very well established by the time he started treatment at age 6. For the first year of therapy, he would only let me indirectly address his stuttering, resisting my attempts to talk with him about it or to show him how to change it. Our initial work together was mostly through play therapy during which I laced my speech with examples of an easier form of stuttering. Then, gradually, with the use of tangible rewards (Jolly Rancher™ candies), I was gradually able to get David to put easier stuttering into his own speech.

Summary

The development of stuttering is a complex process. As you've seen, it involves the accumulation of classical (increasingly tense stuttering), operant (increasing escape behaviors), and avoidance (increasing avoidances) conditioning. As a child stutters more and more over months and years, a host of cognitive and emotional characteristics become wrapped around the stuttering. The question I will be addressing at great length in this book is: How do we unwind this complicated, attitudinally knotted, and emotionally twisted ball of human behavior?

UNLEARNING

In this section, I will describe the unlearning of the three types of learned behavior discussed earlier—classical, operant, and avoidance. After I describe the general unlearning process for each type of conditioning, I'll briefly depict how the procedure can be applied to stuttering. Note that with stuttering, the unlearning of classical conditioning must be approached differently at different ages because very young individuals will not have been conditioned to the same extent that older individuals have. Moreover, the techniques used with adults will be inappropriate for children, given their differences in linguistic and cognitive skills.

Unlearning Classical Conditioning

People with fears and anxieties about spiders, snakes, and large crowds can be taught to let go of their fears and live without constant worry about these apparent "threats." They can learn that the old conditioned stimulus (the spider) needn't be followed by the unconditioned stimulus (panic and desire to flee). An unexpected encounter with a spider needn't trigger the old response. Uncoupling the link between the conditioned stimulus and the UCS—a link stored in the amygdala—can be achieved if a therapist helps the client experience again and again the conditioned stimulus—via pictures of spiders, stuffed spiders, and live friendly spiders while feeling safe (no UCS).

A good example of this approach when working with anxiety disorders comes from the work of Michelle Craske and her team at UCLA (Craske, Treanor, Conway, Zbozinek, & Vervliet, 2014). Treating a young woman (whom she called Julia) who had developed posttraumatic stress disorder as a result of a sexual assault that occurred at a party, the therapist was able to her help her deal with recurrent traumatic memories and handicapping avoidance behaviors. Craske and her team used exposure therapy that decoupled the CS-UCS link (the connection between stimuli associated with the sexual assault and the experience of threat triggered by the amygdala). A warm and supportive clinician was able to help Julia explore the imagined bad outcomes from leaving her house, attending parties, and dating. Subsequently, the clinician was able to support Julia in participating in more and more of those activities. Julia discovered that when she didn't avoid these opportunities, bad outcomes didn't occur. Gradually, this treatment reduced Julia's threat-based physiological and emotional experiences substantially, and she was able to resume her normal life.

Unlearning Classical Conditioning and Stuttering

With stuttering, as with other classically conditioned behaviors, the aim in treatment is to decouple the link—etched into the amygdala and other areas of the brain—between the CS (conditioned stimulus) and the CR (conditioned response). In stuttering, this is the link between the stuttering (and anticipated stuttering) and defensive reaction and eventually negative emotion (which triggers increased muscle tension—the CR). This decoupling can be done in different ways, depending on the client's age. For example, we work with very young children (ages 2–3.5) to prevent the CS (conditioned stimulus) of multiple repetitions from eliciting negative emotion and the resulting tense muscle co-contractions. Changes in the family environment are made to boost the child's natural fluency and prevent or reverse the child's bad feelings about his early stuttering. It is essential that the family to respond to the child's stuttering with acceptance as part of an overall strengthening of the caregiver-child bond. At the same time, the family is using strategies—like a slow speech rate with many pauses—to facilitate the child's fluency.

When children are slightly older (ages 3.5–6), but still in their preschool years, we use also use a combination of increasing natural fluency and preventing negative emotion from being associated with speaking. This is done through much more structured practice and the use of rewards and very gentle requests for the child to say the word again, followed by praise when he or she repeats it fluently. For us, we may carry out this unlearning by using the Lidcombe Program, but other effective approaches are available. All of these approaches require extensive support and guidance by a speech-language pathologist with expertise in stuttering.

Once the child reaches school age (ages 6–12), treatment can be targeted to elicit the CS (the conditioned stimulus of stuttering) and make sure it is followed not by the CR (the UCS of a defensive reaction or negative emotion) but instead by neutral or even positive emotion. If substantial negative emotion is already associated with stuttering, treatment aims at markedly reducing this. This is done in a very supportive context in which the child engages in games and activities to decouple the link. Treatment provides the child repeated activities in which he experiences the stuttering as being under his control. This leads to reduced negative anticipation of stuttering, which promotes natural fluency. As with all ages, undoing the conscious and nonconscious beliefs about negative listener responses is critical. The clinician should form a warm and accepting relationship with the client. This can be the basis of a "retranscription" of the individual's memory of listener rejection. In other words, a strong relationship with a caring clinician can help the client relearn that listeners will—for the most part—accept the stuttering and even more so if the client accepts it himself.

In adults and adolescents, the decoupling of the CS (conditioned stimulus of stuttering) with the CR (conditioned reaction of defensive reaction and negative emotion) is done much more directly, by educating the client about the likelihood that his stuttering is "kept hot" by negative feelings associated with the anticipation and experience of stuttering, as well as by his avoidance and escape behaviors. These individuals are shown how to go directly into the stutter (without avoidances) and experience it as tolerable, draining away the negative emotion, via coaching and praise by a clinician who has forged a strong relationship with the client (Fig. 5.4).

This therapy is done by gradual desensitization (reducing the fear) of the client to his stuttering, starting in the safe environment of the clinic and moving to more and more challenging real-world situations while keeping up the clinician's support and praise. As the client stops fighting the stutter and is able to reduce the feeling of threat and fear that the stuttering has typically elicited, he discovers that the physical tension in his muscles reduces and he is able to release the word easily. Through repeatedly being able to release the stutter without struggle, the individual stops fearing his stuttering and is able to stop using avoidance and escape behaviors. This sounds simple enough, but most individuals require extensive support and coaching before they can accomplish this.

Unlearning Operant Conditioning

An example of the unlearning of operantly conditioned behaviors is the treatment for drug addiction. Junkies become junkies because of operant conditioning. Heroin and methamphetamine, for example, provide a reward so strong and so immediate that that an addict is willing to forgo food, friends, and family just to get a fix. Some addicts can unlearn their addictive behaviors if operant condition is used to reward healthy behaviors and punishment immediately follows bad behaviors. A partner can provide love and attention to an addicted person who comes home after work "clean." The same partner could also withdraw love and attention by going to her room and locking the door if the addicted person comes home high. Treatment for addiction is notoriously difficult, but the principles of immediately rewarding drug-free behavior with a truly valued activity and strongly punishing addictive behavior can be successful for some addicts in a highly controlled program (Horvath, Misra, Epner, & Cooper, 2016).

Unlearning Operant Conditioning and Stuttering

Most theorists and clinicians do not believe that the core behaviors of stuttering—repetitions, prolongations, and blocks—are caused by operant conditioning. However, there is agreement that much of the abnormality of stuttering—escape behaviors such as facial contortions, eye blinks, head nods, and finger snapping—are maintained by operant conditioning (e.g., Van Riper, 1982). With children, treatment often produces fluency without the need for specific undoing of the escape behaviors. Children learn to speak more fluently, are relieved of the bad feelings tied to stuttering, and stop using the escape behaviors as a happy side effect of learning to talk without stuttering.

The same side effect may occur when older children, adolescents, and adults are taught to stop fighting the moment of stuttering, accept the stuttering, and release the word easily. However, on the way to this goal, the clinician may need to educate the client about why the slow, easy release of a stuttered word is critical: because it stops the tension, struggle, and escape behaviors from being operantly reinforced by the reward of getting the word out.

Unlearning Avoidance Conditioning

In my earlier example of unlearning classical conditioning, I described the treatment of Julia, a young lady who avoided parties, dates, and going out to visit friends and family because she had been sexually assaulted at a party. Thanks to treatment, Julia was able to uncouple the association between the CS (conditioned stimuli that now reminded her of the terrible incident—such as being at a party) and the UCS (the experience of threat and terror). As the therapist helped her gradually feel more and more comfortable leaving the house, she was able to stop avoiding parties and dates and resume her active life.

Unlearning Avoidance Conditioning and Stuttering

I will start this section with a clinical warning about working with older children and adults who stutter: Don't take away avoidance behaviors before you've helped the individual to deal with the stuttering. I learned this lesson the hard way. Once, I suggested to a client on our waiting list that he didn't need the "uh" he was using as an avoidance behavior (a starter) before saying a feared word. He was not scheduled to start treatment for another month. When he did come in for therapy, he had dropped the "uh" but replaced it with "mmm... well, well, well...that is" followed by a mighty head snap that accompanied his attempt to say a word. I had made his stuttering worse because I had taken away his avoidance behavior without helping him first manage his stuttering.

After your clients learn how to handle anticipated stuttering and the fear that often accompanies it, they may

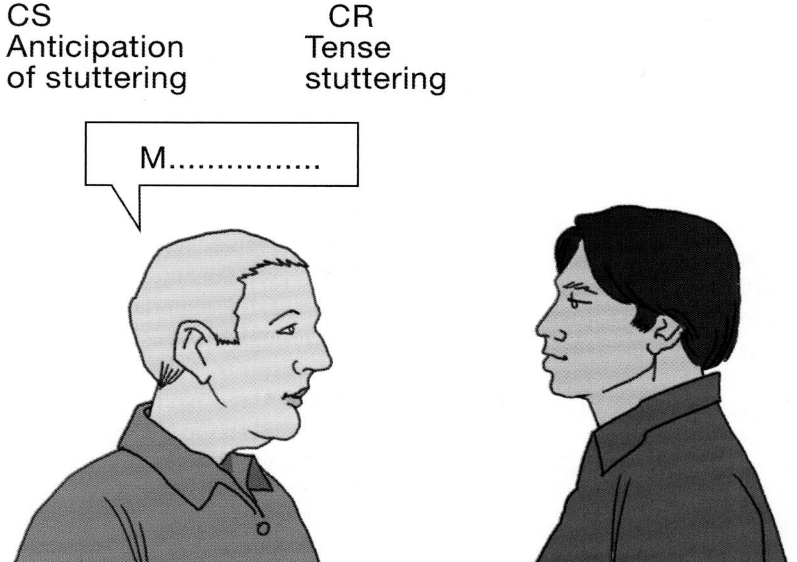

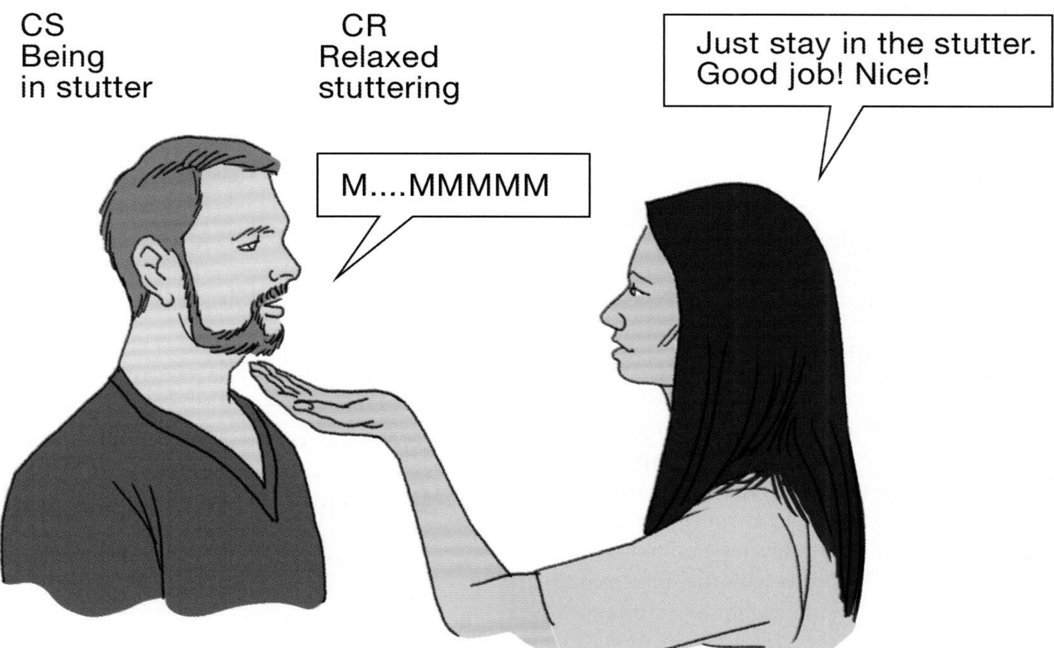

Figure 5.4 Unlearning classically conditioned tense stuttering. CR, conditioned response; CS, conditioned stimulus.

spontaneously drop their avoidance behaviors. In my treatment of older children, adolescents, and adults, after I establish a strong supportive relationship, I teach them first to go right into the sound they fear and stay in it while I help them reduce the negative emotion. A crucial aspect of this is to provide an environment in which stuttering is accepted and the clients' staying in the moment of stuttering is rewarded. As the negative emotion subsides, they find that the physical tension diminishes and they are able to finish the word more easily and slowly. As they gradually master this technique, they can drop the avoidances they have built up over the years and go right into the word they plan to say and feel better about facing down the fear that was the driving force behind their avoidances. For many individuals, this isn't easy. It will take some time before they reduce their fears and learn that actively seeking out difficult situations and using feared words gives them increased fluency and confidence in saying whatever they want to say wherever they want to say it.

In the treatment sections of the book, I will describe other approaches designed to achieve the same outcome.

SUMMARY

- The onset of stuttering in children is typically the result of neurophysiological differences manifesting as multiple part-word and single-syllable whole-word repetitions. These signs of stuttering appear when developmental and/or environmental stresses are strong.
- The development of stuttering—from repetitions to prolongations and blocks with concomitant escape and avoidance behaviors and with attitudinal and emotional overlays—is driven by learning factors.
- Because of classical conditioning, milder stuttering is linked to a defensive state that triggers increased tension. As stutters become increasingly tense, they are transformed into prolongations and blocks.
- As stuttering continues to be experienced as an unpleasant threat, the child will use escape behaviors to terminate the unpleasant experience. An example of an escape behavior is a child being caught in a series of tight repetitions and then squeezing his face to get the word out. Because of operant conditioning, this behavior will occur more frequently; the escape from the unpleasant threat rewards the facial squeezing.
- Children who stutter also learn to avoid stuttering as well as escape from it. If a child has learned to associate particular words or situations with the unpleasant, threatening experience of being caught in a stutter, they will also learn that if they change words or stay away from certain situations, they will not encounter that threatening experience. Both classical and operant conditioning motivate this avoidance learning.
- As suggested in the previous paragraph, the conditioning process gradually spreads to more and more cues, like sounds, words, people, and situations.
- Important individual differences affect the learning process. More rapid conditioning occurs with people who have more anxious temperaments and are therefore more alert to threatening stimuli.
- The conditioning that has caused stuttering to develop can be unlearned or even prevented. (1) In young children who have not experienced their stuttering as threatening, parents can do much to keep this from happening. (2) In slightly older preschool children whose stuttering does create the experience of threat and fear, increased fluency can be learned, and the conditioned negative experiences of stuttering can be undone through positive experiences. (3) In older children, adolescents, and adults who have much fear and many escape and avoidances, new learning can gradually extinguish the tension response and the secondary behaviors and attitudes.

STUDY QUESTIONS

1. Some stuttering experts in the past have suggested that the onset of stuttering is caused by operant conditioning. What ideas could you come up with to explain this suggestion?
2. How would you explain to a parent that classical conditioning has caused their child's stuttering to change from easy, loose repetitions to tightly squeezed blocks?
3. Describe how someone might develop a fear of spiders. Use the classical conditioning paradigm, indicating what are the unconditioned and conditioned stimuli and responses.
4. Add to the above example the concepts of "preparedness" and "anxious temperament."
5. Design a treatment to decrease the fear of spiders in someone.
6. Explain the separate roles of classical conditioning and operant conditioning in avoidance conditioning.
7. If a child learns to decrease her conditioned tension response (and thus learns to stutter easily and loosely) only in a therapy room at her school, what might happen when the child stutters in her classroom?

SUGGESTED READINGS

Bouton, M. (2016). *Learning and behavior: A contemporary synthesis* (2nd ed.). Sunderland, MA: Sinauer Associates, Inc.

This is a clear and lively description of the principles of learning, as well as how these principles can be applied to treatments. Bouton has been called "the leading expert in the study of extinction in animals" (LeDoux, 2015) and presents the latest research and thinking about learning.

Brutten, E. J., & Shoemaker, D. J. (1967). *The modification of stuttering.* Englewood Cliffs, NJ: Prentice-Hall, Inc.

This is a classic book in the field of stuttering. It describes a theory of stuttering that ascribes the initial symptoms of childhood stuttering to the effect of anxiety on fluency and ascribes the later symptoms to learning. The authors go on to suggest therapeutic approaches that derive from their model.

LeDoux, J. (2015). *Anxious: Using the brain to understand and treat fear and anxiety.* New York, NY: Viking.

LeDoux has written two other landmark books, The Emotional Brain *and* Synaptic Self. *This latest book advances LeDoux's views on fear and anxiety and their treatment. From his perspective, fear is not a basic response to threat, but a cognitively synthesized emotion. Fear and anxiety derive from nonconscious responses to threat. These low-level defensive automatic responses include hypertonic behaviors such as freezing. I think our understanding of stuttering may be improved if we take these into consideration.*

6

Theories about Stuttering

Chapter Objectives

After studying this chapter, readers should be able to:

- Explain what a theory is and what hypotheses are
- Identify five theoretical perspectives about constitutional factors in stuttering

- Identify three theoretical perspectives about developmental and environmental factors in stuttering
- Describe the author's integrated two-factor view of stuttering

Key Terms

Anomalous neural organization: Brain structure and function that differ from the typical. This sometimes refers to delayed development in myelination of white matter that interferes with effective intercellular communication. In some cases, the developing brain substitutes other structures or uses other pathways to try to resolve the problem. If other structural subcomponents are substituted, key areas may be located at some distance from each other and neural transmission of information may not be efficient.

Autonomic reactivity: The tendency of the autonomic nervous system to respond quickly and strongly to various stimuli. The sympathetic part of the autonomic nervous system is responsible for the flight-or-fight response and causes the heart, respiratory system, and other organs to be ready for action.

Behavioral inhibition system: A view developed by psychologist Jeffrey Gray (1987) that humans are endowed with a hard-wired protective response to frustration and fear; the body's response in this situation is freezing, flight, or avoidance. Flight occurs if the threatening object (e.g., a predator) is encountered. Avoidance takes place if the individual can detect or predict the threatening object before it is encountered. Then actions can be taken so that the threatening object is not encountered.

Capacities and demands: A view of stuttering (often called the demands and capacities model) that suggests that stuttering results when the demands (e.g., pressure to talk rapidly) put on a child's speech are greater than the child's capacity for fluency (e.g., capacity to manage the complex components of spoken language production at a high rate)

Communicative failure and anticipatory struggle: A view of stuttering that supposes that stuttering begins when a child experiences problems with communication (e.g., having many repetitions or being told he must try harder to say sounds correctly), he may develop a fear of having difficulty, which then causes tension and fragmentation of speech

"Covert repair" hypothesis: An explanation of stuttering suggesting that stuttering occurs as the result of the brain's stopping production of speech when it detects an error in the plan that the brain has made to produce a word

Diagnosogenic theory: A belief that stuttering is caused by the misdiagnosis of typical disfluencies as stuttering

Hemispheric dominance: In general, the phenomenon that one hemisphere of the brain (left or right) takes the lead or is stronger for a particular function. In the context of this chapter, hemispheric dominance refers to the fact that the left side of the brain is usually more specialized for speech and language than the right side.

Hypothesis: A specific and testable proposition derived from a theory. For example, in a theory that proposes that stuttering is caused by lack of hemispheric dominance for speech, a hypothesis might be that, using brain imaging, all individuals who stutter will show equal activity in right and left sides of the brain rather than the expected greater activity in the left side of the brain consistent with hemispheric dominance.

Inverse internal models of the speech production system: A concept about how your brain functions when you learn to talk as a child and as you are talking as an adult. The basic idea is that as a child hears speech in his environment, he stores auditory images of the sounds and words. During babbling, he learns how to send motor commands to his muscles to make those sounds and words. These connections create the internal model for speech production. They are called inverse because they start out as the auditory images or targets but get "inverted" to become the motor commands needed to hit those auditory targets.

Multifactorial dynamic disorder: Stuttering may be seen as multifactorial because many factors (e.g., genetic, emotional, cognitive, social, environmental) interact to create it. It is also dynamic because the overt signs of stuttering are seen as surface manifestations of an ever-changing neurophysiological process underlying the disorder.

Myelination: The development of an insulating sheath around nerve fibers, increasing the speed and integrity of neural transmission. Myelination occurs primarily before age 5 and is achieved in left-hemisphere frontotemporal tracts before the right-hemisphere tracts.

Primary stuttering: Early stuttering, near the onset of the disorder, that is characterized by loose, easy repetitions. For those children who begin stuttering in this fashion, it is assumed that at first they are not aware of their stuttering and do not react to it.

Secondary stuttering: Stuttering characterized by tension and struggle and sometimes by avoidances. In some views, this type of stuttering is thought to be a reaction to primary stuttering, as the child becomes self-conscious and frustrated by her difficulty with speaking.

Sensorimotor modeling: The process of building "maps" that code the motor commands to hit the auditory (and kinesthetic and proprioceptive) targets that the speaker intends; a bidirectional process in which maps that code the motor commands are adjusted if errors are detected in the auditory signal

Sensory targets: These are essentially the auditory targets mentioned in the last definition, but actually the targets contain not only auditory information but also information about the movements of the articulators (kinesthetic and proprioceptive information)

Theory: An explanation of some phenomenon. Regarding stuttering, a theory might explain why some people stutter and others don't. Theories are expected to be quite formal, so I use the term "theoretical perspective" for more informal theories.

What are theories, and what can we learn from them? A **theory** puts together findings in a systematic way so that past phenomena are explained and future ones are predicted. For example, a theory about tsunamis explains that they are caused by earthquakes on the ocean floor, explains the processes by which they are caused, and predicts that when a large undersea earthquake occurs again, another tsunami will occur. A theory about stuttering would take the many facts, findings, and observations that you have been reading about in the first five chapters and put them together to explain why one person stutters and another does not, and why one child recovers from stuttering without/with treatment and another does not. A complete theory would also explain why a person stutters on some words and not others or in some situations and not others and why people who stutter do the things they do when they stutter. When a theory can explain these things well, we believe it can lead to more effective treatments. When we know much about what causes stuttering, we hope to have a better chance of being able to modify it and even prevent it.

Scientists often use the word "theory" to mean a formal set of **hypotheses** that explain the important causal relationships in a phenomenon. These hypotheses are then tested, and the theory may be thrown out, improved, or partially confirmed as a result. The field of stuttering research and treatment hasn't developed far enough to have a formal theory of stuttering, although there are a number of informal theories that might be called "theoretical perspectives" or theoretical models.

In this chapter I present several theoretical perspectives on stuttering as well as my own attempt to integrate research and clinical findings into a two-factor theoretical perspective. I have organized existing theories by the areas covered in Chapters 2 to 5—constitutional, developmental, and environmental factors, and learning processes. These models change every few years as more data are gathered on stuttering and new information is generated in related areas. Without a doubt, the explanations of stuttering I summarize in this chapter, including my own, will be superseded by others in a few years.

THEORETICAL PERSPECTIVES ABOUT CONSTITUTIONAL FACTORS IN STUTTERING

I have chosen several contemporary views of constitutional factors to discuss in the following sections. Although the views differ, they are not mutually exclusive. If linked together, they provide us with some interesting notions about what factors might be inherited or acquired and how that might result in stuttering.

Stuttering as a Disorder of Brain Organization

Many studies of both normal speakers and brain-damaged patients have demonstrated that the left hemisphere is dominant for language in most people. This means that areas in the left hemisphere are specialized for processing language and that the right hemisphere is subservient to the left, playing a less but still important role in the production and comprehension of language.

One early theory of stuttering suggested that it is caused by lack of **hemispheric dominance** (the Orton-Travis theory of stuttering referred to in Chapter 2). The theory came about in the following way: In an atmosphere of intense scientific curiosity and collaboration among researchers at the University of Iowa in the 1920s, Samuel Orton, a neurologist, and Lee Edward Travis, a psychologist and speech pathologist, observed that many stutterers seemed to have been left-handers whose parents changed them into being right-handed (Travis, 1931). They suspected that this change led to conflicts in the control of speech in which neither hemisphere was fully in charge, creating neuromotor disorganization and mistiming of speech, resulting in stuttering. Travis and Orton's treatment derived from this theory was simply to switch stutterers back to being left-handed. This approach, as you might guess, turned out to be fruitless. Furthermore, there was never convincing evidence that high numbers of stutterers were originally left-handed. Consequently, the original cerebral dominance theory of stuttering languished for many years. But in the 1960s, evidence began to accumulate that stutterers may not, after all, have normal left-hemisphere dominance for language. Beginning in the 1970s, more and more studies supported this finding.

In 1985, a new version of the cerebral dominance theory of stuttering was proposed. Two neurologists, Norman Geschwind and Albert Galaburda, suggested that many disorders, including stuttering, dyslexia, and autism, resulted from delays in left-hemisphere growth during fetal development that led subsequently to right-hemisphere dominance for speech and language (Geschwind & Galaburda, 1985). The delay in left-hemisphere growth that resulted in what appeared to be predominantly male disorders was thought to be caused by a male-related factor. Geschwind and Galaburda hypothesized that these delays might result from fetal exposure to excess testosterone during embryonic development. So far, however, no evidence has been found to support their hypothesis about testosterone. In fact, Neilson, Howie, and Andrews (1987) provided some evidence against this hypothesis, but the idea of a delay in left-hemisphere development continues to be of great interest.

Geschwind and Galaburda's hypothesis suggests that a delay in left-hemisphere growth and development may affect speech and language for the following reasons. Various left-hemisphere structures that evolve during embryonic development seem to be especially suited for speech and language functions. As these structures develop, specialized nerve cells that are genetically programmed to sprout the neural connections for speech and language processes disperse from their point of origin in the "neural tube," where the central nervous system is formed. These nerve cells normally migrate to previously developed structures in the left hemisphere that are appropriate for their specialized functions. But if development of left-hemisphere structures is delayed, cells migrating from the neural tube may not receive the "homing beacon" they need to reach the left hemisphere. Instead, these specialized cells receive signals from the more developed right hemisphere and migrate there instead. These specialized cells then organize themselves as "networks" of neural activity in the right hemisphere for processing of speech and language. However, because the right hemisphere is not designed by its architecture and interconnections for this function, speech and language operate inefficiently there, like the Internet search engine Google trying to access information through the postal service. Figure 6.1 shows the result of the inappropriate location of speech networks in the right hemisphere combined with inefficient speech networks in the left hemisphere: poorly timed speech with disruptions.

William Webster proposed another version of the view that stuttering results from anomalous cerebral organization.

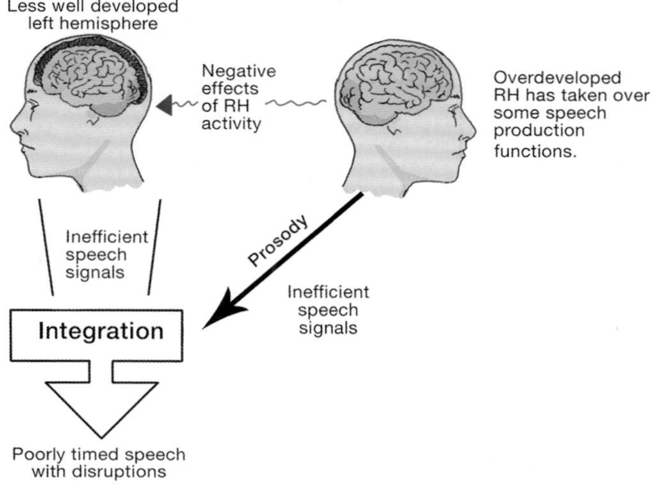

Figure 6.1 Stuttering as a disorder of brain organization. RH, right hemisphere.

As I noted in the discussion of studies of nonspeech motor control in Chapter 3, Webster (1993a) studied the effect of interference on one task (sequential finger tapping) caused by another task (turning a knob in response to an auditory signal) done simultaneously by the other hand. He concluded that people who stutter have normal localization of speech and language in the left hemisphere but that their left-hemisphere structure for speech planning and sequencing, the supplementary motor area (SMA), is especially vulnerable to disruption by activities in other areas of the brain. Webster suspected the SMA because it is strongly connected to the motor cortex as well as to subcortical motor areas and is known to be involved in the initiation, planning, and sequencing of motor activities. The left SMA, located near the corpus callosum, receives input coming across this bridge from the right hemisphere as well as input from the left hemisphere itself. Because of its location and its multiple inputs from both hemispheres, the left SMA might be highly susceptible to disruption by excess activity from either hemisphere. Webster further suggested that individuals who stutter often may have overactive right hemispheres and speculated that overflow of right-hemisphere activation, especially from right hemisphere–regulated emotions (e.g., fear, excitement), would disrupt SMA functions in planning, initiating, and sequencing speech motor output.

Stuttering as a Disorder of Timing

Several authors believe that the known facts about stuttering point toward a disorder of timing (Fig. 6.2). For example, Van Riper (1982, p. 415) stated that "when a person stutters on a word, there is a temporal disruption of the simultaneous and successive programming of muscular movements required to produce one of the word's integrated sounds..." Building on Van Riper's view, Kent (1984) marshaled several lines of evidence to support a hypothesis that stuttering arises from a deficit in temporal programming. He speculated that this deficit reflects the inappropriate localization of speech and language functions to the right hemisphere that results in an inability to create the precise timing patterns needed to perceive and produce speech efficiently. Like a conductor of a symphony orchestra who determines when each section plays, as well as its speed or tempo, mechanisms in the brain control the rate at which we speak and the order of movements for producing sequential sounds. Just as a conductor integrates the timing of an orchestra's several sections, the brain must coordinate complex timing relationships for phonemes, syllables, and phrases of speech.

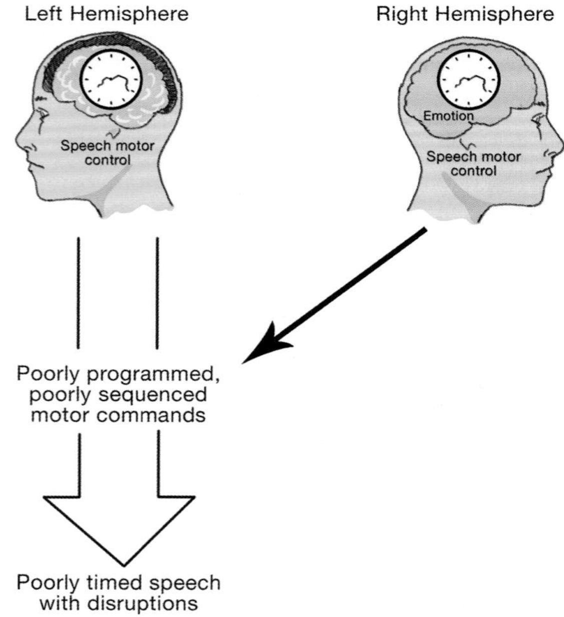

Figure 6.2 Stuttering as a disorder of timing.

Kent (1984) suggested that the inability to perform precise timing functions consistently may stem from the left hemisphere of a person who stutters being less well developed than the right hemisphere (cf., Geschwind & Galaburda, 1985). Because the left hemisphere is specialized for processing brief, rapidly changing events such as those needed for fine motor control of verbal output, a person who stutters may be disadvantaged when trying to process at the speed required for normal speech. This central timing function, Kent points out, not only must regulate left-hemisphere aspects of speech production but also must integrate the production of rapid, left hemisphere–generated speech segments with the slower prosodic elements of speech that are generally functions of the right hemisphere.

Kent also noted that emotion may play an important role in disrupting the timing of the speech of someone who stutters. As I indicated earlier, the right hemisphere is believed to be heavily involved in the regulation of certain negative emotions. The deficit of a person who stutters, then, may be that his timing functions for speech are arranged so that they are (1) less efficient than those of nonstutterers and (2) vulnerable to interference by right-hemisphere activity during increased emotion. How this deficit causes the repetitions, prolongations, and blocks we hear in stutterers' speech is not explained in this theory.

Stuttering as Reduced Capacity for Internal Modeling

Another view of constitutional factors in stuttering was advanced by Megan and Peter Neilson, whose research on stutterers' tracking abilities was reviewed in Chapter 3. The Neilsons proposed that the repetitions of beginning stutterers are the result of a deficit in their ability to create and use "**inverse internal models of the speech production system**" (Neilson & Neilson, 1987). This rather complicated sounding model can be easily understood if we go back to an assumption about how children learn to speak.

During the first year of life, infants store up perceptions of the speech sounds they hear around them and begin to play with speech sounds, trying to imitate what they hear. Gradually, as they grow older, children learn how to make these sounds accurately. Some scientists, like the Neilsons, believe that too much of the brain's neural resources would be required if children had to remember each of the movements needed to produce each sound of their language in every possible phonetic context. Instead, children are thought to develop a mental "model" of the relationship between their speech movements and sounds they hear. Just as someone beginning to play a trombone must learn the relationship between the movements of the trombone "slide" and the sounds that result, experienced trombonists have established mental models of the relationship of their arm movements to the sounds produced and are able to move the slide to produce a desired sound without having to think about it in any deliberate way.

A child, then, develops a mental model of the relationship between speech sounds and motor commands. The mental model in the brain might be called a **sensorimotor model** for speech, which the Neilsons call an "inverse internal model" of how speech is produced. It is an "inverse" model because it transforms or inverts **sensory targets** (i.e., heard speech sounds) into the motor commands needed to produce them. As infants learn to produce the sounds they hear, they constantly use and refine their sensorimotor model for speech. They plan a word or sentence in terms of what it should sound like (the target) and then rely on their sensorimotor model to generate the motor movement commands that will produce the speech targets they are trying to hit.

The process of learning to speak is something like learning to drive a car. At first, keeping the car on the road requires constant vigilance. But as we learn the relationships between turning the wheel, stepping on the accelerator, and going where we want, the linkage becomes automatic, even when driving a stick-shift vehicle in stop-and-go traffic. Moreover, the linkage is refined as we encounter different driving conditions and different cars (e.g., cars with loose steering wheels and sticky accelerators). Just as drivers establish sensorimotor models for driving, children develop sensorimotor models for speaking.

Figure 6.3 is a schematic depiction of how the brain may transform desired sensory (perceptual) targets into motor commands for speech. In the figure, the desired output (the word or phrase, e.g., that a child intends a listener to hear) is fed into the internal inverse model of the speech production system. Here, the desired output is entered as sensory code of its expected auditory and kinesthetic results, which is "inverted" by the model to generate its output as movement codes or motor commands. Experience, practice, and vocal play help the child to acquire these inversions or transformations. Moreover, this internal model is continually updated as a child's speech and language skills mature and the speech production system changes with age. The internal model's

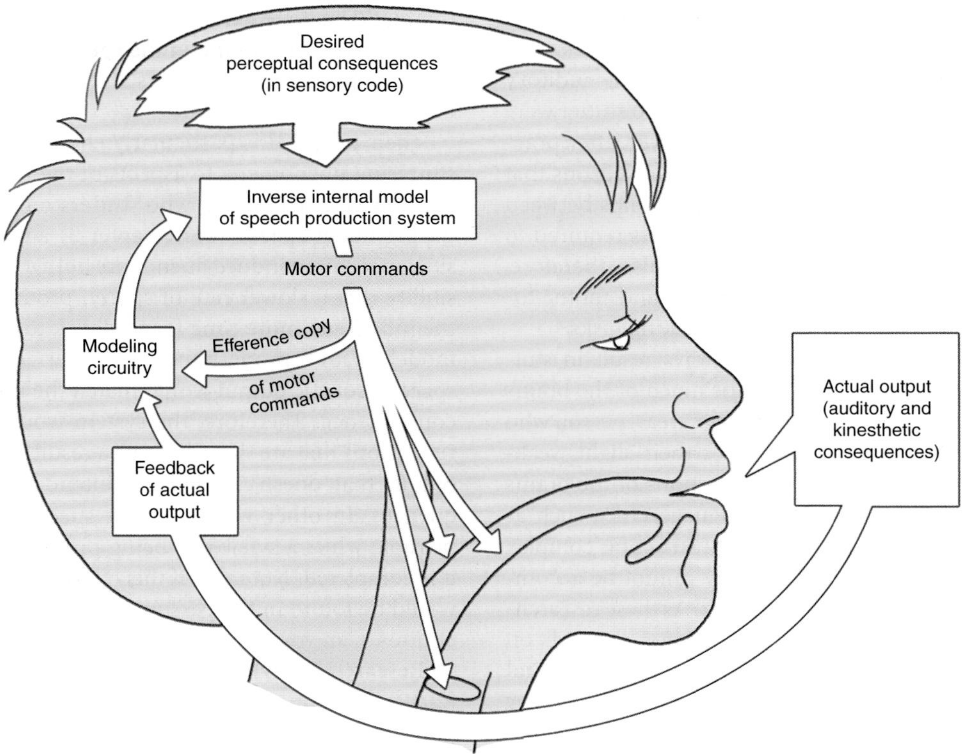

Figure 6.3 Schematic of the inverse internal model theory of speech production.

motor commands are sent to the muscles of the speech production system, whose coordinated contractions produce the acoustic output that result in a planned utterance. Concurrently, ongoing planning and feedback of this process are fed into the modeling circuitry.

Let us retrace our steps for a moment; when motor commands are sent to muscles, a copy of these commands, which is called the "efference copy" by motor physiologists, is also sent to the modeling circuitry. Here, efference copy is transformed into its hypothetical output, which is a model, or template, of the output that should be produced based on the motor commands. This hypothetical output is continuously compared with feedback on the current positions and movements of the speech mechanism so that the inverse internal model can update its ongoing motor commands, if necessary, to produce the desired output more accurately. These components of the speech production process are assumed to involve the corticocerebellar structures and pathways that are commonly described in neural models of speech output (e.g., Neilson & Neilson, 1987, 2005a, 2005b; Neilson, Neilson, & O'Dwyer, 1992).

The Neilsons and their coworkers have used the inverse internal model of the speech production system to understand the performance of stutterers in experiments that tested their ability to track an auditory tone whose pitch changed unpredictably (Neilson, Quinn, & Neilson, 1976). The subjects heard an unpredictably changing "target" tone in one ear and a "cursor" tone, which they could control with a handheld device, in the other ear. Their task was to track the pitch of the target tone with the cursor tone as accurately as possible. The Neilsons' experiments found that person who stutters were poorer than person who doesn't stutter in tracking auditory tones that went up and down in pitch. People who stutter were still poorer than people who doesn't stutter even after practicing the task. These findings suggested to the Neilsons that if stutterers had difficulty learning the relationships between the sounds they want to say and the movements required to produce them as young children, they would also, therefore, have difficulty making the sensory-to-motor and motor-to-sensory transformations required by the tracking tasks.

However, this difficulty would not always result in stuttering. When circumstances don't call for much of the brain's functional capacities in speech and language areas, person who stutters should be able to compensate for their slight weaknesses. On the other hand, when large portions of the brain's functional capacity are allocated for language tasks, such as choosing new or unfamiliar words or constructing complex sentences, the diminished neural capacity cannot be accommodated, and more repetitions would result. As these researchers put it, "whether one will become a stutterer depends on one's neurological capacity for these sensory-to-motor and motor-to-sensory transformations and the demands posed by the speech act" (Andrews et al., 1983, p. 239).

How do these intermittent deficits in available functional neural capacity result in the symptoms of stuttering? This theory attempts to account only for the core behaviors of early stuttering, that is, repetitions and prolongations. According to the theory, repetitions and prolongations result from inadequate transformations of sensory targets, transformations that should generate the motor commands for speech. A speaker with reduced functional neural capacity may begin to speak but be unable to plan and carry out the rest of his utterance without disruption. Repetitions or prolongations may occur if a speaker is attempting to push ahead with speech while his brain is still planning the syllables that follow and how to link them with the initial sound.

Other researchers have also used the concept of inverse internal models to explain the behaviors of stuttering. The Neilsons' view was echoed in the perspective described in Guenther (1994), which was later adapted by Max, Guenther, Gracco, Ghosh, and Wallace (2004) to propose a theoretical model of stuttering based on unstable or insufficiently activated internal models. One of their hypotheses parallels the Neilsons' proposition that some children are predisposed to stutter because of the difficulty learning the relationships between their motor commands and the desired acoustic output. This difficulty would result in an inaccurate inverse internal model of the speech production system (Fig. 6.3), which would generate output that would not match the desired perceptual consequences. The speech production system would then "reset" itself to try again, producing repetitions (one for each mismatch). This resetting process would continue until the child's error-correction process could update the model sufficiently to make the output match the consequences. If this could be done quickly, only one or two repetitions would occur; if not, many repetitions would occur. The Max team's proposal has other hypotheses and an extensive review of the literature to support them.

Their proposal is particularly effective in relating various stuttering phenomena to aspects of the model. For example, the findings that person who stutters movements are slower during fluent speech (see Chapter 3) and the evidence that slow speech can induce fluency are both explained by the possibility that a slower rate of speech production would allow the individual more time for feedback to update the internal model. With a properly updated internal model, the actual speech acoustic output would match the intended perceptual consequence. Therefore, the system would not produce the repetitions that are thought to be a result of inaccurate speech output that doesn't match the intended perceptual consequences. In other words, slower speech makes corrections possible while a syllable is being produced rather than after it is completed. Note that if this hypothesis is accurate, errors would be found in the person who stutters unsuccessful repetitions. Can you devise a study that would investigate this?

Research by Cykowski, Fox, Ingham, Ingham, and Robin (2010) has supported this perspective on stuttering as a deficit in using inverse internal models for speech. Their work suggests that specific pathways in the brain used for sensorimotor integration—within the superior longitudinal fasciculus (SLF III)—are less efficient in adults who stutter compared to adults who do not. This is also shown by Chow and Chang's (2017) study of children who stuttered (those who would recover and those who would become persistent) compared to control children. They found that the children who stuttered who would become persistent had significantly less density (and less growth of density over time) in white matter tracts compared to control children. The most problematic areas appeared to be those that would be critical in an inverse internal model for speech production: white matter tracts responsible for sending motor commands and creating expectations of their auditory and somatosensory consequences, so that the motor commands could be adjusted when errors are detected.

To apply these views to the first signs of stuttering, children's repetitions may be the result of motor commands creating a first syllable of an utterance, but this output may be flawed (or detected as flawed). Repetitions would then occur as corrections are attempted. It is also possible that the first syllable is adequate but the system is not functioning well enough to plan and carry out the following syllables. Hence, the first syllable is uttered again and again while the system awaits the plans and commands for the next.

Stuttering as a Language Production Deficit

Many researchers have been intrigued by the influence of linguistic factors on stuttering. For example, stuttering often begins when a child enters a period of intense language development (e.g., Bloodstein & Ratner, 2008; Yairi & Ambrose, 2005). Similarly, stuttering is most frequent when the load on language functions is heaviest (e.g., in longer utterances, at the beginnings of sentences, and on longer, less familiar words) (Bloodstein, 2002). These factors have prompted several theorists to propose that stuttering reflects an impairment in some aspect of spoken language. I use the term "spoken language" because these theorists believe the major problem is not in the motor execution of speech, but rather in the planning and assembly of language units, such as phonemes, that occur before speech is produced.

Herman Kolk and Albert Postma (1997) developed the **"covert repair" hypothesis** to explain stuttering from a language production point of view. They believe that both stuttering and normal disfluencies result from an internal monitoring process that we all use to check whether what we are about to articulate is exactly what we mean to say. Perhaps this may be clearer if we imagine for a moment that language production is like a factory making bicycles (Fig. 6.4). The factory must monitor the quality of its bicycles by checking them at different stages. Some quality control checks occur after the bicycles leave the factory, when factory workers themselves ride the bicycles and tell the factory about any defects they find. In speech and language production, this

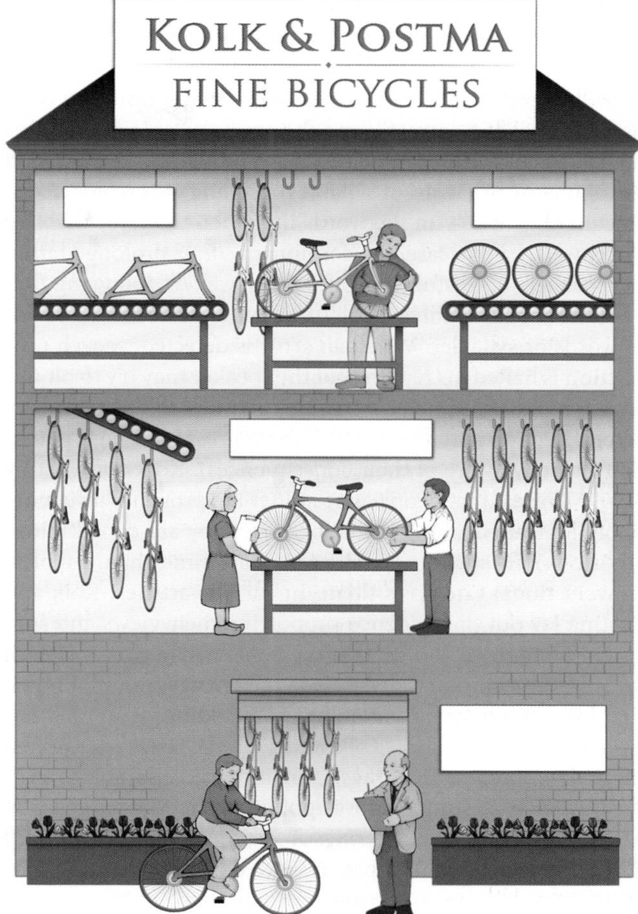

Figure 6.4 Quality control in a bicycle factory as an analogy for part of the language production system in the brain.

is like a speaker's auditory feedback (the sound of your own words as you are speaking them).

The bicycle factory might also use another quality control process, one that occurs inside the factory before the bicycles are shipped out. This is like our internal monitoring process of speech and language. Without being aware of it, we check the "phonetic plan" for what we are about to say before we articulate it. This allows us to detect potential semantic, syntactic, lexical, and phonological errors before they are produced. Just as the production line in a bicycle factory would have to be halted when a defect is detected, speech production is interrupted when our internal monitor detects an error in our phonetic plans. Repairs need to be made before production can continue. Kolk and Postma (1997) believe that the halting of production and the repair process cause the disfluencies of both normal speakers and individuals who stutter.

To Kolk and Postma (1997), the most common stuttering disfluencies (repetitions, prolongations, and blocks) are the result of correcting or "repairing" the phonological (rather than semantic, syntactic, or lexical) errors detected in the phonetic plan before they are spoken. In the case of part-word repetitions, if a speaker detects an error in the final part of a syllable (e.g., the /p/ in "cup"), he restarts the phonological encoding process ("cu-cu-") and keeps going until the phoneme is encoded correctly and the entire syllable can be produced. In contrast, prolongations are thought to occur when the phoneme of a word or syllable preceding the error is a continuant (e.g., the /l/ in the word "lip" when the error involves the vowel). In this case, the continuant, /l/, is prolonged until the speaker successfully encodes the vowel, /i/, following /l/.

Blocks are thought to result from errors in the initial sounds of words or syllables. When an error is detected, speech production is halted for repairs, but the speaker may try to plunge ahead, building up muscle tension, unaware of the automatic error detection and repair that is in progress (although potentially acutely aware of their consequences). Kolk and Postma (1997) suggest that people who stutter are prone to have more phonological encoding errors because they are constitutionally slower in encoding and need more time than a typical conversational rate gives them. In various articles, Kolk and Postma lay out the evidence supporting their views and suggest, among other things, that the benefits of a slower speech rate on stuttering are derived from the greater amount of time that stutterers have for phonological encoding.

Several years before Kolk and Postma (1997) published their covert repair hypothesis, an innovative language production view of stuttering was published by Marcel Wingate in *The Structure of Stuttering: A Psycholinguistic Approach* (1988). In this book, Wingate reviewed linguistic and neurological research on stuttering and hypothesized that stuttering results from a dyssynchrony of functions in the left and right hemispheres, as well as in subcortical structures. These different areas, Wingate suggested, are responsible for different components of language planning and production, such as consonants, vowels, and prosody. He theorized that when speakers produce the initial portion of a syllable, the consonant, vowel, and prosody must be synchronously blended. If some component lags behind at this critical moment, the result is a disruption in speech production that we observe as stuttering. Returning to our imaginary bicycle factory, it is as if the wheels, gears, and frame all must be assembled at the same time on a high-speed assembly line. If one component is delayed, production is halted. However, Wingate does not explain how this halt appears in speech as a repetition, prolongation, or block.

William Perkins, Raymond Kent, and Richard Curlee (1991) proposed another theory of stuttering as a deficit in language production. These authors suggested that stuttering results from a dyssynchrony between two components of language production. The "paralinguistic" component is a right hemisphere–controlled social-emotional process that is responsible for vocal tone and prosodic functions. The other component is linguistic and involves a left hemisphere segmental system that is responsible for the content and structure of language (semantics, syntax, and phonology). The two components must be integrated before spoken language is produced. If one lags behind the other for whatever reason, the resulting dyssynchrony produces disfluency.

Perkins et al. (1991) add two elements to this dyssynchrony that must also be present if the resulting disfluency is stuttering, rather than just a normal disfluency. First, the speaker must experience time pressure from either an outside source or an inner feeling, so that he continues trying to speak even though the dyssynchrony in paralinguistic or linguistic processes has resulted in an incomplete or anomalous speech motor program. Second, the speaker must experience a feeling of "loss of control," which arises from being unaware of why he cannot say the word.

In our imaginary bicycle factory, Perkins, Kent, and Curlee's theory might be characterized as a production line that stops automatically whenever one of the two major subcomponents of a bicycle is not ready for assembly. However, the boss in this factory demands that the production line move rapidly, and the workers panic if the production line grinds to a halt. They frantically keep trying to restart production even though they don't know what the problem is or how to fix it.

Packman, Code, and Onslow (2007) and Packman and Attanasio (2010) have suggested another perspective on the dyssynchrony model. They believe that the challenge of producing variable linguistic stress from syllable to syllable triggers moments of stuttering. The problem, according to these authors, first appears in children's speech as they move from the simple production of single words to the more complex production of phrases. Phrases demand stress contrasts that tax the child's unstable speech production system. Having said the first syllable, the child is unable to move on because he cannot program the needed stress contrast between the first and second syllable. They localize the difficulty in starting utterances to the SMA, a region of the brain involved in initiation of speech. Children are unable to move forward beyond the first syllable because of this problem and, according to Packman and Attanasio, they revert to a babbling-like repetition of the first syllable until brain resources allow the speech production system to move ahead to the following syllables. The authors cite the work of Wingate's theory of stuttering as a deficit in prosody (e.g., 1976, 1981) as an influence in their concept of stuttering as a difficulty in producing contrasting stresses.

Stuttering as a Multifactorial Dynamic Disorder

For almost 25 years, Anne Smith has been carrying out a systematic program of research on stuttering, developing a theory that at the core of stuttering is a motor speech disorder, the appearance and severity of which are influenced by a multitude of cognitive, linguistic, and psychosocial factors (e.g., Smith, 1999; Smith & Goffman, 2004; Smith & Kelly, 1997; Smith & Weber, 2017; Zimmerman, Smith,

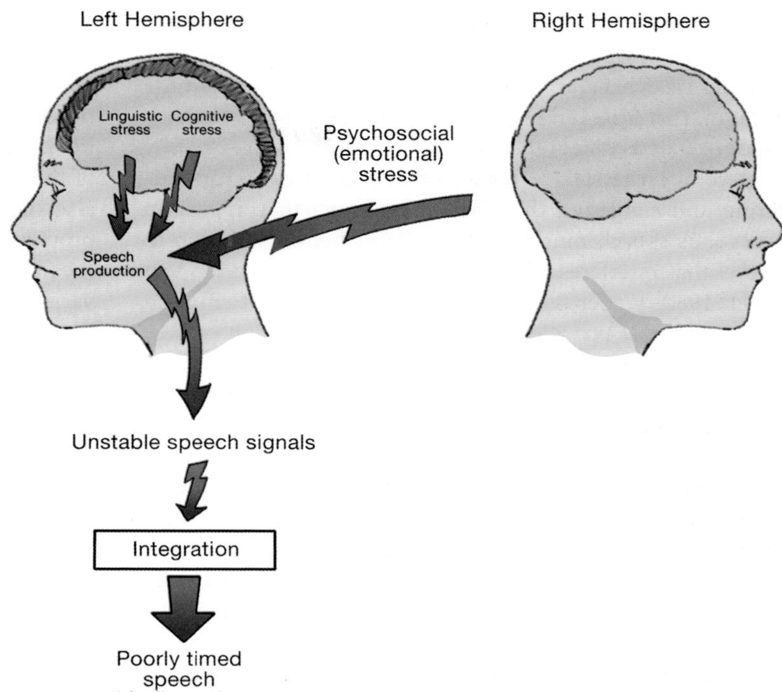

Figure 6.5 Stuttering as a multifactorial dynamic disorder.

& Hanley, 1981). In arguing for the multifactorial nature of stuttering, Smith quotes Van Riper (1982) who makes the point that not only are there multiple factors acting in concert that determine if individuals stutter but that different individuals will have unique combinations of factors—different amounts of various factors—that determine their own stuttering fate.

Portraying stuttering as a **multifactorial dynamic disorder** (Fig. 6.5), Smith thinks it is inappropriate to search for a single underlying "cause" of stuttering but instead thinks it's important to look for which factors interact in stuttering and determine how they interact. A good example of the way this view is manifest in Smith's research is the finding that when individuals who stutter produce utterances that are longer and more linguistically complex, their speech motor coordination becomes more variable (movements of articulators appear less regular when standard deviations—measures of variability—are computed for many repetitions of a phrase), compared to individuals who don't stutter (Smith, Sadagopan, Walsh, & Weber-Fox, 2010). Despite the greater variability in their coordination, the individuals in the stuttering group did not overtly stutter as they produced the utterances in this experiment. Exactly how this greater variability results in stuttering from time to time will probably await further study of other factors that can be manipulated in these experiments, such as psychosocial stress.

The multifactorial, dynamic view characterizes stuttering as a "dynamic" disorder because the "stuttering events" of repetitions, prolongations, and blocks are seen as only the outward manifestation of an underlying, ever-changing process resulting in these events erupting to the surface from time to time. So in the experiment described above, there may be increasing speech motor instability as linguistic load increases, and if psychosocial stress were increased (as part of the underlying, ever-changing process), some stuttering events might surface. Perhaps this would occur in some individuals but not others.

Smith and her colleagues' research on speech motor instability (variability of movements) hints at a substrate that might be related to early or **primary stuttering**, but what can explain the secondary reactions of tension and struggle? What causes stuttering to change from brief, easy repetitions or prolongations of words and syllables that are hardly noticed by the child or listeners to the long, tense blockages that frustrate, embarrass, and upset both the speaker and often his audience?

Smith and her colleagues have done some important research on this aspect of stuttering as well. They have found that some moments of stuttering are characterized by rapid (5–12 Hz), rhythmic, oscillatory neural input to the muscles of speech so that they contract in a rapid, tremor-like way (Smith, 1989). Not every person who stutters muscles show these tremors during stuttering, however, and they may not appear in younger children who stutter but only in older children whose stuttering has persisted for some time. In one study, Kelly, Smith, and Goffman (1995) found that these neural oscillations were present in the stutters of the three older children in their study (ages 10–14 years) but were absent in the stutters of the seven younger children (ages 2–7 years). The researchers noted that such tremors may appear in the stuttering of only those individuals who have stuttered for some time and have developed maladaptive reactions. As Kelly et al. (1995) pointed out, it is also possible that these tremors are evoked or magnified by autonomic arousal or the emotion that arises in response to the expectation or occurrence of speech difficulties.

Several writers have linked emotional stress with stuttering and suggested that the tiny tremors that appear in everyone's speech muscles may be amplified by emotion to a level that interferes with talking (Fibiger, 1971, 1972; Van Riper, 1982; Weber & Smith, 1990). The effects of emotion on tremor may provide a physiological explanation of how the mild disfluencies of young children become the more severe blockages we see as beginning stuttering evolves into advanced stuttering. Even mild disfluencies may trigger emotional responses in some children that result in increased tremors that block speech. Emotional responses may also explain the unusual cases of severe blocks at the onset of stuttering, especially when stuttering begins during conditions of stress and strong emotion. The interaction of very strong emotion with a child's vulnerable speech motor system may create sudden severe stuttering because it amplifies tremors in the speech musculature. Such tremors may be analogous to the quivering lip of a toddler who is about to burst into tears when frightened by a barking dog or by a yelling parent. Just how magnified tremors block or slow the forward movement of speech is not known, but Van Riper's (1982, p. 126) description of tension and tremor may give us some clues. He suggested:

> *What usually seems to happen is that tremors begin when the stutterer creates a fixed closure, invests its antagonistic musculatures with tension, and then suddenly produces an increase of air pressure behind or below the closure. At the moment this increase occurs, the antagonistic musculatures become suffused with a sudden burst of further tension and the stuttering tremor comes into being. Then it persists…*

Why person who stutters would create fixed closures is a mystery. Perhaps it is one of the body's responses to threat that Gray (1987) described as a behavioral inhibition system, which I discuss later in the section on secondary stuttering and temperament.

THEORETICAL PERSPECTIVES ON DEVELOPMENTAL AND ENVIRONMENTAL FACTORS

The three views presented in this section represent three different conceptualizations of how developmental or environmental stresses (or both) result in stuttering. One view is called the "diagnosogenic" view because it proposes that stuttering begins when parents mistakenly diagnose normal disfluency as stuttering. The other two views look more broadly at circumstances under which stuttering might arise. For example, the **communicative failure and anticipatory struggle** view assumes that some form of communication difficulty precipitates stuttering, whereas the **capacities and demands** view presumes that almost any developmental or environmental pressure may precipitate it. As you read this section, keep in mind that these three views differ not only in their concept of the roles that development and the environment play but also in their specificity. The first view (i.e., diagnosogenic) proposes that specific factors create stuttering; the last view (i.e., capacities and demands) describes how many different variables may interact to produce stuttering. The specificity of the remaining view (i.e., communicative failure and anticipatory struggle) lies somewhere in between the two others.

Diagnosogenic Theory

In the 1930s, Wendell Johnson and other researchers at the University of Iowa began studying the onset of stuttering in children. As Johnson examined the speech of young stutterers and nonstutterers, he noticed a similarity. The most common disfluencies of both groups were repetitions. As Johnson contemplated this observation, he was struck by the possibility that all of these children may have had the same disfluencies to begin with but that those who became children who stuttered developed more serious disfluencies by overreacting to their repetitions. But why? Johnson speculated that perhaps their parents or other listeners mislabeled their repetitions as stuttering and, in so doing, made the children so self-conscious that they tried to speak without any disfluency. Their efforts to avoid all disfluencies may have become what is generally regarded as stuttering (Johnson et al., 1942).

Johnson's hypothesis came to be called the **diagnosogenic theory**, meaning that stuttering was caused by its diagnosis or in this case, misdiagnosis. It was the most widely accepted explanation of stuttering throughout the 1940s and 1950s. It pinpointed environmental factors as the sole cause of stuttering by placing the blame on the negative reactions of parents and other listeners.

Johnson and his associates continued gathering data on the disfluencies of stuttering children and their nonstuttering peers to further support the diagnosogenic theory. The results of several studies were summarized in a landmark book, *The Onset of Stuttering* (Johnson & Associates, 1959). Table 6.1, taken from Johnson's book, gives an overview of the similarities and differences in the disfluencies reported by the parents of children who stuttered and children who didn't. Johnson interpreted these data as showing similarity between the disfluencies of stuttering and nonstuttering children; both groups of children were reported to show at least some of each type of disfluency. He suggested that the same disfluency types that parents of nonstuttering children considered normal were reported by parents of stuttering children as the earliest signs of stuttering. Johnson used this as evidence to support the diagnosogenic hypothesis that the problem was parents' interpretation of their child's disfluencies, or as some often put it, "the problem was not in the child's mouth but in the parent's ear."

TABLE 6.1 Percentage of Parents of Stutterers and Nonstutterers Who Reported Child Was Performing Each Speech Behavior When They First Thought Child Was Stuttering

Group	Repetition			Other Nonfluency			
	Syllable	Word	Phrase	Prolonged Sounds	Silent Intervals	Interjections	Complete Blocks
Control (Nonstutterers)							
Fathers	4	59	23	3	36	30	0
Mothers	10	41	24	4	41	21	0
Experimental (Stutterers)							
Fathers	57	48	8	15	7	8	3
Mothers	59	50	8	12	3	9	3

From Johnson, W., et al. (1959). *The onset of stuttering*. Minneapolis, MN: University of Minnesota Press. Copyright © 1959 by the University of Minnesota. © 1987 Edna Johnson. Reprinted with permission of the University of Minnesota Press.

It should be noted that later authors interpreted the data in Table 6.1 quite differently than Johnson did. The data were seen as evidence that the two groups of children were different at the onset of stuttering. McDearmon (1968), for example, as we pointed out earlier, argued that these findings showed that the disfluencies of normal children were notably different from those in the stuttering children. Syllable repetitions, sound prolongations, and complete blocks were reported to have occurred much more frequently in the stuttering children, whereas phrase repetitions, pauses, and interjections were reported more frequently in the nonstuttering control group. This reinterpretation of Johnson's evidence and new findings about genetic and constitutional factors in stuttering have caused the diagnosogenic view of stuttering to be largely abandoned.

To illustrate the diagnosogenic view, I take an example from a master's thesis that Johnson directed (Tudor, 1939). At that time, the diagnosogenic theory had not been formally proposed, but undoubtedly Johnson and others must have entertained the possibility that labeling a child as a person who stuttered would create more hesitancy in his speech. This thesis was an exploration of that idea. Johnson's student, Mary Tudor, screened all the children, at a nearby orphanage, for speech and language disorders. Tudor selected six children who were normal speakers, but she told these children that they should speak more carefully because they were making errors when they talked. She warned them that they were showing signs of stuttering. She also cautioned caregivers that these children should be watched closely for speech errors and corrected when they slipped up. After several months, Tudor went back to the orphanage and found that a number of these children showed stuttering-like behaviors. Although she tried to treat them, at least one child was reported to have continued stuttering for some time thereafter (Silverman, 1988). Tudor was remorseful about these results and regretted conducting this experiment (P. Zebrowski, personal communication, January 2001). Nonetheless, it reinforced Johnson's strong conviction, which he held throughout his career, that if a child is made self-conscious about his normal disfluencies, he may begin to stutter.

Communicative Failure and Anticipatory Struggle

The theoretical view of communicative failure and anticipatory struggle, developed by Oliver Bloodstein (1987, 1997; Bloodstein & Ratner, 2008), proposes that stuttering emerges from a child's experiences of frustration and failure when trying to talk. The child's original difficulty in talking may be the typical disfluencies of childhood, but other frustrations might instead be the provocation for stuttering. Many types of communication failure may lead the child to anticipate future difficulty with speech and thus increase tension. It is common, Bloodstein noted, to find delays in the development of articulation and language, cluttering, and other speech problems in the histories of children who begin to stutter. Table 6.2 lists some of the circumstances that Bloodstein suggested might cause some children to believe that speaking is difficult. If a child cannot make himself understood or is penalized for the way he talks, he may begin to tense his speech muscles and fragment his speech, reactions that become the core behaviors of the child's stuttering. And these behaviors in turn result in more frustration and failure in communication, which the child anticipates with dread.

Other aspects of the child's "internal" and "external" environments and his development also play important parts. The

TABLE 6.2 Experiences That May Make Some Children Believe Speaking Is Difficult

1. Normal disfluencies criticized by significant listeners
2. Delay in speech or language development
3. Speech or language disorders, including articulation problems, word finding difficulty, cerebral palsy, and voice problems
4. Difficult or traumatic experience reading aloud in school
5. Cluttering, especially if listeners frequently say, "Slow down" or "What?"
6. Emotionally traumatic events during which child tries to speak

child's personality may be perfectionistic, or he may harbor the need to live up to parental expectations. His family may have high standards for speech, find any speech abnormality unacceptable, or otherwise pressure the child to conform to standards beyond his reach. The presence or absence of these sorts of developmental and environmental pressures may cause some children to interpret an articulation difficulty, language problem, or disfluency as a failure, whereas other children only shrug it off.

This perspective on stuttering accounts for the wide variability of disfluency among children. Most normal children experience temporary frustration when learning to talk as they produce the mild fragmentations of speech we associate with normal disfluency. Children who stutter for just a few weeks may encounter unusual difficulty when first learning to talk but soon master the fundamentals and feel successful. Children who develop persistent stuttering may be those who repeatedly experience communication failure and grow up in an environment fraught with communicative pressure.

Here is a case—a client of mine—whose experiences illustrate some of the environmental pressures that some children who begin to stutter may experience. Susan grew up in the oil fields of Oklahoma, where her parents set themselves apart from the rest of the community by their aloof manner and precision of speech. They raised their children to feel that they were more cultured than their neighbors; in fact, Susan's father would often say, "We speak better than other people." Unfortunately, Susan's speech development was delayed. When she did begin talking in sentences at about age 3, she began to stutter with mild repetitions. When she started school, she worried that her father was embarrassed by her speech. Then she tried to speak better and began to push out the words instead of repeating the first parts of them. She soon developed severe secondary stuttering.

Although we have no way of knowing for sure, Susan's critical father may have been a major factor in the onset of her stuttering. However, many children who grow up in families that are critical of speech don't develop stuttering. Perhaps both a constitutional deficit, which led to her delayed speech development, and family pressure for perfect speech were necessary to produce Susan's stuttering. Neither may have been sufficient by itself to create stuttering, but together they may have been enough to tip the balance.

Capacities and Demands

A third interactional view of stuttering onset is proposed by the capacities and demands theory. Others have called this a "demands and capacities" view, but I prefer to put capacities first, because they exist in children before demands are placed on them. This view suggests that disfluencies as well as real stuttering emerge when a child's capacities for fluency are not equal to speech performance demands. Earlier in this chapter, I briefly discussed a narrow version of this view in describing the reduced capacity for internal modeling theory of stuttering. Andrews and colleagues (1983) stated that "whether one will become a stutterer depends on one's neurological capacity … and the demand posed by the speech act" (p. 239). These authors indicated that some demands come from the rapid development of language between ages 3 and 7 years. Other demands may come unintentionally from fast-talking parents, whose speech rates may be hard for a child to keep up with. Demands for speech performance sometimes come from within the child, sometimes from outside stimuli, and sometimes from both.

Joseph Sheehan (1970, 1975) expressed an early variation of the capacities and demands view when he wrote that "a child who has begun to stutter is probably a child who has had too many demands placed on him while receiving too little support" (Sheehan, 1975, p. 175). The demands that Sheehan pinpointed were primarily those of parents who have high standards and high expectations for their child's behavior. The support he refers to appears to be the environment's capacity to provide love, care, and encouragement. In addition, he believed that "there are persisting reasons for retaining the possibility that some kind of physiological predisposition for stuttering exists" (Sheehan, 1975, p. 144). Thus, Sheehan, who is best known for a theory that stuttering is learned, professed the view that stuttering is precipitated by the demands of the environment interacting with a predisposition to stutter.

Starkweather (1987) added considerable detail to the concept of capacities and demands as an explanation of stuttering onset and development. The normal child's capacities, he points out, include the potential for rapid movement of speech structures in well-planned sequences that are coordinated with the rhythms of his language. Demands on the child include those of her internal environment, such as her increasingly complex thoughts to be expressed, which require more sophisticated phonology, syntax, semantics, and pragmatic skills. The external environment often places demands on the child's fluency through parents' interactions. Parents may ask questions rapidly, interrupt frequently, and use complex sentences choked with big words. They may show impatience about the child's normal disfluencies and may make the child feel that she meets their expectations only when she performs at high levels. These kinds of interactions can stress any child but are likely to push a slowly developing child to try to speak beyond her capacity for fluency.

Because a child's capacities develop in spurts and environmental demands fluctuate, stuttering may wax and wane in cycles. A child may be highly fluent for a day or a week when he has mastered new speech and language skills and when external demands are low. But his stuttering may suddenly flare up if his capacities become strained by his efforts to use more advanced syntax or if the demands of the external environment suddenly increase when his fast-talking, interrupting, big-city cousins arrive for the Fourth of July holiday weekend.

The capacities and demands view provides a way to account not only for the day-to-day variability of stuttering within an individual but also for the great differences between one individual who stutters and another. As Adams (1990) pointed out, some children may grow up in an environment with normal levels of demand but have limited speech production capacities. Others may have normal capacities for speech production but grow up with excessive demands for rapid, fluent speech.

Treatment based on this model would begin with a careful evaluation of the child's capacities and the demands in her environment. Therapy would be designed to enhance capacities, decrease demands, and provide support for the child and her family while these changes are taking place. Starkweather and his colleagues have used this approach to formulate a sensible and effective program of stuttering prevention (Gottwald, 2010; Gottwald & Starkweather, 1984, 1985; Starkweather & Gottwald, 1990; Starkweather, Gottwald, & Halfond, 1990). Figure 6.6 depicts the ratios of capacities and demands in a child predisposed to stutter. In one view, the demands are greater than the child's capacities and stuttering occurs. In the second, the demands are lessened, and although capacities stay the same, stuttering is diminished.

To illustrate the capacities and demands view more fully, the following case is from my own experience. Gina was a bright, happy 7-year-old. Her mother had been a severe stutterer as a child, but through treatment and her own perseverance, she had largely recovered. When Gina began the second grade, she had no history of stuttering or any problem with school. Some time before Christmas that year, however, when her class was learning to read, Gina began to dislike school, and her mother soon discovered that she was having problems academically. After testing, it was discovered that she had a learning disability that had not been apparent before; however, once reading was required, it became obvious. As Gina struggled to cope with her reading problem throughout the rest of the second grade, she began to stutter. Over the course of the next 2 years, she stuttered noticeably but did not receive therapy. She was, however, given extra help for her reading disability. By the fourth grade, Gina was making headway with reading, and her stuttering had diminished to an inconsequential level without treatment.

Although there are various ways to account for the onset of Gina's stuttering and recovery, a capacities and demands view would see it this way: Gina was predisposed to stutter, but it lay dormant until she was faced with the challenge of reading. Reading, at least when first learned, involves a highly conscious use of linguistic processes, in contrast to the more automatic linguistic processing used in listening and speaking. Consequently, learning to read puts a heavy demand on the pool of available resources that are also used for speech and language processing. Such demands may result in a reduced capacity (i.e., fewer available resources) for speech production, which may result in disfluency for a vulnerable child. In this case, Gina did not seem to develop a persistent fear of speaking as a result of her stuttering. Thus, when she overcame her initial reading difficulty and reading became more automatic (i.e., demanded fewer resources), her available capacity for speech processes increased, and she "outgrew" her stuttering.

Once again, the reader is reminded that the capacities and demands view is a model for describing relationships that appear again and again but are not well understood. As such, its major function is to help students and clinicians organize the complex interrelationships of variables associated with stuttering into a set of principles that may guide its treatment and suggest hypotheses for research.

INTEGRATION OF PERSPECTIVES ON STUTTERING

In this section I draw together some of the theoretical views just described coupled with my own speculations to provide a description of the etiology and development of stuttering that can guide your assessment and treatment. Figure 6.7 depicts the major components of this perspective.

A Two-Stage Model of Stuttering

Many years ago, a child psychiatrist who stuttered, Charles Bluemel, observed that stuttering begins in most children as repetitions, of which they are hardly aware and to which they don't react. He thought that over time, many of these children become aware of their disfluencies and react to them by increasing the tension and tempo of their repetitions. These repetitions then become fast, irregular, and halting as children are bothered by them and do what they can to stop them. As they tense further, the repetitions become blocks and sometimes prolongations. This can happen overnight in some children and over a period of months for others. Bluemel (1932) called the beginning behaviors "primary" stuttering and the later reactions "secondary" stuttering. Brutten and Shoemaker (1967) also described stuttering as

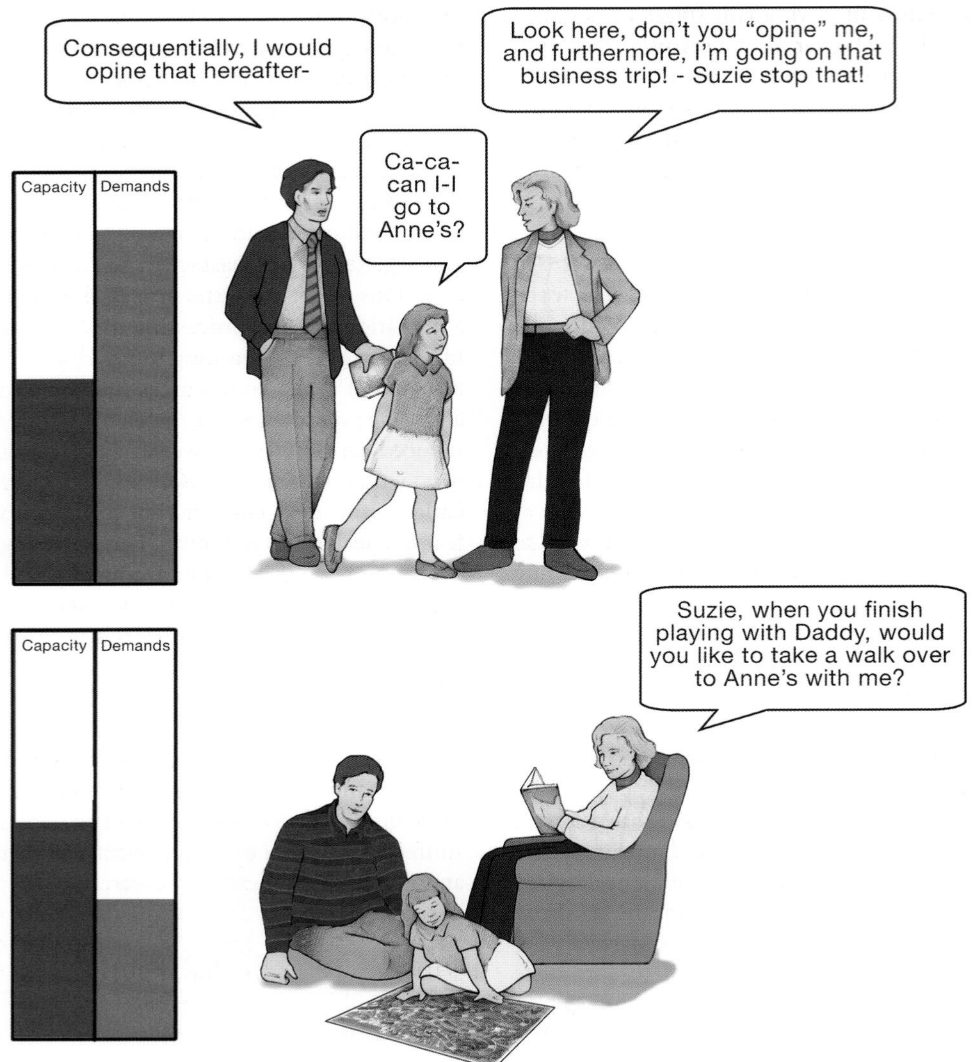

Figure 6.6 Two different ratios of capacities and demands and their hypothesized effects on fluency.

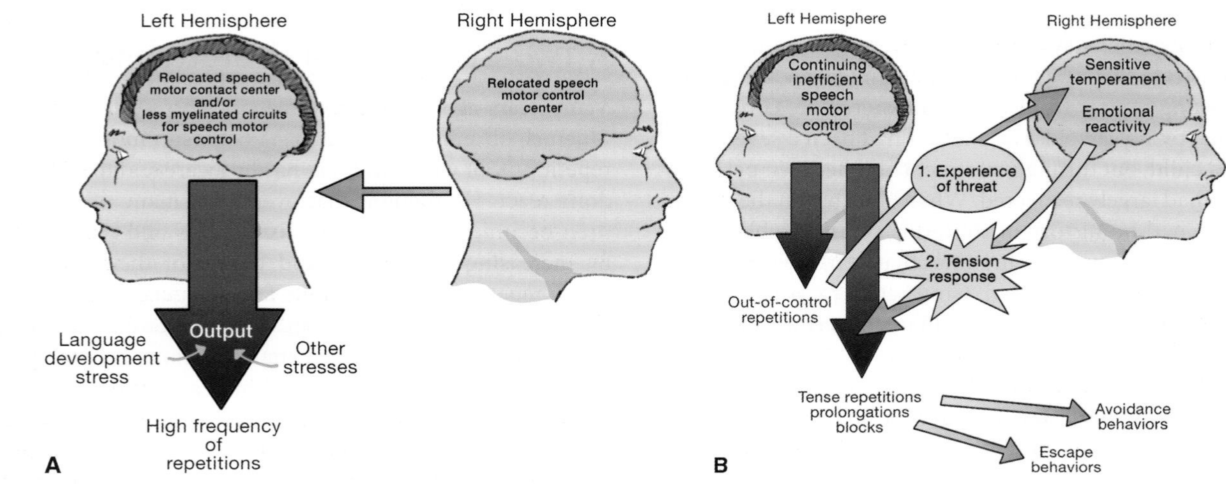

Figure 6.7 A two-factor view of stuttering: primary stuttering **(A)** and secondary stuttering **(B)**.

deriving from two factors or having two stages of development, as I mentioned in Chapter 5 on Learning. This view of stuttering as having two separate stages or components seems useful to me also and suggests the possibility that each component may have a different etiology. Understanding the nature of each stage may help us choose the most appropriate treatment—which may be different for each stage—for each individual who stutters.

There are reasons to be cautious about embracing this apparently simple view. For example, primary and secondary stages of stuttering may overlap in children because the forces that create these stages wax and wane and make it hard to place children clearly in one stage or another. Moreover, there is evidence that some children begin stuttering in the secondary stage—or at least with tense blocks (Van Riper, 1982; Yairi & Ambrose, 2005). Despite these exceptions, I will lay out out an integrated view of stuttering on the presumption that there are, for most children, two stages of stuttering, and I describe how the exceptions themselves can be explained in this view.

A Perspective on Primary Stuttering

In Chapters 2 and 3, I reviewed studies of genetics, brain structures and functions, and sensorimotor function. These studies support the view that individuals who stutter have differences in the way their brains process sensory information and produce motor output. Many of the brain imaging studies point to structural and functional anomalies in the language- and speech-generating areas of the left hemisphere with possible compensatory activity in homologous areas of the right.

The source of these differences in people who stutter appears to be the result of genetic inheritance or early brain damage. Either of these factors would affect how the brain grows during embryonic development or how the brain responds to injury. Let's look more closely at this process.

The development of speech and language networks in the brain begins—soon after conception—with the proliferation, migration, and differentiation of neural cells, a process guided by genetic predisposition and affected by external events, such as experience, injury, and disease (Chase, 1996). As neural cells continue to proliferate and differentiate, millions of synapses are formed, and pathways of communication emerge when clusters of cells send information back and forth in response to stimulation. Cells that communicate readily among themselves become self-organizing, functional neural circuits that perform various tasks. For example, after birth as an infant interacts with the outside world, groups of circuits and systems in the infant's brain bind together to form "maps" or representations of the outside world to help the infant process incoming sensory information and produce appropriate motor responses (Edelman, 1992).

If there are anomalies in speech and language areas of the left hemisphere due to inheritance or injury, the developing brain will deal with them in a number of different ways. The most common is by extensive anatomical reorganization, including growth of new fibers, new synapses, and entire new cortical tracts (Hadders-Algra & Forssberg, 2002). This reorganization would attempt to establish the functional circuits necessary for the development of spoken language in whatever structures are available. If reorganization involves relocation of these circuits to areas that have not naturally evolved to serve these circuits, or if reorganization entails neuronal groups being placed at an unusual distance from each other, these circuits will be both inefficient and vulnerable to disruption by other brain activities occurring in nearby areas. Vulnerability to disruption may occur if new circuits or even the original ones are insufficiently myelinated (insulated by a protective sheath), an outcome that would result in less-efficient transmission of neural signals. In fact, several researchers (Chang, Zhu, Choo, & Angstadt, 2015; Chow & Chang, 2017; Cykowski et al., 2010; Karlin, 1947) have suggested that inadequate **myelination** itself may be the reason why neural circuits for speech and language are inefficient or vulnerable to disruption in the brains of those who stutter.

Which neural circuits underlying spoken language may be inefficient or vulnerable to disruption? One of the functions that often seems to be atypical in stuttering is sensorimotor processing, particularly auditory-motor processing. Because auditory processing plays a major role in infants' use of the sounds of adult speech and the sounds of their own babbling, a dysfunction in this area would obviously have an influence on the development of interacting neuronal circuits for speech and language production. The sounds of adult speech give infants auditory targets to aim for when they are learning to speak. The sensorimotor activity in babbling helps a child develop internal models that specify what articulatory gestures are needed to produce desired auditory targets (Guenther, Ghosh, & Tourville, 2006; Hickok, Houde, & Rong, 2011; Hickok & Poeppel, 2007; Neilson & Neilson, 1987, 2005a, 2005b). Moreover, the auditory information from babbling allows the child to adapt his internal auditory-articulatory model to his rapidly growing speech production mechanism (Callan, Kent, Guenther, & Vorperian, 2000). Because these circuits are self-organizing, they may develop a variety of solutions to the auditory processing problem. Some individuals may use homologous right-hemisphere structures for auditory processing, others may continue to use inefficient areas of the left hemisphere, and still others may try to do both.

Many of the brain imaging studies described in Chapter 2 suggest problems in the very pathways that would be expected to support sensorimotor modeling for speech. The findings of Sommer, Koch, Paulus, Weiller, and Buchel (2002), Chow and Chang (2017), Chang, Erickson, Ambrose, Hasegawa-Johnson, and Ludlow (2008), Watkins, Smith, Davis, and Howell (2008), and Cykowski and colleagues (2010) suggest that individuals who stutter have less dense bidirectional fiber tracts between sensory and motor areas. If these fiber tracts are less dense, they are probably less efficient for rapid transmission of signals. Let's step through the process of speech production to see why this matters. Remember that according to the inverse internal model theory of speech production, when individuals plan to generate a word or phrase, they use the inverse internal model system (see Fig. 6.3) to generate motor commands (including making an efference copy—a copy used to rapidly produce a hypothetical output of the motor commands for error-correction purposes) based on the sensory target they are trying to produce. However, this inverse internal modeling system depends on continuous back-and-forth communication between sensory and motor areas. Sensory areas supply information about the current tension in muscles and positions of speech structures, while motor areas use this information to plan and carry out the motor commands to speech system muscles to produce speech output. Then sensory areas analyze both the efference copy of the motor plans as well as the actual speech output to correct errors and update the internal model (Guenther, 1994; Max et al., 2004; Neilson & Neilson, 1987).

Rapid information flow between sensory and motor areas is critical for accurate and fluent speech. If there is a delay in the information needed to generate the motor plans and execute them, repetitions may occur. This often happens after the speaker produces the first sound, syllable, or word. This sound, syllable, or word is usually fluent because it can be based on already obtained sensory information about the resting state of the speech system structures. But new information is needed to go forward—information required for production of the next sound, syllable, or word. However, that information is often delayed because it depends on rapid updating of information about the new state of the speech system (sensory analysis) and the rapid analysis of the sound just produced (comparison of efference copy of motor commands and feedback of actual output). Again, see Figure 6.3 for a description of the process.

This description of dyssynchrony in the assembly of components of speech and language production is intended only as a possible explanation of primary stuttering, which is a stage of stuttering usually characterized by relatively relaxed repetitions and occasional prolongations that typically occur, as Bloodstein (2001, 2002) and Bloodstein and Ratner (2008) have suggested, at the beginnings of phrases or sentences. As indicated in the paragraph above, the first sound or syllable may be fluent but the second is often a repeat of the first, li-like this. Most children who begin to stutter outgrow their disfluencies as their speech and language systems mature or as they develop effective ways to work around the problem. The work of Chow and Chang (2017) suggests that at least some of the children who do not outgrow their stuttering but persist in it have a slower growth rate in the myelination of white matter tracts interconnecting speech motor areas. This, they suggest, continues to interfere with the feedforward and feedback needed for fluent speech production in the inverse internal model of speech production described earlier.

Another factor that may be operating to make some children persist in stuttering as well as become more severe is the child's reactions to her primary stuttering. Why do some children react to their primary stuttering by increasing the speed and tension of their disfluencies? Why do they go on to develop the characteristics of secondary stuttering: blocks, escape behaviors, and avoidance reactions? The answer, I think, can be found in the temperament of these children, interacting with the processes of learning.

A Perspective on Secondary Stuttering

In earlier sections I mentioned that several authors (e.g., Brutten & Shoemaker, 1967) have suggested that the speeding up, tension, struggle, escape, and avoidance behaviors of **secondary stuttering** are a reaction to the simple repetitions and sometimes prolongations of sounds and syllables that often characterize stuttering when it first begins. I now want to make the case that the child's general temperament and his in-the-moment emotional responses interacting with learning can explain the behaviors of secondary stuttering.

Temperament

This section focuses on the personality or temperament of children and uses both "sensitive" and "reactive" to refer to the same thing: a behavioral and emotional style characterized by being easily aroused by novel stimuli, as well as a tendency to withdraw when confronted by unfamiliar people or situations. Kagan (1994a, 1994b) and Kagan, Reznick, and Snidman (1987) often use "inhibited" to describe the same traits. There is evidence, which was discussed in Chapter 3, that individuals (even adults) who stutter tend to have more sensitive or reactive temperaments (Anderson, Pellowski, & Conture, 2001; Eggers, 2012; Embrechts & Ebben, 1999; Fowlie & Cooper, 1978; Guitar, 2003; LaSalle, 1999; Ntrourou, Conture, & Walden, 2013; Ntrourou, DeFranco, Conture, & Walden, in review; Oyler & Ramig, 1995; Wakaba, 1998). If so, such reactivity may explain why some children who stutter eventually respond to their disfluencies by tightening their muscles, a reaction indicative of a response to a perceived threat, as I described in Chapter 5. Research on even nonstuttering children who are typically developing and have sensitive temperaments suggests that they respond to novel, threatening, or unfamiliar events by increasing their physical tension in the larynx—as measured acoustically in terms of decreased fluctuations in pitch (Coster, 1986; Kagan et al., 1987). The same has been shown with adults who stutter. As long ago as 1925, Lee Edward Travis assessed the effects of emotion on laryngeal tension in individuals who stutter (Travis, 1925). Using 19 subjects who stuttered and 18 who did not, Travis measured pitch fluctuations under two emotional conditions. First, he had subjects prolong an "ah" while relaxed. Then Travis induced emotional upset by questions and suggestions, followed by his firing a gun, after which he administered an electric shock. In the nonstuttering subjects, the emotional upset produced fluctuations in pitch, but in the subjects who stuttered, pitch changes over the few seconds of "ah" were markedly reduced during the emotional condition, suggesting to Travis that this was caused by "muscular fixation" in the larynx. We have seen similar results in our lab, but without firing guns or shocking our subjects.

If children who stutter have more sensitive temperaments than their peers, they may be more likely to increase their laryngeal tension (as well as elsewhere) in response to primary stuttering, which they experience as threatening because it seems out of their control and thus emotionally upsetting. This may be the mechanism that causes many children's disfluencies to change from easy, relaxed repetitions to tense repetitions and progressively more tense prolongations and blocks.[1]

Laryngeal tension as a result of threat has been indirectly suggested by a researcher interested in species-specific defense reactions. Fanselow (1994) indicates that in animals experiencing threat, the amygdala sends a signal to the periaqueductal area of the brain that triggers physically tense immobility (freezing). The periaqueductal area is known to be richly connected to laryngeal muscles (Jurgens, 1994) and is active for expression of emotion in animals (Jurgens, 1979). In Chapter 1, in my discussion of the types of core behaviors that characterize stuttering, I mentioned that many researchers believe that excess laryngeal tension occurs once stuttering blocks appear. I think it may occur to some extent in repetitions and prolongations as well.

The just-mentioned increases in physical tension may be part of a larger defensive response that is triggered more easily in individuals with reactive temperaments. In describing his **behavioral inhibition system**, Gray (1987) proposes that when individuals experience fear, their innate response is freezing (i.e., widespread muscular contractions that produce tense and silent immobility), flight (i.e., speeded up activity to escape), or avoidance. Gray (1987) indicates that these unconditioned responses may occur rapidly without intervening autonomic arousal, arising from the central nervous system substrate underlying the increased muscle tension, increased tempo, and escape behaviors and avoidance behaviors (that characterize secondary stuttering). It is notable also that Gray suggests that the way an individual's behavioral inhibition system affects behavior is influenced by temperament. The more reactive individuals are, the more they will engage in freezing, flight, or avoidance responses when experiencing fear. LeDoux (2015), commenting on Gray's behavior inhibition system, suggests that, in his view, rapid defensive responses are made to nonconscious threat rather than conscious fear. LeDoux makes this distinction because he believes that the response is nonconscious, whereas responses to fear are conscious. Nonconscious responses are part of the individual's innate repertoire to enable survival and are thus very rapid. Conscious fear responses, which take longer because they require conscious processing, can create anxiety when there is uncertainty about a threat.

Further evidence of a neurological substrate underlying the characteristics of secondary behavior is provided by the research of Davidson (1984), Kinsbourne (1989), and Kinsbourne and Bemporad (1984), which was described in Chapter 3. They propose that the right hemisphere is specialized for emotions that accompany avoidance, withdrawal, and arrest of ongoing behavior, whereas the left hemisphere is specialized for emotions that are associated with approach, exploration, and release of ongoing behavior. Thus, it can be argued that individuals who stutter and are more reactive are more prone to behaviors regulated by right-hemisphere emotions. This argument is supported by the findings of Calkins and Fox (1994) and Davidson (1995) who reported that sensitive children (nonstutterers) are right hemisphere dominant for emotion. Their research may also explain why secondary behaviors develop in the forms they do in many stutterers. Those beginning stutterers who develop tension responses may be more sensitive individuals whose innate defensive mechanisms are triggered more easily because of their right-hemisphere dominance for emotions. It is possible that some of the excess activity seen in the right hemisphere of those who stutter, described in Chapter 2, may be related to activation of behavioral inhibition. Some support for this idea comes from brain imaging research by Neef et al. (2017). These researchers demonstrated that the nucleus accumbens in the right hemisphere is larger in individuals who stutter than in matched controls. Because the nucleus accumbens is considered a bridge between limbic and motor systems (Mogenson, Jones, & Yim, 1980), the larger nucleus accumbens in those who stutter could be a link between reactive temperament and motor dysfunction in stuttering—as either a precipitator or consequence of experiences of stuttering.

The notion of greater emotional reactivity in children who stutter is supported by a study of 65 children who stuttered and 56 children who did not by Karrass and colleagues (2006). Those researchers found that compared to nonstuttering children, children who stutter have greater emotional reactivity, less emotional regulation, and poorer attention regulation. These authors suggest that this combination of traits contributes to the development of stuttering in a "reverberant" fashion. Reacting to what I would term "primary stuttering," these children have a strong emotional response to their primary stutters and they are unable to regulate this emotion. This in turn makes them stutter more (and more severely), and they have even stronger emotional responses to the more severe stutters and on and on.

The importance of emotion in secondary (persistent) childhood stuttering is also supported by genetic evidence. As I indicated in Chapter 2, mutations in several genes, including GNPTG, have been linked to persistent stuttering, and it

[1]The non-stuttering, sensitive children in the study by Coster may have retained their fluency because the threat in their situation was not related to speech, but was induced by separating them from their parents.

is also known that this same gene influences the development of the cerebellum and the hippocampus (Kang et al., 2010). The cerebellum is known for its role in motor control and in emotional regulation (e.g., Schmahmann & Caplan, 2006). The hippocampus is also a structure that influences emotion and is a key component of Gray's behavioral inhibition system, described previously. Thus, many lines of evidence converge on the link between secondary stuttering and emotion.

I've described many of the temperamental and emotional factors related to secondary stuttering as though they were completely within the child. But of course the child interacts with a complex environment, and this influences temperament and emotion, which in turn influence stuttering. An example that comes to mind is a girl and her mother in a study of parent-child interaction that we published many years ago (Guitar, Kopff-Schaefer, Donahue-Kilburg, & Bond, 1992). We computed correlations between several variables in the mother's talking and the girl's primary stuttering and secondary stuttering. What we found led us to surmise that different aspects of the mother's conversation affected the two types of stutters differentially. The mother's speech rate was highly correlated with the girl's primary stutters but not with her secondary stutters. On the other hand, the mother's nonaccepting comments were highly correlated with the girl's secondary stuttering but not her primary stuttering. We speculated that when her mother made nonaccepting comments to her, the girl reacted with negative emotion (nonconscious response to threat), triggering secondary stuttering. We also speculated that when the mother talked fast, the girl tried to keep up, but because of an inefficient speech processing system, she stuttered with the easy repetitions of primary stuttering.

Learning

Even though I described learning factors in stuttering in Chapter 5, here here I will recap the role of learning to include it in this theoretical perspective on stuttering.

The preceding information on temperament suggested that some children who begin to stutter are more reactive or sensitive than others. This reactivity may contribute to why learning affects some individuals more than others. For all of us, emotional arousal enhances learning. Emotional events are etched into the brain more strongly than neutral ones. Think about how well you can remember what you were doing when you found out about a very exciting or upsetting event. For example, many people can remember vividly what they were doing when they heard about the planes crashing into the twin towers of the World Trade Center in New York City on September 11, 2001. The strength of emotional memories is enhanced even further in people with more reactive limbic systems, which may account for why some people suffer posttraumatic stress syndrome and others do not (e.g., LeDoux, 2002, 2015).

This link between reactivity and learning has been shown in adults who stutter. A small but important study by Arenas and Zebrowski (2013) demonstrated the link between emotional reactivity, classical conditioning, and effects on speech production. Three individuals who stuttered were compared with three who were typical speakers in a paradigm that assessed the **autonomic reactivity** of subjects (skin conductance response) and their susceptibility to classical conditioning (reaction to stimuli linked to a loud noise). The individuals who stuttered had a significantly greater autonomic response to the aversive stimulus and they showed significantly greater susceptibility to classical conditioning. Moreover, the subjects who stuttered (but not the typical speakers) demonstrated speech production anomalies in acoustic measures taken in speech probes during the conditioning. These findings suggest that individuals who stutter may be emotionally reactive, highly conditionable, and likely to show disturbances in their vulnerable speech production systems.

Returning to children just beginning to stutter, it seems to me that children with reactive temperaments are more likely to respond to the multiple repetitions of primary stuttering with tension, escape, and avoidance and are also much more likely to store their stuttering memories indelibly. Such reactions and memories can snowball. The child's natural defensive response to a repetition that feels out of control (or to parent reactions that are perceived as negative) is to tense his muscles. This increased tension soon makes the stutter last longer, which increases his feeling that he is helpless and then triggers a bigger threat response that includes more tension. The child's reactive amygdala mediates the storage of unpleasant memories of stuttering, largely on a nonconscious level. At the same time, another part of the limbic system, the hippocampus, stores information about the situations in which stuttering occurs (e.g., whom the child was talking to, what word was being said, where it happened). These contextual cues cause stuttering to spread rapidly from isolated experiences to more and more repeated experiences in similar contexts and eventually to many other situations.

I suggest that children with reactive temperaments are not only more likely to learn to increase tension when they anticipate or experience stuttering but are also more likely to engage in other components of the behavioral inhibition system. These include increases in tempo, other aspects of escape behaviors, and a wide array of avoidances. Thus, these children quickly develop secondary symptoms, such as eye blinks and changing words, to escape from the moment of stuttering or to avoid anticipated stuttering.

Classical conditioning occurs rapidly in these children, but unlearning is a much slower and more difficult process. There is evidence that emotional memories are stored permanently, and even when new behaviors replace them, the original emotions and learned behaviors may reappear under stress (Ayres, 1998). When clinicians work with individuals who have secondary stuttering, they need to keep in mind the strength and persistence of behaviors learned through classical conditioning. They should also keep in mind that learning is highly contextual (e.g., Bouton, 2016). New behaviors will have to be learned as new responses to the stimuli that elicited the old responses. And new behaviors will have to be carefully generalized to many different contexts.

Two Predispositions for Stuttering

This is a recap to remind you that primary and secondary stuttering may have two constitutional predispositions: one for primary stuttering and one for secondary stuttering. As may be evident, the most common occurrence is for a child to have a predisposition for primary stuttering that is resolved through neural maturation or reorganization—this accounts for the 70 percent or so of children who recover naturally. It is also possible for a child's primary stuttering to continue into adulthood and for secondary behaviors never to emerge. Think about the evidence that some individuals have great delays in myelination of white matter tracts in speech production areas of the brain. But some of them may have very nonreactive temperaments. These adults may simply be considered highly disfluent, rather than people who stutter. But other individuals who develop stuttering instead of high levels of typical disfluency may have been born with more reactive temperaments, and thus may respond strongly to primary stuttering are at the mercy of classical conditioning, increased tension in their stutters, and the vagaries of the environment. The increased stuttering leads to the operant and avoidance conditioning underlying escape, and avoidance behaviors that characterize secondary stuttering. I believe that neither of these predispositions is "all or nothing." I think that a child may have a little or a lot of either. For instance, an adolescent may have a substantial amount of repetitions in his speech but only occasionally show tension, escape, or avoidance behaviors. Or a child may start stuttering suddenly at age 3, with severe repetitive stutters that quickly result in struggle, tension, escape, and avoidance. Perhaps that child has only a little predisposition for primary stuttering but a substantial predisposition for secondary stuttering. This continuum for stuttering agrees with most clinicians' observations that we see a wide range of severity, from mild to very severe, with some who stutter having little avoidance and others having a great deal. I also notice that outside the clinic, there are many individuals whose "stuttering" is so mild that they don't recognize it in themselves and other lay persons don't notice it either.

The possibility of two predispositions for stuttering may also shed light on such phenomena as neurogenic stuttering, which are the disfluencies that sometimes appear in persons with neurological diseases or injuries. The changes in the brain that may occur as part of a neurological problem may give rise to a dyssynchrony in speech and language production processing that is similar to that of primary stuttering. On the other hand, the changes in temperament that sometimes occur with brain injury (e.g., Kinsbourne, 1989) may, in a few cases, give rise to disfluencies that are more characteristic of secondary stuttering.

There is support in genetic research for two (or more) predispositions in individuals who do not naturally recover from stuttering. After an analysis of many children who stutter for some period of time in their lives, Ambrose, Cox, and Yairi (1997) concluded that persistent and recovered stuttering are not two different forms of the disorder. Both persistent and recovered stutterers appear to have genetic factors related to the onset of stuttering. Those children who persisted in stuttering (i.e., continued to stutter for more than three years), however, have additional genetic factors, related to the persistency of the disorder. The additional genetic contributions may be related to the delayed rate of maturation in the white matter tracts interconnecting speech motor areas. But also, the additional genetic factors may give rise to a reactive temperament, making it more likely that these children will become frustrated, have other emotional reactions to their stuttering, and thus develop secondary/persistent stuttering. This connection between a child reacting to his stuttering and the persistence of the stuttering is reflected in Van Riper's beliefs that "... most children who begin to stutter become fluent perhaps because of maturation or because they do not react to their ... repetitions, or prolongations by struggle and avoidance ... [while] those who struggle or avoid because of frustration or penalties will probably continue to stutter all the rest of their lives no matter what kind of therapy they receive" (Van Riper, 1990, p. 317).

Indeed, as Ambrose et al. (1997) suggest, there may be more than two predispositions in stuttering. The factors that cause a child to have a threat-based defensive reaction (tension response) to primary stuttering may also cause another child to react the same way to lack of intelligibility or difficulties in word finding, for example. Communicative failures may lead to anticipatory struggle (Bloodstein & Ratner, 2008), as described earlier in this chapter. However, no matter how many predispositions a child may have, the chance of his actually developing primary or secondary stuttering may be enhanced or diminished by both developmental and environmental factors.

Interactions with Developmental Factors

In this section, I describe three ways in which aspects of children's development may interact with the two predispositions to trigger or exacerbate stuttering. You will see elements of the capacities and demands theory of stuttering in this section.

The first interaction is with the demands of language development and a predisposition for primary stuttering. Consider a child who begins to acquire speech with dysfunctional or inefficient speech and language networks. The functional plasticity of the child's brain may allow these pathways to reorganize or repair themselves so that the child processes spoken language more efficiently as he strives to communicate. However, the exponential growth of the child's speech and language at this very time may compete for cerebral and other brain resources, straining or exceeding the child's capacity to handle the demands of both reorganization and advancing language, at the same time. To see what this may be like, imagine yourself as a student who has let part of the semester slip by without studying. After bombing the first two exams, you resolve to reorganize your study habits and catch up, but just then, your professors decide to pile on even more work than before. Like the child, you may or may not be able to accommodate the professor's increasing demands at the same time you are spending energy to reorganize.

A second interaction will be the maturation of the brain with a predisposition for primary stuttering. Some individuals will have an earlier maturation of the brain or a natural flexibility to respond to anomalies in the wiring for spoken language. Girls, for example, are more likely to recover from early stuttering—either naturally or with treatment, probably because of their inherently greater organizational plasticity and their more widely distributed language centers (Guitar et al., 2015; Shaywitz et al., 1995). Some males may also be genetically endowed with more flexibility than average for reorganizing their cerebral circuitry and thus may recover more readily than others.

The third type of interaction will occur when a child has normal neural circuitry for spoken language but has a constitutionally inhibited temperament. Typical developmental challenges for most children include some frustration at not being able to speak as fast or with the same complexity as adults and older children in the family. The child may not only be frustrated but embarrassed at his inability to produce more advanced speech and language. Social-emotional development takes the child through some stressful times. All of these typical experiences may produce increased tension, escape, and avoidance behaviors associated with speech. Based on my clinical experience, I suspect that some children fitting this description might be hesitant to speak and may be referred for a stuttering evaluation but would not manifest the typical signs of stuttering. Their hesitancies may consist of long pauses, phrase repetitions, or both when their right-hemisphere proclivity toward avoidance, withdrawal, and arrest of ongoing behavior manifests itself while they are speaking. Such hesitancies may diminish in time as myelination of neural circuits and systems serving speech production continues.

Interactions with Environmental Factors

Here I consider the influence of the environment on anomalous speech and language neural networks (predisposition for primary stuttering) and on constitutional predispositions for inhibited temperaments and their effect on learning (predisposition for secondary stuttering).

Interactions of Anomalous Neural Networks with Environmental Factors

As a child's developing central nervous system adapts to the inherited or acquired differences in her neural substrates for speech and language, the environment plays a role through various listeners' responses to the child's emerging speech and language skills. Obviously, a child's family will have the most opportunities to provide acceptance and support. The accommodations they can provide, such as accepting reactions toward the child's stuttering, using slower speech rates, fewer interruptions, and dedicated one-on-one listening time, may foster adaptations of the child's inefficient, dyssynchronous neural networks. At least this environment will not stress the child's speech and language production system and will probably enable the child to develop her own adapted rate of speech and language output. In contrast, an environment with evident disapproval of the child's stuttering, many interruptions, rapid conversational give and take, demands for recitations, and little time for the child to talk may "overdrive" the child's immature speech and language production system, produce an excess of disfluencies, and inhibit the successful adaptation of the child's system to its original anomalous wiring.

Interactions of Temperament with Environmental Factors

The work of Calkins (1994), Kagan and Snidman (1991), and others suggests that families can have a strong influence on temperament. As Calkins and Fox (1994) expressed it, "the child's interactions with a parent provide the context for learning skills and strategies for managing emotional reactivity." In addition, the environmental factors that I have called "life events" can also influence the development of temperament. As noted earlier, Kagan (1994b) suggested that certain life events could cause a child who is not particularly reactive to become more reactive and inhibited.

Implications for Treatment

In some ways, this section will mirror the implications for treatment described in Chapter 5 where I discussed the unlearning that must take place for treatment to be effective. However, here we also consider treatment of primary stuttering that is not so much unlearning as it is prevention of the learning that creates secondary stuttering.

Preschool Children

Preschool children often have a milder form of stuttering—or at least stuttering that has not been subjected to years of learning. Much of stuttering at this age is primary stuttering that results from the dyssynchronies in brain development described earlier.

The first aim of treatment for this age should be to maximize these children's fluent speech, by creating an environment filled with models of slower speaking rate, including pauses. Additionally, the environment should also reduce pressure on the child's speech by asking fewer questions, not interrupting, and giving the child adequate attention when he's speaking. These strategies can help the child take the time needed to coordinate the elements of speech with the components of language to produce a fluent utterance.

The second aim in treating preschoolers is to prevent the child from having a defensive reaction to his disfluencies. Such a reaction would trigger the tension response. Preventing this should be done by helping both the parents or caregivers and the child to be comfortable with and accepting of the repetitive stuttering. The parents can be guided to understand that most children recover from their stuttering and that even those children who don't recover completely can be given treatment that will minimize its effect. Parents, in turn, can reassure the child, if he seems frustrated or upset by his stuttering. Just a casual comment like "It's ok. Lots of kids get stuck sometimes on words" may be enough. Parents' demeanor at this moment can be relaxed and convey, "It's no big deal."

School-Age Children

Treatment for a school-age child should begin with an assessment of how much tension the child has added to her stuttering. Are her moments of stuttering often characterized by tense postures and physical struggle that are the result of her reacting to the threat of runaway repetitions to fear of being "trapped" in a stutter? Does she use extra movements or sounds to break free of her stutters? Do you hear and see "starters" or other behaviors before stutters or does she talk "all around Robin Hood's barn" to dodge possible stutters? Excess physical tension, as well as escape and avoidance behaviors, suggest that the child is reacting to her stuttering, probably with both nonconscious defensive reactions and conscious fear of stuttering. If this is the case, treatment should focus on (1) reducing the fear of stuttering to reduce reactions to it and (2) practice talking fluently so that the child develops confidence that she will be fluent. On the other hand, if the child's stuttering is mostly tension free and there are few, if any, escape or avoidance behaviors, treatment can help the child practice fluent speech and develop confidence in herself as a fluent speaker. In both cases, generalization of new responses must be assiduously pursued to ensure that increased fluency is maintained.

Adolescents and Adults

An adult or adolescent who needs treatment will probably stutter with excess physical tension, accompanied by escape and avoidance behaviors. At some point these individuals benefit from training in being aware of and increasing their fluent speech. However, the first goal must be to diminish their defensive reactions and fear that trigger the excess tension and the escape and avoidance behaviors. In the context of an accepting and strong clinical relationship, the individual must confront and explore his stuttering behaviors, attitudes and feelings. He must understand that what he does, thinks, and feels about stuttering is essentially learned behavior and can be unlearned. The clinician guides the adolescent or adult to stutter easily, without avoidances prior to the speech attempt, without the excess physical tension, and without trying to "blast out" of the moment of stuttering but instead remain relaxed as he eases the word out. The clinician also helps the client learn that most listeners are patient rather than rejecting. Some of this learning occurs when the clinician accepts whatever stuttering happens as they are working on it together. Some occurs because the clinician accepts the client as he is. And some occurs when the clinician pseudo-stutters in public and the client can see for himself that listeners are able to accept stuttering and that the person stuttering can be calm as he stutters. Much more detail is given in Section 2 on treatment.

Accounting for the Evidence

Let us now turn to the research findings and clinical observations for which these views of stuttering must account.

Stuttering Occurs in All Cultures

The fact that stuttering is universal should not be unexpected because it depends less on culture than on basic biological variations of the human brain. Many other disorders, such as dyslexia and specific language impairment, as well as such personality differences as sensitive temperament, are associated with atypical activity of the central nervous system and are also universal. Children's responses to their primary stuttering may be slightly different in cultures that are more or less accepting of differences. Nonetheless, children in most cultures would show reactions when their articulators suddenly go out of control.

Stuttering is a Low-Incidence Disorder

The fact that the prevalence of stuttering is relatively low may be a consequence of chronic stuttering resulting from a combination of at least two biological predispositions, the co-occurrence of which does not happen frequently. In addition, evidence suggests that the predisposition related to the development of neural circuitry for speech often resolves because of neural growth.

Stuttering Does Not Begin with the Onset of Speech

Why does stuttering usually begin only after fluency at the one- and two-word stage has been achieved? Most researchers agree that stuttering emerges first from disruptions caused by a child's inefficient neural networks for speech and language processing. Perhaps these networks can handle the relatively simple processing required for simple words and phrases. But once children begin to reorganize their language functions from a lexical to a grammatical-rules basis and try out more complicated syntax, their inefficient neural organization breaks down. An added demand on their planning system is that the shift from one- to two-word utterances requires the use of a more complex prosody that is a bigger challenge to those inefficient networks (Kent, 1984; Packman & Attanasio, 2010; Perkins et al., 1991; Wingate, 1988).

Stuttering Sometimes Begins with Tense Blocks, but Often with Repetitions

There are children who begin to stutter with tense blocks that did not follow a period of repetitions and occasional prolongations. With a few children, the act of speech becomes so threatening that a dramatic tension response (blocks) is the first sign of stuttering. In other cases, repetitions change so quickly to tense blocks that listeners don't remember that the repetitions occurred first. I have recently been working with a 2-year-old girl who showed excessive squeezing and tension in her stutters after only a few hours of stuttering in a repetitive pattern. But in general, the first sign of stuttering is repetition of sounds, syllables, or single-syllable words. As we have said earlier, these repetitions appear to be the result of anomalies in the neural networks for speech production that are not able to have the next syllable or word ready "to go out the door." Thus, the preceding unit is repeated until the system is ready to produce the following one.

Stuttering Severity Changes over Time

The course of development of stuttering seems to be determined in part by the biological responses of the child to uncontrollable repetitions and the classical and operant learning that follow. In more severe children, there may be a neuroanatomical basis for more frequent and persistent disfluencies (Chow & Chang, 2017) to which these responses are made. Details on the development of stuttering are discussed in Chapter 7.

Stuttering Appears as Repetitions, Prolongations, and Blocks

Very often, the earliest signs of most childhood stuttering are relatively loose repetitions of syllables. These may arise from a breakdown in the function of neural circuits for sensorimotor control of speech output. Repetitions may occur simply because there is a lag in the readiness of the next part of a word or sentence, although the impulse or pressure to continue speaking is strong. The repetitions sometimes become more rapid and end in prolongations, as the child responds to the threat of being unable to speak with increases in speed and tension. As the child tries to cope—consciously and nonconsciously—with being unable to continue speaking, tension increases and prolongations begin to show increases in pitch. Not long after, the tension results in momentary blockages of speech altogether.

In those cases in which the earliest signs of stuttering are characterized by tension and blocking (Van Riper, 1982), an emotional response may be primary. As Van Riper suggested, these may be children whose onset is very sudden, resulting usually after an emotionally difficult period or traumatic emotional stress.

Not All Stutterers Have Relatives Who Stuttered

How do we account for both the genetic transmission of stuttering and that evidence of genetic transmission is lacking in some cases? Genetic transmission of stuttering in many cases may be through the two factors I just described: **anomalous neural organization** for speech and sensitive temperament. In some cases of childhood stuttering, genetic transmission may seem unlikely because no other family members seem to be affected. However, it may occur because persistent stuttering appears to require both predisposing factors. Some family members may inherit one factor and some the other, but unless both factors are inherited by the same individual, persistent stuttering may not develop. Another reason for the absence of stuttering in other family members may be that the predisposing factors were the result not of genetic inheritance but of environmental factors affecting fetal or early childhood development that created the neural substrate for stuttering. Moreover, such anomalous speech and language circuitry may create language, learning, or phonological problems in other family members. Remember that the unfolding of the genetic blueprint is extensively influenced by environmental factors and by chance. Thus, the anomalous circuitry in one child may result in stuttering, but in an uncle or grandmother, it may have resulted in an articulation disorder or learning problem.

Stuttering Is More Common in Boys Than in Girls

I suspect that the reason more boys stutter than girls is that the genetic blueprints for neural organization of speech and language differ between boys and girls and may be more flexible in females (Burman, Bitan, & Booth, 2008; Shaywitz et al., 1995). Neuroplasticity of the human brain is greatest in the first few years of life, and this neuroplasticity probably diminishes after puberty. Neuroplasticity permits reorganization of neural pathways and, in many cases, recovery. Karlin (1947) advanced another explanation of why more girls recover early from stuttering. He postulated that delayed myelinization of nerve fibers in speech processing areas was a possible explanation of stuttering and cited research that myelinization of nerve fibers is more advanced in girls than in boys of the same age. The research by Choo et al. (2016) confirms Karlin's hypothesis, demonstrating a relationship between deficiencies in language performance and less dense white matter tracts in the left hemisphere (less myelination) in boys who stutter but not girls.

Many Conditions Reduce or Eliminate Stuttering

Conditions that temporarily ameliorate stuttering, such as singing or speaking in a rhythm, probably improve fluency by giving speech and language processes more time or an external organizing stimulus to aid speech production. These conditions may also involve other parts of the brain rather than those anomalous networks used inefficiently for typically spoken language. Research using neuroimaging has shown that speech-language areas of the brain that are typically dysfunctional during stuttering actually function normally during conditions that ameliorate fluency (e.g., Chang, Kenney, Loucks, & Ludlow, 2009; Toyomura, Fujii, & Kuriki, 2011).

Individuals Who Stutter Often Have Poorer Performance on Sensory and Motor Tasks

How about differences in performance between groups of stutterers and nonstutterers? As suggested earlier in this chapter, the wide range of performance on language tests, school achievement tests, and tests of sensorimotor ability by groups of stutterers may reflect the generally lower, but wide range of delays and deviations in the neural substrates for these abilities that led to their inefficient processing of speech and language. In fact, the neural substrates of these performance differences were demonstrated to be associated with poorer white matter integrity (less myelination) in left hemisphere auditory-motor areas (Choo et al., 2016).

Other Research Findings and Clinical Observations That Should Be Accounted for

Other characteristics of stuttering that I have said should be explained by any view of stuttering, such as the influence of developmental and environmental factors, are explicitly addressed in earlier parts of this chapter. Some characteristics, findings, and observations are explained more easily than others. Those that are not accounted for in detail (such as the strong effect of rhythmic stimuli on stuttering) should not be ignored. They are a reality and are hard-edged facts that should reshape any theoretical view until it is more fully explanatory. Can you think of any more?

SUMMARY

- Several theoretical perspectives have been proposed to account for constitutional factors in stuttering. They include views of stuttering: (1) as an anomaly of how the brain is organized for speech and language; (2) as a disorder of timing of the sequential movements for speech; (3) as a result of deficits in the internal modeling process used to control speech production; (4) as a disorder of spoken language production; and (5) as a result of physiological tremor in speech musculature. The first four of these views focus on dysfunctions of cortical and subcortical mechanisms that control the planning and production of speech and language to produce the initial repetitions and prolongations of early stuttering; the fifth view targets neuromuscular malfunctions that may explain the tension and tremors of secondary stuttering.
- Theoretical perspectives concerning developmental and environmental factors include (1) the diagnosogenic theory, which implicates the listener's response to the disfluencies of the child; (2) the anticipatory struggle theory, which suggests that a child may develop stuttering as a result of negative anticipation of speaking after he has had frustrating or embarrassing experiences in communicating; and (3) the capacities and demands theory, which postulates that stuttering arises when the child's capacities for rapid, fluent utterances are unequal to the demands within the child himself or within the environment.
- In this chapter, I elaborated a two-stage etiological model of stuttering that I first proposed in a chapter on children's stuttering and emotions (Guitar, 1997) and that owes much to Bluemel (1957) and Brutten and Shoemaker (1967). The first stage is primary stuttering, which involves repetitions that are frequently the first signs of stuttering. These signs are thought to be the result of a constitutional factor: a dyssynchrony at some level of the speech and language production process. The second stage is secondary stuttering, which involves the tension, struggle, escape, and avoidance behaviors that are often present in persistent stuttering. These behaviors are proposed to be the result of a separate constitutional factor—a reactive temperament that triggers a defense response from the behavioral inhibition system and that makes the individual more emotionally conditionable than the average speaker.

STUDY QUESTIONS

1. What are the differences between the Geschwind and Galaburda (1985) theory of stuttering and the Webster (1993a) view?
2. Compare Kent's (1984) view of stuttering as a disorder of timing with the Geschwind and Galaburda (1985) theory.

3. Both Neilson and Neilson's view of stuttering and one of Max and colleagues' (2004) hypotheses about stuttering suggest that repetitions occur because of a problem with the internal models used for speech production. What is the difference between the cause of repetitions in each view?
4. The study by Kelly et al. (1995) reviewed in this chapter suggested that tremors don't appear in younger children who stutter but do appear in older children. Why would this be?
5. Table 6.2 lists experiences that may generate stuttering in some children because the experiences have led children to believe speaking is difficult. Add as many other hypothetical experiences as you can to this list.
6. A capacities and demands view of stuttering in children would lead to a therapy strategy of enhancing a child's capacities. What are some examples of what capacities in a child you could strengthen to reduce stuttering? Describe how you would do this.
7. What is the relationship between a sensitive temperament and a high ability to be conditioned?
8. I have suggested there may be two predispositions for persistent stuttering—one for primary stuttering and one for secondary stuttering. How, according to this view, would primary stuttering lead to secondary stuttering?
9. There is strong evidence that girls are more likely than boys to recover from stuttering and are therefore less likely to become persistent stutterers. Is this because girls are more likely to recover quickly from primary stuttering or because their primary stuttering is less likely to trigger secondary stuttering?
10. In this chapter I suggested that there are two stages of stuttering—primary and secondary. What are the signs and symptoms of each, and what is the suggested etiology of each?

SUGGESTED PROJECTS

1. The view of stuttering as a problem of the "internal modeling" process in speech production is a complex idea. Read the article by Max and colleagues (2004) and make a class presentation about their full theoretical model, explaining it in as clear and simple a way as possible.
2. Read the article entitled "Resources—A Theoretical Stone Soup" (Navon, 1984) and use the arguments in it to evaluate the capacities and demands theory in this chapter.
3. Wendell Johnson's "diagnosogenic" view of stuttering led to a master's thesis that tried to create stuttering in orphans in 1939. In 2003, this thesis was the topic of a controversy that centered on the ethics of trying to induce stuttering in children. Using the Internet, research this controversy, using "Monster Study" as a keyword. Make a presentation or write a paper on the ethics of this research, given the fact that it was conducted more than 50 years ago when the ethical climate was markedly different than it is now.
4. Pick a theory of stuttering—either one described in the first two sections of this chapter or one you have found elsewhere—and evaluate how it can account for the basic facts about stuttering enumerated in Chapter 1.
5. Go to Guitar and McCauley (2010) and read two chapters concerning specific interventions related to a specific age group of people who stutter. Identify which theories addressed here are cited and how they appear to impact the developers of each intervention approach.

SUGGESTED READINGS

Brutten, E. J., & Shoemaker, D. J. (1967). *The modification of stuttering*. Englewood Cliffs, NJ: Prentice-Hall, Inc.

This is a classic book in the field of stuttering. It describes a theory of stuttering that ascribes the initial symptoms of childhood stuttering to the effect of anxiety on fluency and ascribes the later symptoms to learning. The authors go on to suggest therapeutic approaches that derive from their model.

Gray, J. A. (1987). *The psychology of fear and stress* (2nd ed.). Cambridge, UK: Cambridge University Press.

Gray's experimental work and his theoretical model of a behavioral inhibition system are clearly described here. Some of the book (those parts dealing with the effects of pharmacological agents on the brain) is for specialized readers. Much of it, however, is a readable exposition on the biological basis of learning, stress, and fear. Because this is the second edition of a popular book, I hope a new edition will be available soon.

Guitar, B., & McCauley, R. (2010). How to use this book. In B. Guitar, & R. McCauley (Eds.), *Treatment of stuttering*. Baltimore, MD: Lippincott Williams & Wilkins.

This chapter describes in user-friendly language what a theory is and how it can help researchers and clinicians.

Kagan, J., Reznick, J. S., & Snidman, N. (1987). The physiology and psychology of behavioral inhibition in children. *Child Development, 58*, 1459–1473.

This article discusses the findings of Kagan and his colleagues that behaviorally inhibited children show high levels of laryngeal tension. Neurophysiological mechanisms are also discussed, as well as possible genetic and environmental contributions. This article is recommended for those interested in the hypothesis that behavioral inhibition may be a component in some stuttering.

LeDoux, J. (1996). *The emotional brain: The mysterious underpinnings of emotional life.* New York, NY: Simon & Schuster.

LeDoux, a highly respected brain researcher, brings together a great deal of evidence about how the brain processes experiences that we consider emotional. His explanations of emotional learning are very clear and relevant to stuttering.

LeDoux, J. (2015). *Anxious: Using the brain to understand and treat fear and anxiety.* New York, NY: Viking.

Although I listed this book in Suggested Readings for the previous chapter on learning, I think it is important enough to suggest it again here for this chapter on theories. LeDoux's latest book advances his views on fear and anxiety and their treatment. From his perspective, fear is not a basic response to threat, but a cognitively synthesized emotion. Fear and anxiety derive from nonconscious responses to threat. These low-level defensive automatic responses include hypertonic behaviors such as freezing. I think our understanding of stuttering may be improved if we take these into consideration.

Packman, A., & Attanasio, J. (2017). *Theoretical issues in stuttering* (2nd ed.). New York, NY: Routledge Press.

The authors review current and past theories of stuttering and evaluate them in terms of testability, explanatory power, parsimony, and heuristic power. This book effectively teaches the reader what a theory should be expected to do.

7

Typical Disfluency and the Development of Stuttering

Chapter Objectives

After studying this chapter, readers should be able to:

- Describe and explain the typical (a) core behaviors, (b) secondary behaviors, (c) feelings and attitudes, and (d) underlying processes for the following age and developmental levels, as well as exceptions and variations:
  - ☐ typical disfluency
  - ☐ stuttering in younger preschool children: borderline stuttering
  - ☐ stuttering in older preschool children: beginning stuttering
  - ☐ stuttering in school-age children: intermediate stuttering
  - ☐ stuttering in older teens and adults: advanced stuttering

Key Terms

Advanced stuttering: This level is characteristic of older teens and adults who have been stuttering since childhood. Their stuttering pattern, especially behaviors associated with avoidance and ways of coping with blocks, is quite ingrained.

Age/developmental levels: These levels reflect both the age of the individual (e.g., younger preschooler, older preschooler, etc.) and the severity of the stuttering (e.g., borderline, beginning, etc.)

Antiexpectancy devices: An unusual way of speaking or acting that seems to reduce stuttering, like laughing and pretending that most things said were a joke. Another example is speaking with an accent that the speaker pretends to have. An avoidance.

Avoidance conditioning: A type of learning that occurs when a person avoids something he or she thinks will be unpleasant. The avoidance is rewarded by the fact that the unpleasantness doesn't happen. Avoidance conditioning is important in thinking about stuttering development and interventions because it can be difficult to combat. See Chapter 5, on learning, to read more about avoidance conditioning.

Beginning stuttering: This level of stuttering is usually seen in children between ages 3.5 and 6, although it may occur before and after those ages. It is characterized by more tension and hurry in disfluencies than that seen in borderline stuttering. Stuttering at this level usually consists of repetitions and prolongations, but some children will also exhibit blocks. Escape and even some avoidance behaviors appear in this level of stuttering.

Borderline stuttering: This is the earliest or lowest level of stuttering, usually seen in children ages 2 to 3.5. This type of stuttering is characterized by more frequent part-word and single-syllable whole-word repetitions than children who are developing typically have, but without awareness or concern on the part of the child.

Circumlocutions: Rather than stutter on a word, a person who stutters might use a different way of saying something, such as "My father was in the N...n...he served aboard ships in the armed forces." Again, another avoidance.

Dysrhythmic phonation: A sound prolongation, broken word, or other instance of ongoing phonation being stopped, extended, or distorted

Intermediate stuttering: Typical of children in their school-age years, this level of stuttering will abound in repetitions and prolongations, but blocks will also be frequent. In addition to escape behaviors, avoidances will be frequent at this level because there is fear of being "stuck" in a stutter and fear of listener reactions.

Postponements: This is like a starter, but usually it just involves waiting a few beats before saying a feared word as in "Back then I use to drink a lot of ...... soda." An avoidance.

Starters: Words or sounds used by someone who stutters to get started speaking when blocked or when anticipating a block. For example, a person who stutters might say "My name is, uh, Barry." Starters are a type of avoidance behavior because they are used before the individual is in a moment of stuttering.

"Stuttering-like" disfluencies: Short-segment repetitions (i.e., part-word and monosyllabic whole-word repetitions), as well as sound prolongations, and blocks. These are disfluencies that are more typically judged by listeners as stuttering.

Substitutions: The substitution of an "easier" word for a "harder" word on which a stutterer expects to stutter. For example, a stutterer who often stuttered on words beginning with "p" and who had a dog named "Pluto" might generally substitute "my dog" for the dog's name when talking about him. These are a type of avoidance.

Typical disfluency: These are the disfluencies in the speech of individuals who do not have stuttering or other speech problems. They are more prevalent in younger children (e.g., ages 2–4), but still appear in the speech of all talkers. Some examples are multisyllable word repetitions, revisions, incomplete phrases, and interjections.

Underlying processes: These are speculations about the process that may cause disfluencies or stuttering at each developmental level. For stuttering, these processes help us understand why stuttering often changes from borderline to beginning to intermediate to advanced levels.

"Within-word" disfluencies: Disfluencies that occur within a word boundary such as repetitions of parts of words, prolongations, or blocks. Stuttered speech is said to contain a higher proportion of within-word disfluencies (as opposed to disfluencies that happen between words or across words, such as hesitations, fillers, and repetitions of whole words) than typical disfluency. Note that some disfluencies of children who are developing typically may also include within-word disfluencies.

OVERVIEW

This chapter describes the development of stuttering and what it is like at various ages. It is designed to help you understand why, once stuttering has emerged, it often (but not always) progresses from a few relaxed repetitions in preschool children to frequent stuttering accompanied by tension, avoidance, and many negative feelings and beliefs in older children or adults. This chapter will also help you understand how to match treatment procedures to the underlying dynamics of stuttering, as well as to the age of the client. To accomplish these goals, I have organized the content into five levels that reflect not only age groupings but also stages of development of stuttering and important characteristics of each stage of stuttering to guide your selection of a therapy approach (Fig. 7.1).

The five age groupings/developmental levels are given in Table 7.1, along with the four subcategories of stuttering characteristics. The first three subcategories—core behaviors, secondary behaviors, and feelings and attitudes—were described in a general way in Chapter 1. The fourth, **underlying processes**, explains why symptoms change from level to level. My explanations are hypotheses based on evidence from studies of animal and human behavior that may help us understand how stuttering behaviors become more severe and complex. The material in the "underlying processes" subcategory should help you understand the nature of the symptoms as well as the rationales for the treatments presented in the second section of this book.

Specific age groupings (younger preschool, older preschool, school age, and teens and adults) are used because age is often critical in selecting the appropriate treatment. Let me give two examples. No matter how severely a preschool child stutters, treatment should always involve his or her parents, and in my experience, it should focus primarily on increasing fluency rather than modifying stutters. Conversely, a school-age child—whether stuttering is mild or severe—needs an approach that involves teachers and classmates as well as parents. Also, treatment helps children of this age to discuss their stuttering and their feelings about it. In general, the cognitive-emotional level of clients at different ages should be considered when choosing a therapy strategy. In other words, younger preschool children don't need extensive work on their feelings about stuttering; their parents or caregivers can reassure them when needed. Adolescents and adults, however, may need some focus on what they think and feel about their stuttering.

Exceptions and Variations

The **age/developmental levels** presented in this chapter do not characterize absolutely everyone who stutters. For example, some older preschool children may be stuttering so mildly and be so relatively unaware of it that they might best be treated by an approach described for younger preschool children. Clinicians should feel free to borrow or combine treatment strategies if an individual's stuttering does not fit the pattern described for his age. Apart from a few exceptions, however, clinicians should stay with a specific approach if it appears to be working. In my experience, it is rarely beneficial to haphazardly take procedures from several different approaches.

Another qualification of the hierarchy presented here concerns the implication that all individuals who stutter pass through each stage in sequence. This is generally true, but there are exceptions. A child may show only typical disfluencies one day and beginning or intermediate stuttering on another day. She may stop stuttering without apparent reason a week later, or she may continue stuttering unless treated. One 3-year-old boy I knew changed overnight from borderline to severe beginning stuttering after a change in his allergy medication. As soon as he resumed taking his original prescription, he became a borderline stutterer again and then recovered completely without treatment. There are many unsolved mysteries in stuttering.

Two clinical researchers who wrote extensively about the development of stuttering, Van Riper (1982) and Bloodstein (1960a, 1960b, 1961a), agreed that a simple sequence of stages could never capture every individual's pattern. Bloodstein (1960b) proposed a series of four stages of stuttering development, which he described as "typical, not universal" (Bloodstein & Ratner, 2008, p. 36). He also cautioned that although stuttering near onset is often characterized by repetitions without awareness or by a lack of concern, some

Age Groupings/Developmental Levels
Typical Disfluency
Da - Da - Dad
Younger Preschool Child: Borderline Stuttering
Wa - Wa - Wa - Wa - Watch my car go
Older Preschool Child: Beginning Stuttering
C-C-C... Can I go out to p-p-p... play?
School-age Child: Intermediate Stuttering
I-I-I, uh, uh, don't, uh, know.
Adult and Adolescent: Advanced Stuttering
C... C... Could y... you make a ph... ph... phone call for me?

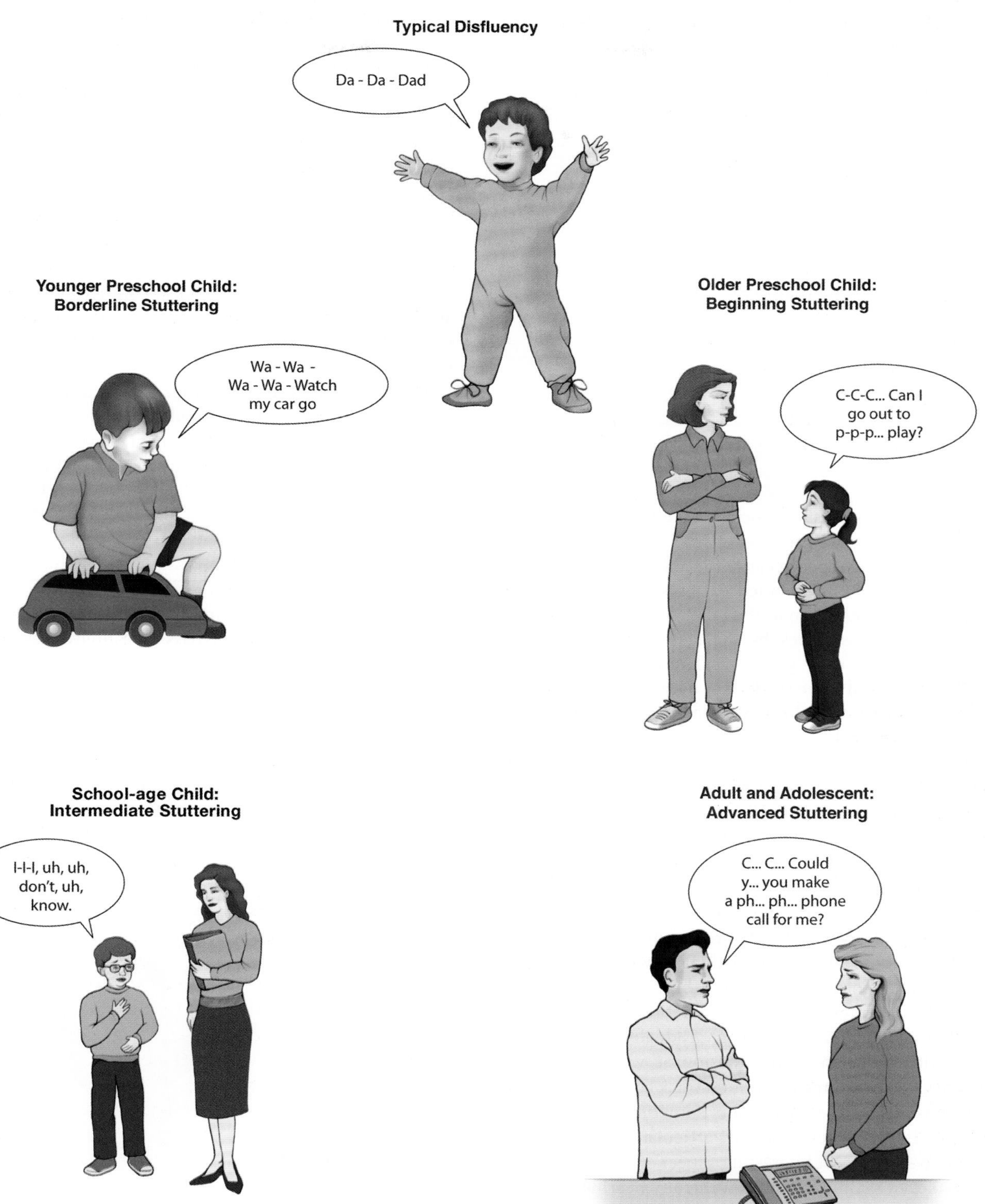

Figure 7.1 Overview of Chapter 7.

TABLE 7.1 Developmental/Treatment Levels of Stuttering

Developmental/ Treatment Level	Typical Age Range (Years)
Typical disfluency	1.5–6*
Younger preschoolers: borderline stuttering	1.5–3.5
Older preschoolers: beginning stuttering	3.5–6
School age: intermediate stuttering	6–13
Older teens and adults: advanced stuttering	≥14

*A small amount of typical disfluency continues in mature speech.

children at this stage show considerable effort and strain in their stuttering as well as crying from frustration at their inability to produce speech easily (Bloodstein, 1960a).

Van Riper (1982) also noted the presence of forcing and struggle in some children at the onset of stuttering, and like Bloodstein, he was struck by the fact that most children, especially in their early years, oscillate between remissions and recurrences of their stuttering, between mild stuttering and **typical disfluency**, or between more advanced and less advanced stages of development.

In addition to such swings in the progression of stuttering development, there may also be different paths of development, which different individuals may follow. After searching his clinical files on many individuals whom he had followed for several years, Van Riper (1982) found that his data suggested there are subgroups of individuals who stutter. These subgroups are characterized by different onsets and different trajectories of development. He proposed that there are four distinctive "tracks" that an individual may follow. The most common track consists of children between 2 and 4 years of age whose stuttering begins as repetitions, progresses to include prolongations, and then gradually develops into blocks with more and more tension as well as fears and avoidances. The next most common track comprises children whose onset is a little later and is sometimes accompanied by delayed speech development, articulation problems, or very rapid speech. An interesting aspect of this track is that these children seem to have had difficulty hearing their own speech, perhaps as a result of auditory processing problems. This is particularly interesting in light of findings from brain imaging studies of adults who stutter (e.g., Foundas et al., 2001), indicating that some have anatomical anomalies that might produce difficulty with higher-level auditory processing. A third track—far less common that the first two—includes children who have a sudden onset of stuttering with a great deal of tension that results in tight, laryngeal blocks. Finally, a fourth track consists of individuals whose disfluency appears to have psychogenic components. (An expanded discussion of psychogenic disfluency is presented in the chapter on neurogenic and psychogenic stuttering and cluttering.) This track is characterized by late onset, a stereotyped pattern of stuttering that is accompanied by few avoidances and that changes very little with age.

Van Riper's four tracks serve as a warning to us that there is much diversity in the evolution of stuttering. Yairi (2007) reviewed past attempts to subtype individuals who stutter. Yairi discussed Van Riper's tracks of stuttering development as well as other authors' attempts to identify subgroups of individuals who stutter, including variations in the progression of symptoms.

Keeping these variations, exceptions, and limitations in mind, I will now begin a detailed description of the levels of stuttering development and treatment, starting with a group of behaviors that is really not stuttering at all but a part of typical speech.

TYPICAL DISFLUENCY

Children vary a great deal in how disfluent they are as they learn to communicate. Some pass their milestones of speech and language development with relatively few disfluencies. Others stumble along, repeating, interjecting, and revising as they try to master new forms of speech and language on their way to adult competence. Most are somewhere between the extremes of exceptional fluency and excessive disfluency, such as the 2-year-old shown in Figure 7.2.

A video clip with an example of a child with typical disfluency is available on www.thepoint.lww.com (Video 7-1: Normal Disfluency and the Development of Stuttering. She

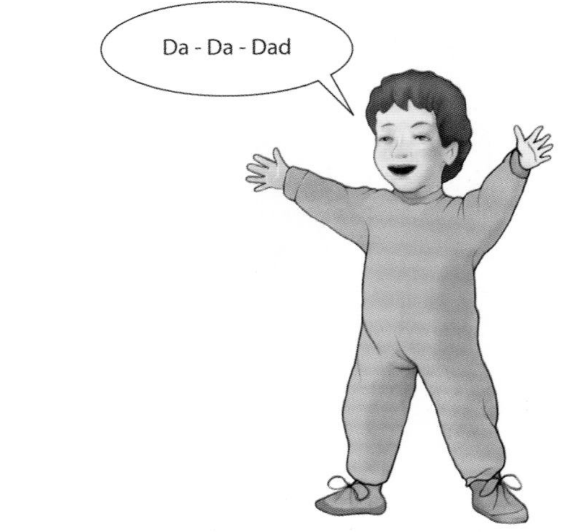

Figure 7.2 Child who may be typically disfluent.

is the first child on this video, Annie). Notice the many different types of disfluencies in her speech, as well as her lack of concern and happy demeanor even during her disfluencies. I have selected a portion of her conversation that has an unusually large amount of disfluency to show that some moments of a typically disfluent child's speech can seem a lot like stuttering.

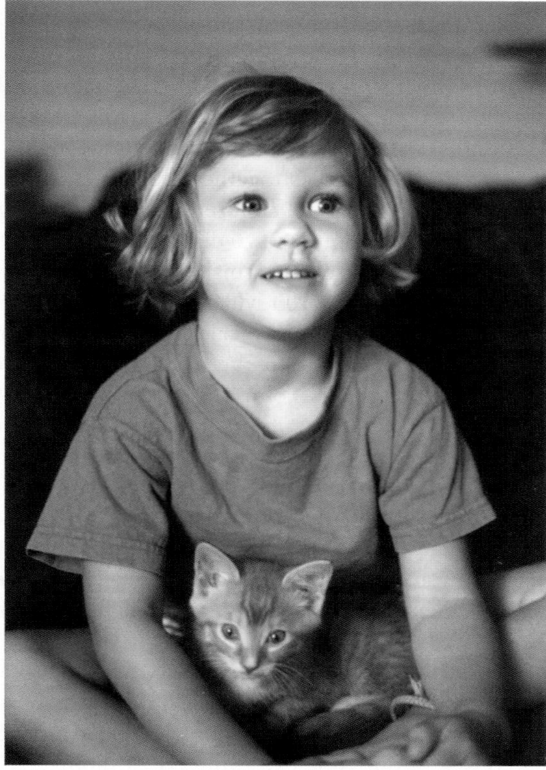

Typically disfluent children swing back and forth in the degree of their disfluency. Some days they are more fluent and other days less fluent. Such swings in disfluency may be associated with language development, motor learning, or other developmental or environmental influences mentioned in the preceding chapters. In the following sections, I discuss factors that may influence disfluency, specific behaviors that I categorize as typical disfluency, and the reactions that some children may have to their disfluency. I also highlight aspects of typical disfluency that distinguish it from early stuttering, because one of my aims in this chapter is to prepare you to make this distinction.

Core Behaviors

Typical disfluencies have been cataloged by several authors who generally agree about what constitutes disfluency (Bloodstein, 1987; Colburn & Mysak, 1982a, 1982b; Juste & Furquim de Andrade, 2011; Williams, Silverman, & Kools,

TABLE 7.2 Categories of Typical Disfluencies

Type of Typical Disfluency	Example
Part-word repetition*	"mi-milk"
Single-syllable word repetition*	"I...I want that"
Multisyllabic word repetition	"Lassie...Lassie is a good dog"
Phrase repetition	"I want a...I want a ice-ceem comb"
Interjection	"He went to the...uh...circus"
Revision-incomplete phrase	"I lost my...Where's Mommy going?"
Prolongation*	"I'm Tiiiiiiiimmy Thompson"
Tense pause*	"Can I have some more (lips together, no sound) milk?"

*Stutter-like disfluency.

1968; Yairi, 1982, 1983, 1997a; Yairi & Ambrose, 2005). Table 7.2 lists eight commonly used categories of disfluency. The first two (part-word repetitions and single-syllable whole-word repetitions) and the last two (prolongations and tense pauses) have been labeled "stuttering-like disfluencies" (Yairi & Ambrose, 2005). "Tense pauses" are moments when the child is not producing speech but shows muscle tension in those parts of the speech mechanism that can be observed, such as the lips or jaw. The other categories (multisyllable word repetitions, phrase repetitions, interjections, and revision-incomplete phrase) are believed, by most experts, to be not stuttering disfluencies but more typical disfluencies. Note that some typically fluent children will have a few stuttering-like disfluencies mixed in with their greater number of non–stuttering-like disfluencies.

The speech of typically fluent children has other characteristics (besides these categories). These include the amount of disfluency and the number of units of repetitions and interjections, especially in relation to the age of the child.

Let's begin with the amount of disfluency. This is often measured as the number of disfluencies per 100 words or syllables, rather than "percentage disfluencies." "Percentage disfluencies" implies that the disfluencies are associated with the production of particular words. For example, if you said that a child had 10 percent disfluent words, it would be assumed that 10 percent of the words spoken were spoken disfluently. However, many disfluencies, such as revisions, interjections, or phrase repetitions, are composed of several words or occur between words. For example, a child may say "Mommy, can you … can you … um … can you buy me that?" It's inaccurate to say that some of these words were spoken disfluently, because the disfluencies were the repetition of the phrase "can you" and the interjection of "um." Were the disfluencies on the words actually spoken, or did they (e.g., a phrase repetition) occur because the child was having trouble formulating the remainder of the sentence? In this case, we say that the child spoke six words ("Mommy can you buy me that?") and had two disfluencies (a phrase repetition and an interjection). Hence, we calculate the number of disfluencies that occur when the child speaks 100 words. More details on counting disfluencies are given in Chapter 8.

Although many researchers have measured disfluencies per number of words spoken, a good argument can be made for measuring disfluencies per number of syllables spoken. Andrews and Ingham (1971) first recommended the practice of assessing frequency of stuttering in relation to syllables spoken because some multisyllabic words may have more than one disfluency, like "S-S-S-Sept-te-te-tember" or "di-dinosa-sa-saur." These examples would be one disfluency each if disfluent words were counted, but two if disfluent syllables were counted. In line with this, Yairi (1997a) noted that as children get older, they are more likely to use multisyllable words. To keep the count equitable between younger and older children, Yairi has assessed disfluencies in children as the number per 100 syllables attempted (Hubbard & Yairi, 1988; Yairi & Ambrose, 1996; Yairi & Lewis, 1984).

When the frequency of all of a child's disfluencies is measured, we need to know how many disfluencies are typical disfluencies. Some of the earliest research on disfluency was conducted by Wendell Johnson at the University of Iowa. He assembled a team of researchers in the 1950s to examine the evidence for his "diagnosogenic" theory of stuttering. As indicated in Chapter 6, Johnson hypothesized that at the time a child is first "diagnosed" as stuttering by his or her parents, the child's disfluencies do not differ from those of children who do not stutter. One of the research team's projects was to record children identified by their parents as children who stutter and compare the disfluency in their speech with that of children who do not stutter (Johnson & Associates, 1959). One part of this study compared 68 male children who stuttered with 68 male children who didn't. The results showed that although there was some overlap, the stuttering children had more than twice the amount of disfluency (on average, 18 disfluencies per 100 words) than did the children who did not stutter (only 7 disfluencies per 100 words). Johnson interpreted the findings as showing that the two groups were essentially the same because there was so much overlap in both amount and type of disfluency. Researchers following Johnson (e.g., McDearmon, 1968) have reinterpreted these data as indicating there are two different groups, as I discussed in the last chapter.

Other researchers who have examined the disfluencies in children who do not stutter put the amount of their disfluencies at about the same level as Johnson and his colleagues reported (DeJoy & Gregory, 1985; Hubbard & Yairi, 1988; Wexler & Mysak, 1982; Yairi, 1981; Yairi & Ambrose, 1996; Yairi & Lewis, 1984; Zebrowski, 1991). A study by Tumanova, Conture, Lambert, and Walden (2014) examined the conversational speech of 244 children who did not stutter (ages 36–71 months) and found that the mean number of total disfluencies (both nonstuttered and stuttered disfluencies) was 4.28 (SD = 2.3) per 100 words. This figure may be lower than those in other studies because these researchers did not include children younger than 36 months (e.g., between 24 and 36 months) when disfluencies could be quite high.

Bringing all these studies together, we can estimate that normally speaking preschool children, if you include ages 2 to 3, have on average about 6 to 10 disfluencies for every 100 words spoken. If measured in terms of syllables, it would be closer to 5 disfluencies per 100 syllables.

The range in frequency of typical disfluency is important to note also, especially if the frequency of disfluency is used to make clinical decisions. Johnson and Associates (1959) and Yairi (1981) found that, although many children who do not stutter have only one or two disfluencies per 100 words, at least one child in their samples had slightly more than 25 disfluencies per 100 words. All of these nonstuttering children were categorized as typically speaking children by their parents and by an experienced speech-language pathologist. Thus, the frequency of disfluencies is not a definitive clinical measure by itself.

Another distinguishing characteristic of typical disfluency is the number of units that occur in each repetition or interjection. Yairi's (1981) data suggest that typical repetitions usually consist of only one extra unit. For example, a child might say "That my-my ball." Interjections are likely to be just a single unit, such as "I want some … uh … juice." Instances of multiple repetitions were occasionally observed in these children, but they were the exception. The rule of thumb is that in typical disfluencies, there is one and sometimes two units per repetition or interjection. This agrees with the findings of Johnson and Associates (1959) that children who do not stutter have one- or two-unit repetitions.

Another major characteristic of typical disfluency is the type of disfluency that is most common. Johnson and Associates (1959) found that interjections, revisions, and whole-word repetitions were the most common disfluency types among the 68 nonstuttering males, who ranged in age from 2.5 to 8 years of age. Yairi's (1981) study of 33 typically developing 2-year-old children found that there were two clusters of common disfluency types. One cluster involved repetitions of speech segments of one syllable or less (one-syllable words or parts of words were repeated). The second cluster consisted of interjections and revisions.

The most common disfluency type seems to change as a child grows older. In a follow-up to his earlier study, Yairi

TABLE 7.3 Characteristics of Typical Disfluency in the Average Nonstuttering Child

1. No more than 10 disfluencies per 100 words
2. Typically one-unit repetitions; occasionally two
3. Most common disfluency types are interjections, revisions, and word repetitions. As children mature past age 3, use of part-word repetitions will decline

(1982) found that as typically disfluent children matured between 2 and 3.5 years, they gradually increased their frequency of revisions and phrase repetitions but decreased their frequency of part-word repetitions and interjections. He suggested that these data indicate that as children who do not stutter mature, part-word repetitions decline, even if other disfluency types increase. Thus, an increase in part-word repetitions as a child is observed longitudinally may be a sign that warrants concern.

Although the research is far from complete, we can characterize typical disfluency types as follows:

- Revisions are common in typical development and may continue to account for a major portion of their disfluencies as children grow older.
- Interjections are also common, but usually decline after 3 years of age.
- Repetitions may also be a frequent type of disfluency around 2 to 3 years of age, especially single-syllable word repetitions having fewer than two extra units. Repetitions are also more likely to involve longer segments (e.g., phrases) as a child grows older.

Table 7.3 summarizes the major characteristics of typical disfluency.

Secondary Behaviors

A child who is typically disfluent generally has no secondary behaviors. He has not developed any reactions to his disfluencies, such as escape or avoidance behaviors. Although research suggests that some typical children occasionally display "tense pauses" (some muscle tension evident during the pause), such tension does not appear to be a reaction to their disfluencies. If a child shows what appears to be typical disfluencies, such as single-word repetitions, but consistently displays pauses or interjections of "uh" immediately before or during disfluencies, he should be carefully evaluated for possible stuttering.

Feelings and Attitudes

A typically disfluent child rarely notices his disfluencies, even though they may be apparent to others. Just as a child may stumble when walking but regains his balance and continues walking without complaint, a child with typical development who repeats, interjects, or revises usually continues talking after a disfluency without evidence of frustration or embarrassment.

Underlying Processes

First, let's review the behaviors for which we are trying to account. Typical disfluency occurs throughout childhood and adulthood. It may begin earlier than 18 months of age and peak between ages 2 and 3.5 years. It slowly diminishes, thereafter, but also changes in form. Some types of disfluency, such as repetitions, decrease after 3.5 years, but other types, such as revisions, may increase. Episodic increases and decreases in disfluency are also common throughout childhood. What causes these changes? Why are there ups and downs and changes in form? Like most natural phenomena, multiple forces probably have an impact on fluency at any given moment, but specific forces may predominate at certain times. In Chapter 4, I talked about developmental and environmental influences on stuttering and typical disfluency, and I will review these influences as I discuss studies of children with typical disfluencies.

The integrated perspective on stuttering described in Chapter 6 has implications for typical disfluency as well. This view suggests that breakdowns in speech fluency may occur when some of the neural pathways critical for sensorimotor control of speech production are immature or inefficient, perhaps because of delayed myelination. Serious delays may result in stuttering, but minor delays may result in typical disfluencies, especially when a child is learning to integrate all the subcomponents of spoken language at increasingly faster rates with increasingly greater options for vocabulary, syntax, and prosody.

These rapid developments in language are—as I've said many times—the context in which disfluencies often first appear. As you have learned, children tend to be most disfluent at the beginning of syntactic units (Bernstein Ratner, 1981; Bloodstein, 1974, 1995; Silverman, 1974) and when the length or complexity of their utterances increases (DeJoy & Gregory, 1973; Gordon, Luper, & Peterson, 1986; Hall, Wagovitch, & Bernstein Ratner, 2007; Pearl & Bernthal, 1980; Zackheim & Conture, 2003). Bloodstein and Ratner (2008) have an excellent summary and discussion of the loci of disfluencies in typically disfluent children. Taken together, these findings suggest that disfluency is greatest when a child is busy planning long or complex language structures. Typically, a child will begin speaking even before all the planning for the phrase is finished. This puts a heavy load on cerebral resources. It seems likely that producing newly learned language structures would be hardest of all because more attention must be devoted to them. It would follow then that disfluencies occur more frequently on a child's most recently acquired forms. However, evidence gathered from four children between 2 and 4 years of age suggests that typical disfluency may be greatest on structures that have been learned but perhaps not fully automated, thereby requiring more cerebral resources for their production. These extra resources may not be readily available—hence disfluencies occur (Colburn & Mysak, 1982a, 1982b).

Pragmatics may influence disfluency, too. Studies by Davis (1940), Meyers and Freeman (1985a, 1985b), and Newman and Smit (1989) indicate that children's disfluency increases under certain pragmatic conditions, such as when interrupting, when directing another's activity, or when responding to requests/demands to change their own activity, and when the listener's response time is very fast. Mastering such pragmatic skills, especially those involving more complex social interactions, creates yet another challenge for a developing child. The pressures of language acquisition, interacting with other factors, can be seen as competing for cerebral resources, which leaves fewer remaining resources available for fluent speech production.

In addition to language acquisition, another likely influence on disfluency is speech-motor control. Most children—as they mature between ages 2 and 5—learn to produce almost all the segmental and supersegmental targets of their native language, as well as to increase their speech rates as they produce longer and longer utterances. These maturational changes must keep the average child fairly busy, although the demanding nature of these changes may not be obvious. The child is automatically scanning his parents' and older siblings' speech, acquiring information about talking. He is also continuously modifying his own productions to make them more and more like the speech he hears. This period—from 2 to 5 years—also encompasses an intensive refinement of nonspeech-motor skills. It is at this age that children are learning to skip, run, jump, and take part in numerous games requiring skill and speed (Gabbard, 2016). Thus, children are mastering a myriad of other motor tasks at the same time they are acquiring the ability to speak in rapid, complex, fluent sequences. With all these competing demands, no wonder that almost all children have disfluencies.

Besides the continuing demands of typical development, there are also episodic stresses in a child's environment that may temporarily increase typical disfluency. An experiment by Hill (1954) demonstrated that conditioned fear could elicit disfluency in typical adults' speech. It is easy to imagine, therefore, that there are many psychological stresses in a child's life that would also increase disfluency. Clinically, I have observed many situations that seem to increase typical disfluency. Among them are the stress of a move from one home to another, parents' separation or divorce, the birth of a sibling, and other events that may decrease a child's sense of security.

We have also seen increases in typical disfluency during periods of excitement, such as holidays, vacations, and visits by relatives. Disfluency increases especially when excitement combines with competition to be heard, such as during dinner table conversations when everyone is talking at once or after school when several children are competing to tell Mom what happened during the day. As we speculated in Chapter 6, emotions may have an especially strong influence on fluency in young children. This happens after interactions between right and left hemispheres develop during the child's first 2 years (Fox & Davidson, 1984), and overflow activity from emotional arousal in the right hemisphere may disrupt vulnerable, immature language production networks in the left.

Summary

Between ages 2 and 5, most children pass through periods of increased disfluency. Repetitions, interjections, revisions, prolongations, and pauses are commonly heard during this period. When the average child is between 2 and 3.5, disfluencies reach 6 per 100 words spoken and may occur even more frequently in some typically disfluent children.

Repetitions are probably the most common type of typical disfluency in younger children, whereas revisions are a more common type of typical disfluency in older children.

Despite the fact that children's disfluencies may occasionally attract some adult attention, typically disfluent children seem generally unaware of the disfluencies in their own speech and don't react to them or engage in secondary behaviors to escape or avoid them as a consequence.

Some factors thought to contribute to increases in typical disfluencies include the demands of language acquisition, inefficient speech-motor control skills, interpersonal stress associated with growing up in a typical family, and threats to security from such events as relocation, family breakup, or hospitalization. Disfluencies may also increase under the ordinary daily pressures of competition and excitement while speaking.

YOUNGER PRESCHOOL CHILDREN: BORDERLINE STUTTERING

Stuttering in preschool children between the ages of 2 and 3.5 resembles typical disfluency, but differs in several important ways. The most obvious—the thing that gets parents' attention—is that these children have more disfluencies (e.g., Tumanova et al., 2014). We will discuss other key differences in the following sections. Sometimes diagnosis is difficult, because a child may drift back and forth between typical disfluency and borderline stuttering over a period of weeks or months. Most children with borderline stuttering gradually lose their stuttering and grow up without a trace of it. Others develop more stuttering symptoms and progress through levels of beginning, intermediate, and advanced stuttering. Still others may continue to show **borderline stuttering** throughout their lives but may never seek treatment because their disfluency is so mild. A speech sample of a younger preschool child with borderline stuttering is depicted in Figure 7.3.

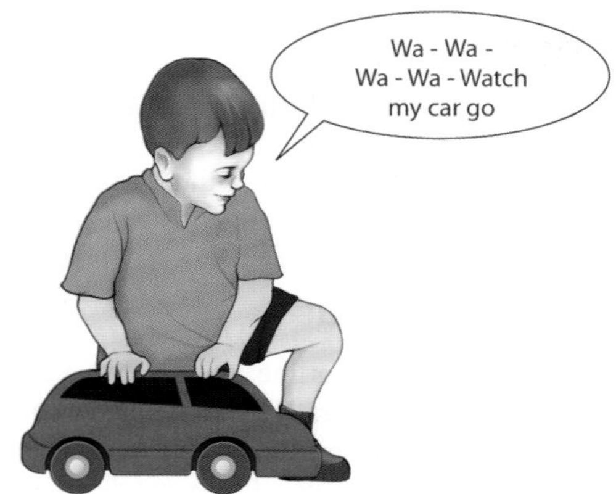

Figure 7.3 Child who may be a borderline stutterer.

A video clip of a child with borderline stuttering is available on *thePoint*. (Video 7-1: Normal Disfluency and the Development of Stuttering. Watch the clip of the second child on the video, Ashley.) Note that although Ashley has fairly relaxed repetitions and seems relatively unaffected by them, she does stop in the midst of saying "coo-coo-coo-coo-coo-cookie" and just continues on with the rest of her utterance without finishing the word. This is a mild escape behavior. Ashley received indirect therapy soon after this clip was filmed and has made a full recovery.

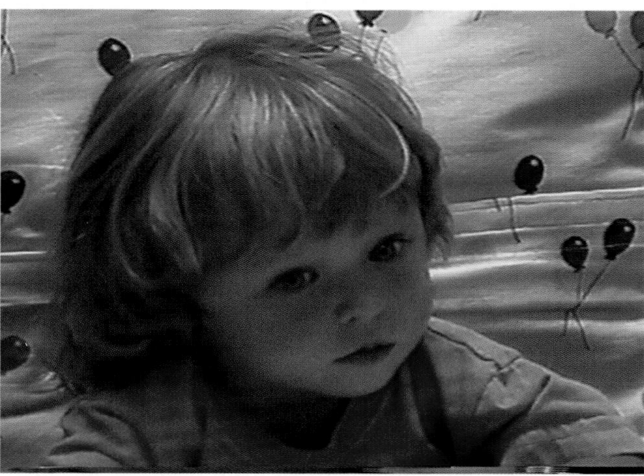

In describing the behaviors of borderline stuttering, I will begin to define my view of how stuttering differs from typical disfluency. The distinction between stuttering and typical disfluency has been of great interest to theorists for many years. Some theorists (e.g., Johnson, 1955; Johnson et al., 1942) suggested, as was noted previously, that a stuttering child developed symptoms only after his parents mislabeled his typical disfluencies as stuttering. That is, a child's first "stuttering" symptoms were actually just typical speech disfluencies.

An opposing view maintains that there are objective differences between the speech of a typically disfluent child and the speech of a child who is stuttering, even before a parent or someone else labels behaviors as stuttering. Although I hold this latter view, I also agree that there is much overlap between the disfluencies of stuttering children and the disfluencies of typically disfluent children. Moreover, as previously stated, these children often go back and forth between stuttering and typical disfluency over a period of months. For this reason, we use the term "borderline" to indicate that these children are neither entirely normally disfluent nor undeniably stuttering.

Core Behaviors

No single core behavior distinguishes borderline stuttering from typical disfluency. However, many researchers and clinicians have suggested three elements that are useful for making this distinction. The frequency of disfluencies is one important aspect to consider. As we indicated in our description of typical disfluencies, children who do not stutter between 2 and 5 years may go through periods of increased disfluency. Even so, their level of disfluency averages about 6 per 100 words. Typically, if children have many more disfluencies per 100 words (e.g., 10 or more), we consider them borderline.

Another feature that can help identify borderline stuttering rather than typical disfluency is the proportion of certain types of disfluencies. The study we cited earlier by Johnson and colleagues (1959) suggested that compared to children who don't stutter, those who stutter had significantly more sound and syllable repetitions, single-syllable word repetitions, broken words (i.e., phonation or airflow is abnormally stopped within a word), and prolonged sounds. There were no significant differences between the groups in their number of interjections, revisions, or incomplete phrases.

More information on types of disfluencies was provided by Young (1984), who reviewed a large number of studies that had assessed which types of disfluencies were identified as stuttering and which were not by the researchers who published the studies. His summary impression was that repetitions of parts of words, and to a lesser extent prolongations, are the disfluency types that are most likely to be classified as stuttering. Bloodstein and Ratner (2008) and Conture (1982, 1990, 2001) generally concurred with other writers, suggesting that **"within-word" disfluencies** (i.e., part-word repetitions and audible as well as inaudible prolongations including blocks) are the types of disfluencies most frequently heard in children who stutter.

Yairi and colleagues (e.g., Yairi, 1997a, 1997b; Yairi & Ambrose, 1996) proposed that children who stutter can be distinguished from children with typical disfluencies using a grouping of **"stuttering-like" disfluencies**. Included in this grouping were short-segment repetitions (part-word and monosyllabic word repetitions); tense pauses (stoppage of speech with evident muscular tightening both within and between words); and a category introduced by Williams, Silverman, and Kools (1968) called "**dysrhythmic phonation**" (any distortion, prolongation, or break in phonation within a word). Yairi (1997a, 1997b) notes that when many previous studies of children who stutter and children who do not stutter are reanalyzed using this grouping, the proportion of stuttering-like disfluencies in children who do not stutter is always less than 50 percent of the total number of disfluencies. Thus, if a child has more than 50 percent stuttering-like disfluencies, he might well be considered to be stuttering.

In summary, we can say that one measure that will help us distinguish a child with borderline stuttering from a normally disfluent child is a higher proportion of part-word and monosyllabic whole-word repetitions and prolongations compared with multisyllabic word and phrase repetitions. In the next section, we will see that children who show regular tension in their disfluencies that lead to abrupt repetitions, pitch rise, blocks, broken words, and dysrhythmic phonations are beginning rather than borderline stutterers.

The number of times a word or sound is repeated in a part-word or monosyllable word repetitive disfluency appears to be another sign that distinguishes children who stutter from their normally disfluent peers. In Yairi's (1981) sample of 33 children who did not stutter, repetitions typically involved only one or two extra units of repetition (e.g., one extra unit would be li-like this). Other studies comparing children who stutter and children who do not stutter (Ambrose & Yairi, 1995; Johnson & Associates, 1959; Yairi & Lewis, 1984; Zebrowski, 1991) have found that the repetitive disfluencies of nonstuttering children average 1.13 extra units and that of stuttering children 1.51. Thus, the frequent occurrence of repetitions having more than one extra unit is a warning sign of borderline stuttering. Of course, when there are many repetition units, li-li-li-li-li-li-li-like this, it is much more likely the child is demonstrating stuttering rather than typical disfluency.

We have said that borderline stuttering consists primarily of effortless repetitions and occasional prolongations. However, as Van Riper (1971, 1982) and Bloodstein (1995) note, these young children are often highly variable in their stuttering. Although they usually show the core behaviors of borderline stuttering, they may have brief periods of fluency as well as days when they show signs of slightly more advanced stuttering.

Secondary Behaviors

A younger preschool child with borderline stuttering has few, if any, secondary behaviors. The degree of tension may sometimes seem to be slightly greater than normal, but these children generally don't increase tension and struggle like older preschool children do when they stutter. Children with borderline stuttering also do not exhibit accessory movements before, during, or after stutters. In fact, there is often nothing in their behavior to indicate that they are aware of their stutters. Some children with predominantly borderline stuttering may go through periods in which their stuttering suddenly escalates to the level of beginning stuttering, with tension and some other secondary behaviors, but then it falls back again to the borderline level.

Feelings and Attitudes

Because children with borderline stuttering seem to have little awareness of their stutters, they do not show concern or embarrassment. When they repeat a sound or a syllable, even five or six or more times, they usually go on talking as though nothing has happened. One exception, however, is that once in a while, children with borderline stuttering might appear surprised or frustrated when they are repeating a syllable several times and are unable to finish a word. Then, they may stop and cry out, "Mommy, I can't say that word," or otherwise demonstrate brief alarm or surprise. But in general, these younger preschool children show little or no evidence of awareness that they have disfluencies that are different from those of their peers. Moreover, at this age (2–3.5 years), peers usually don't react to the child's stuttering. Table 7.4 summarizes the major characteristics of younger preschool children's borderline stuttering.

Underlying Processes

I hypothesize that the symptoms of borderline stuttering result from the constitutional, developmental, and environmental factors described in Chapters 2, 3, and 4. The constitutional factors associated with borderline stuttering (anomalies in the development of neural pathways for speech) often first show their effects as an excess of typical disfluencies. As I mentioned earlier, environmental and developmental pressures may be great between 2 and 3.5 years, and it is during this period that borderline stuttering typically emerges. The converging demands of expressive language and motor speech development ordinarily peak about this time "when an explosive growth in language ability outstrips a still-immature speech motor apparatus" (Andrews et al., 1983, p. 239). This age is also filled with psychosocial conflicts as a child copes with security needs as an infant

TABLE 7.4 Characteristics of Borderline Stuttering in a Younger Preschool Child

1. More than 6–10 disfluencies per 100 words
2. Often more than two units in repetition
3. More repetitions and prolongations than revisions or incomplete phrases
4. Disfluencies loose and relaxed
5. Rare for child to react to his or her disfluencies

while striving to become more independent as a toddler. The child may be ready to explore but is also fearful. The birth of a new brother or sister may trigger the child's insecurity with the threat of being overlooked. A still older sibling (e.g., a preteen) may turn belligerent toward him because of the older child's own need to express aggression as a prelude to puberty. Just as these stresses wax and wane in strength during preschool years, so does the child's stuttering.

As children mature, certain developmental stresses may taper off. After age 5, children may feel more integrated within themselves and within their families. Articulation and language skills, although still not at adult levels, have been mastered sufficiently for most children to say what's on their mind and to be understood. They have also mastered other motor skills, such as walking and running, as well as riding a tricycle or a bike with training wheels. They may have adjusted to a new, younger sibling as well and made at least temporary peace with an older one.

By now, the capacities of many of the children who had modest predispositions to stutter can easily meet most environmental demands. Therefore, many of those who were borderline stutterers will have acquired typical fluency skills by the time they are 4 or 5 years old. Others may still have many disfluencies at this age, but will eventually outgrow them. This may happen because neural pathways will have matured enough to allow the child to speak fluently. These children may also have relatively robust (rather than reactive) temperaments and do not respond to disfluencies by increasing physical tension or speaking rate. In general, they are functioning well, feel accepted, and can use their resources to compensate for whatever difficulties in speaking remain.

Some children, of course, do not outgrow borderline stuttering. They may continue to stutter, and their symptoms may worsen. They may be children who have substantial predispositions to stutter, which cannot be offset by a "good enough" environment (Winnicott, 1971). Their ability to produce speech and language at the rate and level of complexity used by parents and peers may be insufficient. And their continuing efforts to meet advanced speech and language targets may result in excess disfluency that does not diminish as they pass their third and fourth birthdays. Their frustration tolerance for the repetitions that 2- and 3-year-olds have may be low, as a result of a reactive temperament. Rather than shrugging off their disfluencies, they may begin struggling to produce flawless speech, thereby placing greater demands on their speech production and emotional resources. Still other children may continue to stutter because environmental and developmental stresses do not diminish. Their insecurity may continue from sibling rivalry, breakup of the family, or a parent's death. They may have language or articulation problems, as well as stuttering, which limit their communication abilities throughout their preschool years.

Deficits in the processes underlying speech and language development, plus the frustration of being unable to communicate easily, may be devastating to fluency. This may result in the increased tension we see in older preschool children with beginning stuttering. A child in this situation is unlikely to outgrow stuttering unless parents and professionals provide extensive support.

Summary

Younger preschool children with borderline stuttering usually exhibit a greater amount of disfluency than do typical children—more than 6 disfluencies per 100 words. Using another measure of frequency, the proportion of stuttering-like disfluencies relative to all disfluencies may be greater than half. Children with borderline stuttering are also likely to repeat units more than once in many of their part-word and monosyllabic word repetitions and to have many more part-word and monosyllabic word repetitions and prolongations than multisyllabic word and phrase repetitions, revisions, and interjections.

At the same time, their disfluencies, like those of children who do not stutter, are usually loose and relaxed appearing. Also, like children who do not stutter, children with borderline stuttering show little or no awareness of their speaking difficulty. Only rarely do they express frustration about it. Among the underlying processes behind borderline stuttering are probably some of the neural speech and language-processing anomalies described in the earlier chapter on constitutional origins of stuttering. Such deficits in resources may interact with the demands of speech and language development, the pressure from higher rates of speech, more complex language, competitive speaking situations, and other attributes of a typical home. In addition, some of the psychosocial conflicts described earlier that increase typical disfluency are likely to be active in creating borderline stuttering.

OLDER PRESCHOOL CHILDREN: BEGINNING STUTTERING

In the older preschool child (Fig. 7.4), stuttering usually has more tension and hurry than stuttering in a younger child. It may have evolved over a period of months or a year or two from the borderline stuttering that the child manifested earlier. Or it may appear suddenly in an older preschool child during a time of stress or excitement. The tense and hurried stuttering may alternate with looser, easier disfluencies. Gradually, this more advanced type of stuttering will become commonplace. I described this change as the appearance of "secondary stuttering" in Chapter 6. Both temperament and learning play a major role as the child responds defensively to his multiple repetitions, increasing tension and hurry. Soon, the child becomes impatient with his stuttering as it is happening—perhaps even embarrassed—and may begin to use a variety of escape behaviors as a consequence. For example, he may try to end long repetitions by using an eye blink or head

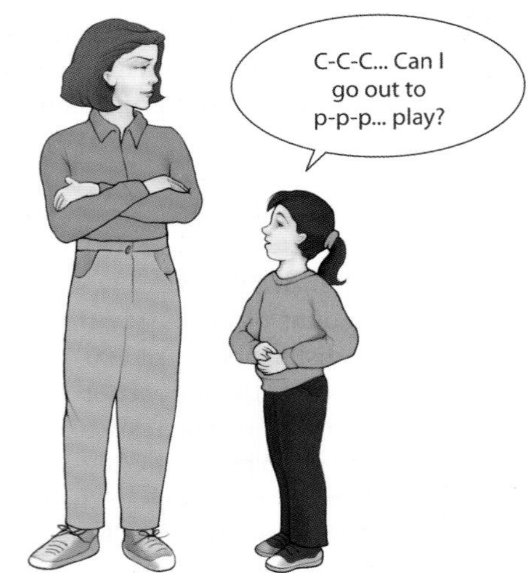

Figure 7.4 Child who may be a beginning stutterer.

nod. Or the child may respond to being stuck in a block by going back to an earlier word in the sentence and starting the phrase over. Periods of increased stuttering may last for several months, but periods of fluency may last only a few days. As these signs occur more consistently, tension increases and struggle is more evident. Classical and operant conditioning processes increase the frequency of struggle behaviors, complicate the child's pattern of stuttering, and spread the symptoms to many more situations.

As mentioned, some children exhibit **beginning stuttering** at onset, without passing through a stage of borderline stuttering. Van Riper (1971, 1982) described several different profiles of stuttering with tense blockages at onset. Many of the children he depicted as more severe at onset were relatively older (e.g., 4, 5, or 6 years old) when their stuttering first appeared. Onset in these children seemed to be related to one of two factors: delayed language development or emotional events. In a study of the onset of stuttering, Yairi and Ambrose (1992b) described onsets of stuttering that were characterized by the signs I described for beginning stuttering in 28 percent of their sample of 87 children. Many of these children had relatively sudden onsets, with typical disfluency changing to beginning stuttering within 1 day or at most 1 week.

A video sample of a child with beginning stuttering is available on *thePoint* (Video 7-1: Normal Disfluency and the Development of Stuttering). The third child on this video, Katherine, has severe beginning stuttering. She shows tense blocks as well as escape behaviors. One escape maneuver is stopping in the middle of a block and restarting with the word preceding the stuttered word ("...yes, yes, I want to put it back in [block on "here"]...i-i-iiin here"). Another escape behavior that Katherine uses is to hit her mother several times to try to release the block. This sample is limited to her more severe stutters and is not entirely representative of her overall speech at this time. She received treatment beginning shortly after the video was made. Because her stuttering was severe, treatment took longer than usual—almost a year. She recovered completely and showed no sign of stuttering in her 5-year follow-up.

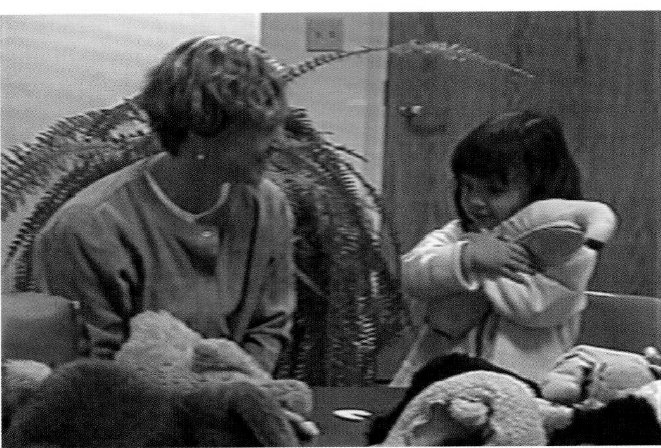

Core Behaviors

The core behaviors of beginning stuttering differ from those of borderline stuttering in several ways. Repetitions begin to sound tense, rapid, and irregular. The final segment of a repeated syllable often sounds abrupt; if it is a vowel, it will sound as if it were suddenly cut off or were a neutral or schwa vowel ("uh") that had been substituted for the appropriate one, as in "luh-luh-luh-like" instead of "li-li-li-like." Repetitions are also produced more rapidly, sometimes with an irregular rhythm. Rather than patiently repeating a syllable as a borderline stutterer does, a child with beginning stuttering hurries through repetitive stutters, as though juggling a hot potato.

As symptoms progress, a child with beginning stuttering increases tension throughout her speech mechanism. Stuttering is sometimes accompanied by a rise in vocal pitch, resulting from increased tension in the vocal folds. Rising pitch may first appear toward the end of a string of repeated syllables, but over time will appear earlier in the repetitions. Rising pitch both within the stuttered iterations (liii-li-like this) and between them (li-li-li-like this) seems to be a more definitive sign of beginning stuttering (Hertsberg, 2010). A child with beginning stuttering sometimes prolongs sounds that she would have previously repeated. Initially, she may prolong the first sounds of syllables, but as stuttering grows more severe, she may also prolong middle sounds, and they too may be accompanied by an increase in pitch.

As beginning stuttering progresses, blocks begin to replace repetitions and prolongations. These are significant landmarks, which indicate that a child is stopping the flow of air or voice at one or more places (Van Riper, 1982). She may inappropriately jam her vocal folds closed or wide open, interrupting or possibly delaying the onset of phonation (Conture, 1990). Shutting off the airway is usually heard as a momentary stoppage of sound in a child's speech and is sometimes accompanied by visual cues; the child may seem momentarily unable to move his mouth or may make groping movements with his mouth as he tries to get air or voice going again. When the stoppage of movement, voice, or airflow first begins, it may be so fleeting that we don't notice it unless we are listening and watching carefully. As these blocks worsen, they become so obvious that they may overshadow the repetitions and prolongations that may remain.

Secondary Behaviors

As these older preschool children's symptoms progress, secondary behaviors are added. They are called secondary because they appear to be responses to the runaway repetitions and increased muscle tension that have emerged. It is not clear how voluntary they are. Many begin as almost reflexive responses, like the common eye blinks or eye squeezing that occur when a child is stuck in a stutter. They may disappear when treatment helps the individual reduce his fear of stuttering. If they don't disappear, the individual may reduce or eliminate them as they become more and more conscious as a result of treatment. A client in one of Van Riper's therapy groups told me that he had a habit of pursing his lips when he thought he would stutter. It somehow gave him a start on getting the word out. Van Riper made him go to a pet store and stand in front of the goldfish tank and purse his lips while watching the goldfish do the same as they breathed. That experience made his lip-pursing "starter" so embarrassing that he soon got rid of it.

Among the earliest of the secondary symptoms are "escape" behaviors, which are maneuvers used to end a stutter and finish a word. Children with beginning stuttering often show escape behaviors after several repetitions of a syllable. They may nod their heads, squint their eyes, or blink just as they try to push a word out. This extra effort often seems to help—in the short run. For the moment, they escape from the punishing repetition, prolongation, or block. Alternatively, they may insert a filler, such as "uh" or "um," after a string of fruitless repetitions. The "um" seems to release the word, perhaps by relaxing the tightly squeezed larynx or by unlocking the lips. The "um" can usually be said fluently, and once uttered, phonation and movement for the word often begin. The fillers work like a little push you might give your sled if it were stuck in the snow as you start down a hill; the "um" gets the child going again when he is stuck in a stutter.

A child with beginning stuttering starts to use escape behaviors earlier and earlier in stutters. The first appearance of these behaviors is usually after a child has repeated a sound quite a few times and is thoroughly frustrated about it. It may sound this way: "Luh-Luh-Luh-Luh-Luh-umLet's go!" Soon, however, the child will not wait until she has tried to say the sound five times. She finds herself about to say a word, feels convinced it won't come out, and then perhaps instinctively uses escape behaviors when she is first starting to stutter: "L-umLet's go!" Such "starters" may even appear before the first sound of the word, in this fashion: "umLet's go!" This is really an avoidance behavior (because it is deployed to avoid a stutter before being stuck in one); they are more common among children with intermediate stuttering, even though these avoidances occasionally appear in the speech of a child with beginning stuttering.

Feelings and Attitudes

An older preschool child with beginning stuttering has stuttered many times. She is aware of stuttering when it happens. The feelings a beginning stutterer has just before, during, and after stutters are often strong. Frequently, frustration is a major feeling. The child may stop in the middle of a stutter and say, "Mommy, why can't I talk?" However, such momentary frustration grows into fear when a word or sound is stuck for several seconds, and the child feels helpless and out of control.

Although a child with beginning stuttering is conscious that she has some "trouble" when she talks, she has not yet developed a belief that she is a defective speaker. This lack of a negative self-image may be attributed, as Bloodstein (1987), Zebrowski (2003), and Van Riper (1982) have suggested, to the "episodic" nature of stuttering. Sometimes it's there; sometimes it's not. Sometimes a child feels that he has problems when he talks; other times he forgets about it. The essential characteristics of beginning stutterers are presented in Table 7.5.

Underlying Processes

The signs and symptoms of beginning stuttering in the older preschool child can be recognized by any experienced clinician. But the processes underlying these behaviors are

TABLE 7.5 Characteristics of Beginning Stuttering in an Older Preschool Child

1. Signs of muscle tension and hurry appear in stuttering. Repetitions are rapid and irregular with abrupt terminations of each element.
2. Pitch rise may be present toward the end of a repetition or prolongation.
3. Fixed articulatory postures are sometimes evident when the child is momentarily unable to begin a word, apparently as a result of tension in speech musculature.
4. Escape behaviors are sometimes present in beginning stuttering. These include, among other things, eye blinks, head nods, and "ums."
5. Awareness of difficulty and feelings of frustration are present, but there are no strong negative feelings about self as speaker.

not so easy to see. In Chapters 5 and 6, I suggested that beginning stuttering may result from the interplay between constitutional and environmental factors, especially in a child with a reactive temperament. In the next sections, I review my speculations about the core behaviors of beginning stuttering as well as the learning processes that are likely to perpetuate the core behaviors and a child's secondary reactions.

Increases in Muscle Tension and Tempo

One of the first signs of beginning stuttering in older preschool children is the appearance of excess muscular tension in repetitions and prolongations and increased tempo or rate in repetitive stutters (Boey, Wuyts, Van de Heyning, DeBodt, & Heylen, 2007; Van Riper, 1982). Why do these changes occur? Oliver Bloodstein (Bloodstein, 1987; Bloodstein & Ratner, 2008) suggests that facial tension and strained glottal attacks in the speech of young children who stutter may reflect the extra muscular effort that emerges when they anticipate difficulty. Edward Conture (1990) offered a related view. He sees the increased articulatory and laryngeal muscle tension as a child's attempt to control sound-syllable repetitions, which are so distressing to him and to some listeners. We have described such tension as a child's effort to control a frustrating and scary behavior of his own body, an attempt to stiffen the speech muscles and brace himself against the perturbations of seemingly involuntary, runaway repetitions (Guitar, Guitar, Neilson, O'Dwyer, & Andrews, 1988). One can imagine this taking place in the same way that a child who is learning to skate may respond to the threat of falling by stiffening and assuming a less than ideal stance for continued forward movement. I've speculated in Chapters 5 and 6 that the initial increases in tension are nonconscious.

The other early sign of beginning stuttering—increases in the rate of repetitive stutters—is cited by a number of authors as an indication that stuttering is worsening. Van Riper (1982), in describing the developmental course of the majority of children whose stuttering persists, stated "the tempo changes as the disorder develops. The repetitive syllables become irregular and are often spoken more rapidly than other fluent syllables." Starkweather (1987) explained this increase in the speed of repetitions as a product of the pressure that children feel as they become more aware of the extra time it takes them to produce an utterance.

But why are these increases in tension and tempo so common in the development of stuttering, and why are they so difficult to change in therapy? In Chapter 6, I described my view that children in whom stuttering persists may be especially sensitive to certain kinds of experiences. Faced with frustration or fear, they react defensively with a type of freezing or flight response, increasing muscle tension or hurry, turning their frustrating or frightening repetitive disfluencies into abrupt, tense repetitions, blocks, or prolongations. As I have mentioned, some children appear to show tense blocks at the onset of their stuttering. These may be children who have high degrees of emotional sensitivity and whose very first manifestation of stuttering (tense blocks) may result from defensive responses mediated by the amygdala.

Research bears out the speculation that at least some adults who stutter contract their muscles in such a way that movement and phonation are immobilized. Freeman and Ushijima's (1978) and Shapiro and DeCicco's (1982) studies indicate that stuttering is associated with abnormal muscle co-contraction of adductor and abductor muscles in the larynx. Such co-contraction could produce stiffening of the phonatory structures and silencing of vocal output. Other studies of stuttering have demonstrated co-contraction in articulatory structures (Fibiger, 1971; Guitar et al., 1988; Platt & Basili, 1973), which could also produce immobility and silence.

Unfortunately, little research directly supports the notion that the increased rate of repetitions reflects the flight response. We have some preliminary evidence that stutterers have more rapid productions during repetitions than do children who do not stutter. An unpublished study (Allen, 1988) carried out in our clinical laboratory indicated that the durations of beginning stutterers' repeated segments and the silences between them were shorter than the durations in similar disfluencies of children who did not stutter matched for age. This finding has been confirmed in the work of Throneburg and Yairi (1994), who replicated our work and found that the silent intervals and the total durations of repetition disfluencies were significantly shorter in stuttering children compared with those of children who did not stutter. Such shortening of segments results in a faster speech rate, at least for the stuttered elements, and may reflect the "great increase in activity" seen in the flight response, although these particular data do not exclude the possibility that stuttering children were more rapid speakers to begin with. It may be relevant at this point to note that Kloth, Janssen, Kraaimaat, and Brutten (1995) found that rapid speaking rate was a predictor of which young children who were fluent at the time of testing but had family histories of stuttering would eventually stutter. The rapid rate in these children might be related to a reactive limbic system, although no evidence indicates that speech rate is related to such reactivity.

The possibility that increased muscle tension and rapid repetitions are a result of biologically based freezing or flight responses is highly speculative at this time. If these responses are part of humans' neural wiring designed for survival, this may be a potential explanation of why some children develop stuttering so rapidly and why tension responses are so difficult to change. The work of Bolles (1970) and Le Doux (2015) has influenced my thinking on this.

Effects of Learning on Stuttering

I presented a detailed account of the effect of learning on the development of stuttering in Chapter 5. Here is a quick overview: Once the child with beginning stuttering reacts repeatedly to his repetitions with increased tension because they are threatening to him, the repetitions themselves elicit the tension response. Through classical conditioning, the repetitions themselves become a conditioned stimulus that elicits the conditioned response of tension. The repetitions then become more abrupt and more rapid and gradually turn into prolongations and blocks, as tension increases. Classical conditioning also generalizes the tense stuttering to any stimuli that are paired with the child's stuttering. People, places, words, sounds, and the pragmatics of speaking situations become conditioned stimuli that elicit the tense stuttering.

As classical conditioning continues its work, operant conditioning becomes important as well. When a child is frustrated or embarrassed by a moment of stuttering, she will often employ an escape behavior (such as facial squeezing or eye blinking) to get out of the stutter and finish the word. Because escaping the stutter and finishing the word reward the behavior, it is likely to increase in frequency. Soon, the child with beginning stuttering is using a variety of "moves" to get out of the stutter. These should be enumerated during a diagnostic evaluation. They don't necessarily need to be addressed directly in treatment, however. If all goes well, they will disappear as the child replaces stuttering with fluency.

Avoidance conditioning may occur to some extent in beginning stuttering but will be more evident in intermediate and advanced stuttering (school age, adolescent, and adults). This learning process combines classical and operant conditioning. Classical conditioning turns cues—both nonconscious and conscious—into conditioned stimuli. These cues may be proprioceptive information from muscles that are beginning to tighten as a stutter looms ahead. Or they may be conscious knowledge that "words beginning with/b/are hard to say." Because these cues have been followed repeatedly by the experience of stuttering with all its attendant threat and fear, they induce threat and fear. When a child senses these cues, he experiences threat and fear. But if she substitutes another word for the feared word or refuses to talk, the threat and fear are reduced and she is rewarded. Several years ago, I saw avoidance conditioning in a two-and-a-half-year-old. For a week after the onset of her repetitions, she kept trying to talk despite a high frequency of stuttering. But, in the second week, she'd had enough. She then refused to talk and only pointed to what she wanted. In very young children like this, avoidances will usually disappear after a few months of treatment. Hers did.

Summary

Borderline stuttering seen in younger preschool children and beginning stuttering common in older preschool children show five principal differences:

1. The older child with beginning stuttering shows more tension and "hurry" in his stuttering. This is often manifested in abruptly ended syllable repetitions, irregular rhythms of repetitions, evident stoppages of phonation, and momentarily fixated articulatory postures. Older preschool children also evidence such secondary behaviors as escape devices and starters (a type of avoidance). In addition, children with beginning stuttering sometimes see themselves as persons who have trouble talking. This comes and goes, but as their stuttering becomes a constant fact of life for them, the more their self-image is that of someone who can't talk right.
2. A major factor underlying beginning stuttering appears to be a child's sensitivity to stress, which may result in frustration, triggering tension responses.
3. Classical conditioning then links such unconditioned response sensitivity to disfluency. When the child is disfluent, he feels threatened, frustrated, or afraid, and this in turn leads to the rapid, tense disfluencies that appear in beginning stuttering. After repeated pairings, disfluency itself, rather than the emotion, elicits increased tension and rate. Classical conditioning also links a child's disfluency to more and more people and places.
4. A third factor in beginning stuttering in older preschool children is operant conditioning, which increases and then maintains the use of escape devices. These escape behaviors are negatively reinforced by reduction in frustration and positively reinforced when the child is then able to complete her communication.
5. Avoidance conditioning can also appear in beginning stuttering. Using "um" or a similar extra sound as a "starter" is one example.

SCHOOL-AGE CHILDREN: INTERMEDIATE STUTTERING

The school-age child with **intermediate stuttering** (Fig. 7.5), who is typically between ages 6 and 13 years, is consciously aware of his stuttering and may have strong feelings about it. Frustration, embarrassment, and fear during the moment

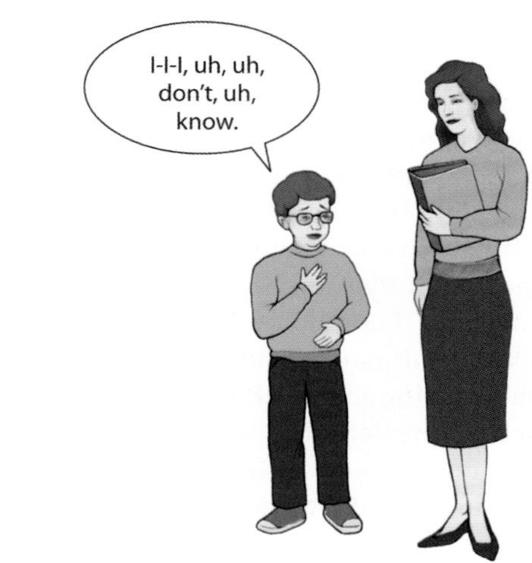

Figure 7.5 Child who may be an intermediate stutterer.

of stuttering become stronger as stuttering develops and persists. These feelings motivate escape and avoidance behaviors. Both behaviors can be seen in the video clip of "David" on *thePoint* (he is the fourth individual on Video 7-1 Normal Disfluency and the Development of Stuttering). In this clip, David is explaining a board game to his clinician. It starts with him just ending a sentence, saying, "...land here. He-he-he goes home auto..." (voicing cuts out, perhaps as the larynx abducts or adducts, then a silent block occurs on /m/ and David rocks back in his chair and comes forward in an escape behavior to help him finish the word "automatically." He continues, "...matically because...um...("tsk" sound made with tongue)...because he he i...is on the shortcut." Note that the "um" and perhaps the "tsk" sound are starters (avoidances). His repetition of "he" is also a starter. All these starters are probably motivated by his fear of stuttering on "is."

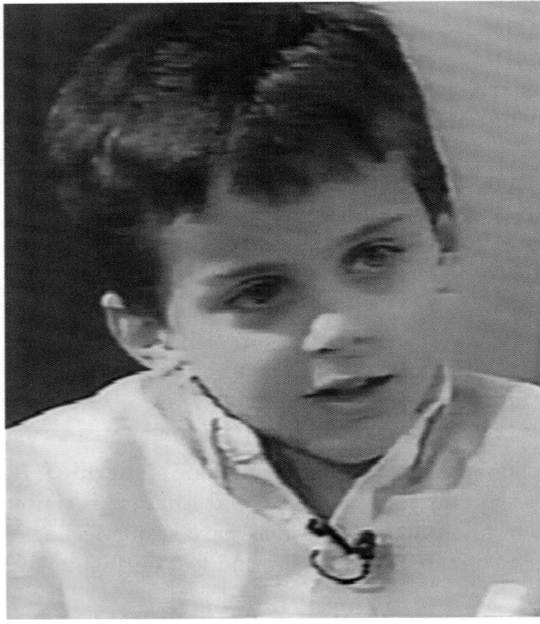

The fear felt by a student with intermediate stuttering may be attached at first to the sounds and words on which he stutters most. He becomes convinced that these sounds are harder for him. Then he begins to scan ahead to see whether he might have to say them. When he anticipates the sounds he may stutter on, he tries to avoid them. For example, he may say, "I don't know" to questions his teacher asks him in class, or he may substitute "my sister" for his sister's name when talking about her. Sometimes, he may start a sentence, realize a feared word is coming up, then switch the sentence around to avoid stuttering, and end up producing a maze of half-finished sentences. With tactful questioning, the clinician can verify these avoidances. She can also explore his escape behaviors—those things he does to finish a word he's stuttering on. It is essential that as the clinician talks to the student about his pattern of core behaviors, escapes and avoidances, she adopts an approach that helps the student feel accepted, "warts and all." Much will be conveyed by an accepting tone of voice. It's as if she says, "Yes you do have some things you've learned to do to try to deal with your stuttering. It's ok. But we'll work together to try to make talking easier so you don't have to use all these extra things to talk."

The fear of stuttering felt by most students with intermediate stuttering may be associated not only with sounds and words he often stutters on, but with situations as well. The youngster may find that he stutters more in some situations than in others. At first, he approaches these situations with dread, but later, he may go to great lengths to avoid them. Van Riper (1982) suggested that the development of such situational fears and avoidances depends on listener reactions. I think peer reactions may be particularly important. Over the course of therapy, the student can be helped to deal with peer reactions, by learning to be open about his stuttering with his class, his peers, and by talking with the clinician about some people's reactions. Sometimes a small group of students who stutter can be formed and can share their wounds inflicted by unhelpful or even belligerent peers.

With this overview in mind, we'll now get into the details of intermediate stuttering in school-age children.

Core Behaviors

What are these students' moments of stuttering like—when they don't avoid them? What are the core behaviors?

These students still have plenty of repetitions and prolongations. Many of these have pitch rise, indicating increasing tension. One of the big differences between beginning and intermediate core behaviors is the frequency of blocks. The blocks of students with intermediate stuttering seem to grow out of the cycle of fear → tension → longer, more struggled blocks → more fear → more tension. An individual at the intermediate level often stutters by stopping airflow, voicing, movement, or all three, and then struggling to get his speech going again. His stutters seem to surprise him less than when he was a beginning stutterer. Instead, as evidenced by his voice and manner in certain situations, he anticipates stutters.

I have the impression that the blocks in intermediate stuttering are frequently characterized by excessive laryngeal tension (Van Riper, 1974). Of course, tension is often seen elsewhere as well. The student may squeeze his lips together, jam his tongue against the roof of his mouth, or hold his breath. Even though he is not highly conscious of just what he's doing during a block, he has a vivid awareness that he is stuck, that he feels helpless, and that the word he wants to say just won't seem to come out. Because this happens when he is talking to someone, the connection to that person seems to be fractured when he gets stuck. As a result, the student often projects his own worst thoughts on the listener and imagines rejection.

A school-age child described his feeling of being blocked as like "a rock stuck in my throat." When he was lucky, he said, a little army of men would come into his throat and break the rock into little pieces, breaking the block so that sounds would come out. He was describing the experience of first being totally stuck and then rapidly repeating the first segment of the sound as he fought his way out of the block. A common example is the "...uh-uh-uh-I" that you will hear when someone is blocked on "I" and tries to push through it. At first, there is a moment of silence and then the rapid, staccato first segment of the sound as the child who stutters gets his larynx vibrating while maintaining a static articulatory posture. The larynx is still very tense; vibration stops and starts again and again. The vowel—either at the beginning or end of the syllable—is often the "schwa" or neutral vowel. In fact, it is only the first, brief segment of the intended vowel, which is cut off too abruptly to be perceived as the sound normally used in the word. Inexperienced clinicians sometimes mistakenly categorize these repeated parts of blocks as repetitions, not realizing the stuttering has advanced from repetitions to blocks.

In addition to repetitions of parts of sounds, blocks can have prolongations in them. Sometimes, as he is pushing through a block, a student will momentarily prolong a continuant sound as in "[m]...mmm...mmmm...my." Again, this probably results from the individual's larynx vibrating momentarily, then seizing up again, and then vibrating again. I categorize these events as blocks rather than prolongations, because I think the core behavior is a complete stoppage of speech, even though it is mixed with momentary releases of laryngeal vibration. This confusing situation probably results from the fact that the sequence of repetitions, prolongations, and blocks reflects basically similar behaviors along a continuum of increasing tension, particularly in the larynx, as stuttering progresses. When you analyze the speech of a school-age child with intermediate stuttering, try to discriminate which stutters are really repetitions and prolongations on their own, versus parts of the struggle behavior in blocks. The presence of blocks may mean that the young person's stuttering behaviors are affected by fear, and this must be dealt with in treatment.

Secondary Behaviors

The blocks just described can be devastating to a student who stutters. He is frustrated not only with his inability to make a sound, but he is often faced with surprised and uncomfortable listeners as well. Even patient listeners may not know what to do. They may interrupt, look away, or fidget, leaving the child to conclude that he is doing something wrong and should try to escape or avoid these painful moments.

The escape behaviors that a speaker uses to free himself from stutters are present in preschool children with beginning stuttering, but they occur far more frequently in school-age children with intermediate stuttering. They are often more complex, too. A child with intermediate stuttering may blink his eyes and nod his head in an effort to escape a block. Sometimes, he may do both, and if he is still unable to say the word, he may resort to yet another device, such as slapping his leg. As these patterns grow more complex, they may also become disguised to look like natural movements and are performed more rapidly.

A video clip of Richard, showing an escape behavior, is available on www.thepoint.lww.com. The clip is in the Chapter 7 videos. Notice that when Richard is first talking with the clinician, you can see movement of his right arm as he speaks. Later, when he answers the clinician's question "Where do you usually fish?" Richard brings his arm up near his mouth. What is he doing to escape from his moments of stuttering? Do you think his gesture becomes an avoidance behavior when he seems to bring his arm up before beginning the first word in his reply? Richard is now in his 30s and is Operations Manager for one of the largest automobile auction companies in the country. He uses his speech extensively to work with many employees who work for him, and he is constantly on the phone with dealers despite some residual stuttering.

In addition to escape behaviors, a student at the intermediate level develops both word and situation avoidances, as previously mentioned. Word avoidances appear after he has had repeated difficulty with a particular word or sound and has discovered how to take evasive action before he has to say it. For example, a young client in our clinic had been asked his name by a particularly stern teacher. He blocked severely on it and subsequently became fearful of saying his name, as well as other words starting with the same sound. He could usually think up synonyms for other words but what could he substitute for his name? So he learned to get a running start in saying his name by beginning with "My name is..." whenever he was asked his name. This permitted him to avoid stuttering about half of the time. It is a subtle form of avoidance that many clinicians call "starters." More obvious examples of avoidances are given in the following paragraph.

Van Riper's (1982) catalog of word avoidance techniques included **starters** (beginning a word by saying another word or sound, such as "well" or "uh" just before saying it); **substitutions** (substituting a word or phrase for another when stuttering is expected, as in "he's my unc-unc-unc ... my father's brother"); **circumlocutions** (talking all around a word or phrase when anticipating stuttering, as in "well, I went to ... yes, I really had a good time there, I saw the Empire State Building"); **postponements** (waiting a few beats or putting in filler words before starting a word on which stuttering is expected, as in "My name is......... Bill"); and **antiexpectancy devices** (using an odd manner or funny voice to avoid stuttering when it's anticipated). I had a client when I worked in Australia who could only tell jokes fluently if he put on an accent that sounded like he came from Mississippi or Alabama.

Like escape behaviors, word avoidance techniques often become more rapid and more subtle with time. Indeed, some individuals can disguise word avoidances to look like typical behavior. For example, they may put on pensive facial expressions and appear to search for a word while postponing their attempt to say a feared sound. Experienced clinicians learn to pick up subtle cues in the rate and manner of speaking that tip them off to the use of such avoidances. These avoidances can be explored by the clinician and client at the appropriate moment in treatment.

Situational fears and avoidances are also common in the school-age child with intermediate stuttering. Past stuttering in specific places or with specific people are the seeds from which situational fears grow. In school, students who stutter usually have trouble reading aloud or giving oral reports. Most people who stutter, and even many who don't, dread those classes in which teachers call on students by going up and down the rows. As in an earlier example, the students' fears steadily mount as a teacher goes down the row, getting closer and closer to calling on them. Then, if called on, they may say "I don't know" even when they do. Or they may take a failing grade rather than give the oral report. In contrast, other school situations, especially casual ones like gym class or lunch period, are likely to hold little fear or expectation of stuttering for them.

Situational fears quickly generate situation avoidances. The student who fears talking aloud in class may try to slouch low in his seat in hopes of being overlooked. A person who stutters who is afraid of making introductions will contrive ways of having other people make them. In junior high school, I coped with my fear of ordering in restaurants by ducking into the bathroom when the waitress approached our table, asking my friends to order a cheeseburger for me. Every person who stutters has his or her own pattern of situation avoidances, which may provide an important focus for therapy.

Feelings and Attitudes

Students with intermediate stuttering have gone well beyond the momentary frustration and embarrassment experienced by those with beginning stuttering. They have felt the helplessness of being caught in many blocks and runaway repetitions. The anticipation of stuttering and subsequent listener penalties has been fulfilled many times. These experiences pile up like cars in a demolition derby to create an entanglement of fear, embarrassment, and shame that accompanies stuttering. These feelings may not be pervasive or dog a stutterer all the time. However, stuttering has now changed from an annoyance to a serious problem.

A major influence on such a student's feelings is increased cognitive maturity, starting at age 3 or 4, that enables him to compare himself with his peers. Once he begins school, peers have a greater and greater influence on him. He may stutter more as he encounters new people and new situations, and, as he does, peers may begin to ask him why he talks the way he does and to make comments about his stuttering or tease him about it. As a result, increasingly negative self-awareness about his speech leads to feelings of embarrassment, shame, and guilt.

The Stuttering Foundation publication "Kids Letters" (Spring 2017) has several comments by school-age children that vividly depict their feelings about stuttering: "When I stutter, I feel like I am an idiot and dumb." "I stutter a lot and when I stutter I feel like I am trapped in a box with no door. I am trying to break down the walls with an axe." "My stuttering feels like a volcano." On the bright side, many of the students who made these comments also expressed very positive feelings about their progress in treatment. They also expressed their own growing confidence as they work on their speech: "I am a stuttering hero!" "Stuttering has never stopped me from being who I am." And they appreciate the help they get: "I love my speech teacher!"

For those who aren't able to get therapy, negative feelings may grow and soon affect behavior. The student may look away from listeners when he is stuttering and flush with embarrassment immediately afterward. He may become stiff and uneasy at the prospect of speaking. His stuttering pattern includes an increasing number of avoidance devices, and he is beginning to evade situations in which he feels he may stutter. These are all signs that his feelings and attitudes are becoming suffused with fear. Table 7.6 gives the characteristics of intermediate stutterers.

The emotions I have described, especially embarrassment and shame, may be mixed with hope as treatment begins. Figure 7.6 was drawn by a young man in his first few weeks of therapy. It reflects his extensive negative feelings on the left side—he has drawn himself in a jail cell with tears/rain falling around him and the key just out of reach. On the right side of the drawing, he shows himself as he hopes he will be after therapy, escaping from jail, running in the sunshine with grass underfoot and a flower in the background.

Underlying Processes

Many of the symptoms of intermediate stuttering result from the same processes that underlie those of beginning stuttering. There are important differences, however. In intermediate stuttering, classically conditioned tension responses are more evident, conditioned emotion is now turning into a more intense conscious fear reaction, and avoidance conditioning has become a big factor in shaping stuttering behaviors.

TABLE 7.6 Characteristics of Intermediate Stuttering in a School-Age Child

1. Frequent core behaviors are blocks in which the child shuts off sound or voice. He or she will also probably have many repetitions and prolongations.
2. Child uses escape behaviors to terminate blocks.
3. Child appears to anticipate blocks, often using avoidance behaviors prior to feared words. He or she also anticipates difficult situations and sometimes avoids them.
4. Fear before stuttering, embarrassment during stuttering, and shame after stuttering characterize this level, especially fear.

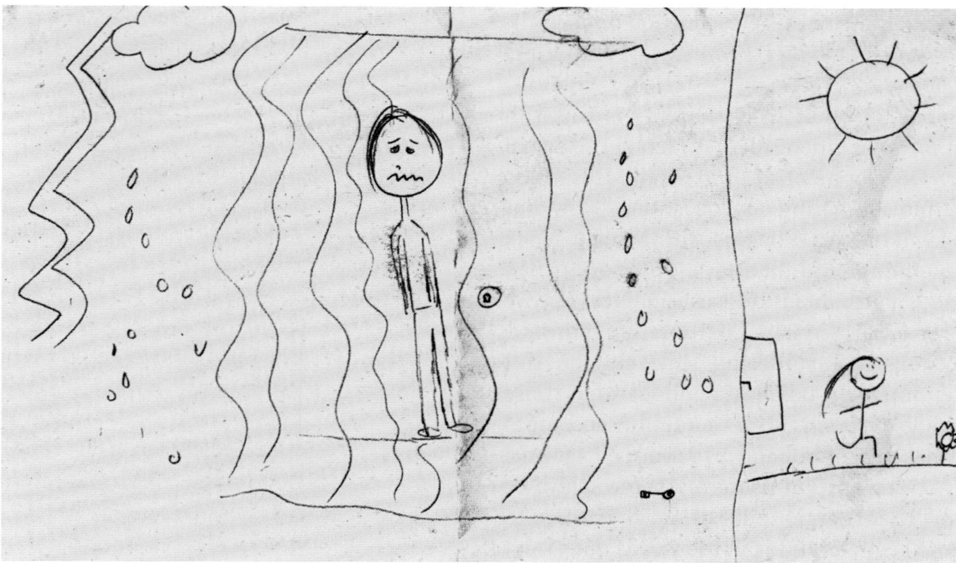

Figure 7.6 A young man's drawing of himself as he begins therapy (*left side*) and his hopes for a happy outcome (*right side*). (Drawn by Marcel Etienne.)

Avoidance conditioning transforms escape behaviors, such as the use of "um" to escape from a stuttering block, into avoidances, such as saying "um" before saying a word on which stuttering is expected. This learning process also leads students with intermediate stuttering to avoid words, to change sentences around, and to avoid speaking situations entirely. Avoidance learning also generalizes from one word to another and from one situation to another.

Avoidance conditioning may proceed very quickly in people with persistent stuttering because they may have a genetic or congenital bias toward right-hemisphere, emotionally based behaviors, as we described in Chapters 2, 3, 5, and 6. The threat of stuttering may elicit "prepared" defensive reactions, such as avoidances of words or situations. Such avoidances are strongly maintained because individuals who have developed them use them when they anticipate stuttering, which decreases or eliminates the fear. Thus, avoidances are maintained by negative reinforcement. By avoiding the stuttering, individuals who stutter never have the opportunity to discover that stuttering is not so painful after all. Therapy must do two things to reduce avoidance. First, the clinician must structure situations to help the student learn that the moment of stuttering can be tolerated and fear can be reduced by resisting the impulse to push through the stuttering—a behavior that rewards tension and struggle. Second, the clinician should help the student learn new behaviors to substitute for the old avoidances. Specific strategies such as easy onsets and slow pullouts, combined with reduction of fear and tension, can provide the student with new tools that will increase confidence. What better feeling for the student to have about his stuttering than "Bring it on!"

Summary

Three characteristics differentiate intermediate stuttering in school-age children from beginning stuttering in preschool children:

1. There are increasingly tense blocks, repetitions, and prolongations. The increased tension results from feelings of frustration, fear, and helplessness. These feelings trigger further tension responses, which interfere with fluency and in turn produce more frustration, fear, and feelings of helplessness. As tension mounts, this vicious cycle continues. Blocks are longer and more noticeable, more listeners react with surprise and impatience, and the student's fear increases in response to these reactions.
2. The increasing presence of fear and anticipation of bad experiences spurs the student to develop avoidance behaviors in addition to the escape behaviors he is already using. Avoidance conditioning is difficult to undo. Unless the fear that underlies avoidance is markedly reduced, relapse lurks close by.
3. The child with intermediate stuttering increasingly feels embarrassment, shame, and guilt as he realizes that his speech is markedly different from that of his peers.

OLDER TEENS AND ADULTS: ADVANCED STUTTERING

Individuals whose stuttering has persisted into older adolescence and adulthood (Fig. 7.7) typically have a deeply ingrained pattern of core and secondary behaviors. Often, stuttering is a major player in their school, work, and social lives. They may avoid talking in class, decline job opportunities, and limit their social activities from fear of stuttering. This described me at age 20.

A clip of "Sergio"—an adult who stutters—is the fifth and last sample on *thePoint* video titled "Video 7-1: Normal Disfluency and the Development of Stuttering." This video clip starts with Sergio answering my question, "How has your speech been lately?" Sergio begins with a silent block accompanied by jaw tremor and then says, "A lot of my bad habits are back." He is fairly fluent on this sentence, but we see some eye closures associated with his Tourette syndrome, which he has had, along with stuttering, since childhood. I then suggest, "Why don't you talk a little about what those bad habits are." Sergio responds with "uuuuuh," accompanied by a facial grimace used probably to release a laryngeal block. He then says, "I'm-I'm-I'm using mu-(note schwa or truncated vowel)-my (here Sergio makes a facial grimace to escape from the block) eyes to uh to get the words out."

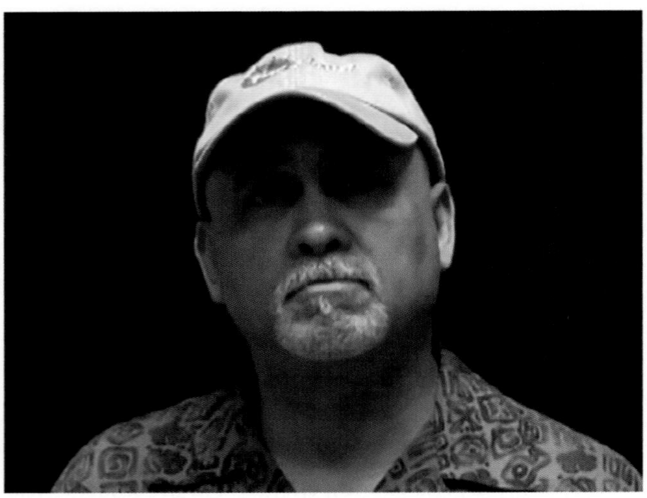

As you view the remainder of Sergio's clip, make a transcript and analyze what his stuttering behaviors are. This clip represents relatively severe stuttering in an adult.

In contrast to Sergio, some older teens and adults stutter only mildly or aren't bothered by their stuttering. They carry on their lives seeing it as a minor annoyance. These individuals often don't seek treatment—unless their stuttering suddenly gets in the way of something they want to do. One of my clients who had relatively mild stuttering was in the Air Force and wanted to move up from navigator to pilot. This was during the Vietnam War, and I worried that this promotion would put him more at risk. Nevertheless, we worked hard together for 6 months, and he made the grade.

Treatment of older teens and adults differs from treatment of younger stutterers because the client can take much of the responsibility for therapy including substantial work outside the clinic. An older teen or adult's increased capacity for independent work may compensate for another characteristic of

C... C... Could
y... you make
a ph... ph... phone
call for me?

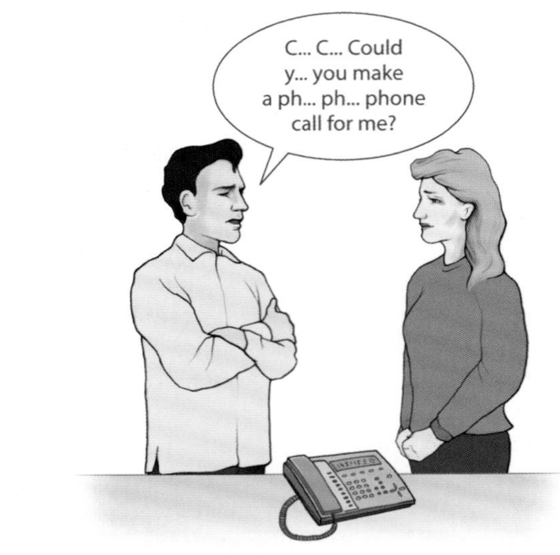

Figure 7.7 Individual who may be an advanced stutterer.

this level—a long history of stuttering. Patterns of stuttering with tension, escape, and avoidance behaviors are now firmly established. Emotions such as frustration, fear, guilt, and hostility have built up over many years of being unable to speak like other people and many bad experiences with thoughtless, uninformed, or momentarily startled listeners. Beliefs are usually distorted by the conviction that other people are impatient or disgusted by the speaker's stuttering.

After many years of stuttering, adults and adolescents who stutter increasingly think of themselves as "stutterers" rather than as people who have occasional difficulty speaking. Except for a few safe situations in which they may be relatively fluent, they have some fear of most speaking situations, and they shape their lives accordingly. They may believe that their stuttering is as noticeable to others as though they had two heads—and nearly as unacceptable.

Core Behaviors

Core behaviors in **advanced stuttering** include repetitions and prolongations, but are often distinct in the struggle and tension of blocks—stoppages of sound and movement. Advanced stutterers may block and then release a little sound only to fall back into the block again. It might sound like this: "[silence]... m-m-m...[silence]...m-m-muh...[silence]...my [said with a sudden effort]...name is Barry." Such behaviors may be longer and display more struggle in clients with advanced stuttering than in school-age youngsters who have intermediate stuttering, but they are essentially similar. However, blocks now may be associated with tremors. During blocks, tremors of the lips, jaw, or tongue may be apparent. Tremors appear in those who have been stuttering for several years and may occur when stuttering is accompanied by strong emotion. The video clip of "Sergio" referred to earlier has examples of tremors, such as when he makes his first attempt to say "patience."

In a few advanced stutterers, blocks are hardly evident. These individuals may have honed their avoidances to such a fine edge that core behaviors are scarcely noticeable. If stuttering does occur, it usually feels devastating to them. Consequently, much of their energy is spent anticipating blocks that never happen and mustering avoidances to keep anxiety at bay. One such individual, a delightful woman I knew and whom I'll call "Lenore," said she had stuttered since childhood. Yet, she almost never had a repetition, prolongation, or block that I could see. Lenore was highly competent at everything she did, but severely limited her life because of her fear that she would stutter. In particular, she often felt she came across as far less articulate than she might have because of the frequency with which she substituted words to avoid stuttering.

Older teens and adults with advanced stuttering, like school-age youngsters at the intermediate level, have repetitions as well as blocks. These are usually not the easy, regular repetitions of borderline stuttering, but are more like those of beginning stuttering—tense, with a rapid, irregular tempo. They may be repetitions of syllables, luh-luh-luh-like this, or words, like I-I-I-I. As I've indicated earlier, some apparent repetitions are actually components of blocks. The latter look as if the speaker recoils from a momentary fixation and then gets stuck again. In an evaluation, and throughout therapy, be sure to distinguish relatively easy repetitions that emerge from anomalies in neural pathways for speech from those that are recoil reactions to hitting up against the hard wall of a block. An example of the latter is Sergio's "mu-mu-my eyes."

Secondary Behaviors

Advanced stuttering in older teens and adults involves many of the same word and situational avoidances that are seen in intermediate stuttering, but the avoidances are likely to be more extensive. Some behaviors are more obvious than others. When I was in high school, I used several avoidance devices that often didn't work, such as "uh ... well ... you see" and a gasp of air, followed by a block of long duration filled with unsuccessful escape attempts before I finally released the blocked word with great effort. Other advanced stutterers may approach feared words cautiously and use subtle mannerisms, such as appearing to think just before saying them, so that most listeners don't realize they are stuttering. These stutterers are usually on guard much of the time, scanning ahead with their verbal early-warning systems.

Many individuals with advanced stuttering also control their environments carefully so that they can avoid situations in which they are likely to stutter. They may feign sickness when they have to give a speech, use answering machines rather than answering the telephone, or arrange to have their spouses or children deal with store clerks. Often, with careful questioning of individuals with advanced stuttering who use avoidances a great deal, you can learn what occurs when avoidances don't work. Even the most skillful avoiders are sometimes caught with their defenses down and become stuck in a block. Core behaviors may also be elicited by asking some stutterers to stutter openly without using secondary behaviors. Individuals who can do this, especially those who can do it without excessive discomfort, are more amenable to change.

Feelings and Attitudes

The feelings and attitudes of older teens and adults, like their stuttering behaviors, have been shaped by years of conditioning. Over and over, they have learned that much of their stuttering is unpredictable. When it is predictable, it comes when they want it least—when they want more than anything to be fluent. As a result, they often feel out of control. Figure 7.8 reflects one individual's depictions of his own feelings of being "locked up" and out of control when stuttering. Note the iron band clamping his head, his jammed up teeth, and clenching of his abdomen.

These uncomfortable feelings are often buttressed by an individual's perceptions of how others see him. Listeners' reactions look overwhelmingly negative to him. Even when listeners say nothing, their faces appear to say everything. It is as though stuttering is a rattletrap car that always stalls in heavy traffic amid honking drivers. Such experiences gradually shape the attitudes of those with advanced stuttering toward feelings of helplessness, frustration, anger, and hopelessness.

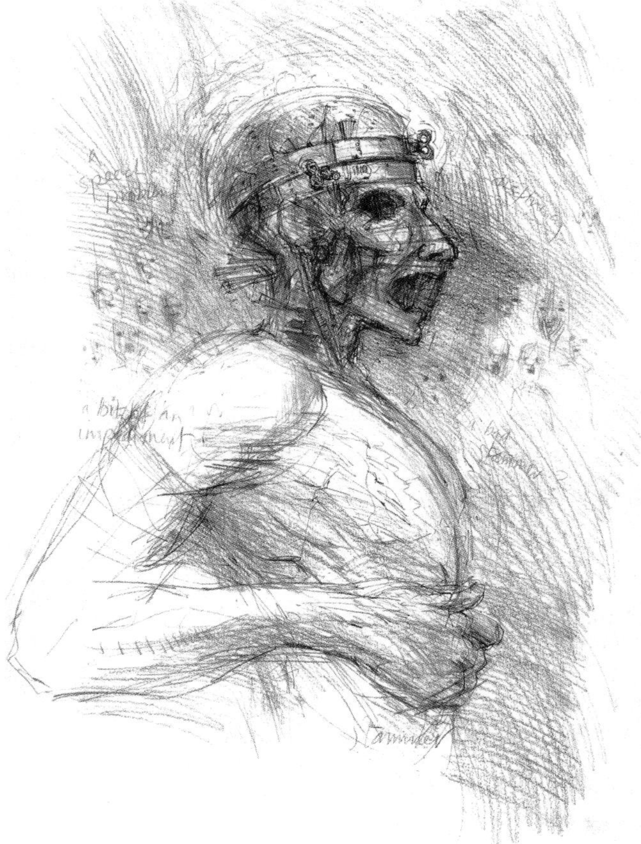

Figure 7.8 "How I feel when I stutter" by Mike Peace. (Courtesy of Dr. Trudy Stewart.)

Of course, individuals' responses to stuttering vary greatly. If a person who stutters has many talents and abilities for which he is recognized and if he has an assertive personality, he may be less devastated by stuttering. The former CEO of General Electric, Jack Welch, is a good example. But if the individual has a highly sensitive nature, his feelings and attitudes about stuttering may be an important component of his problem. The movie "The King's Speech" suggested that Bertie, who was to become the King of England, George VI, was a sensitive soul who was debilitated by his stuttering until he received some very confidence-building treatment from Lionel Logue, his unorthodox Australian clinician.

The point is that by the time a person who stutters is an adult, he has had years of experiencing stuttering, feeling frustrated and helpless, and has developed techniques to minimize pain. Unless he has strong attributes to compensate, he is likely to feel that stuttering is a big part of who he is to other people. It is a part that he hates, a part on which he blames many other troubles, and a part he wants desperately to eliminate.

Some people who stutter, however, who reach the advanced level have become reconciled to their stuttering. If they are in their 20s, 30s, or beyond, there may be some natural resistance to treatment, because stuttering has become part of their identities. After years of doubt and turmoil, they've grown accustomed to themselves as someone who stutters. To consider treatment is to reject a part of themselves, to open old wounds. Those who risk change, enter treatment, and succeed will find the risk to have been worthwhile. But those who enter treatment and do not succeed may suffer twice from the pain of failure as well as the loss of the denial or reluctant acceptance of stuttering that had been in place before the attempt at treatment but was given up.

Table 7.7 lists the major characteristics of advanced stutterers.

TABLE 7.7 Characteristics of Advanced Stuttering in Older Teens and Adults

1. Most frequent core behaviors are longer, tense blocks, often with tremors of the lips, tongue, or jaw. Individual will also probably have repetitions and prolongations.
2. Stuttering may be suppressed in some individuals through extensive avoidance behaviors.
3. Complex patterns of avoidance and escape behaviors characterize the stutterer. These may be very rapid and so well habituated that the stutterer may not be aware of what he does.
4. Emotions of fear, embarrassment, and shame are very strong. Individual has negative feelings about himself as a person who is helpless and inept when he stutters. This self-concept may be pervasive.

Underlying Processes

Advanced stuttering, unlike lower levels of stuttering, is influenced less by its original constitutional, developmental, and environmental factors than by the older teen or adult's reactions to his stuttering. That is not to say that anomalies in neural pathways are having no effect. It is likely that individuals with more inefficient neural pathways will still experience the effect on their speech. However, it seems likely that the effects of home environments and developmental pressures of speech and language have been somewhat diminished by maturation and learning. But conditioned responses that were learned in reaction to disfluencies caused by constitutional factors are stronger than ever. Their effects have been magnified by years of experience, and the way the brain operates in speech has probably been modified as a consequence. Moreover, an individual's characteristic patterns of tension, escape, and avoidance have become almost automatic through years of practice. For example, the individual with advanced stuttering may exhibit a string of avoidance and escape behaviors but only remember that "the word got stuck."

The older teen and adult's stuttering is affected by higher-level explicit learning as well. He has developed a self-concept as an impaired speaker, which carries highly negative connotations for most. Self-concepts begin to be formed during preschool years and are based initially on what one can do, rather than what one is (Clarke-Stewart & Friedman, 1987). More enduring traits are added as a result of social interactions in later childhood, adolescence, and beyond (Roessler & Bolton, 1978). Thus, the self-concept of someone who stutters is determined, in part, by his perception of how he talks. In a child's early years, his impression of stuttering may be a fleeting awareness that he sometimes has difficulty talking. In later levels of development, the reactions of significant listeners—parents, peer group, other adults—have a major impact. Now, his self-concept may become filled with relatively enduring negative perceptions as a result of listeners' impatience and rejection. A negative self-concept is formed not only by perceptions of listeners' reactions, but, in a continuing spiral, the negative self-concept also affects those perceptions.

To return to research, studies of the psychology of disability suggest that "one's perception of self influences one's perception of others' views of oneself, rendering social interaction more difficult" (Roessler & Bolton, 1978). Applied to clients with advanced stuttering, this suggests that they are likely to project their own rejections of stuttering onto listeners, thereby affecting their interactions with them. This vicious cycle can only be stopped when an outsider helps a person who stutters test the reality of his perceptions.

In addition to working on cognitive aspects of the problem, therapy for advanced stuttering also must deal directly with the avoidances that such clients have learned so well. As mentioned in the discussion of intermediate stuttering, as avoidance conditioning progresses, individuals fear not only words and situations but also stuttering itself. By reducing this fear and changing avoidances, treatment enables individuals who stutter to stutter with less fear by associating the clinician's approval and their own successes with a calmer, more relaxed way of stuttering. Gradually, tension and hurry fade from disfluencies, they feel more in control, and their fears diminish even further as a result.

Summary

The category of advanced stuttering in older teens and adults describes a developmental level and implies a particular treatment orientation as characterized by the following:

1. Treatment may be easier because the client can assume much of the responsibility for generalization beyond the clinic.
2. On the other hand, treatment is more challenging because the client with advanced stuttering has more deeply habituated patterns of behavior than at earlier levels. The individual's core behaviors often consist of long blocks with considerable tension and at times visible tremors. Secondary behaviors may consist of long chains of word avoidance and escape behaviors. Situational avoidance is common.
3. Some older teens and adult stutterers may hide and disguise their stuttering well enough to avoid detection by many listeners, but this is at the cost of constant vigilance. If this behavior is pervasive, it is sometimes called "covert stuttering." It can be difficult to treat because the individual may strongly resist bringing the stuttering out into the open so that they may modify it.
4. Feelings of frustration and helplessness usually accumulate over the years, leading to coping behaviors and a lifestyle that may be highly constrained. Such responses create a self-concept of an inept speaker whose stuttering is unacceptable to listeners. This in turn affects the stutterer's perceptions of the listener's reactions.

TABLE 7.8 Characteristics of Five Developmental/Treatment Levels

Developmental/ Treatment Level	Core Behaviors	Secondary Behaviors	Feelings and Attitudes	Underlying Processes
Typical disfluency	10 or fewer disfluencies per 100 words; one-unit repetitions; mostly repetitions, interjections, and revisions	None	Not aware; no concern	Typical stresses of speech/language and psychosocial development
Borderline stuttering	≥11 disfluencies per 100 words; more than two units in repetitions; more repetitions and prolongations than revisions or interjections	None	Generally not aware; may occasionally show momentary surprise or mild frustration	Stresses of speech/ language and psychosocial development interacting with constitutional predisposition
Beginning stuttering	Rapid, irregular, and tense repetitions may have fixed articulatory posture in blocks	Escape behaviors such as eye blinks, increases in pitch, or loudness as disfluency progresses	Aware of disfluency, may express frustration	Conditioned emotional reactions causing excess tension; instrumental conditioning resulting in escape behaviors
Intermediate stuttering	Blocks in which sound and airflow are shut off	Escape and avoidance behaviors	Fear, frustration, embarrassment, and shame	Above processes, plus avoidance conditioning
Advanced stuttering	Long, tense blocks; some with tremor	Escape and avoidance behaviors	Fear, frustration, embarrassment, and shame; negative self-concept	Above processes, plus cognitive learning

SUMMARY

- Table 7.8 summarizes the characteristics of the five developmental/treatment levels described in this chapter.
- Each individual who stutters will have his own course of development, influenced by the interaction of constitutional and environmental factors.
- The clinician needs to use her understanding of the underlying processes to design procedures to treat each individual's core behaviors, secondary behaviors, and feelings and attitudes.

STUDY QUESTIONS

1. In the "Exceptions and Variations" section of the Overview, different types of stuttering onset and development are described. What factors might cause these differences?
2. In discussing typical disfluency, it is suggested that "if a child shows what appears to be typical disfluencies, such as single-word repetitions, but consistently displays pauses or interjections of 'uh' immediately before or during disfluencies, he should be carefully evaluated as possibly stuttering." What might be going on? What might these pauses or interjections signify?
3. The idea of a dyssynchrony in the timing of the elements of spoken language production is suggested as an underlying process of typical disfluency. It is also used to account for primary stuttering. How can both types of disfluency be accounted for by the same process?
4. What is the difference between core behaviors and secondary behaviors?
5. At what ages is typical disfluency likely to be most frequent?
6. Name three influences that may cause typical disfluency to increase.
7. What are three ways in which core behaviors of typical disfluency differ from those of borderline stuttering?
8. Describe the core behaviors of the beginning stutterer.
9. What causes greater muscle tension in beginning stuttering compared to borderline stuttering?
10. Describe why an escape behavior is used by a stutterer. Give examples.
11. What is a major secondary behavior that differentiates the intermediate from the beginning stutterer?
12. Compare the feelings and attitudes of the borderline, beginning, and intermediate levels of stuttering.
13. Describe the role of the listener in the development of the advanced stutterer's self-concept.

SUGGESTED PROJECTS

1. Visit *thePoint* and watch the video clips of speakers who are representative of each level of stuttering (typical disfluency, borderline, beginning, intermediate, and advanced), and play them in random order for your class. See how many of your fellow students can correctly identify each level.
2. Make audio or video recordings of a number of nonstuttering students in a class, and determine which of them are more disfluent and which are less disfluent. Is there a gradual continuum between more disfluent and less disfluent, or are there two distinct groups? Do any of the "typically disfluent" students who show a high frequeny of disfluencies actually showing borderline stuttering? Should the term "borderline stutterer" be used only for preschoolers?
3. Read Yairi and Ambrose's (2005) chapter on the development of stuttering (see Suggested Readings), and compare that perspective with the view presented in this chapter.

SUGGESTED READINGS

Bloodstein, O., & Ratner, N. (2008). Symptomatology. In: *A handbook on stuttering* (pp. 1–38). Clifton Park, NY: Tomson-Delmar Learning.

The subsection titled "Developmental Changes in Stuttering" in this chapter describes four stages similar to our levels of stuttering development. Other schemas of developmental changes are also discussed in a clear and logical style.

Gray, J. A. (1987). *The psychology of fear and stress.* Cambridge, UK: Cambridge University Press.

This is a very readable exposition of findings about innate fears, conditioning, and brain processes involved with escape and avoidance learning. Gray also describes his concept of the "behavioral inhibition system," a model of the role of conditioning, language, the limbic system, and anxiety on behavior.

Luper, H. L., & Mulder, R. L. (1964). *Stuttering: Therapy for children.* Englewood Cliffs, NJ: Prentice-Hall.

An excellent treatment text that describes four developmental levels of stuttering similar to the levels described here. Although out of print, this book is available for under $10 at http://www.AbeBooks.com.

Starkweather, C. W. (1983). *Speech and language: Principles and processes of behavior change.* Englewood Cliffs, NJ: Prentice-Hall.

This book describes the principles of instrumental, classical, and avoidance conditioning that underlie much of stuttering behavior. It gives a clear account of how these principles create stuttering behavior and how conditioning is used in treatment.

Stuttering Foundation. (Autumn, 2017). *Kids' letters and drawings. Magazine.* Memphis, TN: Stuttering Foundation.

Stuttering Foundation has an electronic magazine called Letters and Drawings from Kids. You can access it at www.stutteringhelp.org/drawings-and-letters-kids. The Web site invites kids to submit letters and drawings to their Web site so they can be shared with a wide audience.

Van Riper, C. (1982). The development of stuttering. In: *The nature of stuttering* (pp. 88–110). Englewood Cliffs, NJ: Prentice-Hall.

In this chapter, Van Riper describes four developmental tracks of stuttering, three of which depart substantially from our stages of stuttering development. This chapter gives the reader a good sense of individual variability in stuttering.

Williams, D. F. (2006) *Stuttering recovery: Personal and empirical perspectives.* Mahwah, NJ: Lawrence Erlbaum Associates.

This book is an informal compendium of essays about the experience of stuttering, information about stuttering, and personal anecdotes about the things that happen to you when you stutter.

Yairi, E., & Ambrose, N. G. (2005). The development of stuttering. In: *Early childhood stuttering: For clinicians by clinicians* (pp. 141–195). Austin, TX: Pro-Ed.

This chapter reviews other authors' descriptions of the development of stuttering and presents a different perspective on the changes that occur in stuttering from onset to recovery or persistence. The data provided support the view that 75 to 85 percent of children who begin to stutter will recover without treatment and that stuttering typically decreases in severity and frequency after onset.

Compare the description of stuttering development in this chapter with those of three other popular textbooks on stuttering:

1. Conture, E. (2000). *Stuttering: Its nature, diagnosis, and treatment.* New York, NY: Allyn & Bacon.
2. Shapiro, D. (1999). *Stuttering intervention.* Austin, TX: Pro-Ed.
3. Manning, W., & DiLollo, *A.* (2017). *Clinical decision making in fluency disorders.* San Diego, CA: Plural Publishing.

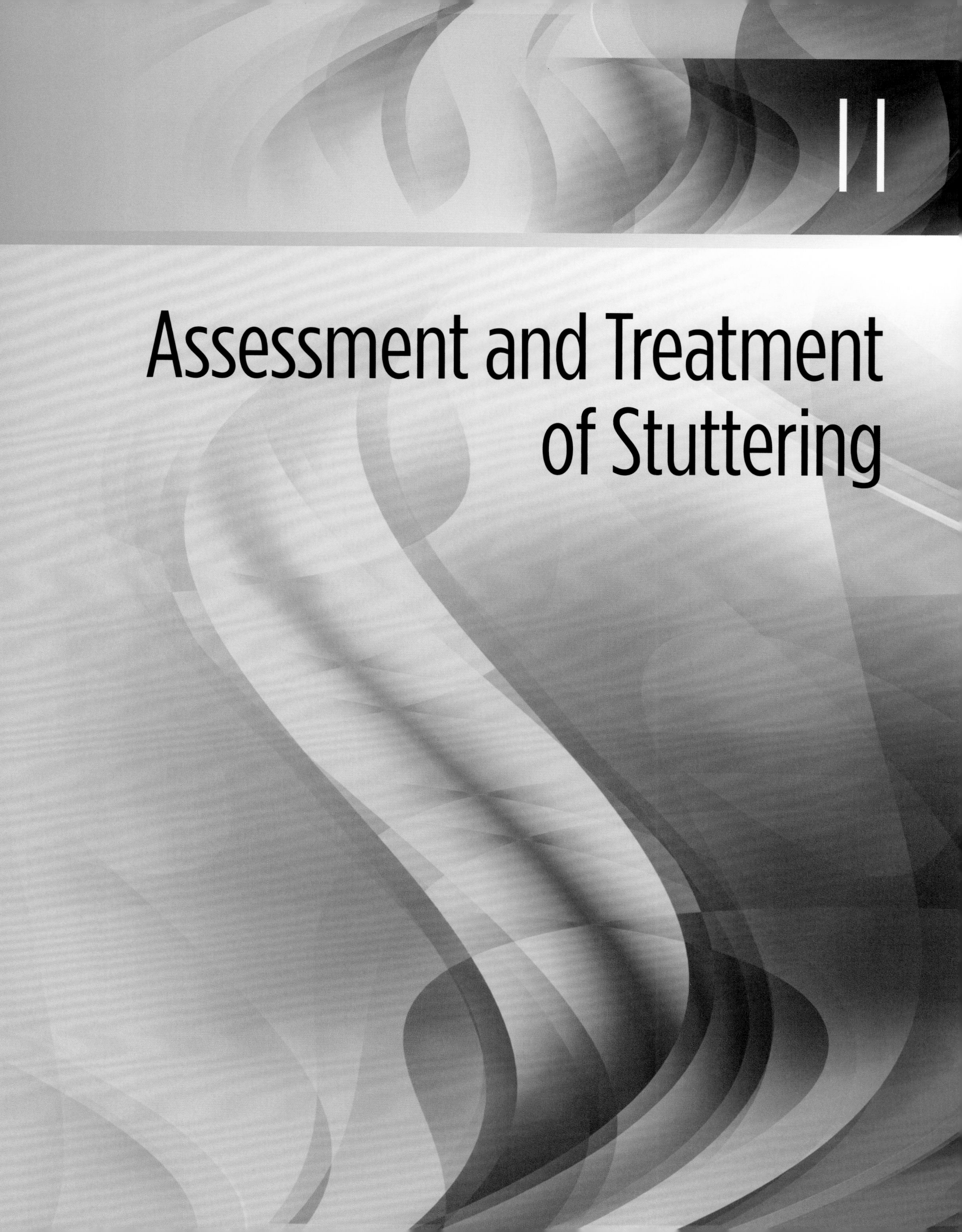

II

Assessment and Treatment of Stuttering

8

Preliminaries to Assessment

Chapter Objectives

After studying this chapter, readers should be able to:

- Understand how to discern the client's needs and plan treatment around them
- Describe how to protect the client's right to privacy and how awareness of the client's right to privacy can facilitate trust
- Explain why multicultural awareness is so important when working with clients from different cultural and linguistic backgrounds
- Describe how a clinician can demonstrate her expertise about stuttering in a way that will engender trust and motivation
- Explain why reliability in a measurement procedure is important and how reliability may be assessed
- Discuss the need for obtaining appropriate speech samples when assessing stuttering
- Explain the advantages and disadvantages of assessing frequency of stuttering and how frequency can be assessed effectively
- Explain why it can be useful to assess different types of stutters that a client may have
- Describe how duration of stutters may be important and how this can be assessed
- Discuss assessment of secondary stuttering behaviors
- Describe four tools to assess stuttering severity and explain when each might be used
- Explain why speech naturalness can be a useful measure related to fluency
- Explain why assessment of speaking rate may be important

- Discuss at least three ways in which feelings and attitudes can be assessed in each of these age groups: preschool, school-age, and adolescents and adults
- Talk about the need for continuing assessment of clients in treatment

Key Terms

Confronting stuttering: Talking about stuttering, emulating it, and being aware of what's happening during the moment of stuttering. These activities can be engaged in by either the clinician or client, when appropriate. These activities and others are thought to reverse the tendency to run away from stuttering that may make stuttering worse.

Continuing assessment: Measurement and evaluation of changes the client is making/has made over the short and long term

Duration: The length of time, usually in seconds, that a stutter lasts. From my perspective, this includes the time when forward movement of speech is halted; therefore, the moment of the actual block, prolongation, or repetition is measured as well as the time taken by various starters, postponements, and other secondary behaviors.

Empathy: The capacity to understand another's perspectives, beliefs, and emotions. Having this capacity to some degree allows the clinician to undertake appropriate treatment and to develop trust between herself and the patient—a prerequisite for change.

Evidence of reliability: Data suggest that a procedure or measurement tool produces approximately the same result when used by different individuals or the same individual at different times

Feelings and attitudes: Feelings are the transient emotions experienced by the person who stutters, especially regarding the experience of stuttering and perceived listener responses. They can vary from one time to the next. Attitudes are more long-lasting; they reflect the stutterer's beliefs about how people perceive him and how he perceives himself in regard to his stuttering.

Health Insurance Portability and Accountability Act of 1996 (HIPAA): Legislation that created national standards to protect the privacy of patient information and still allow access to that information for the safety and proper treatment of patients

Interrater reliability: Comparison of results by different individuals using a measurement tool

Intrarater reliability: Comparison of results by an individual using a measurement tool at two or more different times

Multicultural perspective: An awareness by the clinician of differences in cultures regarding speech, language, and hearing issues as well as differences in styles of interaction between men and women, elders and younger individuals, family and strangers

Percentage of syllables stuttered: A common measure of frequency of stuttering obtained by counting the total number of syllables spoken and dividing it into the number of syllables that are stuttered

Severity: Generally a measure of the impediment to communication caused by the stuttering. This may be an overall impression or a compilation of stuttering frequency and duration as well as other behaviors that impede communication.

Speaking rate: How fast a person talks, usually with short pauses included. (Articulation rate is with the pauses removed.) Speaking rate is most often measured in syllables per minute.

Speech naturalness: The extent to which speech sounds like that of a typical speaker who doesn't stutter. This measure is useful because sometimes treatment leaves the individual technically "fluent" but sounding overly slow or otherwise odd, for example, due to altered intonation patterns.

Types of stutters: The different ways in which an individual may stutter. These include the categories of repetitions, prolongations, and blocks.

Assessment operates on many levels. On one level, there is information gathering, such as interviewing, measuring speech fluency, and administering tests and questionnaires. This requires careful planning, good observation, and thorough analysis. It begins with clients seeking help and often ends with a plan for treatment. On another level, assessment is a personal encounter. It involves getting to know another person and sometimes his family as well, trying to connect to him, and tuning your antennae to pick up the subtle signals he may be sending out about his needs and how you might help him. On this more subjective level, you are becoming aware of the entire person and family, not just the stuttering. Your clients are also getting to know you and sizing up your ability to help them; thus, this first meeting may be the most critical. Although you will want to show an individual client or family that you know about stuttering and understand its treatment, you will want to spend most of your time listening to their concerns and demonstrating your desire to understand them. The two hats you will wear—that of the humanist and that of the scientist—will become a natural part of your wardrobe as you gain more experience.

THE CLIENT'S NEEDS

It is easy to say we must always consider a client's needs, but it can sometimes be hard to put this into practice. One reason for this being a challenge is that we can develop expectations that function as blinders. Such expectations affect our perceptions of what our clients want, what caused or precipitated their stuttering, what their priorities are, and many other things. Although I know intellectually that every client is different, I have found a tendency in myself, perhaps increasing as I have become more experienced, to jump to conclusions. I sometimes think, "Ah, yes, I understand this kiddo. So much like that child I saw last month." You will find this true for yourself too as you work with more and more clients. We must try to listen carefully to what each client says and see each person with fresh eyes.

We must also be cautious about letting referral information, past experience, and biases cloud our ability to see all aspects of the person clearly. We must be wary of simple explanations and quick judgments about which factors are critical for a client. For instance, if parents tell us that they often ask their child to stop and start again when she stutters, that both parents work long hours outside the home, and that dinner is a noisy and confusing time, we should try not to assume that these pressures at home are a major problem for the child. They may or may not be, and other things may be more critical. We need to ask more questions and explore how the child responds in these and other situations before we decide how to begin helping the child and her family.

Sometimes individuals' or families' requests differ from what we think they need. An adult may say that she wants "completely fluent speech," but we know this is not a likely outcome for a person who has been stuttering for 20 or 30 years. Or a family may want us to treat their 3-year-old child without their having to take part in therapy, although our preferred approach for a child this age involves parent participation. I have found it best not to feel I have to resolve such issues during a single session. I make no promises but do make a concerted effort to understand what clients and families want and why. My experience has been that after I work with a family or individual for several sessions, we build up enough trust to work together to make the changes that we mutually decide are appropriate. I vividly remember a young school-age child brought to me by his mother after years of previous therapy had failed. When we started therapy, this mom was troubled by the approach I took for therapy with her son. As I adjusted the therapy so that it was less objectionable to her but still moving in the right direction to help her son, I also spent a considerable amount of time listening to her concerns about her son's future and his difficulty being teased in school. Over the ensuing months, my graduate student and I also went to the child's classroom to help his peers understand the child's stuttering. Gradually, the mother began to trust us and became a stronger ally in the treatment of her son.

One way to begin to understand an adolescent or adult client's needs is to ask him directly about what he would like from therapy. Rebecca McCauley and I (Guitar & McCauley, 2010) developed a questionnaire to gather this information from clients. It has been improved by Hilda Sønsterud and her colleagues at the National Support System for Special Education in Norway. The form is illustrated in Figure 8.1. It should be used as a basis for discussion of what the client's hopes and desires are in therapy, rather than to gather the information to simply decide upon what to focus on in treatment. With adolescents and adults, the course of therapy is a mutually determined process.

In this regard, I remember seeing a young man who came to our clinic from some distance away for intensive therapy. We didn't have the questionnaire for discussing aims at that time, but during the evaluation, he said he didn't want a kind of therapy he'd heard about where the person who stutters is treated like a rat in a cage; in other words, he wanted no talk of conditioning, reinforcement, or shaping. In responding to his concerns, I talked about his stuttering with him in terms of what he felt about it, what he believed his listeners thought, and why he did some of the things he did when he stuttered. Together, we designed an intensive treatment program for him that included plenty of "fluency shaping" and "maintenance" but that made him feel respected as a human being and not treated like a laboratory animal. In the process, I also explored with him his concerns about therapy that was too "behavioral."

In trying to meet a client's needs, I consider the person as well as the problem. The client, no matter what age, will sense quickly whether a clinician is seeing him as an individual or is only seeing his stuttering. An effective clinician is genuinely interested and empathetic; she accepts failures and reversals into older habits as well as victories and progress. The initial evaluation session with a school-age child, a teen, or an adult provides the clinician with her first opportunity to show the client that she accepts him just as he is, without rejection or fear of his stuttering. This atmosphere helps the client begin to accept himself and his stuttering. A change takes place in the client's feelings of frustration and fear when the clinician shows genuine curiosity and interest in what the client does when he stutters and how he feels about it. You can see this happening right before your eyes as you encourage your client to stutter, as you both try to collect a good sample to analyze together. As Van Riper (1982) observes, "....in this collecting and analyzing process, the [person who

Personal aims for the stuttering treatment

I would like treatment to focus on:

[ ] the physical aspects of stuttering

[ ] the feelings associated with stuttering

[ ] both physical and emotional aspects

How important are the following goals for you?	(Rank from 1 = not important to 5 = very important)				
Very fluent speech	1	2	3	4	5
Feeling of control of stuttering	1	2	3	4	5
More positive feelings associated with stuttering	1	2	3	4	5
Ease of participation in most or all speaking situations	1	2	3	4	5
Other: ______________________	1	2	3	4	5
<u>In which situations would you particularly like to speak more easily?</u>					
Talking on the telephone	1	2	3	4	5
Introducing myself to others	1	2	3	4	5
Conversations with family members	1	2	3	4	5
Conversations with friends	1	2	3	4	5
Conversations with strangers	1	2	3	4	5
Conversations with colleagues	1	2	3	4	5
Talking to supervisor	1	2	3	4	5
Other situations: ______________________	1	2	3	4	5
Motivation and expectations	(Rank from 1 = not at all/nothing, to 5 = very much, completely)				
<u>Answer the questions based on your personal views:</u>					
How persistent are you at seeing tasks through, in general?	1	2	3	4	5
How motivated are you to work on your stuttering?	1	2	3	4	5
How much time can you set aside for independent training?	1	2	3	4	5
How much support or help do you expect during the treatment?	1	2	3	4	5
What is your anticipation of the success of the treatment?	1	2	3	4	5

Figure 8.1 Personal Aims for Stuttering Treatment. This is a questionnaire filled out by a client that can provide a basis for understanding clients' hopes and desires for treatment. (Reprinted from Guitar, B., & McCauley, R. J. (2010). *Treatment of stuttering: established and emerging approaches*. Philadelphia: Lippincott Williams & Wilkins, a Wolters Kluwer business, with permission.)

Describe, using your own words, your goals and wishes for the treatment (both short- and long-term)

____

____

____

____

What do you need in order to achieve these goals?

____

____

____

____

Other factors that are important for you in this collaboration, or that you wish to highlight:

____

____

____

____

Name of a close friend or relative who can take a role of "training partner":

____

Your name: ______________________ **E-mail:** ______________________

Phone: ______________ **Date for filling out this form:** ______________________

Figure 8.1 *(Continued)*

stutters] soon discerns that the therapist does not reject or punish his stuttering but instead welcomes it as necessary for the analytic confrontation. Identification aids desensitization" (p. 246).

INSURANCE CONSIDERATIONS

An issue that might come up when you first talk with a client is whether their insurance will cover their stuttering evaluation and treatment sessions. You may help them get the best information about how to approach the problem by doing an Internet search using the phrase "insurance coverage for stuttering." Excellent advice is available online from the Stuttering Foundation, the American Speech-Language-Hearing Association, the National Stuttering Association, and other sites.

Among the tips that these sources provide are that (1) clients should read their insurance policy and talk with a representative on the phone to get details on coverage for stuttering evaluation and therapy; (2) clients should provide the insurance company with information about the neurological and genetic basis of stuttering (some Web sites provide examples) and that stuttering is not an educational issue or a developmental issue but a medical problem, with its onset in childhood; (3) some insurance companies require a referral for treatment from a physician; and (4) there are steps to follow to respond to a denial of coverage, via an appeal process.

THE CLIENT'S RIGHT TO PRIVACY

All clients should feel they can trust you to protect their privacy and confidentiality. Trust is a vital element of client-clinician relationships. It enables the client to feel that she can safely reveal personal information to you that will help you plan and carry out appropriate treatment. In many cases, the act of expressing feelings in an accepting, secure environment can be therapeutic. For example, a mother whose school-age child was not making progress told her clinician that she was feeling resentment and impatience about her child's stuttering. She talked at some length about this over several sessions, and the clinician listened empathetically. Once this mother had released these feelings, her child made remarkable progress. Although creating an accepting atmosphere for the child is the most important outcome in this scenario, this example illustrates that the parent had to trust the clinician to accept her feelings without judgment, as well as not to share this information inappropriately with other family members or the child, or, just as inappropriately, with others not involved in the child's care.

Federal and state legislation, such as the Health Insurance Portability and Accountability Act of 1996 (**HIPAA**), helps clinicians follow best practices for protecting clients' privacy. Clinicians should familiarize themselves with these laws and guidelines and ensure that clients give their consent for video recording and observation and for sharing information about them. You can learn more from the Web site http://www.hhs.gov/ocr/privacy/. When clients perceive that we are scrupulous in guarding their privacy and confidentiality, we gain a level of trust that enhances therapy. This confidentiality extends to children as well. The bond between a child and clinician will be enhanced if the clinician discusses what information the child is willing to have shared with her parent and what not to share. This is especially relevant for school-age children, who should also be consulted about the extent to which they would be comfortable having their parents involved in treatment.

I should mention that there are a few rare circumstances in which confidentiality may be broken. These are the unusual situations when a client discloses plans to hurt self or others and instances of child abuse disclosed by the child.

MULTICULTURAL AND MULTILINGUAL CONSIDERATIONS

Let me begin this discussion of stuttering in other cultures and other languages by introducing you to a former client of mine, Sergio Torres. Sergio grew up in New York City in a Latino household (the term "Latino" includes Latin American countries, not just those speaking Spanish). His parents were from Puerto Rico, and Sergio said that his father embraced an attitude of "men don't cry" and was intolerant of Sergio's stuttering. In fact, Sergio's father regularly hit him on the head with his fist when Sergio stuttered. Sergio thus learned to fear stuttering in the presence of his father, and soon his fear of stuttering generalized to most other listeners. When he came to us for treatment, we worked with him both individually and in a group. In both settings, Sergio talked at length about his father and his growing up in an environment where he was teased for his stuttering and treated badly by schoolmates. He dropped out of school at an early age and supported himself working as a musician—singing and playing a guitar. In his therapy, clinicians and group members were empathetic listeners, and, as time went by, Sergio seemed to forgive his father, explaining that his hitting him was a result of ignorance and frustration in a culture that valued manliness and regarded stuttering as weakness. Sergio gradually learned to stutter more easily and became an inspiration to students and other clients, helping out in the classroom and in our support group. Sergio is now employed as a group leader in a rehabilitation setting and also works as a musician with his own band. In a brief video clip, Sergio first demonstrates his old stuttering and then changes to a more fluent form of stuttering, as he talks about his recent visit with his parents and relatives. This is available on *thePoint* in a clip named "Chapter 8: Sergio."

When people who stutter grow up in other cultures, our task of deeply understanding them requires an understanding of their culture as well as how that culture regards stuttering. This understanding is vital and increasingly important as the world changes. The 21st century will be a time of more and more migration among people from different cultures and countries. For example, my own state of Vermont has recently become home to immigrants and refugees from 23 different countries, and yet it ranks as only the 48th in diversity. Other states like California, Texas, Hawaii, and New Jersey have much larger and more diverse populations. Many other countries besides the United States have hugely diverse populations. Some of the diversity comes from refugees who have resettled in countries other than their own. Many have experienced serious trauma that, in some cases, may have precipitated or worsened stuttering. Thus, it is vital for clinicians working with communication disorders to develop a **multicultural perspective** on assessment and therapy.

An underlying principle of this perspective is becoming sensitive to differences in communicative style in other cultures and learning how other cultures view speech and language disorders and, especially for our purpose here, stuttering. You can improve your multicultural sensitivity by reading about cultural issues related to communication disorders in general (Battle, 2012; Coleman, 2000; Goldstein, 2000; Taylor, 1994) and to stuttering in particular (Conrad, 1996; Cooper & Cooper, 1993; Culatta & Goldberg, 1995; Tellis & Tellis, 2003; Watson & Kayser, 1994). Insights into cultural difference can change the way treatment is organized. For example, Tellis and Tellis (2003) report that families from India often feel that stuttering is a reflection on the entire family. This perception may strongly influence family members' responses to a child's stuttering. It would be important to listen to family members' perspectives on stuttering and, in the process, gently let them know about the latest scientific findings about stuttering, about high-achieving individuals who stutter, and about remediation for stuttering. This may lead to the family being more accepting of a family member's stuttering. Tellis and Tellis suggest that the clinician ask "open-ended culturally specific questions that address the beliefs, attitudes, and values of the client" (p. 23), in ascertaining how best to work with the client or family.

The Stuttering Home Page—an information source about fluency disorders for the public and professionals—has a wide variety of interesting papers accessible from a Web page titled "Stuttering in Other Countries/Cultures" (http://www.mnsu.edu/comdis/kuster/nonenglish.html). There is also a series of monographs about working with people with disabilities from other cultures, available from http://cirrie-sphhp.webapps.buffalo.edu/culture/monographs/.

In addition to these readings, a special issue of *Perspectives on Fluency and Fluency Disorders*[1] contains several articles on multicultural issues in stuttering. In that issue, Daniels (2008) and Ramos-Heinrichs (2008) suggested that, as we have said before, finding out about the client's and/or family's attitudes about stuttering is crucial. Many of the questionnaires to assess attitudes and feelings that will be presented later in this chapter can tap into perceptions of the stuttering behaviors and how much stuttering impedes an individual's communication, but these questionnaires don't plumb the client's culture's views of stuttering. To help clinicians learn about a Hispanic American client's beliefs about stuttering, Tellis (2008) created a questionnaire that taps into many cultural values that may be different from those in the mainstream culture. The Stuttering Inventory for Hispanic Americans (SIHA) may be adaptable for cultures other than Hispanic, with minor changes. Culturally sensitive questionnaires should be administered in a way that makes the client feel safe in responding honestly and fully. Right from the beginning, the clinician should begin to establish a relationship in which the client feels accepted for who he is and trusts that the clinician is open-minded and genuinely curious about the client's culture.

As you work with clients from other cultures, here are a few issues that may be important as you explore the client's stuttering and help him become more fluent:

1. *Eye contact.* Most treatments for stuttering encourage clients to improve their eye contact when speaking. A major reason for this is that many people who stutter look away from the listener when they stutter, increasing the perceived abnormality of the symptom and further disrupting communication. This is only true in some cultures, however. In contrast, in some cultures, eye contact with a listener may be inappropriate, depending on the status of the listener and the context. Among some Native Americans, for example, not looking at the listener is a sign of respect. Thus, a person from such a culture who stutters may look away from listeners but not necessarily because of shame or embarrassment. The clinician should become aware of situations in which eye contact while speaking is appropriate and when it is not.
2. *Physical contact.* During an evaluation or in treatment, many clinicians may touch clients to help them identify points of tension or to signal them to make a change in their stuttering as it is happening. However, many individuals may regard being touched during an evaluation as an invasion of their personal space. It is important to ask permission before touching someone. You might say, for example, "I'd like you to try to catch a stutter and keep it going without finishing the word. Is it OK if I touch your arm to signal you to stay in the stutter?"
3. *Nature of reinforcers.* Some approaches to treatment use praise as a reinforcer that is given immediately after a child has spoken fluently. Cultures differ in the amount and type of praise they give children. A clinician I know working in a suburb of Sydney, Australia, a city rich in new immigrants, adapts her treatment contingencies to fit many different cultures. One family from the Middle East was adamantly against giving verbal praise to their child. Instead, they developed a special signal that the father gave to his son to reinforce fluent speech.
4. *Family interactions.* Children with borderline stuttering are often helped when families change their interaction patterns. One such change that families can make is to speak more slowly and pause between conversational turns when speaking with the child (e.g., Stephanson-Opsal & Bernstein Ratner, 1988, and our own treatment of borderline stuttering described in Chapter 11). However, in some cultures, particularly in urban areas of the eastern United States, families speak quickly and often overlap each other while talking. For these families, slowing speaking rate and not interrupting each other may seem so unnatural that they are unable to sustain this new interaction pattern. For their children, an operant conditioning approach in daily one-on-one conversations with a parent may be more appropriate.
5. *Intentional stuttering.* Sometimes I ask the person I am working with in therapy to stutter on purpose, thereby decreasing her tendency to avoid and be afraid of stuttering. But in some cultures, stuttering is regarded so negatively that stuttering on purpose would be unthinkable, at least in the early stages of treatment. It is important for you to become aware of how stuttering is viewed in different cultures and to understand when and where voluntary stuttering might be helpful and acceptable to your clients. Sometimes, the cultural stigma of stuttering makes it difficult for individuals and families to even discuss it.

[1]This is a publication by the Fluency and Fluency Disorders Special Interest Group 4 of the American Speech-Language-Hearing Association.

Our clinic recently treated a young man from China because he wanted to reduce his accent. Only after months of accent reduction treatment was he willing to talk about his greater problem, stuttering. Until we discussed it, he thought he had been successful in disguising it, even though his stuttering was obvious to most of his listeners.

6. *Conversational style.* Sensitive evaluations and treatment take into consideration not only the culture's view of stuttering but also the culture's style of verbal and nonverbal interaction. Orlando Taylor (1986) described a number of cultural differences in communication style that are relevant to evaluations of stuttering. For example, interruptions of one speaker by another may be expected among African Americans, so trying to change that style of interaction in a family may meet with resistance. In addition, people from African American and Native American cultures may feel uncomfortable responding to the personal questions often asked in an initial interview, and people from a Hispanic culture may feel it is rude to get down to business before greetings and pleasantries are exchanged.
7. *Modes of address.* The clinician should find out how to address individuals involved in the assessment and treatment, including proper pronunciation. Also, discuss how they'd like to address you. A family from India that I am working with now prefers to address me as "Dr. Barry."

These cultural considerations are summarized in Table 8.1. It may not be possible for a clinician to know all relevant aspects of each new client's culture. But clinicians can be aware of the importance of culture in a person's response to stuttering, as well as the differences in communication styles between their own cultures and those of their clients. Such awareness can come from reading about a client's culture and discussing it with the client, if appropriate.

Similar sensitivity should be extended to different social classes within the clinician's own culture. Understanding

TABLE 8.1 Cultural and Interpersonal Considerations in Assessment and Treatment

Issue	Cultural or Interpersonal Concern	Possible Solution
Eye contact is sometimes a target of treatment.	In some cultures, direct eye contact may be disrespectful.	Discuss with client the appropriateness of eye contact in his culture.
Clinician may touch a client to make a point.	For some individuals, physical contact is unwelcome.	Ask permission before touching a client.
Clinician may use or advocate reinforcers such as candy or praise.	Some families do not choose to use these reinforcers.	Explore with the family what would be acceptable reinforcement for the child.
Clinician may try to change family interaction style.	Family may value their interaction style and not welcome changing it.	Clinician should talk with family about rationale for suggesting change but should accept that family may prefer not to change interaction style.
Clinician may try to teach client to use voluntary stuttering.	Some clients or their families may find stuttering so unacceptable that they will terminate treatment rather than use voluntary stuttering.	Clinician should proceed slowly and tactfully in helping client learn and adapt voluntary stuttering. Some clients will never use it, which is reasonable but may require a work-around.
Clinician may not use appropriate conversational style with client.	Some mode of conversational style (such as asking personal questions) may offend some clients.	Clinician should become aware of conversational style preferences when client is from a different culture than her own.
Clinician may not use appropriate mode of address.	Clients may be offended by insensitive mode of address (use of first name) or mispronunciation of name.	Clinician should become sensitive to client's preferred way of being addressed and proper pronunciation of client and family names.

and respecting class differences in such areas as vocabulary and values are crucial. Sometimes, working with people from other cultures increases our respect for class differences within our own culture. When I worked in Australia, I often attended grand rounds in a Sydney hospital. One particular case presentation involved a working-class Australian woman who had been mutilating herself with needles. Some of the staff and medical residents were highly unsympathetic to her condition, but a psychiatrist, renowned for his work in other cultures, shifted their attitudes. He spoke passionately about how we fail to understand people when we are blinded by our own values and beliefs and that trying to learn about this woman's circumstances would go a lot further in helping her than our simple condemnations of her self-mutilating behavior.

Some clients will not only be from a different culture or different social class, but they will also speak a different language, one that the clinician may not understand. In this case, an interpreter is necessary, if a referral to a clinician who speaks that language is not available. Because interpreters are often from the same culture as that of the client, they may help not only in translating but also in providing information about important aspects of the culture to aid the clinician's understanding. In the process of translating sensitive or complex messages, interpreters sometimes need to change the clinician's message to the client. When a message is rephrased by an interpreter to a more culturally appropriate style, therapeutic interaction will be facilitated. However, if an interpreter doesn't understand the intent of a question or statement, he may inadvertently convey wrong information. A friend of mine who was working with non-English–speaking Haitian immigrants in Boston understood just enough French to realize that the interpreter was providing wrong information to a client. She rectified the situation by giving the interpreter a brief overview of what she wanted to discuss with the Haitian family and why certain elements were vital, which immediately improved communication.

Special considerations apply when clients are both bicultural and bilingual. Bilingual clients, in fact, are not uncommon; there is evidence of an increased risk for stuttering in bilingual individuals (Howell & Van Borsel, 2011; Karniol, 1992; Mattes & Omark, 1991; Roberts & Shenker, 2007; Van Borsel, Maes, & Foulon, 2001). In these cases, one challenge for clinicians is to determine if the "stuttering" is really stuttering or is simply an increase in disfluency as a result of limited proficiency in a second language. Making this determination may be aided by careful observation of whether there are secondary symptoms (such as eye blinks or signs of increased tension) and cognitive or emotional responses to the suspected stuttering. For example, does the client feel ashamed of her disfluencies? Does she anticipate them? Are they consistently on the same words or same sounds? Another clue is that the disfluencies may be stuttering if there is a history of stuttering in the client's family.

There is some debate in the literature about the extent to which stuttering occurs in one or more languages of a bilingual speaker. The excellent review of stuttering and bilingualism by Van Borsel et al. (2001) discusses the evidence on this issue, concluding that although stuttering may occur in one or both languages, it is more likely to occur in both. In some speakers, stuttering may be more severe in one language than another, so that careful analysis of stuttering in both languages will enable the clinician to decide whether to apply treatment to both. Analysis of stuttering in a language not spoken by the clinician is likely to be more accurate if a native speaker of that language, such as a family member or friend of the client, can work with the clinician to identify stutters. In adults, the client herself will be able to help identify stuttering in the language unfamiliar to the clinician. This topic is more thoroughly discussed in the many good chapters on multilingual aspects of stuttering in Howell and Van Borsel (2011).

In terms of treatment of bilingual speakers, Findlay and Shenker (2014) demonstrated that bilingual/bicultural children take essentially the same amount of time to achieve fluency as monolingual children. It should be kept in mind, however, that there are probably widely different bilingual/bicultural groups of individuals. Some have grown up in an environment where their dual language and culture are the norm and the individuals feel accepted. The children in the study by Findlay and Shenker may be an example of that: the children were from Montreal where many children grow up in bilingual homes. In other cases, children may be refugees and are learning a new language and may not feel part of the new environment, thus being perhaps more anxious and insecure and more at risk for stuttering, and may take longer in treatment.

THE CLINICIAN'S EXPERTISE

During an assessment, the clinician has a chance to demonstrate not only her **empathy** with a client's feelings but also her mastery of evaluating and treating stuttering. Adolescents and adults who stutter and their family members often come into treatment with feelings of frustration, fear, and helplessness. They are looking for someone they can trust and someone who can successfully guide them through the often difficult process of recovery. One of the first things a clinician can do to establish trust and credibility is to show that she not only knows about stuttering but is comfortable asking questions about it, duplicating it in her own speech and exploring it empathetically. This provides both clients and family members with an ally, someone who is unafraid of the problem that is so troubling to them.

This process can begin with the clinician asking an older school-age, adolescent, or adult client how they feel about their stuttering and then indicating that those feelings are very normal for people who stutter. The clinician may also speak about other clients she has seen who have similar feelings, and describe those feelings. In some cases, the clinician may ask the client specific questions about avoidance behaviors and explain to the client why they use them and why they may be only temporarily helpful. This same credibility can be achieved in the evaluation of a preschool child if the clinician asks her family about the types of stutters that the child has and demonstrates various possible types such as repetitions, prolongations, and blocks. With a younger school-age child, once the clinician has gotten to know the child a little—this may take a few sessions of working together—the clinician can tell the child she has worked with other kids who stutter but needs to learn about her particular way of stuttering. Then she can ask him if it's OK if she interrupts him when he stutters to have him show her how to stutter like him. This requires tact, a sense of timing, and even humor to be sure the child feels comfortable **confronting stuttering**, but it can convey the clinician's expertise and thus engender trust.

The clinician's statements and questions also convey her expertise. For example, as she interviews an older child, she can show that she knows about stuttering by making empathetic comments, such as "Giving reports in front of class can sometimes be hard for kids who stutter." This allows the child to respond without the pressure of a direct question but also lets the child appreciate that the clinician is someone who has experience with stuttering. When talking with families, the clinician can intersperse questions with such statements as "When children keep repeating a sound that won't come out, their voices sometimes rise in pitch as the repetition continues." The family can then confirm whether or not they have noticed this in their child's speech and at the same time recognize that the clinician is knowledgeable about children's stuttering. Obviously, these kinds of comments and questions are easier for experienced clinicians, but even beginning clinicians can rely on their reading, their all-too-brief practicum experiences, and their intuition to convey their interest and understanding.

Because it has risks as well as rewards, the approach to interviewing clients and families that was just described should be used carefully. By making comments based on past experience, we may inhibit some individuals and families from telling us about experiences that differ from those offered by the clinician. It is an art to find the balance between showing understanding and leading the witness. As your clinical judgment develops, you will learn which clients will be helped by this approach and when.

I also caution that demonstrating your expertise should be secondary to acquiring an understanding of clients' needs. A clinician's first task is to discern what an individual or family would like from the clinician. The second task is to understand the stuttering problem. In the normal course of accomplishing these two tasks—with attentive listening, empathetic comments, and perceptive questions—the clinician's expertise will emerge naturally.

ASSESSING STUTTERING BEHAVIOR

Assessment of stuttering behaviors is a broad area that can be divided into several different targets for evaluation, such as frequency, type, duration, and severity. In some situations, it may also be important to assess **speech naturalness**, speech rate, and concomitant or associated behaviors. The importance of each of these is slightly different, depending on the age of the client and the type of treatment you expect to use. Before describing how to assess stuttering, I will clarify what behaviors are considered stuttering. As I mentioned in Chapter 7, a number of authors (e.g., Conture, 2001; Yairi & Ambrose, 1992a) have discussed which types of disfluencies distinguish stuttering from nonstuttering children. Borrowing from their discussions, I have concluded that the following behaviors should be counted as stutters: part-word repetitions, monosyllabic whole-word repetitions, sound prolongations, and blockages of sound or airflow. The latter category (blockages of sound or airflow) can sometimes be quite subtle, occurring in the middle of a word (as in "cooo-kie" in which a glottal stop appears to break the word in half) or before a word. I also count successful avoidance behaviors as stutters if they are unequivocally an avoidance. See the section on assessing frequency for a further description of deciding on unequivocal avoidances.

Reliability

Whenever a procedure is used to assess a behavior or a trait, it is important to know how reliable the procedure is. For example, if a police officer pulls you over for speeding because the radar gun has clocked you going 40 mph in a 25-mph zone, you might want to know how reliable the radar gun was. When this happened to me several years ago, I went to court to contest the ticket. Many factors, I figured, could affect the accuracy of the radar gun's measurement of my speed: the weather, the age of the gun, and whether it was adjusted properly. Fortunately, the judge asked the officer for **evidence of reliability** of the radar gun to prove that it could repeatedly, dependably, and consistently measure the speed of a car. Unfortunately, the officer was able to provide the judge with evidence of the gun's recent reliability check, and I shelled out $85 for the fine.

Reliability is obviously an important characteristic of a procedure to measure stuttering. Many factors affect the measurement process, and some of these influences may result in data that are not representative of a client's true performance. In addition, it appears that stuttering is a particularly changeable behavior, making it difficult to be sure you have a really representative sample—or that a single sample even can be representative. This phenomenon and its consequences are described by Cordes (1994) in her seminal article about reliability:

> *Perceptions, judgments, and observations are affected by variables attributed to the observers, to the instrumentation or coding procedures, to the situation or conditions of observation, to the subjects being observed, and to interactions among all of these. Consequently, researchers using direct observation methods are currently expected to provide evidence that their findings are not simply the results of situational influences or observer idiosyncrasies. They are expected, in other words, to provide evidence that their data are reliable (p. 264).*

The same caveat is true for clinical work. Despite our good intentions, observations of clients' stuttering before and after treatment may be influenced by our desires to see them improve. Measurements may also be affected by random fluctuations in stuttering apart from treatment effects, by the setting in which the client is assessed, by length and type of sample taken, and by the particular dimension of stuttering, such as frequency, severity, duration, or type that is chosen for assessment. It is important for clinicians to learn to assess stuttering reliably and to provide evidence that they have done so. It is also part of the clinician's responsibilities to know the reliability of the standardized measures used to assess stuttering and to choose those measures that are most reliable.

When human judgment is involved, as it always is with measures of stuttering, reliability is checked first by demonstrating that the observer makes the same judgment when observing the same behavior a second time from a video recording, usually several weeks later so that the second observation is fresh and not affected by memories of the earlier judgment. This is called **intrarater reliability**. Reliability is also checked by comparing the original judgment with the judgment of a second observer who rates the sample independently of the first observer. This is called **interrater reliability**.

Remeasurement of the data does not have to include the entire sample that is used, although doing so would certainly be the most rigorous approach (e.g., O'Brian, Packman, & Onslow, 2004). It is common for clinical researchers in stuttering to remeasure a randomly selected portion (10–25 percent) of samples taken (e.g., Hakim & Bernstein Ratner, 2004; O'Brian et al., 2004). When reliability of judgments is to be established for measurements made on clients who increase their fluency over the course of a treatment regimen, samples should be randomly selected from various points in therapy to include both less fluent and more fluent samples.

Measures of reliability are usually selected according to what behavior is being measured. In situations where evaluation and treatment depend on accurate identification of stuttering moments (such as whether a word or syllable is stuttered or not), reliability can be measured using what is commonly called "point-by-point agreement." A videotaped sample (e.g., 400 syllables of conversational speech) can be transcribed, and each stutter can be identified and marked on the transcript by an original judge or rater. Sometime later, the rater can return to the sample and again identify stutters by marking a fresh copy of the transcript. The two transcripts are then compared syllable by syllable, and the rater determines how many syllables are agreed upon as stuttered and how many are agreed upon as fluent. This total is termed "number of agreements." The number of disagreements (syllables that were determined to be stuttered in the first rating but not stuttered in the second rating or vice versa) is totaled and termed "number of disagreements." The reliability measure is then the number of agreements divided by the total number of agreements plus disagreements multiplied by 100. Cordes (1994) notes that 80 percent agreement is commonly thought of as the lower limit for a sample to be considered reliable. Figure 8.2 gives an example of a point-by-point assessment of reliability.

Point-by-point agreement is appropriate when it is important to judge whether stuttering is present or absent on each syllable. It is also a good tool for new clinicians to use to assess their ability to accurately judge stuttering. However, other procedures are called for when assessment requires quantification rather than presence or absence. An example would be measurement of the duration of stutters. An appropriate measure of reliability would be percent error, obtained by remeasuring at least 10 percent of the data. In this case, it is appropriate to begin by (1) obtaining the absolute differences between each first judgment and each second judgment (change all negative numbers to positive), (2) summing those absolute differences together, (3) dividing by the total number of them to get the average, and finally (4) dividing the average absolute difference by the average of the first judgments. Table 8.2 shows an example.

A third method of assessing reliability can be used when measuring the amount of stuttering in cases when point-by-point agreement is not critical. One example would be when you are assessing frequency of stuttering as a measure of week-by-week progress. This procedure involves calculating both the correlation between the first rating and a second rating for multiple samples, as well as a test of significant differences between the means of the ratings, such as a paired sample *t* test. Correlations and *t* tests should be done for both intrarater and interrater reliability. Correlations should be above 80 percent, and *t* tests should show no significant difference between the samples. Table 8.3 depicts correlations and *t* tests for a sample of 12 original and rerated samples.

As a final comment about reliability, I would suggest that although different measures of reliability can be used for different purposes, beginning clinicians should establish their reliability using a point-by-point agreement procedure, both during their initial training and to recheck their reliability periodically as they gain more experience. This may help them develop relatively consistent and agreed-upon definitions of what a stutter is and is not.

A summary of reliability measures is given in Table 8.4.

Observer 1:
You wish to know all about my grandfather. Well, he is nearly ninety-three years old; yet he still thinks as swiftly as ever. He dresses himself in an old black frock coat, usually several buttons missing. A long beard clings to his chin, giving those who observe him a pronounced feeling of the utmost respect. When he speaks his voice is just a bit cracked and quivers a trifle. Twice each day he plays skillfully and with zest upon our small organ. Except in the winter when the snow or ice prevents, he slowly takes a short walk in the open air each day. We have often urged him to walk more and smoke less, but he always answers, "Banana oil!" Grandfather likes to be modern in his language.

Observer 2:
You wish to know all about my grandfather. Well, he is nearly ninety-three years old; yet he still thinks as swiftly as ever. He dresses himself in an old black frock coat, usually several buttons missing. A long beard clings to his chin, giving those who observe him a pronounced feeling of the utmost respect. When he speaks his voice is just a bit cracked and quivers a trifle. Twice each day he plays skillfully and with zest upon our small organ. Except in the winter when the snow or ice prevents, he slowly takes a short walk in the open air each day. We have often urged him to walk more and smoke less, but he always answers, "Banana oil!" Grandfather likes to be modern in his language.

There are approximately 14 syllables upon which the observers did not agree. There are approximately 156 syllables upon which they agreed were either stuttered or were fluent. The simple point-by-point agreement (rather than the kappa statistic) would be calculated as agreements (156) divided by agreements plus disagreements (170), or 92 percent.

Figure 8.2 An example showing how to calculate point-by-point agreement. An initial observer has marked the reading passage by underlining syllables on which stuttering was judged to occur. A second observer has marked the second passage. Point-by-point agreement can be calculated by comparing the total number of agreements with the agreements plus disagreements.

Speech Sample

The size and number of samples depend on the purpose of the assessment. In a first assessment, it would be wise to have at least two samples: one recorded in the clinic and one recorded in the client's typical environment. Before I see a preschool child for an evaluation, I ask the parents to send in a video of the child in conversation at home. Video recording is common in some homes so that the presence of a video camera will probably not make most children self-conscious. I sometimes ask parents to leave the camera on a tripod in a familiar place for several days so the child is used to it when the recording is actually done. When video recording is not possible, audiotaping is still useful. With a school-age child, a sample collected in the school would be important. Practically speaking, of course, a sample could be most easily recorded in the therapy room at school. A second sample from home would also be very helpful, but it is not always obtainable. When evaluating an adolescent or adult, I recommend that a sample be taken in the treatment room and a sample be taken from work or home. It is often convenient for adolescents or adults to audiotape telephone conversations. I often urge clients to buy a small digital audio recorder for recording work done outside therapy; Sony has a digital voice recorder for about $20. I ensure that the client knows how to record only his own voice and not that of the listener, unless he has gotten permission.

TABLE 8.2 An Example of Assessment of Reliability by Calculating Percent Error of Duration Measurements

	Time 1	Time 2	Absolute Difference
	3.5	3.0	0.5
	4.0	4.0	0.0
	0.5	0.7	0.2
	0.4	0.3	0.1
Mean	2.1		0.2

Duration of stuttering (in seconds) measured by an observer at Time 1 and remeasured at Time 2. Percent error = 0.2/2.1 = 9.5 percent.

An important consideration in obtaining samples is that stuttering varies. It differs in frequency and severity from month to month, week to week, day to day, and situation to

TABLE 8.3 Assessing Interrater Reliability by Calculating Correlations and *t* Tests

Observer 1	Observer 2
12	11
10	9
15	10
4	6
8	5
2	2
14	12
7	9
3	4
6	6
5	3
1	3

Measures are percentages of syllables stuttered measured by observer 1 and observer 2.
Pearson $r = 0.90$; paired $t = 0.92$; df = 11; $p = .38$. These calculations suggest that substantial interrater reliability exists because the ratings are highly correlated, and no significant difference is observed between the means.

situation within the same day. Such variability affects both children and adults but is most apparent with young children who stutter. Sometimes, a preschool child is stuttering severely, and then 3 weeks later during the evaluation, the child is entirely fluent. Therefore, it is important to discuss with the client or family whether the sample you have obtained is representative of the stuttering and if not, whether more samples should be taken, maybe in other situations and at other times.

After the initial sample, when further assessment is done to measure progress in therapy, it is crucial to ensure that any reduction in stuttering is not confined to the therapy room. Thus, ongoing assessments should include measures taken in the client's real world, outside the treatment situation.

For any sample in which severity of stuttering is to be rated or any sample for research purposes, videotaping is essential. Many subtleties of stuttering would be missed if only an audiotape were used; thus, video recording allows better assessment of observer reliability than audio recording. Sometimes online (while the client is talking), scoring can be done without either video or audio recording. For example, online scoring is appropriate when the clinician samples severity of stuttering at the beginning of every session for clinical rather than research purposes.

The length of the sample must be long enough for it to be representative of the speaker's typical stuttering. A sample that's too short won't include enough stuttering to see the range of severity and types of stuttering, and a sample that's too long would take time away from other assessment activities and would be tedious to score. For a client who reads, I usually like to take a sample of 300 to 400 syllables of conversational speech (where there is likely to be more variability) and 200 syllables of a reading passage (where there is likely to be less variability).

TABLE 8.4 Measures of Reliability

Type of Reliability	Brief Description	When to Use
Point by point	Transcript of speech sample made; original judge and another observer mark whether a syllable is stuttered. Reliability is assessed by counting the number of syllables that were agreed upon by both observers as stuttered and dividing that number by the total number of syllables in the sample (agreements plus disagreements).	Use when it is important to ascertain whether stuttering has occurred on each individual syllable, as in an experiment that consequates individual stutters. Also useful for new clinicians to assess their accuracy at judging stuttering.
Percentage error	Experimenter assesses the difference between the first observer's judgment and the second observation on at least 10 percent of the sample. Expressed as absolute difference (all numbers made positive). Then these differences are averaged (average absolute difference), and this figure is divided by the average of the first observer's measures.	Use when assessing reliability of a continuous variable like duration of stutters.
Correlation and *t* test	Pearson product-moment correlation used to see the extent to which initial observations of behavior are related to second observations. In addition, the *t* test is used to assess whether the mean of the second observations is significantly different from the mean of the initial observations.	Use when an overall measure of variable (e.g., percent syllables stuttered) is used and when it is not important to show agreement on individual syllables.

Using a typical figure of 1.5 syllables per word (Williams, Darley, & Spriestersbach, 1978), these samples would be equivalent to approximately 200 to 265 words and 130 words, respectively.

When obtaining a reading sample, it is important to ensure that the reading passage is at or below the client's reading level. A client's stuttering is likely to worsen when reading a passage that is difficult, giving a false impression of typical stuttering during reading. Reading passages in the Stuttering Severity Instrument-4 (SSI-4) (Riley, 2009) are designed for third, fifth, and seventh grade levels, as well as for an adult reading level. You can also write your own passages and check them for grade level using the Tools option on Microsoft Word, which uses the Flesch-Kincaid Reading Level statistics, or you can use the Fry Readability Graph (find this graph through an online search for the phrase "Fry readability"). When obtaining a speaking sample, it would be wise to select topics that are not emotional unless it is desirable to elicit a maximal amount of stuttering, as you might do with a client who says she stutters but is not demonstrating any during the evaluation. I usually ask children and adolescents to talk about their favorite weekend or after-school activities, sports, hobbies, or pets. With adults, I ask them to talk about their favorite activities, sports, hobbies, work, or school.

When making a formal assessment or when first learning to assess stuttering, it is very useful to make a written transcript of the spoken material, including all words and even those non-meaningful utterances, such as "uh." However, you should not indicate on the original transcript which syllables are stuttered, so that you, at a later date, or another rater, on a separate occasion, can rescore a copy of the transcript to check for reliability without being influenced by the notations indicating which syllables were stuttered. Using your recording of the spoken material and an unmarked transcript, you can note where the stutters are, with details of how the individual stuttered. Write out each element of a repeated sound or syllable, the sounds that were prolonged, and the sounds on which blocks occurred. Describe escape and avoidance behaviors accompanying each moment of stuttering. Mark those moments of stuttering that seem longer than most. For a complete assessment, you will want to return to the longer stutters and time how long each one was to determine the average length of the three longest stutters. You will also want to count the words or syllables spoken, although it is often most accurate to count syllables from recordings because some speakers omit syllables in longer words. This can be done with software, such as the Computerized Scoring of Stuttering Severity (CSSS) software that accompanies the SSI-4.

Assessing Frequency

Frequency of stuttering is a simple, reliable measure (Andrews & Ingham, 1971) that can be used for a variety of purposes. It is important in an initial assessment to help distinguish a normally disfluent child from a child with borderline stuttering. It is a vital part of composite ratings, such as the SSI-4 (Riley, 2009), that provide a multidimensional view of stuttering. Frequency of stuttering is also useful as a "snapshot" measure of progress during treatment. In the first place, it is highly correlated with severity (Young, 1961). If used alone, however, frequency has the limitation that it doesn't reflect the duration of stutters or physical tension associated with stuttering. Decreases in these variables are often signs of improvement.

Frequency of stuttering is most commonly reported as percentage of syllables stuttered, although some use percentage of words stuttered or number of stutters per 100 words. I prefer to use **percentage of syllables stuttered**, following the logic of Minifie and Cooker (1964), because it can capture instances when a speaker stutters on more than one syllable of a multisyllable word. Moreover, when counting syllables and stutters online, syllables can be counted more easily than words by counting the syllable beats as the client talks.

Here are some guidelines for counting stutters:

Each syllable can be counted only once. Thus, multiple repetitions, like "Where is my ba-ba-ba-basketball?" are counted as only one stutter.

The total number of syllables are only those that would have been produced if the speaker had been fluent. Thus, "Where is my ba-ba-ba-basketball?" is totaled as six syllables. Each syllable that would have been produced if the speaker had been fluent is counted as either stuttered or fluent.

Don't count interjections that you judge to be part of the stutter as syllables or as separate stutters. In the sentence "Where is my...my...uh...well ba-ba-ba-ba-basketball?" there would be a total of six syllables and one stutter.

If a speaker seems to be using a particular word or sound as an avoidance behavior, I will count a word as stuttered even if no overt stuttering occurred. For example, a speaker may say "Where is my...uh...uh...uh basketball?" In this case, the speaker seems to be using "uh" to postpone starting the word "basketball" on which he anticipates stuttering. And he keeps saying "uh" until he feels he can say "basketball" fluently and then rushes to say "basketball" after saying the last "uh." When I am fairly certain that a speaker has used a sound or word as an (successful) avoidance behavior like this, I count the word as stuttered. Note that I do not count each utterance of the sound or word that is used as an avoidance; instead, I count the next word in the utterance as stuttered. When I am in doubt about whether an avoidance has occurred on a word, I count it as fluent.

When assessing the speech of someone who can read, I find it helpful to compare the frequency of stuttering in reading to that in speaking. If stuttering is markedly greater in the reading task, this may be because the speaker is avoiding words he expects to stutter on in the speaking task, but he can't do this when reading. In most cases, I talk about my hypothesis with the client to see if he agrees.

A variety of instruments designed for counting stutters are available. A free online counter that counts stuttered syllables and fluent syllables and calculates percent syllables stuttered and speech rate is available at http://www.natke-verlag.de/silbenzaehler/index_en.html/.[2]

Assessing Types of Stutters

When assessing the speech of preschool children, it is often useful to count the total number of disfluencies, both those that are considered **types of stutters** and those considered normal. As you will remember from Chapter 7, disfluencies that are not considered stutter-like include multisyllable word repetitions, phrase repetitions, interjections, and revisions in which a phrase is incomplete. When both types of disfluencies (stutter-like and not) are counted, you can use the proportion of total disfluencies that are stutter-like to help you decide whether a child is stuttering or normally disfluent. As I indicated in Chapter 7, Yairi (1997a, 1997b) surveyed a number of studies and proposed that if less than 50 percent of a child's disfluencies are stutter-like, the child is more likely to be normally disfluent. Caution must be used with any single measure used alone. Conture (2001) noted that a child he had recently evaluated was, in his opinion, stuttering severely even though the child's proportion of stutter-like disfluencies was only 34 percent of the total disfluencies. Clearly, Conture had relied on several other measures of stuttering in concluding that the child was a severe stutterer.

Another measure involving the type of disfluencies that a child produces is the number of stutter-like disfluencies per 100 words. In summarizing his findings on disfluencies in stuttering and nonstuttering children, Yairi (1997b) noted that children who stutter have more than three stutter-like disfluencies per 100 words, whereas normally disfluent children have fewer. In this same chapter, Yairi reviewed research about the gradual decline in some types of disfluencies as children grow older. Perhaps the most important finding is that part-word repetitions show a steady decline in normally disfluent children by age 4 and thereafter. Thus, if a child shows a plateau or increase in part-word repetitions in later preschool years, the child may be showing stuttering rather than normal disfluency.

Assessing Duration

In a thorough assessment, measures of the **duration** of a client's longest stutters can give us important information about how much stuttering may be interfering with communication. Van Riper (1982, p. 208) noted in his inimitable prose that "The duration of the individual moments of stuttering is one of the basic components of any adequate index of severity. Like tapeworms, longer stutterings are worse than shorter ones."

A common practice is to average the duration of the three longest stutters in a speech sample (Myers, 1978; Preus, 1981; Riley, 2009; Van Riper, 1982). One way to do it is to use a digital stopwatch while watching a videotape of the client speaking. With a little practice, you can turn the stopwatch on at the moment the stutter begins and turn it off when it ends and measure the moment of stuttering to the nearest half-second. Any delays in starting the stopwatch at the beginning of stutters are compensated for by similar delays when you stop it at the end. I recommend using duration as part of a more complete assessment of severity, such as the SSI-4 (Riley, 2009), when making an initial assessment of a client's progress and when you want to give a detailed description of a client's stuttering in a report. The software accompanying the SSI-4 provides a means to automatically calculate the mean of the three longest stutters by holding down the mouse key for the duration of each stutter as it is being counted.

Many applications are available on the Internet to assess stuttering using your cell phone or other connected devices. But buyers beware: read the reviews of various apps before purchasing. In a later section of this chapter, I'll discuss a free Web site for assessing stuttering that is part of FluencyBank (http://fluency.talkbank.org).

Assessing Secondary Behaviors

Stuttering feels like being in the grip of an unseen hand damming up the flow of your speech. Or as one of my young clients said, it is like having "a rock jammed in your throat." You struggle to keep going, squeezing your lips, blinking your eyes, and twisting your shoulders in the process. Such behaviors add to the abnormality of stuttering and reflect an important aspect of its development. Reducing or eliminating these behaviors may be a vital goal for therapy.

Secondary behaviors are also referred to as "concomitant," "associated," or "accessory" behaviors. They are most often escape behaviors that are used to break out of a stutter once it has started, but secondary behaviors may also be avoidance behaviors that are used in an attempt to keep from stuttering (see Chapters 1, 5, and 7 for further discussion of these terms). These behaviors may be physical movements (e.g., eye blink), extra sounds (e.g., "uh"), or changes in the way speech is produced (e.g., pitch rise). They are often signs that stuttering has progressed to a more advanced stage (e.g., escape behaviors distinguish beginning from borderline stuttering), but they may in a few cases appear very close to the onset of stuttering.

Conture (2001) briefly reviewed the limited research on secondary behaviors and noted that most are just more frequent and more exaggerated versions of behaviors seen in normal speakers. Zebrowski and Kelly (2002) suggested that the most common behaviors involve the eyes, particularly blinking, squeezing, lateral and vertical eye movements, and loss of eye contact. These authors and Shapiro (2011) also pointed out that the presence of secondary behaviors can be an important diagnostic sign that may distinguish normally disfluent children from those who are beginning to stutter.

[2]I thank Julie Pera for recommending this online tool.

Some clinicians enumerate these secondary behaviors as part of their assessment, particularly when they will use a treatment approach that helps the client gradually modify her stuttering behaviors. Standardized measures, such as the SSI-4 (Riley, 2009), include ratings of these behaviors as part of an overall severity assessment. We will consider this assessment next.

Assessing Severity

Measures of **severity** may be the most clinically relevant assessment of overt stuttering behaviors. Severity reflects an overall impression that listeners may have when they listen to an individual who stutters. Thus, it is an important measure for assessing the outcome of treatment. It is also an important yardstick of progress during therapy because many treatments gradually reduce the severity of stuttering rather than eliminate it.

The most commonly used measure of severity is the Stuttering Severity Instrument (SSI), which was first published in the Journal of Speech and Hearing Disorders (Riley, 1972). A recent version, the SSI-4, is illustrated in Figure 8.3. It is available with forms and a manual from PRO-ED (http://www.proedinc.com). In my mind, it is the best measure of severity available, but like its predecessors, the SSI-4 has some drawbacks. The sample of children and adults on which it

Stuttering Severity Instrument–4

SSI–4

Examiner Record Form

Glyndon D. Riley

Identifying Information

Name ______ Female ☐ Male ☐
Grade ______ Date of Birth ______
Date of testing ______ Age ______
School ______ Examiner ______
Preschool ☐ School Age ☐ Adult ☐ Reader ☐ Nonreader ☐

Frequency (Use Readers Table or Nonreaders Table, not both)

Readers Table: 1. Reading Task %SS	Task Score	Readers Table: 2. Speaking Task %SS	Task Score	Nonreaders Table: 3. Speaking Task %SS	Task Score
1	2	1	2	1	4
2	4	2	3	2	6
3–4	5	3	4	3	8
5–7	6	4–5	5	4–5	10
8–12	7	6–7	6	6–7	12
13–20	8	8–11	7	8–11	14
21 & up	9	12–21	8	12–21	16
		22 & up	9	22 & up	18

Frequency Score (use 1 + 2 or 3) ☐

Duration

Average length of three longest stuttering events timed to the nearest 1/10th second		Scale Score
Fleeting	(.5 sec or less)	2
Half-second	(.5–.9 sec)	4
1 full second	(1.0–1.9 sec)	6
2 seconds	(2.0–2.9 sec)	8
3 seconds	(3.0–4.9 sec)	10
5 seconds	(5.0–9.9 sec)	12
10 seconds	(10.0–29.9 sec)	14
30 seconds	(30.0–59.9 sec)	16
1 minute	(60 sec or more)	18

Duration Score ☐

Physical Concomitants

Evaluating Scale
0 = none
1 = not noticeable unless looking for it
2 = barely noticeable to casual observer
3 = distracting
4 = very distracting
5 = severe and painful looking

Distracting Sounds:	Noisy breathing, whistling, sniffing, blowing, clicking sounds	0 1 2 3 4 5	____
Facial Grimaces:	Jaw jerking, tongue protruding, lip pressing, jaw muscles tense	0 1 2 3 4 5	____
Head Movements:	Back, forward, turning away, poor eye contact, constant looking around	0 1 2 3 4 5	____
Movements of the Extremities.	Arm and hand movement, hands about face, torso movement, leg movements, foot-tapping, or swinging	0 1 2 3 4 5	____

Physical Concomitants Score ☐

Total Score

Frequency ____ + Duration ____ + Physical Concomitants ____ = ☐ Percentile ____ Severity ____

©1994, 2009 by PRO-ED, Inc.
2 3 4 5 6 7 8 9 10 17 16 15 14 13 12 11 10 09 08

Additional copies of this form (#13027) may be purchased from PRO-ED, 8700 Shoal Creek Blvd., Austin, TX 78757-6897 800/897-3202, Fax 800/397-7633, www.proedinc.com

Figure 8.3 The Stuttering Severity Instrument-4. (From SSI-4 Stuttering Severity Instrument-4: Examiner Record Form (p. 1-2), by G. D. Riley, 2009, Austin, TX: PRO-ED. Copyright 2009 by PRO-ED, Inc. Reprinted with permission. No further duplication may be made without written permission from PRO-ED, Inc.)

Table 2.2

Percentile Ranks and Severity Equivalents of SSI–4 Total Scores for Preschool-Age Children (*N* = 72)

Total score	Percentile rank	Severity equivalent
0–8	1–4	Very mild
9–10	5–11	
11–12	12–23	Mild
13–16	24–40	
17–23	41–60	Moderate
24–26	61–77	
27–28	78–88	Severe
29–31	89–95	
32 and up	96–99	Very severe

Table 2.3

Percentile Ranks and Severity Equivalents of SSI–4 Total Scores for School-Age Children (*N* = 139)

Total score	Percentile rank	Severity equivalent
6–8	1–4	Very mild
9–10	5–11	
11–15	12–23	Mild
16–20	24–40	
21–23	41–60	Moderate
24–27	61–77	
28–31	78–88	Severe
32–35	89–95	
36 and up	96–99	Very severe

Table 2.4

Percentile Ranks and Severity Equivalents of SSI–4 Total Scores for Adults (*N* = 60)

Total score	Percentile rank	Severity equivalent
10–12	1–4	Very mild
13–17	5–11	
18–20	12–23	Mild
21–24	24–40	
25–27	41–60	Moderate
28–31	61–77	
32–34	78–88	Severe
35–36	89–95	
37–46	96–99	Very severe

Figure 8.3 *(Continued)*

was normed is not well described, its reliability is not strong, and its validity has not been convincingly demonstrated (McCauley, 1996). Despite these limitations, the SSI is easy to use and captures the severity of overt stuttering behaviors as a composite of three important dimensions: frequency, duration, and physical concomitants. In addition, because there are no perfect measures, the goal in choosing a measure is to choose the one that seems to have the best evidence of those available. The SSI-4 is one of the few measures of stuttering for a broad age range that has standardized procedures for gathering and scoring speech samples and is the only measure that includes the three dimensions just cited.

The total overall score for the SSI is the sum of the three subcomponents measured.

1. *Frequency* is assessed as the percentages of syllables stuttered on a speaking task and a reading task. For nonreaders, the speaking task is given twice the weight in the scoring procedures. Riley originally used percentage of words stuttered but currently uses the percentage of syllables stuttered, which is converted to a "task score" on the form which is the Frequency Score.
2. *Duration* is assessed by measuring the length of the three longest stutters, calculating their mean duration, and finding the appropriate "scale score" on the form for the Duration Score.
3. *Physical concomitants* are assessed by adding the scale values of each subcomponent (i.e., distracting sounds, facial grimaces, head movements, and movements of the extremities) and deriving a Physical Concomitants Score.

The values for frequency, duration, and physical concomitants are then added together to provide a total overall score. Percentiles and severity ratings (e.g., mild, moderate, and severe) based on total overall scores are given on the form. Clinicians should carefully read Riley's directions in the manual of the SSI-4 before administering this measure.

Clients should be video recorded, and the SSI should be calculated from the recording because duration measures and assessment of physical concomitants cannot be done easily online and the frequency count will be more accurate if equivocal stutters are replayed repeatedly until a decision can be reached. The CSSS software accompanying the SSI-4 allows computer-aided calculation of stuttering frequency and duration for the overall severity score.

Another measure of severity, the Test of Childhood Stuttering (TOCS) (Gillam, Logan, & Pearson, 2009), can be used with children ages 4 to 12. It can be obtained from PRO-ED (http://www.proedinc.com). The TOCS consists of several subparts:

1. A Speech Fluency Measure, which is based on scores obtained during 4 tasks: (1) rapid picture naming, (2) modeled sentences, (3) structured conversation, and (4) narration
2. An Observational Rating Scale to be used by the clinician, teacher, or caregiver. This component provides information from the observer about (1) how often the child has various stuttering behaviors and (2) how often the child has negative responses to his own stuttering, such as showing such secondary reactions as concomitant physical behaviors and avoidance of speaking.

3. A Supplemental Clinical Assessment, which allows a more detailed analysis of the stuttering frequency, duration, types, and associated behaviors, as well as speech naturalness. This measure can help to decide if the child stutters and how severe the child is. It can also be used for assessment before and after treatment.

In a review of TOCS in *Mental Measurements Yearbook*, Shapely and Guyette (2010) commented favorably on the instrument's validity and reliability but suggested caution in interpreting the test's index scores and percentile ranks because of limited sample sizes used in standardization and in validity and reliability assessment.

Another measure of severity, which captures frequency, duration, and perhaps secondary behaviors, is the Scale for Rating Severity of Stuttering (Johnson, Darley, & Spriestersbach, 1952; Williams, 1978). This early scale, shown in Figure 8.4, is more subjective than the SSI, relying on an overall impression of a speech sample to rate the sample with one of eight values (0–7). Raters are encouraged to treat each of the eight intervals between the scale values as equal, although there is some debate about whether this is truly an equal-interval scale (Berry & Silverman, 1972). Although it has been shown to be reliable when a group of raters is used, the reliability of the Scale for Rating Severity of Stuttering for use with single raters is questionable. Williams (1978)

Scale for Rating Severity of Stuttering

Speaker________________________ Age ___ Sex___ Date_________

Rater __________________________ Identification ____________________

Instructions:

Indicate your identification by some such term as "speaker's clinician," "clinical observer," "clinical student," or "friend," "mother," "classmate," etc. Rate the severity of the speaker's stuttering on a scale from 0 to 7, as follows:

0 No Stuttering

1 Very mild–stuttering on less than 1 percent of words; very little relevant tension; disfluencies generally less than one second in duration; patterns of disfluency simple; no apparent associated movements of body, arms, legs, or head.

2 Mild–stuttering on 1 to 2 percent of words; tension scarcely perceptible; very few, if any, disfluencies last as long as a full second; patterns of disfluency simple; no conspicuous associated movements of body, arms, legs, or head.

3 Mild to moderate–stuttering on about 2 to 5 percent of words; tension noticeable but not very distracting; most disfluencies do not last longer than a full second; patterns of disfluencies mostly simple; no distracting associated movements.

4 Moderate–stuttering on about 5 to 8 percent of words; tension occasionally distracting; disfluencies average about one second in duration; disfluency patterns characterized by an occasional complicating sound or facial grimace; an occasional distracting associated movement.

5 Moderate to severe–stuttering on about 8 to 12 percent of words; consistently noticeable tension; disfluencies average about two seconds in duration; a few distracting sounds and facial grimaces; a few distracting associated movements.

6 Severe–stuttering on about 12 to 25 percent of words; conspicuous tension; disfluencies average three to four seconds in duration; conspicuous distracting sounds and facial grimaces; conspicuous distracting associated movements.

7 Very severe–stuttering on more than 25 percent of words; very conspicuous tension; disfluencies average more than four seconds in duration; very conspicuous distracting sounds and facial grimaces; very conspicuous distracting associated movements.

Figure 8.4 Scale for Rating Severity of Stuttering. (Reprinted from Sherman D. (1952). Clinical and experimental use of the Iowa Scale of Severity of Stuttering. *Journal of Speech and Hearing Disorders*, *17*, 316–320, with permission.)

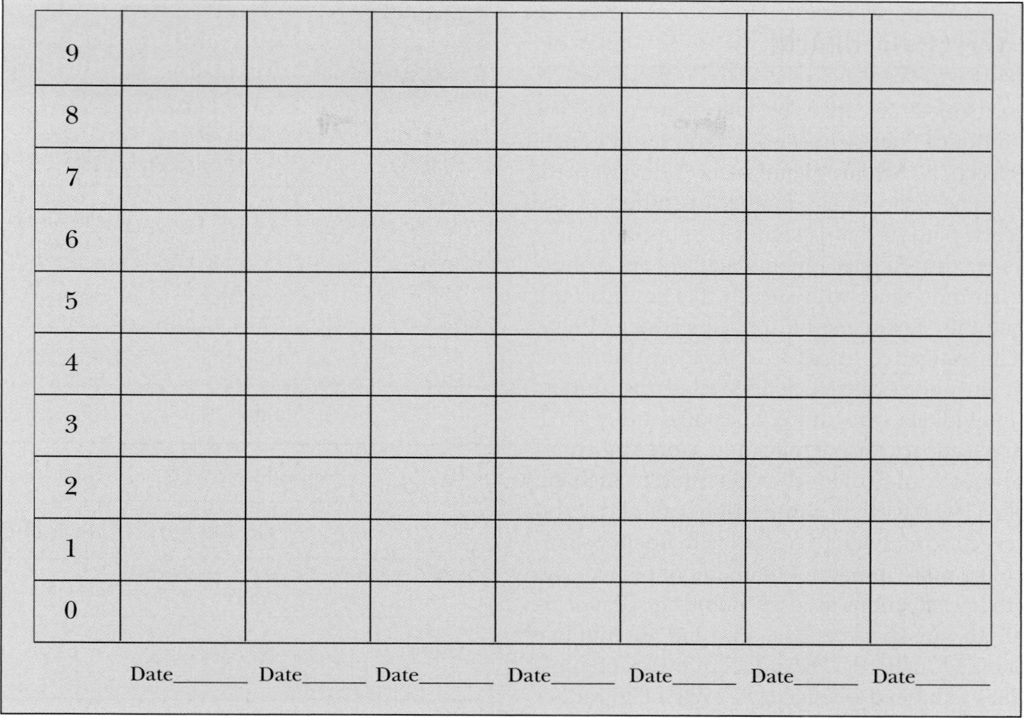

Figure 8.5 The Severity Rating Scale. Rate the speaker on a 9-point scale, where 0 = no stuttering and 9 = extremely severe stuttering (the worst stuttering the speaker has produced) for the entire day. Put an X in the appropriate box at the end of each day. (Reprinted from The Australian Stuttering Research Centre, http://lidcombeprogram.org, with permission.)

cautioned that the scale gives only a rough measure of severity because of its limitations. But he also noted that it has clinical utility because it captures the listener's impression of a client's speech and may therefore convey information about what the client faces every day when he is speaking. Ratings by a number of real listeners in the client's environment, as well as the client herself, would increase the value of this information. Any scale, including this one, has real risks if used as a single measure of therapeutic progress by a clinician. Unconscious bias and familiarity with the client may lead to improved ratings in the absence of change. Progress should be assessed with a variety of tools, including the SSI-4.

A fourth measure of severity in children is the Lidcombe Program's Severity Rating (SR) Scale, which was developed by Onslow, Costa, and Rue (1990) as part of a direct treatment program for preschool children. This is simply a 0-to-9 scale that parents use to make daily ratings of their child's stuttering (0 = no stuttering, 1 = extremely mild stuttering, through 9 = extremely severe stuttering). The scale, in a format that allows for a week's ratings, is shown in Figure 8.5. At the beginning of treatment, parents are trained to accurately rate their child's severity using observations of the child's speech in the clinic. The clinician and parent compare their ratings and discuss any differences between them until the parent's ratings are within one scale value of the clinician's. Throughout treatment, a sample of the child's speech that is long enough to ensure that any stuttering is observed is taken at the beginning of each clinic meeting. Both the clinician and the parent rate this sample, ensuring continued agreement.

This severity rating scale has also been used with school-age children who stutter. These older children often rate themselves in a version of the Lidcombe Program developed for older children. Research on this severity rating scale has shown it to be a valid and reliable tool for conveniently obtaining information on a child's stuttering outside of the treatment environment (Onslow, Andrews, & Costa, 1990; Onslow, Harrison, Jones, & Packman, 2002). In a recent article, a cohort of clinical researchers has published a strong argument espousing use of the SR scale for clinical research (Onslow et al., 2018). They suggest that the SR scale is easier to use than measuring frequency of stuttering using percent syllables stuttered (%SS). In my own mind, both measures are useful, but the SR scale is far easier to use for constant assessment (i.e., daily ratings) of a child's progress or problems in treatment. Assessing stuttering severity with detailed measure, such as the SSI-4 or the 9-point stuttering severity scale used by the Lidcombe Program, can be important for assessing progress, comparing scores at the beginning and end of treatment.

ASSESSING SPEECH NATURALNESS

Many years ago, clinical scientists became concerned that treatments that produce fluency may not always result in natural-sounding speech. As Schiavetti and Metz (1997) warned, "Some stutterers may reduce their number of stutters at the expense of a speech pattern that is stutter-free but not really fluent." Thus, some stuttering treatments may get rid of stuttering but leave an individual with speech that sounds odd, unusual, or unnatural. Martin, Haroldson, and Triden (1984), one of the first investigative teams to report on this problem, found that unsophisticated listeners rated the stutter-free speech of individuals who stutter speaking under DAF (delayed auditory feedback) as significantly more unnatural than the general speech of people who don't stutter. Ingham, Gow, and Costello (1985) used the same rating scale and found that the fluent speech of individuals treated with fluency shaping was judged to be more unnatural than that of people who don't stutter. Both investigations used a 9-point, equal-appearing interval scale to rate speakers based on judges' intuitive sense of what sounded "natural." The judges in these and most subsequent studies exhibited satisfactory levels of intrarater reliability and agreement, although between-rater reliability (interrater) was only marginally satisfactory.

Clinically, we need to be sure that clients sound as natural as possible after treatment. Otherwise, they are likely to abandon their fluency skills in favor of old, familiar stuttering patterns because of their own and listeners' negative reactions to their posttreatment speech. Can we rate our clients' naturalness reliably? Schiavetti and Metz (1997) indicated that clinicians who have learned to be consistent raters of speech naturalness may rely on the relative values of their ratings. Thus, they can judge when a client sounds less natural than other clients they have treated and take appropriate steps to improve that client's naturalness before releasing her from treatment. The SSI-4 incorporates a naturalness rating as part of the assessment.

ASSESSING SPEAKING AND READING RATE

Many clinicians believe that **speaking rate** often reflects the severity of stuttering (e.g., Shapiro, 1999, 2011; Starkweather, 1985, 1987). Van Riper (1982) described studies that found correlations that ranged from 0.68 to 0.88 between reading rate and severity. If a client's speaking rate is well below average for their age, communication will be affected; listeners may become impatient or lose the thread of what the speaker is saying. Speech rates that are too fast will also affect communication. A subgroup of individuals who stutter also has the disorder of cluttering, which is rapid, often unintelligible speech (see Chapter 15). Thus, it is useful to measure the client's rate in standard speaking and reading tasks. Table 8.5 gives average speaking rates in syllables per minute for children and adults.

TABLE 8.5 Average Speaking Rates for Children and Adults

Age (y)	Syllables per Minute (Range)	Reference
3	116–163	Pindzola, Jenkins, and Lokken (1989)
4	117–183	Pindzola et al. (1989)
5	109–183	Pindzola et al. (1989)
6	140–175	Davis and Guitar (1976)
8	150–180	Davis and Guitar (1976)
10	165–215	Davis and Guitar (1976)
12	165–220	Davis and Guitar (1976)
Adult	162–230	Andrews and Ingham (1971)

Rate can be measured as either words or syllables per minute, depending on the clinician's preference. Some clinicians find it easier to calculate rate by using words per minute because words are easily observable units on the page. Others note that syllables per minute can be calculated more rapidly than words because clinicians can use the "beat" of syllables to count them online (i.e., while a speaker is talking). The syllables-per-minute approach also accounts for the fact that some speakers use more multisyllabic words than others and might be penalized because such words take longer to produce than one-syllable words. I recommend using syllables for these reasons.

No matter which method is used, the following rules can be used for counting words or syllables. Count only those words or syllables that would have been said if the person had not stuttered. Thus, if a person says, "My-my-my, uh, well my name is Peter," this should be counted as four words or five syllables because it is apparent that the extra instances of "my," the "uh," and the "well" are part of the stuttering. If a person says, "When I went to Boston, I mean when I went to New York...," and it does not appear that the person was postponing or using a "trick" to avoid stuttering, this would be counted as 13 words or 14 syllables because stuttering did not interfere with the utterance. Only true words (or syllables in true words) are counted; "uh" or "um" is not counted. "Oh" or "well" is counted, unless they are used as a postponement, starter, or other component of stuttering. These distinctions may seem difficult to remember, but the main rule of thumb you should use is that you are counting syllables or words that convey information to the listener.

When syllables per minute are calculated, it is often easiest to use an inexpensive calculator to count syllables cumulatively as they are spoken, although this takes some practice. Before the speaker begins, push the "1" key and then the "+." When the speaker starts speaking, press the "=" key for each syllable spoken or read, and the cumulative total will appear in the readout window. It is easier to count syllables by reading a transcript of the conversational sample aloud slowly and pushing the "=" key for each syllable spoken; inexperienced raters should learn to count syllables first from a transcript. Experienced raters can assess conversational speech rate directly from recordings by pressing the "=" key for each syllable spoken. Some calculators will count cumulatively when the "1" is pressed, followed by repeated presses of the "+" button; I have not found an expensive calculator that will count cumulatively (a cheap one will), but the calculator that came with my PC laptop and also the one in my Mac will count cumulatively with the 1, +, = maneuver.

Some clinicians have found that they are able, with practice, to count syllables per minute as the client is speaking by using graph paper with small boxes. As the client is talking, they put a dot in each box for each syllable spoken. They also use this method to assess frequency of stuttering, by putting a check instead of a dot for each syllable stuttered.

When words per minute are calculated, a transcript is made of a client's 5-minute sample of conversational speech, and her 5-minute reading sample is marked to indicate where she finished. The total number of words is counted, and this figure is divided by 5 to give a per-minute conversational or reading rate.

It is important to measure these samples accurately with a stopwatch or another timing device. In measuring the amount of speaking time in a conversational sample, I stop the stopwatch whenever the client is not talking but allow it to run during moments of stuttering. Short pauses of less than 2 seconds are incorporated into the 5 minutes, but formulation pauses longer than 2 seconds are excluded. With a little practice, starting and stopping a stopwatch during pauses and turn-switching become easy and natural.

The CSSS software that comes with the SSI-4 allows the clinician to count number of stutters and number of fluent syllables and assess total sample duration in seconds. By totaling the stuttered and fluent syllables and dividing that total by the sample duration in minutes, you can get overall speech rate in syllables per minute.

FLUENCYBANK

FluencyBank is a Web site that contains programs for analyzing samples of stuttered (and fluent) speech from your clients and research subjects. The site was developed by Nan Bernstein Ratner and Brian MacWhinney, extending the original child language platform to include stuttering and cluttering (Bernstein Ratner & MacWhinney, 2018). To access the site, go to talkbank.org and, then under the "Clinical Banks" heading, choose "FluencyBank." You will see a myriad of links to help you learn to use the FluencyBank tools. FluencyBank also invites you to send audio and video samples of stuttering so that they may be used by clinicians and researchers around the world.

For our purposes, I would like to introduce you to the tools you can use to make a transcript of a speech sample from your client and then analyze it. The result of the "instant" analysis will be many bits of information that will, among other things, be helpful in deciding if a young child is normally disfluent or is stuttering. Of particular interest is the weighted stuttering-like disfluency (SLD) index. The publication by Ambrose and Yairi (1999)—particularly Figure 1—suggests why this index may be important. As I will describe in Chapter 9, I used FluencyBank to analyze a child's speech during a parent-child interaction to show how strong the quantitative evidence was that the child was stuttering rather than normally disfluent. But it should be noted that when you watch the parent-child video, your qualitative judgment should bring you to the same conclusion.

To use FluencyBank, go to www.talkbank.org and choose (under Clinical Banks) FluencyBank. On that Web page, see SLP's Guide to CLAN that explains many programs but, for our purpose, tells you how to use FluencyBank to create a transcript and have it analyzed via FLUCALC. Also on the FluencyBank Web page, see the two tutorial screencasts that also describe how to use FLUCALC. It takes some careful reading, viewing, and listening to digest all the steps needed to get an output, based on the transcript that you have marked with codes for various kinds of stutters. The output will be an Excel sheet that details total numbers and percentages of various stuttering behaviors and typical disfluencies. As I indicated, the weighted SLD output may be very helpful indeed.

ASSESSING FEELINGS AND ATTITUDES

The feelings or emotions of individuals who stutter, as well as their beliefs and attitudes about themselves, about communication, and about stuttering, are all components of stuttering. For most people who stutter, the experience of stuttering and the reactions of others to their stuttering have a notable effect on their behavior and on their response to therapy. Therefore, assessment of these aspects of stuttering is important. In this section, I will focus on formal measures of **feelings and attitudes** that can be administered throughout therapy to assess progress. As clinicians gain more experience, they will develop informal procedures to supplement formal measures. I will describe informal measures in the next chapter, as well as in appropriate treatment chapters.

Assessing Preschool Children

Clinical researchers have developed several instruments to assess feelings and attitudes of preschool children who stutter. Guttormsen, Kefalianos, and Næss (2015), in their review of 18 studies of communication attitudes of children (ages 3–18 years) who stutter, concluded that children who stutter had more negative attitudes than children who did not. These greater negative attitudes were present in preschoolers and became increasingly negative with age. One of the early measures designed for use with preschool children is the KiddyCAT (Hernandez, 2001; Vanryckeghem, Brutten, & Hernandez, 2005; Vanryckeghem, Hernandez, & Brutten, 2001). The KiddyCAT consists of 12 yes/no questions asked by the clinician after some practice items. An example is "Do you think that Mom and Dad like the way you talk?" The questions are asked in a play environment, such as putting a marble in an egg carton after each response. Higher scores indicate more negative attitudes about speech. In a sample of 45 children who stutter (ages 0–3 to 5–6) and 63 children who don't (ages 2–3 to 3–6), the mean scores were 4.35 (SD = 2.78) for children who stutter and 1.79 (SD = 1.78) for children who don't. This difference was statistically significant ($p < .001$) (Vanryckeghem et al., 2005). I would only use the KiddyCAT when I am sure the child is consciously aware of their stuttering, so the assessment procedure does not make them aware when they were not.

Another assessment tool for attitudes and feelings of preschool children who stutter takes an indirect approach by surveying parents about the impact of stuttering on the child and themselves (Langevin, Packman, & Onslow, 2010). The survey—The Impact of Stuttering on Preschoolers and Parents (ISPP)—consists of 20 questions covering (1) child-related questions (e.g., "Has your child ever been frustrated when stuttering?"); (2) questions about playmates (e.g., "Has your child ever been teased by other children about his stuttering?"); and (3) parent-related questions (e.g., "Has your child's stuttering ever affected you emotionally?"). One of the purposes of this tool, according to the authors, is to help decide whether to enroll the child in treatment or to delay treatment to see if stuttering resolves itself. This survey awaits further testing to assess validity and reliability. The ISPP is shown in Figure 8.6.

Abbiati, Guitar, and Hutchins (2013) presented preliminary results of a measure that was designed to assess awareness of stuttering in preschool children who stuttered without making them self-conscious about their speech. A video of two puppets talking (one of whom stutters) is shown to a child, and he is asked several questions about the puppet's speech (e.g., how hard is it for the cow puppet to talk?) and then several questions about the child's own speech. Responses were made by selecting 1 of 3 faces (frowny, neutral, and smiley) representing 3 possible answers (e.g., speaking is really hard, not hard at all, somewhere in the middle). This was given to 16 preschool children who stutter and 11 children who did not. Results showed that the children who stuttered rated their own speech not significantly different from their rating of the stuttering puppet's speech. On the other hand, the children who did not stutter rated their own speech significantly different from the puppet's speech (e.g., much easier, not worried about, etc.). This suggests the children who stuttered were aware of their stuttering and even worried about it. These results are based on a small sample, and we would like to enlist SLPs who have preschool children who stutter on their caseloads to help collect more data.[3]

A number of clinicians have suggested that a preschool child's sensitivity or reactivity to new situations may be an important consideration in therapy and possibly predictive of chronicity (Conture, 2001; Guitar, 1998). I have found that the Behavioral Style Questionnaire (BSQ) (McDevitt & Carey, 1978, 1995), which is administered to parents, provides some information on this dimension. Some research indicates that the BSQ may be able to identify those children who have a more inhibited, sensitive temperament (Anderson, Pellowski, Conture, & Kelly, 2003; Conture, 2001). The BSQ has relatively high mean test-retest reliability for the 3- to 7-year scales (0.81) and a moderate internal consistency for this age range (0.70) (McDevitt & Carey, 1995).

A 7-item scale to measure sensitive temperament in children via parent report was developed by Oyler several years ago for her doctoral dissertation (Oyler, 1996). Recently, the scale (Short Behavioral Inhibition Scale or SBIS) has been shown to be a valid and reliable assessment of behavioral inhibition—a characteristic of children that is similar to sensitive temperament (Ntourou, DeFranco, Conture, & Walden, in review). Ntourou et al. also found that the scale demonstrated significantly greater behavioral inhibition in a group of children who stuttered (n = 183) compared to a group who did not (n = 201) (p = .038). Further analysis showed that children who stuttered who were more behaviorally inhibited showed significantly greater stuttering frequency and stuttering severity, as well as significantly more negative speech-related attitudes. This scale, which is both simple to administer and easy to interpret, can provide clinically relevant information when used in an evaluation. First, it can identify children who are highly behaviorally inhibited. In my experience, these children are less likely to benefit from highly structured, direct treatments (such as the Lidcombe Program) but may do better with an indirect approach (such as parent-child interaction therapy). And the converse is true (also, in my experience but without objective data to support my impressions): less behaviorally inhibited children thrive in programs such as Lidcombe. Second, as Ntourou et al. point out, there is evidence that more behaviorally inhibited individuals are more susceptible to classical conditioning (cf. Arenas & Zebrowski, 2013; Holloway, Allen, Myers, & Servatius, 2014), which as readers may recall plays

[3]If you are interested in participating, please email Claudia.abbiati@med.uvm.edu.

THE IMPACT OF STUTTERING ON PRESCHOOLERS AND PARENTS (ISPP) QUESTIONS

Response options were (a) "Yes," "No," and "Don't Know" for questions 1–10 and 11–14, and (b) "Yes" or "No" for questions 16–19. For "Yes" responses, more information was most often solicited.

Part I. Child-related questions:

1. Has stuttering ever caused any changes in how easy it is for your child to talk with other children? If you answered YES, was it easier or more difficult?
2. Has stuttering ever caused any changes in your child's self-confidence? If you answered YES, did your child gain or lose self-confidence?
3. Has stuttering ever caused any changes in your child's general talkativeness? If you answered YES, did your child become more or less talkative?
4. Has stuttering ever caused any changes in how much your child plays with other children? If you answered YES, did your child play with other children more or less?
5. Has stuttering ever caused any changes in the way your child plays with other children? This question refers to a broad range of possible changes in the way children play. For example, a child may change from being more or less assertive, may use gestures to communicate in play, or may give up when he/she can't get or keep a playmate's attention. If you answered YES, please comment on the way your child's play changed.
6. Has stuttering ever caused any changes in your child's general mood? If you answered YES, please comment on how your child's general mood changed.
7. Has stuttering ever caused any changes in your child's quality of life? If you answered YES, please comment on the changes.
8. Has your child ever been frustrated when stuttering?
9. Has stuttering ever caused your child to become withdrawn?
10. If you think stuttering has affected your child in any way other than in the ways referred to above, please summarize.

Part II. About playmates:

11. Has your child ever been teased by other children because of his/her stuttering? If you answered YES, can you please describe what children do or did when they tease(d)?
12. Has stuttering ever caused a change in how much children play with your child? If you answered YES, did children play more or less with your child?
13. Has stuttering ever caused a change in the way children play with your child? Again, this question refers to a broad range of possible changes in the way children play with your child. For example, playmates may become more empathetic and watch out for your child, they may not wait for your child to say what he/she wants to say, or they may become more bossy or directive. If you answered YES, please describe the change.
14. Have other children ever reacted in any other way to your child's stuttering? If you answered YES, please describe how the children react(ed).
15. Is there anything else about how children react to your child or your child's stuttering that you wish to share?

Part III. Parent-related questions:

16. Has your child's stuttering ever affected you emotionally?
17. Has your child's stuttering ever affected how you communicate with your child?
18. Have you ever not known what to do or say when your child was stuttering?
19. Has your child's stuttering ever affected the relationship between you and your child insofar as it would be affected by a breakdown in communication?

Figure 8.6 The Impact of Stuttering on Preschoolers and Parents. (From Langevin M, Packman A, Onslow M. (2010). Parent perceptions of the impact of stuttering on their preschoolers and themselves. *Journal of Communication Disorders, 43*(5), 407–423, with permission.)

a role in the development of stuttering (see Chapters 5 and 6). In short, using the SBIS may help a clinician pinpoint those children who will be most susceptible to conditioning and then implement steps to minimize/counter the effects of negative responses by listeners or the child himself.

Assessing School-Age Children

Several tools are available for assessing attitudes about speaking or about stuttering in school-age children. Figure 8.7 depicts a scale that a graduate student and I developed many years ago, called the A-19 Scale (Guitar & Grims, 1977). It consists of questions that we have found will distinguish between children who stutter and children who do not. Further research needs to be conducted on this tool, but it can provide the basis for discussion with a school-age child.

In addition to the A-19, the Communication Attitude Test (CAT), which was developed by Brutten and his colleagues, has been shown to be a reliable and appropriate tool to measure the attitudes of children and adults who stutter. This was done in a series of studies from 1991 to 2001. Initially, in 1991, in a study of 341 children between the ages of 7

Establish rapport with the child, and make sure that he or she is physically comfortable before beginning administration. Explain the task to the child, and make sure he or she understands what is required. Some simple directions might be used:

"I am going to ask you some questions. Listen carefully, and then tell me what you think: true or false. There is no right or wrong answer. I just want to know what you think." To begin the scale, ask the questions in a natural manner. Do not urge the child to respond before he or she is ready, and repeat the question if the child did not hear it or you feel that he or she did not understand it. Do not reword the question unless you feel it is absolutely necessary, and then write the question you asked under that item.

Circle the answer that corresponds to the child's response. Be accepting of the child's response because there is no right or wrong answer. If all the child will say is "I don't know," even after prompting, record that response next to the question. For the younger children (kindergarten and first grade), it might be necessary to give a few simple examples to ensure comprehension of the requited task:

a. Are you a boy? Yes No

b. Do you have black hair? Yes No

Similar, obvious questions may be inserted, if necessary, to reassure the examiner that the child is actively cooperating at all times. Adequately praise the child for listening, and assure him or her that a good job is being done.

It is important to be familiar with the questions so that they can be read in a natural manner.

The child is given 1 point for each answer that matches those given below. The higher a child's score, the more probable it is that he or she has developed negative attitudes toward communication. In our study, the mean score of the K through fourth grade stutterers (N = 28) was 9.07 (S.D. = 2.44), and for the 28 matched controls, it was 8.17 (S.D. = 1.80).

Score 1 point for each answer that matches these:

1. Yes	11. No
2. Yes	12. No
3. No	13. Yes
4. No	14. Yes
5. No	15. Yes
6. Yes	16. No
7. No	17. No
8. Yes	18. Yes
9. Yes	19. Yes
10. No	

Figure 8.7 A-19 Scale of Children's Attitudes by Susan Andre and Barry Guitar (University of Vermont). (Reprinted from Susan Andre, with permission.)

A-19 SCALE

Name________________________ Date __________

1.	Is it best to keep your mouth shut when you are in trouble?	Yes	No
2.	When the teacher calls on you, do you get nervous?	Yes	No
3.	Do you ask a lot of questions in class?	Yes	No
4.	Do you like to talk on the phone?	Yes	No
5.	If you did not know a person, would you tell your name?	Yes	No
6.	Is it hard to talk to your teacher?	Yes	No
7.	Would you go up to a new boy or girl in your class?	Yes	No
8.	Is it hard to keep control of your voice when talking?	Yes	No
9.	Even when you know the right answer, are you afraid to say it?	Yes	No
10.	Do you like to tell other children what to do?	Yes	No
11.	Is it fun to talk to your dad?	Yes	No
12.	Do you like to tell stories to your classmates?	Yes	No
13.	Do you wish you could say things as clearly as the other kids do?	Yes	No
14.	Would you rather look at a comic book than talk to a friend?	Yes	No
15.	Are you upset when someone interrupts you?	Yes	No
16.	When you want to say something, do you just say it?	Yes	No
17.	Is talking to your friends more fun than playing by yourself?	Yes	No
18.	Are you sometimes unhappy?	Yes	No
19.	Are you a little afraid to talk on the phone?	Yes	No

Figure 8.7 *(Continued)*

and 14 years—70 children who stuttered and 271 children who did not stutter—De Nil and Brutten (1991) found that the children who stuttered had significantly more negative communication attitudes ($p < .01$) and that this difference increased with age. Vanryckeghem and Brutten (1997) replicated this finding with children (age 6–13). In 1993, Vanryckeghem and Brutten affirmed the CAT's test-retest reliability using 44 school-age children; results indicated correlations of 0.86, 0.81, and 0.76 for retesting after 1, 11, and 12 weeks, respectively, indicating that it is appropriate to administer it to a child several times. In a study of 143 children who stuttered (ages 7–13), Vanryckeghem, Hylebos, Brutten, and Peleman (2001) examined the relationship between negative attitudes as measured by the CAT and negative emotions elicited by the questions on the CAT, as measured by a 1-to-5 scale filled out by the children. The authors found a high positive correlation ($r = 0.89$) between negative attitudes and negative emotions. Both negative attitudes and negative emotions increased with age. In summary, the CAT is a well-researched tool that can be used to determine the presence of negative attitudes in individuals ages 6 and older. It is now part of a larger assessment battery (Behavior Assessment Battery for School-Age Children Who Stutter, Brutten, & Vanryckeghem, 2007), which also contains the Speech Situation Checklist that evaluates a child's reactions to a range of situations, as well as the Behavioral Checklist which assesses a child's coping responses to his disfluency. It is important that a trusting relationship with the child has been developed before administering either the A-19 or the CAT to a school-age child.

The Overall Assessment of the Speaker's Experience of Stuttering (OASES) is a questionnaire designed to assess the impact of stuttering on a person's life. It is based on the World Health Organization's International Classification of Functioning, Disability and Health (World Health Organization, 2001; see Web site for updates, 2018) and focuses on feelings about stuttering, reactions to stuttering, communication in daily situations, and the extent to which stuttering interferes with daily living. Two new versions were adapted for use with children ages 7 to 12 (OASES-S) and ages 13 to 17 (OASES-T) (Yaruss & Quesal, 2010). A more detailed description is given in the next section on adolescents and adults, and a sample for adults is shown in Figure 8.13.

Although not strictly a measure of attitude, the Teachers Assessment of Student Communicative Competence (TASCC) (Smith, McCauley, & Guitar, 2000), which is depicted in Figure 8.8, is useful in assessing a child's communicative functioning in the classroom. I have listed it here because one of the subscales purports to measure approach/avoidance in the classroom based on questions about the child's class participation and volunteering to talk. Other areas that the teacher rates the child on include intelligibility, comprehension, appropriateness of communication, and pragmatic/nonverbal communication skills. I have found the TASCC to be helpful in getting information about how a child's communication is changing over the course of treatment. The measure was tested on 69 students in grades 1 through 5 in Maine, Vermont, Texas, Virginia, and Idaho and showed high internal consistency. Cronbach's coefficient alphas (a measure of a test's reliability) for the five subscales ranged from 0.77 to 0.95, respectively, suggesting that the TASCC items were related measuring a similar construct (Smith et al., 2000). Redundancy analysis was used to remove redundant items and combine some that were similar, leaving a 50-item scale.

Further pilot work on the TASCC was conducted with 14 children who stuttered, paired by gender and ethnic background with 14 who did not stutter (Sequin, 1999). Scoring of each pair of participants was obtained from teachers of children in grades 1 to 5; the participants included eight Caucasian pairs, two Hispanic pairs, and four African American pairs. Three of the pairs were females and 11 were males. The children who stuttered had significantly lower communicative competence scores ($p = .0001$) than the control children; the "approach/avoidance attitude" subscale showed the greatest difference between the groups. A second pilot study (Pierson, 2004) compared TASCC ratings of eight children who stuttered and eight children who did not (grades 1–5) matched for age, gender, grade, cultural background, and academic performance. Again, the children who stuttered had significantly lower communicative competence scores ($p = .002$). The approach/avoidance attitude subscale was not found to be significantly different between the groups, but the following three scales were, with the differences between the groups in this rank order: intelligibility > appropriateness of communication > clarification/repair (of output)/comprehension (of input) > pragmatic/nonverbal communication. Clinically, I have found it useful to know what subscales are most deviant for a child in a classroom. In one instance, a child who was rated deviant on the intelligibility subscale benefited from learning to speak more slowly and loudly, even when he stuttered.

As the preceding section indicated, there are several tools for assessing attitudes in schoolchildren. Those measures with the best evidence for validity and reliability are OASES and CAT. Assessment of classroom performance is best done using the TASCC. The A-19 can be used as a brief measure that will provide information about attitudes toward communication situations and is most appropriate for stimulating a discussion of stuttering with the child.

Assessing Adolescents and Adults

A variety of questionnaires can be used to assess various aspects of a person who stutters' feelings and attitudes about communication and stuttering. I typically use the Modified Erickson Scale of Communication Attitudes (S-24) (Andrews & Cutler, 1974) to obtain information about a client's communication attitudes (Fig. 8.9). This questionnaire has been normed on both individuals who stutter and individuals who don't stutter. A colleague and I (Guitar & Bass, 1978) studied a sample of 20 individuals treated by a fluency-shaping program and found that if communication attitude as measured by the S-24 does not change during treatment, the likelihood of relapse within 12 to 18 months increases. Ingham (1979) disputed this finding, but Young (1981) confirmed it using a reanalysis of the original data. Later data by Andrews and Craig (1988) also supported the relationship between normalizing attitudes on the S-24 and long-term treatment outcome.

I also use a questionnaire to assess a client's tendency to avoid stuttering, which is the avoidance scale of the Stutterer's Self-Rating of Reactions to Speech Situations (SSRSS) (Johnson et al., 1952); this questionnaire assesses a client's tendency to avoid specific speaking situations (Fig. 8.10). Research suggests that clients with avoidance scale scores higher than 2.56 before treatment may be more likely to have appreciable levels of stuttering 1 year after treatment with fluency-shaping therapy than clients with lower scores (Guitar, 1976). Thus, I suggest that clinicians use a client's avoidance scale score to guide them in choosing whether to focus more on ways of enhancing fluent speech or to combine enhancing fluency with an approach that modifies stuttering as well as the fears and avoidances associated with stuttering.

Sometimes I also use the Perceptions of Stuttering Inventory (PSI) (Woolf, 1967) to examine a stutterer's perception of the presence of struggle, avoidance, and expectancy of stuttering (Fig. 8.11). Woolf suggests that the PSI can be used to help a person who stutters view her problem more objectively, to develop treatment goals, and to assess progress. I find that the avoidance section of the PSI complements the avoidance scale of the SRSS because the SRSS focuses more on situations, whereas the PSI deals more with stuttering behaviors.

Another measure of attitude that has been shown to predict long-term outcome is the Locus of Control of Behavior Scale (Craig, Franklin, & Andrews, 1984), which assesses the extent to which a client believes he controls his own behavior

TEACHER ASSESSMENT OF STUDENT COMMUNICATIVE COMPETENCE (TASCC)

Student's Name ____________________ **Age** ____ **Gender** _____ **Ethnicity** _________

Below are a series of items that describe a student's communicative competency. Use the following scale to rate a student in your grade whom you consider to have communication competency issues. For each item, circle the number that best describes the student's communication. Please answer each item as well as you can, even if the item does not seem to apply to the student.

1 = Never **2 = Seldom** **3 = Sometimes** **4 = Often** **5 = Always**

Item					
1) Student remains attentive when others communicate with him/her	1	2	3	4	5
2) Student verbally relates thoughts in an age-appropriate meaningful manner to adults	1	2	3	4	5
3) Student adjusts style and content of speech according to communication partner and situation	1	2	3	4	5
4) Student appears to nonverbally relate feelings in an age-appropriate meaningful manner (e.g., facial glare, smile)	1	2	3	4	5
5) Student demonstrates age-appropriate nonverbal requests for message repetition (e.g., makes a "puzzled" face)	1	2	3	4	5
6) Student participates in age-appropriate turn-taking in conversations and class discussions	1	2	3	4	5
7) Student demonstrates age-appropriate verbal requests for message repetition (e.g., "Could you say that again?" or "What?")	1	2	3	4	5
8) Student uses appropriate voice inflection when speaking (e.g., intonation with questions)	1	2	3	4	5
9) Student uses appropriate eye contact when speaking to adults	1	2	3	4	5
10) Student gets the listener's attention before the student introduces a topic	1	2	3	4	5
11) Student uses age-appropriate opening and closing communication comments in conversations with peers (e.g., "Hello, see you later.")	1	2	3	4	5
12) Student's speech is understandable even when the topic is unknown	1	2	3	4	5
13) Student participates in story-description/retell interactions	1	2	3	4	5
14) Student verbally relates thoughts in an age-appropriate meaningful manner to peers	1	2	3	4	5
15) Student sticks up for his/her own views when confronted by group pressure	1	2	3	4	5
16) Student's overall speech is understandable (e.g., clear voice, clear articulation)	1	2	3	4	5

Figure 8.8 Teacher Assessment of Student Communicative Competence.

17) Student nonverbally expresses frustration toward peers when appropriate	1	2	3	4	5
18) Student responds within an appropriate time frame to remarks, questions, requests	1	2	3	4	5
19) Student joins into conversations with peers easily	1	2	3	4	5
20) Student uses vocabulary that is relevant to the conversation	1	2	3	4	5
21) Student appropriately engages in group discussions	1	2	3	4	5
22) Student uses appropriate rate of speech for situation	1	2	3	4	5
23) Student initiates topics of conversation in one-to-one situations with adults	1	2	3	4	5
24) Student initiates topics of conversation in one-to-one situations with peers	1	2	3	4	5
25) Student adjusts vocal intensity to account for distance and noise variables	1	2	3	4	5
26) Student freely volunteers answers to questions in class	1	2	3	4	5
27) Student uses speech effectively in directing peer's actions when intended	1	2	3	4	5
28) Student's speech is understood by unfamiliar listeners	1	2	3	4	5
29) Student uses appropriate eye contact when speaking to peers	1	2	3	4	5
30) Student uses age-appropriate humor within peer conversations	1	2	3	4	5
31) Student uses age-appropriate verbal communication to gain attention	1	2	3	4	5
32) Student nonverbally expresses frustration toward adults when appropriate	1	2	3	4	5
33) Student uses a variety of age-appropriate (or better) vocabulary	1	2	3	4	5
34) Student seems to understand age-appropriate humor within peer conversations	1	2	3	4	5
35) Student clarifies and/or rephrases when verbal communication is not understood by the listener	1	2	3	4	5
36) Student uses age-appropriate (or better) sentence length when answering questions in class	1	2	3	4	5
37) Student is able to shift to different topics within conversations	1	2	3	4	5
38) Student links his/her words together with age-appropriate (or better) grammatical structures	1	2	3	4	5
39) Student follows three-step instructions with minimal need for repetitions or visual cues	1	2	3	4	5
40) Student's speech is understood even when the speech becomes more complex (e.g., longer sentences, change in topic)	1	2	3	4	5

Figure 8.8 *(Continued)*

41) Student verbally or nonverbally indicates that he/she understands the speaker's message	1	2	3	4	5
42) Student is able to integrate information presented auditorily (e.g., lessons, stories, a sequence of directions) and comprehend the meaning	1	2	3	4	5
43) Student identifies characters/people in conversations	1	2	3	4	5
44) Student uses age-appropriate (or better) sentence length when having a conversation	1	2	3	4	5
45) Student uses the environment to get a message across when the student's verbal communication is not understood (e.g., points to relevant objects or people)	1	2	3	4	5
46) Student seems to understand nonverbal communication (e.g., gestures)	1	2	3	4	5
47) Student uses age-appropriate nonverbal communication to gain the attention of adults	1	2	3	4	5
48) Peers and adults seem to understand what the student says to them	1	2	3	4	5
49) Student interacts with a variety of peers and adults	1	2	3	4	5
50) Student uses age-appropriate nonverbal communication to gain the attention of peers (e.g., wave, gentle tap)	1	2	3	4	5

TASCC SUBSCALES

The TASCC is divided into five subscales. The following information indicates which items, distributed randomly, belong to which subscales.

Subscale	Item #s
I. Intelligibility	8, 12, 16, 22, 25, 40, 48
II. Appropriateness of Communication	2, 3, 6, 10, 11, 13, 14, 18, 20, 27, 30, 31, 33, 36, 37, 38, 44
III. Comprehension (of input) and Clarification or Repair (of output)	7, 34, 35, 39, 41, 42, 43, 46
IV. Pragmatic/Nonverbal	1, 4, 5, 9, 17, 29, 32, 45, 47, 50
V. Approach/Avoidance Attitude	15, 19, 21, 23, 24, 26, 49

Figure 8.8 *(Continued)*

MODIFIED ERICKSON SCALE OF COMMUNICATION ATTITUDES (S-24)

Name: ____________________ Date: __________ Score: __________

Directions: Mark the "true" column with a check (✓) for each statement that is true or mostly true for you and mark the "false" column with a check (✓) for each statement which is false or not usually true for you.

	TRUE	FALSE
1. I usually feel that I am making a favorable impression when I talk.		
2. I find it easy to talk with almost anyone.		
3. I find it very easy to look at my audience while speaking to a group.		
4. A person who is my teacher or my boss is hard to talk to.		
5. Even the idea of giving a talk in public makes me afraid.		
6. Some words are harder than others for me to say.		
7. I forget all about myself shortly after I begin a speech.		
8. I am a good mixer.		
9. People sometimes seem uncomfortable when I am talking to them.		
10. I dislike introducting one person to another.		
11. I often ask questions in group discussions.		
12. I find it easy to keep control of my voice when speaking.		
13. I do not mind speaking in front of a group.		
14. I do not talk well enough to do the kind of work I'd really like to do.		
15. My speaking voice is rather pleasant and easy to listen to.		
16. I am sometimes embarrassed by the way I talk.		
17. I face most speaking situations with complete confidence.		
18. There are few people I can talk with easily.		

Figure 8.9 Erickson S-24 Scale of Communication Attitudes. (Reprinted from Andrews, G., & Cutler, J. (1974). Stuttering therapy: The relation between changes in symptom level and attitudes. *Journal of Speech and Hearing Disorders*, *39*, 312–319, with permission. Copyright 1974, American Speech-Language-Hearing Association.)

19. I talk better than I write.
20. I often feel nervous while talking.
21. I find it hard to talk when I meet new people.
22. I feel pretty confident about my speaking ability.
23. I wish that I could say things as clearly as others do.
24. Even though I knew the right answer, I have often failed to give it because I was afraid to speak out.

Data on the "Modified Erickson Scale of Communication Attitudes"
I. Answers (Andrews & Cutler, 1974)
Score 1 point for each answer that matches this:

1. False	13. False
2. False	14. True
3. False	15. False
4. True	16. True
5. True	17. False
6. True	18. True
7. False	19. False
8. False	20. True
9. True	21. True
10. True	22. False
11. False	23. True
12. False	24. True

II. Adult Norms (Andrews & Cutler, 1974)

	Mean	Range
Stutterers	19.22	9–24
Nonstutterers	9.14	1–21

Figure 8.9 *(Continued)*

STUTTERER'S SELF-RATING OF REACTIONS TO SPEECH SITUATIONS

Name______________________________ Age________ Sex ____________
Examiner __________________________ Date ______________________

After each item put a number from 1 to 5 in each of the four columns.

Start with the right-hand column headed "Frequency." Study the five possible answers to be made in responding to each item, and write the number of the answer that best fits the situation for you in each case. Thus, if you habitually take your meals at home and seldom eat in a restaurant, certainly not as often as once a week, write the number 5 in the Frequency column opposite item No. 1 "Ordering in a restaurant." In like manner respond to each of the other 39 items by writing the most appropriate number in the Frequency column.

Now, write the number of the response that best indicates how much you stutter in each situation. For example, if in ordering meals in a restaurant you stutter mildly (for you), write number 2 in the Stuttering column.

Following the same procedure, write your responses in the Reaction column and, finally, write your responses in the Avoidance column.

Numbers for each of the columns are to be interpreted as follows:

A. Avoidance

1. I never try to avoid this situation and have no desire to avoid it.
2. I don't try to avoid this situation, but sometimes I would like to.
3. More often than not I <u>do not</u> try to avoid this situation, but sometimes I do try to avoid it.
4. More often than not I <u>do</u> try to avoid this situation.
5. I avoid this situation every time I possibly can.

B. Reaction

1. I definitely enjoy speaking in this situation.
2. I would rather speak in this situation than not speak.
3. It's hard to say whether I'd rather speak in this situation or not.
4. I would rather not speak in this situation.
5. I very much dislike speaking in this situation.

C. Stuttering

1. I don't stutter at all (or only very rarely) in this situation.
2. I stutter mildly (for me) in this situation.
3. I stutter with average severity (for me) in this situation.
4. I stutter more than average (for me) in this situation.
5. I stutter severely (for me) in this situation.

Figure 8.10 Stutterer's Self-Rating of Reactions to Speech Situations. (Reprinted from Johnson, W., Darley, F., & Spriestersbach, D. C. (1952). *Diagnostic manual in speech correction.* New York, NY: Harper & Row. Copyright 1952 by Harper & Row. Copyright renewed 1980 by Edna B. Johnson, Frederick L. Darley, and Duane C. Spriestersbach.)

D. Frequency

1. This is a situation I meet very often, two or three times a day or even more, on the average.
2. I meet this situation at least once a day with rare exceptions (except Sunday perhaps).
3. I meet this situation from three to five times a week on the average.
4. I meet this situation once a week, with few exceptions, and occasionally I meet it twice a week.
5. I rarely meet this situation—certainly not as often as once a week.

	Avoidance	Reaction	Stuttering	Frequency
1. Ordering in a restaurant.	______	______	______	______
2. Introducing myself (face to face).	______	______	______	______
3. Telephoning to ask price, train fare, etc.	______	______	______	______
4. Buying plane, train, or bus ticket.	______	______	______	______
5. Short class recitation (10 words or less).	______	______	______	______
6. Telephoning for taxi.	______	______	______	______
7. Introducing one person to another.	______	______	______	______
8. Buying something from a store clerk.	______	______	______	______
9. Conversation with a good friend.	______	______	______	______
10. Talking with an instructor after class or in his or her office.	______	______	______	______
11. Long-distance phone call to someone I know.	______	______	______	______
12. Conversation with my father.	______	______	______	______
13. Asking someone for date (or talking to someone who asks me for date).	______	______	______	______
14. Making short speech (1–2 minutes).	______	______	______	______
15. Giving my name over telephone.	______	______	______	______
16. Conversation with my mother.	______	______	______	______
17. Asking a secretary if I can see the employer.	______	______	______	______
18. Going to house and asking for someone.	______	______	______	______
19. Making a speech to unfamiliar audience.	______	______	______	______
20. Participating in committee meeting.	______	______	______	______
21. Asking the instructor a question in class.	______	______	______	______
22. Saying hello to friend passing by.	______	______	______	______
23. Asking for a job.	______	______	______	______
24. Telling a person a message from someone else.	______	______	______	______
25. Telling a funny story with one stranger in a crowd.	______	______	______	______
26. Parlor game requiring speech.	______	______	______	______

Figure 8.10 *(Continued)*

27. Reading aloud to friends.	____	____	____	____
28. Participating in a bull session.	____	____	____	____
29. Dinner conversation with strangers.	____	____	____	____
30. Talking with my barber/hairdresser.	____	____	____	____
31. Telephoning to make appointment or to arrange to meet someone.	____	____	____	____
32. Answering roll call in class.	____	____	____	____
33. Asking at a desk for book or card to be filled out, etc.	____	____	____	____
34. Talking with someone I don't know well while waiting for bus, class, etc.	____	____	____	____
35. Talking with other players during game.	____	____	____	____
36. Taking leave of a host or hostess.	____	____	____	____
37. Conversation with friend while walking.	____	____	____	____
38. Buying stamps at post office.	____	____	____	____
39. Giving directions to a stranger.	____	____	____	____
40. Taking leave of a girl/boy after date.	____	____	____	____
Totals	____	____	____	____
Averages (divide total by # of answers)	____	____	____	____

Figure 8.10 *(Continued)*

(i.e., whether the control is "internal" or "external") (Fig. 8.12). Scoring adds the points for each item, and higher scores reflect greater perceived "externality" of control. This scale is given just before treatment and again immediately after treatment. Studies have shown that clients who did not decrease their locus of control scores more than 5 percent from pretreatment to posttreatment are in danger of relapse (Craig & Andrews, 1985; Craig et al., 1984).

Andrews and Craig (1988) reported that two measures of attitude, combined with a measure of stuttering behavior, are useful in predicting relapse after fluency-shaping treatment. They found little relapse among those stutterers who met the following three goals by the end of treatment: (1) no stuttering on telephone calls to strangers, (2) a score of 9 or below on the Modified Erickson Scale of Communication Attitudes, and (3) locus of control score reductions greater than 5 percent. Their assessment of relapse was based on a single telephone call with a stranger 10 to 18 months after treatment, and relapse was considered to be more than 2 percent of syllables stuttered during the call.

As mentioned in the preceding section, the OASES (Fig. 8.13) is an assessment tool based on the WHO's 2001 International Classification of Functioning, Disability and Health. It is a 20-minute paper-and-pencil questionnaire designed to obtain information about the impact of stuttering on a client's life that is not usually gained by other measures. It is divided into four sections: (1) General Information, (2) Reactions to Stuttering, (3) Communication in Daily Situations, and (4) Quality of Life. An "impact score" for each section as well as a "total impact score" can be calculated and then related to normative data so that a clinician can find out how severely stuttering is impacting a client's life.

The developers of the OASES published data on validity and reliability (Yaruss & Quesal, 2006) on the adult version, indicating that internal reliability within each of the four sections was high (Cronbach's alpha coefficient ranged from 0.92 to 0.97), suggesting that questions within a section were tapping into a homogenous area. In addition, Pearson product-moment correlations between total scores for these four sections were low enough (0.66–0.85) to indicate that the different sections were measuring different domains. Criterion-related validity was assessed by comparing an earlier version of the OASES to the Erickson S-24 Scale of Communication Attitudes (Andrews & Cutler, 1974; Erickson, 1969). Correlations suggested one section (Reactions to Stuttering) was positively and highly correlated with the S-24, whereas the other two sections (Communication in Daily Situations and Quality of Life) were moderately correlated. Test-retest reliability was assessed by giving the OASES to 14 individuals two different times, separated by 10 to 14 days without intervening treatment. Responses were identical for 77 percent of responses and within ±1 for 98 percent of responses, suggesting that it is appropriate to administer the instrument repeatedly to an individual (e.g., before, during, and after treatment).

A summary of instruments to assess feelings and attitudes is given in Table 8.6.

CONTINUING ASSESSMENT

Assessment is an ongoing process. As treatment progresses, the clinician should continue to ask herself, "Am I using the best approach with this person? Is there something else or something different I should be doing?" She should also decide what measures of progress are important for a client and apply these measures at regular intervals. My own approach is to assess stuttering behavior at the beginning and the end of each semester. In other settings, I recommend assessing a client after every 10 hours of treatment. Although I don't always succeed in carrying out these periodic assessments, I try to obtain samples of my clients' speech in nonclinical situations, such as in the classroom or at work. I also do **continuing assessment** when I bring a client in for maintenance checkups at increasingly longer intervals after formal treatment is over.

PERCEPTIONS OF STUTTERING INVENTORY (PSI)

The symbols S, A, and E after each item denote struggle (S), avoidance (A), and expectancy (E). In practice, these symbols are not included in the Inventory, but are listed on a separate scoring key.

S A E

Name ______________________ Age ________ # ______________

Examiner ______________________ Date ________ % ______________

Directions

Here are 60 statements about stuttering. Some of these may be characteristic of your stuttering. Read each item carefully and respond as in the examples below.

Put a check mark (✓) under "characteristic of me" if repeating sounds is part of your stuttering; if it is not characteristic, leave the space blank.

"Characteristic of me" refers only to what you do now, not to what was true of your stuttering in the past and which you no longer do, and not what you think you should or should not be doing. Even if the behavior described occurs only occasionally or only in some speaking situations, if you regard it as characteristic of your stuttering, check the space under "characteristic of me."

Characteristic of me

__________ 1. Avoiding talking to people in authority (e.g., a teacher, employer, or clergyman). (A).

__________ 2. Feeling that interruptions in your speech (e.g., pauses, hesitations, or repetitions) will lead to stuttering. (E).

__________ 3. Making the pitch of your voice higher or lower when you expect to get "stuck" on words. (E).

__________ 4. Having extra and unnecessary facial movement (e.g., flaring your nostrils during speech attempts). (S).

__________ 5. Using gestures as a substitute for speaking (e.g., nodding your head instead of saying "yes" or smiling to acknowledge a greeting). (A).

__________ 6. Avoiding asking for information (e.g., asking for directions or inquiring about a train schedule). (A).

Figure 8.11 Perceptions of Stuttering Inventory. (Reprinted from Woolf, G. (1967). The assessment of stuttering as struggle, avoidance, and expectancy. *British Journal of Disorders of Communication*, *2*, 158–171, with permission.)

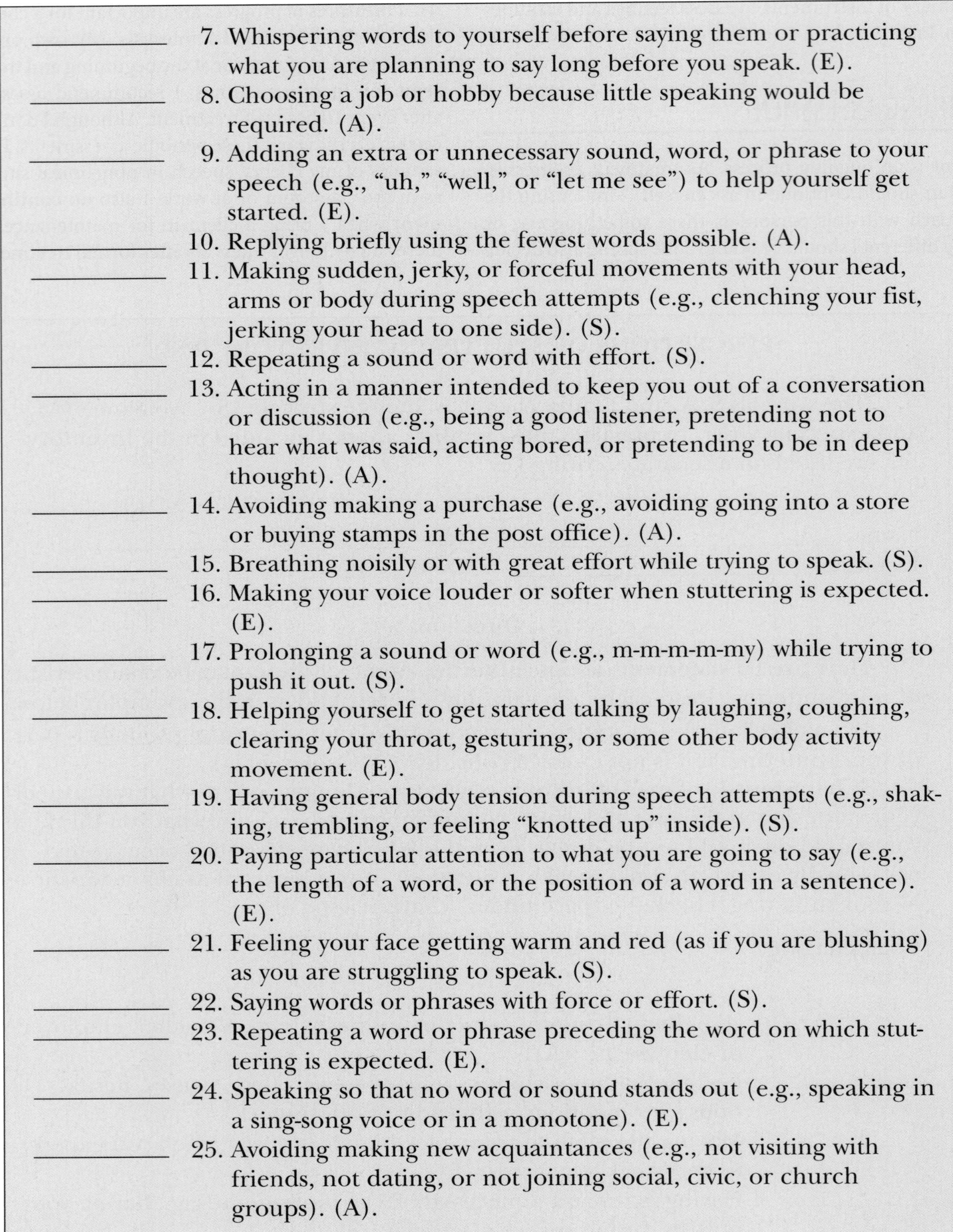

_______ 7. Whispering words to yourself before saying them or practicing what you are planning to say long before you speak. (E).
_______ 8. Choosing a job or hobby because little speaking would be required. (A).
_______ 9. Adding an extra or unnecessary sound, word, or phrase to your speech (e.g., "uh," "well," or "let me see") to help yourself get started. (E).
_______ 10. Replying briefly using the fewest words possible. (A).
_______ 11. Making sudden, jerky, or forceful movements with your head, arms or body during speech attempts (e.g., clenching your fist, jerking your head to one side). (S).
_______ 12. Repeating a sound or word with effort. (S).
_______ 13. Acting in a manner intended to keep you out of a conversation or discussion (e.g., being a good listener, pretending not to hear what was said, acting bored, or pretending to be in deep thought). (A).
_______ 14. Avoiding making a purchase (e.g., avoiding going into a store or buying stamps in the post office). (A).
_______ 15. Breathing noisily or with great effort while trying to speak. (S).
_______ 16. Making your voice louder or softer when stuttering is expected. (E).
_______ 17. Prolonging a sound or word (e.g., m-m-m-m-my) while trying to push it out. (S).
_______ 18. Helping yourself to get started talking by laughing, coughing, clearing your throat, gesturing, or some other body activity movement. (E).
_______ 19. Having general body tension during speech attempts (e.g., shaking, trembling, or feeling "knotted up" inside). (S).
_______ 20. Paying particular attention to what you are going to say (e.g., the length of a word, or the position of a word in a sentence). (E).
_______ 21. Feeling your face getting warm and red (as if you are blushing) as you are struggling to speak. (S).
_______ 22. Saying words or phrases with force or effort. (S).
_______ 23. Repeating a word or phrase preceding the word on which stuttering is expected. (E).
_______ 24. Speaking so that no word or sound stands out (e.g., speaking in a sing-song voice or in a monotone). (E).
_______ 25. Avoiding making new acquaintances (e.g., not visiting with friends, not dating, or not joining social, civic, or church groups). (A).

Figure 8.11 *(Continued)*

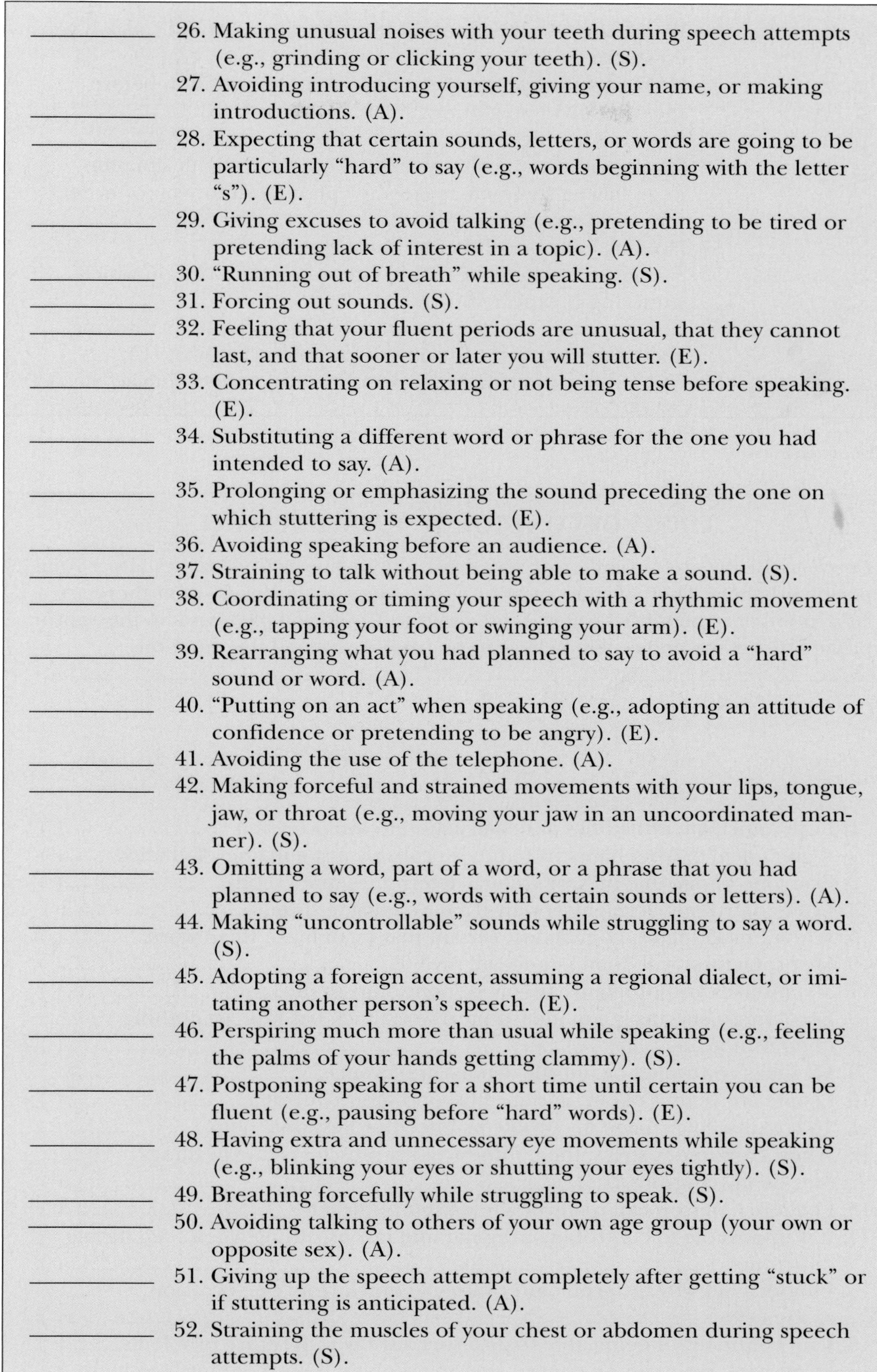

________ 26. Making unusual noises with your teeth during speech attempts (e.g., grinding or clicking your teeth). (S).
________ 27. Avoiding introducing yourself, giving your name, or making introductions. (A).
________ 28. Expecting that certain sounds, letters, or words are going to be particularly "hard" to say (e.g., words beginning with the letter "s"). (E).
________ 29. Giving excuses to avoid talking (e.g., pretending to be tired or pretending lack of interest in a topic). (A).
________ 30. "Running out of breath" while speaking. (S).
________ 31. Forcing out sounds. (S).
________ 32. Feeling that your fluent periods are unusual, that they cannot last, and that sooner or later you will stutter. (E).
________ 33. Concentrating on relaxing or not being tense before speaking. (E).
________ 34. Substituting a different word or phrase for the one you had intended to say. (A).
________ 35. Prolonging or emphasizing the sound preceding the one on which stuttering is expected. (E).
________ 36. Avoiding speaking before an audience. (A).
________ 37. Straining to talk without being able to make a sound. (S).
________ 38. Coordinating or timing your speech with a rhythmic movement (e.g., tapping your foot or swinging your arm). (E).
________ 39. Rearranging what you had planned to say to avoid a "hard" sound or word. (A).
________ 40. "Putting on an act" when speaking (e.g., adopting an attitude of confidence or pretending to be angry). (E).
________ 41. Avoiding the use of the telephone. (A).
________ 42. Making forceful and strained movements with your lips, tongue, jaw, or throat (e.g., moving your jaw in an uncoordinated manner). (S).
________ 43. Omitting a word, part of a word, or a phrase that you had planned to say (e.g., words with certain sounds or letters). (A).
________ 44. Making "uncontrollable" sounds while struggling to say a word. (S).
________ 45. Adopting a foreign accent, assuming a regional dialect, or imitating another person's speech. (E).
________ 46. Perspiring much more than usual while speaking (e.g., feeling the palms of your hands getting clammy). (S).
________ 47. Postponing speaking for a short time until certain you can be fluent (e.g., pausing before "hard" words). (E).
________ 48. Having extra and unnecessary eye movements while speaking (e.g., blinking your eyes or shutting your eyes tightly). (S).
________ 49. Breathing forcefully while struggling to speak. (S).
________ 50. Avoiding talking to others of your own age group (your own or opposite sex). (A).
________ 51. Giving up the speech attempt completely after getting "stuck" or if stuttering is anticipated. (A).
________ 52. Straining the muscles of your chest or abdomen during speech attempts. (S).

Figure 8.11 *(Continued)*

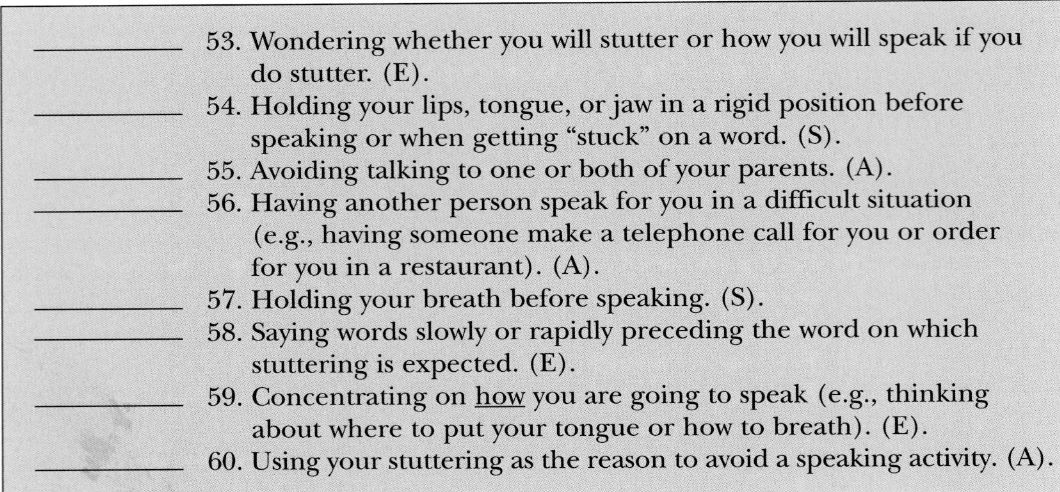

_________ 53. Wondering whether you will stutter or how you will speak if you do stutter. (E).
_________ 54. Holding your lips, tongue, or jaw in a rigid position before speaking or when getting "stuck" on a word. (S).
_________ 55. Avoiding talking to one or both of your parents. (A).
_________ 56. Having another person speak for you in a difficult situation (e.g., having someone make a telephone call for you or order for you in a restaurant). (A).
_________ 57. Holding your breath before speaking. (S).
_________ 58. Saying words slowly or rapidly preceding the word on which stuttering is expected. (E).
_________ 59. Concentrating on <u>how</u> you are going to speak (e.g., thinking about where to put your tongue or how to breath). (E).
_________ 60. Using your stuttering as the reason to avoid a speaking activity. (A).

Figure 8.11 *(Continued)*

LOCUS OF CONTROL OF BEHAVIOR SCALE

Directions: Below are a number of statements about how various topics affect your personal beliefs. There are no right or wrong answers. For every item there are a large number of people who agree and disagree. Could you please put in the appropriate bracket the choice you believe to be true? Answer all the questions.

0	1	2	3	4	5
Strongly disagree	Generally disagree	Somewhat disagree	Somewhat agree	Generally agree	Strongly agree

1. I can anticipate difficulties and take action to avoid them............................. ( )
2. A great deal of what happens to me is probably just a matter of chance.........( )
3. Everyone knows that luck or chance determines one's future.........................( )
4. I can control my problem(s) only if I have outside support............................( )
5. When I make plans, I am almost certain that I can make them work..............( )
6. My problem(s) will dominate me all my life..( )
7. My mistakes and problems are my responsibility to deal with......................... ( )
8. Becoming a success is a matter of hard work; luck has little or nothing to do with it..( )
9. My life is controlled by outside actions and events..( )
10. People are victims of circumstance beyond their control............................... ( )
11. To continually manage my problems I need professional help ....( )
12. When I am under stress, the tightness in my muscles is due to things outside my control..( )
13. I believe a person can really be the master of his fate....................................( )
14. It is impossible to control my irregular and fast breathing when I am having difficulties...( )
15. I understand why my problem(s) varies so much from one occasion to the next..( )
16. I am confident of being able to deal successfully with future problems.........( )
17. In my case, maintaining control over my problem(s) is due mostly to luck....( )

Figure 8.12 Locus of Control of Behavior Scale. (Reprinted from Craig A.R., Franklin J.A., Andrews G. (1984). A scale to measure locus of control of behaviour. *British Journal of Medical Psychology*, *57*, 173–180, with permission.)

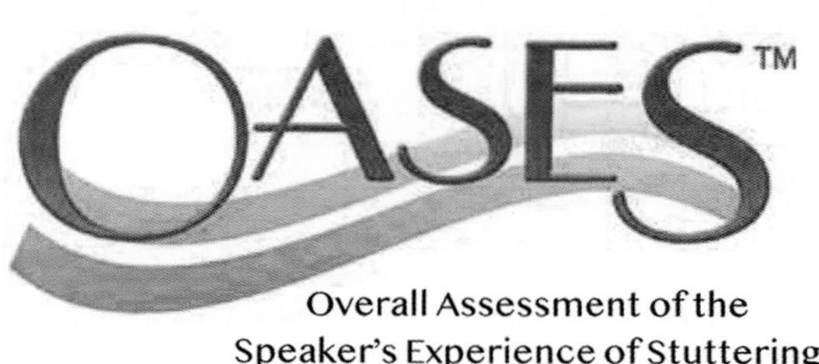

OASES-A
Response Form
Adult: Ages 18 and Above

J. Scott Yaruss, PhD, CCC-SLP, BCS-F, F-ASHA
Robert W. Quesal, PhD, CCC-SLP, BCS-F, F-ASHA

Name: ____________________

Birth Date: ____/____/____ Age: ______ Sex/Gender: ____________

Test Date: ____/____/____ ID Number: ____________

Clinician: ____________________

General Instructions:
This form includes four sections of questions that examine different aspects of your experiences with stuttering. Please complete each question in each section by circling the appropriate number. Please think about how you are *currently* feeling or speaking when answering each question. Some of the questions do not apply to everyone. If one of the questions does not apply to you, please check ❑ N/A for "Not Applicable" and go on to the next question.

Scoring: For Office Use Only

Instructions for Clinicians:

- Calculate Impact Scores for each of the four sections on the OASES–A by first summing the number of points in each section (A) and then counting the number of items completed in each section (B). Divide the total number of points (A) by the number of items completed (B) to obtain the Impact Score.
- Calculate the Overall Impact Score by summing the numbers in columns (A) and (B) at the bottom of each column. Divide the sum of (A) by the sum of (B) to obtain the Overall Impact Score.
- Impact Scores range between 1.0 and 5.0. Circle the Impact Rating that corresponds to the score for each section and for the Overall Impact.

	Impact Score			Impact Rating				
	A Points	B Items Completed	A ÷ B = Impact Score	Score 1.00–1.49	Score 1.50–2.24	Score 2.25–2.99	Score 3.00–3.74	Score 3.75–5.00
Section I: General Information	______ ÷	______ =	______	Mild	Mild-Moderate	Moderate	Moderate-Severe	Severe
Section II: Speaker's Reactions	______ ÷	______ =	______	Mild	Mild-Moderate	Moderate	Moderate-Severe	Severe
Section III: Daily Communication	______ ÷	______ =	______	Mild	Mild-Moderate	Moderate	Moderate-Severe	Severe
Section IV: Quality of Life	______ ÷	______ =	______	Mild	Mild-Moderate	Moderate	Moderate-Severe	Severe
OVERALL Impact:	______ ÷	______ =	______	Mild	Mild-Moderate	Moderate	Moderate-Severe	Severe

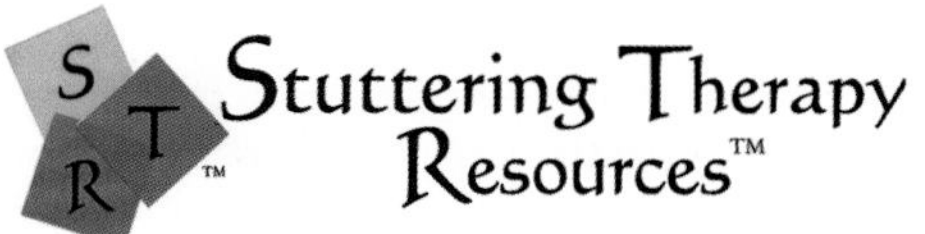

Copyright © 2016 Stuttering Therapy Resources, Inc. All rights reserved.
Do not duplicate. Additional Response Forms available from STR:
8005 Spectrum Drive, McKinney, TX 75070
844-4 STUTTER (844-478-8883)
www.StutteringTherapyResources.com

Figure 8.13 Overall assessment of the speaker's experience of stuttering. (Reprinted from OASES-A, Copyright © 2016 Stuttering Therapy Resources, Inc. All rights reserved. www.StutteringTherapyResources.com, with permission.)

TABLE 8.6 Methods of Assessing Attitudes and Feelings

Age Group	Measure	Comment
Preschool	Children's version of the Communication Attitude Test (KiddyCAT)	A 12-item set of questions that are asked of preschool children about their speech. Vanryckeghem and her colleagues have gathered considerable data comparing children who stutter and children who don't. Our own experience suggests caution lest children give answers they think the examiner wants to hear.
	Impact of Stuttering on Preschoolers and Parents (ISPP)	A 20-item questionnaire for parents about their child's response to his or her stuttering and about parents' own feelings about their child's stuttering.
	Behavioral Style Questionnaire (BSQ)	A broad scale completed by parents, which may reveal children's sensitivity. Children ages 3–7 who stutter have been shown to be more sensitive than typical children, using this scale.
School age	A-19	This is an informal 19-item questionnaire given to children. Although it has been shown to distinguish between children who stutter and those who don't (kindergarten through fourth grade), it has not been extensively tested. Useful for generating discussion about how the student feels about his stuttering.
	Communication Attitude Test (CAT)	This questionnaire, assessing communication attitudes, has been shown to be reliable with individuals who stutter, from school age to adult. It has generated a great deal of research by Brutten, Vanryckeghem, and their colleagues.
	Overall Assessment of the Speaker's Experience of Stuttering (OASES)	Developed as a measure of the overall impact that stuttering has on a person's life, this instrument is very helpful for planning treatment and assessing the effect of treatment on day-to-day functioning.
	Teacher's Assessment of Student Communicative Competence (TASCC)	This is a 50-item questionnaire filled out by teacher(s) to give information about how well the child communicates in his classroom(s). Normed on children in first through fifth grades, it can be helpful in assessing ways in which a student's communication is affected by his stuttering and/or other issues.
Adolescents and adults	Modified Erickson Scale of Communication Attitudes (S-24)	A 24-item questionnaire, shown to be reliable for initial testing and retesting attitudes about communication. Several studies have shown that it can be predictive of outcomes for certain treatments.
	Stutterer's Self-Rating of Reactions to Speech Situations (SSRSS)	This questionnaire assesses the frequency with which an individual encounters speaking situations (like talking on the telephone), his reactions to them, and tendency to avoid them. Also shown to be predictive of outcomes for certain treatments.
	Perceptions of Stuttering Inventory (PSI)	This questionnaire assesses the individual's own perceptions of his own struggle, avoidance, and expectancy related to his stuttering. May be helpful to understand how much the individual is aware of his stuttering.
	Locus of Control	This scale enables the clinician to estimate how much the client believes that he controls his own destiny. May be predictive of treatment outcome.

In addition to periodically measuring client stuttering behaviors, I assess my client's feelings and attitudes at the beginning and end of treatment. Moreover, if progress seems to be slow or plateauing, I may assess them informally on a regular basis, as part of trying to understand any resistance from the client. Van Riper (1982) has suggested that a client's resistance—their objections to doing various assignments and other signs of noncooperativeness—may signal real gains are being made in changing the stuttering. Change can be emotionally challenging, and to unleash further progress, the client may need an opportunity to express his frustration with the process and even anger at the therapist. Good listening, with genuine acceptance on the part of the clinician, can reduce resistance and free the client up to be more accepting of their current level of stuttering and of themselves, both of which are foundations for progress toward more fluent speech. More space will be devoted to the clinical relationship in Chapter 10, "Preliminaries to Treatment."

Sometimes continuing assessment during treatment requires creating a new tool appropriate to a particular client's needs. A student and I were recently working with a developmentally delayed adult. Treatment had started with use of a slower style of speaking and the client's self-rating of his severity. After several weeks, the client's and our own severity ratings began to plateau and were not budging, despite our tweaks to the treatment. We then decided to teach the client to drop his myriad avoidance behaviors and begin feared words with a slow deliberate attempt and remain in the stutter until he was able to lessen the tension and finish the word slowly and loosely. We worked together with him to develop a scale on which he rated his feeling of being in control of his speech, to supplement severity ratings. This proved to be a satisfying and effective approach for him and showed steady progress.

SUMMARY

- In an assessment, the clinician has a variety of tasks. These include
  - ☐ Gathering data from the client
  - ☐ Getting to know the client as an individual
  - ☐ Showing an understanding of the client's point of view and hopes for treatment
  - ☐ Demonstrating an understanding of stuttering
- Clinicians must develop skills and sensitivities in working with clients from cultures other than their own.
- Building a relationship with a client begins in the first meeting, which is usually the assessment. A clinician must take this opportunity to demonstrate that she knows about the disorder of stuttering, is unafraid of it, and is accepting of it. At the same time, she must show that she feels positively about the client's ability to change his stuttering.
- Behaviors counted as stutters include part-word repetitions, single-syllable whole-word repetitions, prolongations, blocks, and unequivocal avoidance behaviors.
- Samples for assessing stuttering should include a variety of situations. The initial sample and samples assessing outcome should be videotaped for more accurate scoring and measurement of reliability. These samples should include speaking and, when appropriate, reading.
- Frequency of stuttering is commonly assessed as the percentage of syllables or words stuttered.
- Different types of disfluencies can be assessed to reveal the percentage of stutter-like disfluencies or number of these disfluencies per 100 words. This information may be particularly useful in helping to decide if a preschool child needs treatment.
- Durations of moments of stuttering are useful in quantifying an aspect of the abnormality of a client's stuttering and the extent to which it may interfere with communication. Speaking and reading rates will also help to quantify this aspect of the impact of stuttering.
- Frequency and severity of secondary or concomitant behaviors associated with stuttering can be important measures of how much these behaviors call attention to themselves and distract listeners.
- Three severity scales are the Stuttering Severity Instrument (SSI-4), the Scale for Rating Severity, and the Lidcombe Program's Severity Rating Scale. The commonly used SSI-4 combines an assessment of frequency of stuttering, mean duration of the three longest stutters, and physical concomitants accompanying stuttering.
- Speech naturalness can be reliably and easily assessed. It is thought to be an especially important measure when evaluating outcomes of treatments that teach a client to use an unnatural speech pattern to initially achieve fluency.
- Various instruments have been created to assess emotions and attitudes associated with stuttering. When combined with measures of stuttering behaviors, these measures provide a multidimensional view of the disorder. In some cases, they can aid the clinician in selecting appropriate treatment and in assessing whether a client is ready for dismissal.
- Assessment is an ongoing activity. Measures of progress are important indicators of whether treatment is effective and should be continued or changed. Measures of outcome are critical for our knowledge of how effective a treatment has been in the long term with each client.

STUDY QUESTIONS

1. What does it mean to suggest that a clinician must play two different roles during an evaluation?
2. Which types of disfluencies are counted as stutters, and which are considered normal?
3. What factors can affect the process of measuring stuttering?
4. Describe the procedures for the two measures of reliability called "point-by-point agreement" and "percent error."
5. Why is it important to obtain several samples of speech from a client when assessing stuttering, whereas a single sample might be adequate for assessing a phonological disorder?
6. Give two reasons why assessment of reliability of measurements of stuttering is important.
7. Describe five dimensions or aspects of stuttering that may be assessed in an evaluation of a client who stutters.
8. To you, what is the most important aspect of stuttering? How a client feels about his stuttering? How much the client's speech deviates from typical fluency? How much the client avoids words and situations? Something else? Defend your choice. How do you measure it?
9. Why is it relevant to assess speech rate for a person who stutters?
10. Discuss the pros and cons of protecting the privacy of conversations between yourself and a teenage client by not sharing their contents with parents.

SUGGESTED PROJECTS

1. Research how different cultures react to stuttering and suggest how evaluation procedures in this chapter need to be changed for individuals from a culture that has very different beliefs about stuttering than those suggested in this text.
2. Make or obtain a video of a conversational and a reading sample of a person who stutters. Use two different methods of measuring the stuttering (such as percentage of syllables stuttered or duration of three longest stutters or speech rate or Scale for Rating Severity of Stuttering) and obtain intraobserver and interobserver reliability assessments for each method. Discuss why one measurement procedure is more reliable than the other.
3. Obtain a videotaped conversational sample of one or more individuals who stutter, and identify moments when you think the client has used an avoidance behavior to prevent stuttering. Discuss whether these avoidances should be counted as stutters.
4. Obtain samples of repetitive stutters from normally fluent children and from children who stutter. Compare the repetitions from both groups in terms of length of silent periods between iterations, pitch, and other acoustic variables.
5. Search the literature on assessment of stuttering to determine whether reliable methods have been developed for clients to assess their own stuttering during the progress of treatment.

SUGGESTED READINGS

Battle, D. (Ed.). (2012). *Communication disorders in multicultural and international populations* (4th ed.). St. Louis, MO: Elsevier/Mosby.

This book provides many descriptions and insights into evaluating and treating communication disorders in many cultures not only in the United States but throughout the world.

Brutten, G., & Vanryckeghem, M. (2007). *Behavior Assessment Battery for school-age children who stutter*. San Diego, CA: Plural Publishing.

This set of assessment tools is designed to measure communication attitudes and reactions to specific speaking situations for school-age children who stutter.

Conture, E. (2001). Assessment and evaluation. In *Stuttering: Its nature, diagnosis, and treatment* (pp. 59–128). Boston, MA: Allyn & Bacon.

This chapter is rich with ideas for assessment of children, adolescents, and adults who stutter. It is particularly good in the breadth of coverage of evaluation of children who stutter, reflecting the years of experience the author has had in working with this age group.

Cordes, A. K. (1994). The reliability of observational data: I. Theories and methods for speech-language pathology. *Journal of Speech and Hearing Research, 37*, 264–278.

This article provides an excellent tutorial on the problems associated with establishing reliability of observational data in stuttering.

Guttormsen, L., Kefalianos, E., & Næss, K. (2015). Communication attitudes in children who stutter: A meta-analytic review. *Journal of Fluency Disorders, 46*, 1–14.

This is a careful review of studies assessing the communication attitudes of children (ages 3–18 years) who stutter. Some clear conclusions are drawn, and directions for future research are suggested.

Howell, P., & Van Borsel, J. (2011). *Multilingual aspects of fluency disorders*. Tonawanda, NY: Multilingual Matters.

An edited book that discusses stuttering in many languages and cultures as well as stuttering and bilingualism.

Rosenberry-McKibbin, C. (2002). *Multicultural students with special language needs: Practical strategies for assessment and intervention* (2nd ed.). Oceanside, CA: Academic Communication Associates, Inc.

This book provides many insights into evaluation of multicultural students.

Wright, L., & Ayre, A. (2000). *The Wright Ayre stuttering self-rating profile*. Chesterfield, UK: Winslow Press Ltd.

This assessment tool was designed to be used by clinicians working with adolescent and adult clients who can participate in assessing their own behaviors and feelings. It is intended to go beyond traditional clinician-based assessments to obtain indications of how clients observe themselves.

9

Assessment and Diagnosis

Chapter Objectives

After studying this chapter, readers should be able to:

- Plan and carry out an evaluation of a preschool child, school-age child, adolescent, and adult
- Understand how to evaluate the stuttering behaviors of a client
- Understand how to evaluate attitudes and feelings of a client (and, when appropriate, the client's family)
- Understand how to determine appropriate follow-up to evaluation of each age level

Key Terms

Accepting environment: Behavior by parents and other family members (and teachers and classmates where appropriate) that convey to the child that they accept the child and his speech

Classroom observation: Time spent in the classroom by the clinician to assess how a child's stuttering may be affecting him in his classes

Clinician-child interaction: Play-based conversation between clinician and child in which clinician observes child's speech and may seek information about child's feelings about his stuttering, as well as information about child's other speech and language skills

Closing interview: A conversation at the end of an evaluation session in which the clinician informs the client or family of her findings, makes recommendations for the future, and elicits questions

Fluency shaping: Ways of speaking designed to induce fluency. Examples are slow rate, easy onset of voicing, and light contact of articulators.

Individualized Education Program (IEP): A plan, mandated by the Individuals with Disabilities Education Act, that describes how a person with a disability will be educated to meet his individual needs

Individuals with Disabilities Education Act (IDEA 1997): A federal law that mandates the procedures for gathering information and deciding on treatment of children in public schools

Parent-child interaction: Play-based conversation between parent(s) and child that is often used to gather a sample of the child's speech and to assess and treat environmental influences on a child's stuttering

Parent interview: A conversation with parent(s) in which parents are encouraged to describe their child's stuttering and express their concerns. In this interaction, the clinician elicits and gives information relevant to the child's stuttering.

Pattern of disfluencies: The types of stuttering and/or typical disfluencies shown by someone who stutters. Examples are whole-word repetitions, part-word repetitions, and prolongations.

Preassessment: The time before the formal assessment, in which the clinician gathers key information needed for the assessment

Risk factors for persistent stuttering: Characteristics within the child or within the environment that are hypothesized to increase probability that the child will not overcome his stuttering naturally—that is—without intervention

Speech sample: A segment of speech used to assess a client's stuttering. A sample may be limited to 300 syllables. It may be spontaneous conversation or written work that is read aloud. It is meant to be representative of a client's speech in general.

Stuttering modification: Ways of managing stuttering that are designed to reduce struggle and tension. Examples are cancellations, pullouts, and preparatory sets.

Teacher interview: A conversation with a child's classroom teacher(s) for the purpose of getting information about the child's speech and performance in the classroom. Such a conversation may also be used to enlist the teacher's help with the child's treatment.

Trial therapy: A brief administration of one or more therapy strategies, used for the purpose of determining the effect on the client's speech in an evaluation

This chapter and the preceding one are bridges between chapters on the nature of stuttering and chapters on treatment. My aim is to show you how to understand a client and/or family and his stuttering problem and then use the information you have gathered to determine a treatment approach. Figure 9.1 has a chapter overview, and Figure 9.2 illustrates the components of assessment and diagnosis.

I've organized the assessment procedures in this chapter by age levels: preschool, school age, and adolescent/adult. I've done this in part because in preparing to evaluate a client, you often know little about him except his age, so you will at least know what section of this chapter to turn to as you plan an evaluation. Another reason for this organization is because each age level requires a different approach and somewhat different procedures. When evaluating preschool children, for example, the clinician must determine whether they are stuttering or normally disfluent and then whether treatment, if warranted, should focus on the family or on the child's speech or both. With school-age children, a clinician often follows procedures that will allow her to provide services that are in line with the state's and the school's hierarchy of intervention. In very serious cases, this may lead to an **Individualized Education Program (IEP)** for children who are eligible for formal services. With adolescents and adults, trial therapy may be a more important part of assessment, and a clinician may more extensively assess emotions and attitudes as well as core and secondary behaviors to determine appropriate treatment.

Within each age level, I have subdivided the sequence of activities you will typically engage in when you evaluate a client. First, under the **Preassessment** sections, I describe the clinical questions guiding the evaluation, as well as preliminary information-gathering activities. Under the Assessment sections, I have described the observations, interviews, and measurements at the heart of the evaluation. Under the "Diagnosis" sections, I discuss how to integrate the information you have gathered to decide on a course of action (whether to recommend treatment and, if so, the type of treatment). Last, under the "Summary and Recommendations" sections, I describe the closing interviews, assignments, and the means to assess progress and outcome.

PRESCHOOL CHILD

Preassessment

In this section, I will present a few ideas to consider before you are in direct contact with the family or caregivers of a preschool-aged child who may be stuttering. These ideas will help you listen effectively to what the family says about the child and perhaps ask some preliminary questions before you even arrange for a face-to-face meeting.

Clinical Questions

When you assess a preschool child, you first want to answer the question, "Is this child stuttering, or is she normally disfluent?" In the process of trying to answer this, I have found that certain other information is critical: what are the amounts and types of disfluency this child shows in various situations? What kinds of risk factors for stuttering does the child have? Is the child reacting to her speech with frustration, fear, or other emotions? Is this something you observe? Do the family members report that the child reacts to her disfluencies? How? This information will also help you determine the developmental/treatment level of the child's disfluency.

To respond to the family's needs and to involve them fully in planning treatment, you need to know the answers to questions like: how are family members responding to the child's disfluencies? Parents would naturally be concerned about their child's disfluencies. Can you tell whether family members show alarm when the child is disfluent? Is the child temperamentally sensitive enough that parents' alarm would influence the child to try to stop his disfluencies? How does the family express their concerns about the child and her stuttering, as well as their preferences, expectations, and availability for treatment?

Once you have gathered this information, you will need to decide among options for the child and family—(1) no treatment, (2) watchful waiting with regular family contact, (3) clinician-guided environmental change and family counseling, and (4) clinician-guided parent- or caregiver-delivered treatment. You will also want to decide if the child is within the normal range for language, phonology, and voice. Finally, you should determine if a referral to another professional (e.g., a family counselor or a learning specialist) is warranted.

Another tool to help you determine whether a child is likely to be stuttering rather than typically disfluent is FluencyBank (Ratner & MacWhinney, 2018). I introduced FluencyBank in Chapter 8 and described how you can access the tutorials to make a transcript of a child's speech and then have it analyzed by the program to produce a spreadsheet that quantifies number and percentage of types of disfluencies. Of particular interest here is the weighted stuttering-like disfluency (SLD) index developed by Amrose and Yairi (1999). Those researchers assessed the disfluencies of 90 children, about half of whom were identified by parents and the authors as stuttering

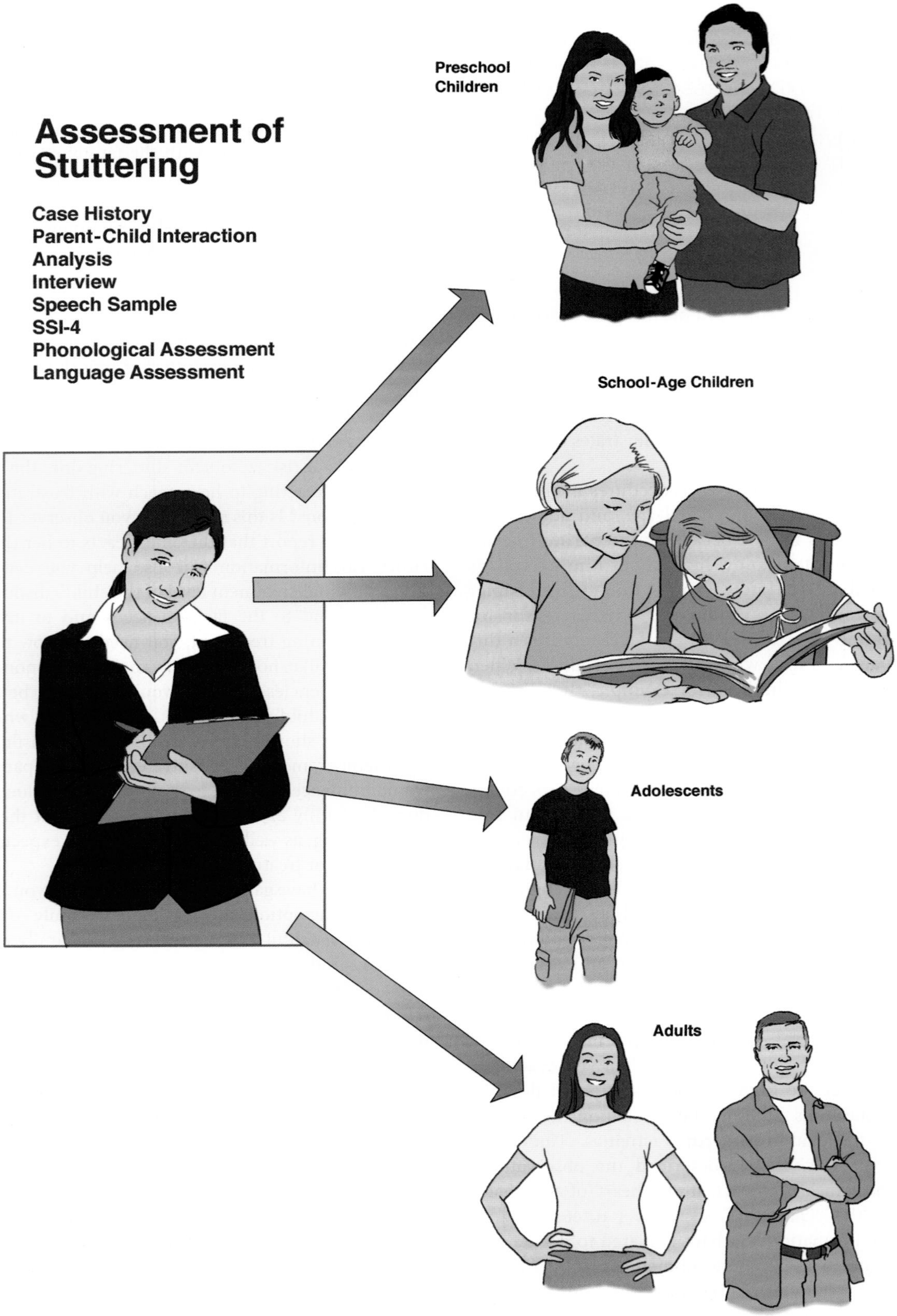

Preschool Children

Assessment of Stuttering

Case History
Parent-Child Interaction Analysis
Interview
Speech Sample
SSI-4
Phonological Assessment
Language Assessment

School-Age Children

Adolescents

Adults

Figure 9.1 Chapter overview.

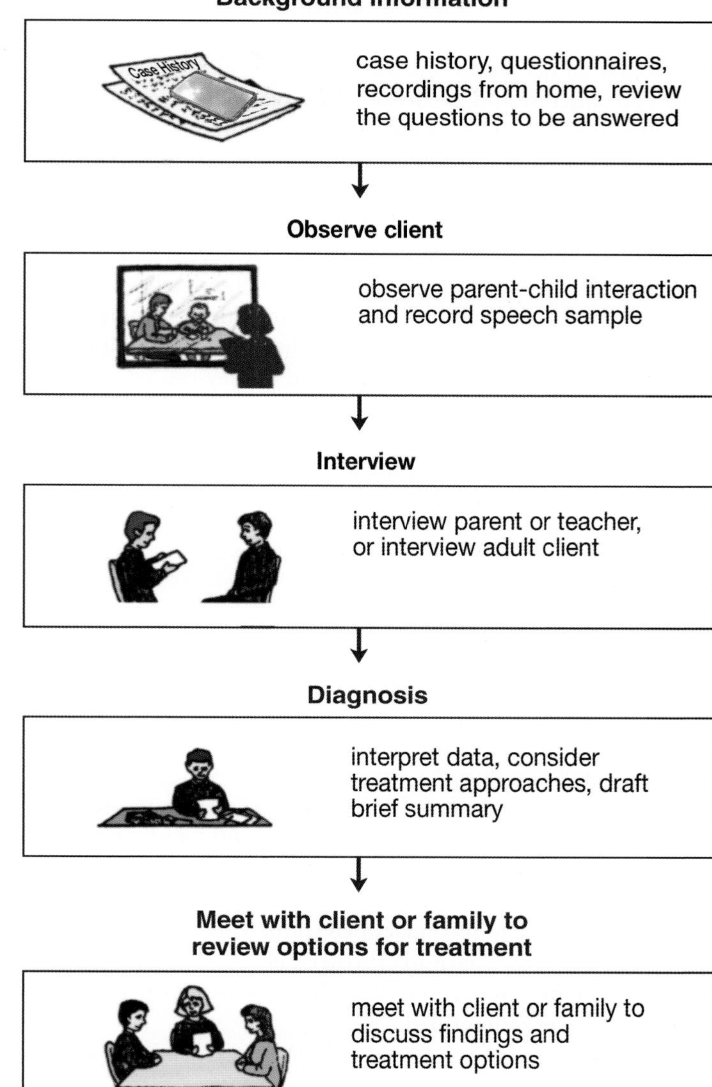

Figure 9.2 Sequence of assessment and diagnosis.

and half who were categorized as typically disfluent. The weighted SLD values for the 90 children were presented in Figure 1 of that article, in which children who were identified as stuttering were, by and large, separated from the typically disfluent children. Elsewhere in this chapter, I suggest you watch a video recording of a parent-child interaction on this book's website (thepoint.lww.com). I used the FluencyBank transcript analysis program, FluCalc, to determine this child's weighted SLD index for her speech in the first part of the interaction. I found the value for her weighted index to be about 21, which was well into the high values of the children identified as stuttering. Ambrose and Yairi suggest that the SLD index for typical children is not greater than 4 and that an index of 21 translates to "moderate stuttering." This child was appropriate for immediate treatment that was started within a few weeks of the diagnostic evaluation. She became fluent within a year and has remained fluent through our last contact, approximately 5 years after her treatment ended.

Initial Contact

In your initial contact, the family member or caregiver who has approached you is forming his or her first impression of you. In many cases, this is the beginning of a therapeutic alliance. You should focus on understanding the other person's point of view, concerns, and hopes. Let them know that you are ready to work with the family member as part of a team who will, together, help the child.

Your initial contact is likely to be on the telephone. If it is, listen to the parent's voice and pay attention to the parent's level of concern. Often, the most helpful thing you can do in this conversation is to listen. As you listen carefully, you may need to ask an occasional question to get clarification and to show your interest and expertise. When you think you have an initial understanding of the problem, set up an appointment, if appropriate. If you cannot meet with the family for several days or longer, I think it is important to give them some suggestions to get started.[1] For example, you may want a parent to rate the child's stuttering using the Severity Rating Scale described in Chapter 8. It also may be helpful to have the family set aside a few minutes every day, in which one parent can play alone with the child and give her special attention. Also, consider letting the family know that they can contact you before the first formal meeting if they have new concerns. Prior to an evaluation, I let the family know what will take place in the evaluation and approximately how long it will take. A discussion of fees and payment may also be appropriate.

Case History Form

The case history form, shown in Figure 9.3, is sent to parents several weeks before their child's assessment. Along with the case history form, we complete an intake form that includes date, name, address, phone number, permission to e-mail, what concerns are, and a note about the insurance we accept. The completed case history informs the clinician about the parents' current perception of the problem, as well as its onset and development, and the child's medical, family, and school history. Considerable detail is obtained about the child's stuttering pattern to help the clinician understand the severity and extent of core and secondary behaviors. This information is used as a starting place for further questions during the **parent interview**. More about this will be discussed when the actual evaluation is described.

Audio/Video Recording

Along with the case history form, I ask the parents of a preschool child to send me an audio or, preferably, a video recording of their child speaking in a typical home situation. I encourage parents to video 5 or 10 minutes of themselves playing with their child so I can preview the child's speech soon after the parents have contacted me. In cases in which several weeks elapse between the parents' contact and the evaluation, the child's stuttering may have diminished substantially, and I may observe only a fluent cycle of the child's speech. In addition to sampling the child's speech, I can learn from the recording a little about this family's parent-child interactions.

[1]It should be noted that some clinicians—for example, those working with direct treatment programs—prefer not to have the family make changes on their own before the evaluation meeting.

Assessment

I begin by greeting the family, introducing myself, and describing the activities we will be engaging in for the evaluation. In our clinic, these involve first our observation of the parents or caregiver interacting with the child and then our interview of the parent(s). This is followed by my interaction with the child, then time for me to pull together the findings, and a wrap-up meeting in which I share my observations and recommendations.

Later in the chapter, I describe how an assessment differs when it is conducted in a school setting or a home visit.

Parent-Child Interaction

When possible, I observe one or both parents (or a caregiver) interacting with the child, preferably at the beginning of the evaluation for several reasons. First, parents may be less affected by my orientation toward stuttering, which they would learn during the parent interview. So, observing the **parent-child interaction** first gives me a more natural sample. Second, this interaction gives me an opportunity to see the child's stuttering firsthand (rather than via a recording). I can try to sense how much the child seems aware of her stuttering, the types of disfluencies the child has, whether or not there are escape and avoidance reactions, and to what extent the child is reacting emotionally to her stuttering. Third, I can observe how the parents or caregivers interact with their child. Do they listen to her and look at her while she's talking? Do they let the child do most of the talking and choose what to play with? Do they talk at a reasonably slow rate with appropriate vocabulary? Do they interrupt? Do they correct? Do they talk at a fast rate or use complex vocabulary or advanced syntax? Fourth, if I began the evaluation by talking with the child, she might not talk much, since she doesn't know me. Thus, the parent-child interaction will give me at least a larger sample of her speech. Then, when I interact with her, I can get a sample of how her speech is with new people. Such observations of the parent-child interaction add to what I have learned from the case history and the audio-video sample that the parents have sent before the assessment. Together, the observation of home and in-clinic samples provides a basis for the parent interview and for developing recommendations for treatment.

The parent-child interaction can be done formally or informally. Some clinicians observe these interactions in the waiting room. Others who work in preschool or early intervention programs may visit a child's home and arrange to observe parent-child interactions while they sit quietly in the same room. Still others, myself included, videotape the parents and child in a play-style interaction in a treatment room supplied with toys and games. When recording these interactions is possible, this sample of a child's speech can be assessed for severity and types of stuttering behavior, as described in Chapter 8.

STUTTERING CASE HISTORY FORM – PRESCHOOL AND SCHOOL-AGE CHILD

Instructions: Please fill out this form in as much detail as possible. You can be assured that this information will be treated as confidential. If information is not available, please specify the reason so that we will know that the question has been considered. **Please return this form prior to your appointment.** Thank you.

Date: ____________________

Child's Name: ____________________ Gender: M F Age: __________ (years: months)

Address: ____________________

____________________ Telephone: ____________________

E-Mail Address: ____________________ Cell Phone: ____________________

Date of Birth: ____________________ Place of Birth: ____________________

Medicaid#: ____________________ Referring Physician: ____________________

Child lives with: Own Parents: __________ Other Relative: ____________________

Foster Parents: __________

If other than own parents, give name/s: ____________________

____

Teacher's Name (if applicable): ____________________

School (if applicable): ____________________

School Placement or Grade Level (if applicable): ____________________

Name of person completing this form: ____________________

Relationship to child: ____________________

FAMILY

Father:

Name: ____________________ Age: __________

Is he living with the family? __________ Occupation: __________

Employed by: ____________________

Education level: ____________________

Telephone (Home): __________ (Work): __________

Social Security#: ____________________

Mother:

Name: ____________________ Age: __________

Is she living with the family? __________ Occupation: __________

Employed by: ____________________

Education level: ____________________

Telephone (Home): __________ (Work): __________

Social Security#: ____________________

Figure 9.3 Case history form for preschool and school-age children.

Brothers and Sisters:

	(Name)	(Age)		(Name)	(Age)
1.	______________________	______	4.	______________________	______
2.	______________________	______	5.	______________________	______
3.	______________________	______	6.	______________________	______

HISTORY OF STUTTERING

Give approximate age at which stuttering was first noticed: ______________________

Who first noticed or mentioned the stuttering? ______________________

In what situation was the stuttering first noticed? ______________________

Describe any situations or conditions that might have been associated with the onset of stuttering:

____

____

Under what circumstances did the stuttering occur after initial onset? ______________________

____

What were the first signs of stuttering (check all that apply):

A. Repetitions of the whole word? (boy-boy-boy) ______________

B. Repetitions of the first letter? (b-b-b-boy) ______________

C. Repetitions of the first syllable? (ca-ca-cat) ______________

D. Complete blocks on the first letter? (b....oy) ______________

E. Prolongations of the vowel? (caaaaaaaat) ______________

F. Visible attempt to speak (i.e., mouth movement) but no sound forthcoming? ________

G. Other ______________________________

Was the stuttering always the same or did it occur in several different ways? ______________

If it occurred in different ways, how were they different from one another? Describe.

____

____

Approximately how long did each block (one word) seem to last? ______________

Was the stuttering easy or was there force at the time when the stuttering was first noticed?

____

Were stuttered words primarily at the beginning of sentences or were they scattered throughout the sentence? ______________________

When stuttering first began, was there any avoidance of speaking (i.e., changing word or stopping mid-stutter, using gestures instead of speech) because of it? Give examples, if any. __________

____

____

Figure 9.3 *(Continued)*

Does or did the child add extra words or sounds to "get started" (i.e., hey mom, hey mom...)?
____

Does or did the child use a lot of "fillers" when they speak (i.e., uh, um)? __________

At the time when stuttering was first noticed, what was your child's reaction?

Awareness that speech was different? ________ Surprise? ________

Indifference to it? ________ Anger or frustration? ________

Fear of stuttering again? ________ Shame? ________

Other? _______________

What attempts have been made to treat the stuttering problem (either at home or with a professional)? _______________
____

Does the child have articulation or pronunciation problems in addition to stuttering? If so, please describe. _______________

Does child have hand preference? Right- or left-handed or use both equally well? ________

Does child have a foot preference for kicking a ball? _______________

Does the child seem to be sensitive or have difficulty adapting to new situations? ________
____

Has the child been diagnosed with ADHD or ADD? _______________

DEVELOPMENT OF STUTTERING

Since onset, has there been any change in stuttering symptoms? Check those that are appropriate.

Increase in number of repetitions per word ________

Change in amount of force used—Increased? ________

Decreased? ________

Increase in amount of stuttering ________

Increase in length of block ________

Periods of no stuttering ________

Longer periods of stuttering ________

More precise in speech attempts ________

Lowered voice ________

Slower speech rate ________

Physical struggle (i.e., facial tension, eye blinks) ________

Looking away from the listener ________

Increase in pitch during stutters ________

Describe any of the above things the child does when he stutters (i.e., eye blinks). ________
____
____

Figure 9.3 *(Continued)*

Were there any periods (weeks/months) when the stuttering disappeared? ______________

Were there any periods (weeks/months) when stuttering increased? ______________

Can you give any explanations for these "worse" periods? ______________

Are there any situations that are particularly difficult? If so, describe: ______________

____

List any situations that never cause difficulty: ______________

____

Does the child stutter when he or she (check those that apply):

Asks questions?	_______	Uses new words that are unfamiliar	_______
Talks to young children?	_______	Uses the telephone?	_______
Says his or her name?	_______	Reads out loud?	_______
Answers direct questions?	_______	Recites memorized material?	_______
Talks to adults, teachers?	_______	Talks to strangers?	_______
Speaks when tired?	_______	Speaks when excited?	_______
Talks to family members	_______	Talks to friends?	_______

Do you know anyone who stutters? ______________ Are they relatives? Friends?

Acquaintances? ______________

Do you feel that stuttering interferes with your child's daily life? ______________

Social relationships? ______________

Success in school? ______________

MEDICAL, DEVELOPMENTAL, AND FAMILY HISTORY

Describe mother's health during pregnancy and birth history (i.e., complications): ______________

____

____

Describe any development problems during infancy or early childhood (i.e., late to walk or talk, feeding problems, food allergies): ______________

____

Do you think the child's speech and language development was unusually rapid or delayed? If so, please describe: ______________

____

List all significant illnesses, injuries, severe fevers, and operations:

	Date	Illness	Complications	Treatment	Physician
1.					
2.					
3					

Figure 9.3 *(Continued)*

List any medications your child is on: ____________________

List all present disabilities: ____________________

Any chronic illnesses, allergies or physical conditions? ____________________

____

Vision normal? ____________ Hearing normal? ____________

Child's eye color? ____________ Hair color? ____________

Do other members of the family have speech, language, reading problems, or learning disabilities?

If so, please describe: ____________________

____

____

____

Are any family members left-handed or use both right and left hands equally well? ____________

____

Does the child or other family members show artistic talent or interest? ____________

____

Do any family members talk very rapidly? If so, who? ____________________

____

SCHOOL AND SOCIAL HISTORY

Favorite subjects or activities in school: ____________________

Difficult subjects: ____________________

Hobbies: ____________ Sports: ____________

Leisure time activities: ____________________

Favorite toys: ____________________

What specific questions do you have about your child that you would like us to try to answer?

(Use back of sheet if necessary) ____________________

____

____

In addition, what goals would you like to see accomplished as a result of this evaluation?

____

____

Signature: ____________________ Date: ____________

Please return these completed forms to us in the envelope provided. Thank you.

Figure 9.3 *(Continued)*

For an example of parent-child interaction with a preschool child who stutters, watch a video clip on the book's website: thepoint.lww.com. You can find it as "Chapter 9: Assessment and Diagnosis, Parent-Child Interaction." As you watch this video clip, notice the interaction style of the mother. How does she react to her child's stutters? Does she give the child adequate time to talk? Is her speech rate slow enough for the child to process easily? Also, observe the child's stuttering. What types of stutters does she have? See if you can categorize them as repetitions, prolongations, or blocks. Are some of the "repetitions" actually responses to feeling stuck and trying to get started (i.e., are they "starters")? How aware of her stutters is this child? Why do you think that?

Parent Interview

I usually talk with the family without the child present, giving them an opportunity to speak about matters that they feel they would like to share in confidence. If I'm working with another clinician or a student, they play with and observe the child while I talk to the parents. If I'm working alone and both parents have come to the evaluation, I talk to each parent separately, while the other is with the child. If only one parent is present, I often arrange to have the child playing by himself in a nearby room with the door open.

I begin by asking parents to describe the problem their child is having. I ask open-ended questions, such as "Tell me about Justin's speech" or "Tell me what concerns you have about Kimberly's speech." Open-ended questions allow parents to describe their concerns in their own words. This provides an opportunity for me to listen carefully, to be nonjudgmental, and to be comfortable with silence so that parents can express themselves fully. Listening attentively and being comfortable with silence require concentration on the clinician's part, so it is worthwhile to remind yourself of this when you are preparing for an evaluation. Often, I sit by myself for a few minutes before meeting with the family, letting my mind become quiet so that I will be open to what they have to say. In the interview, after parents have had a chance to describe the problem and appear to have no more to say at that moment, I ask about the first stages of the child's life (the child's birth and development) and then work up toward the present time. In the ensuing conversation, I try to be sure I get information indicated by the questions in the following paragraphs. This interview is not a strict question-and-answer format, but rather a discussion punctuated by both their questions and mine.

Sometimes, during an initial interview, parents ask direct questions about things they think they may be doing wrong. I let them know that, in my view, stuttering is often the result of many factors acting together and that parents do not cause it. I rarely give advice about what they should change or what they should do until after I have finished interviewing the parents and assessed the child directly. I believe that I am more accurate, and parents are more receptive to my recommendations, if I delay a discussion of what to do until the closing interview when I have the most information possible. On the other hand, there may be "clinical moments" during an initial interview when parents might be most receptive to suggestions. Many times, for example, parents have asked me whether it's a good idea for them to tell their child to slow down whenever the child stutters when excited. My response is usually to ask them how the child responds to this and to build upon their answer so that we can brainstorm the best way to help the child together.

Here are some areas that I touch on during the conversation:

1. **Were there any problems with your pregnancy or the birth of this child?**
   Although there is little evidence that people who stutter as a group have difficult birth histories, there is an increased incidence of stuttering among individuals who have a known history of brain injury (Boehme, 1968; Poulos & Webster, 1991). Thus, I am seeking to determine whether there is the possibility of congenital brain injury. If a difficult pregnancy or birth is reported, I might examine the child's language, motor, and cognitive development more closely. Because it is completed before the evaluation, the case history form provides preliminary information for potential follow-up.
2. **What was the child's speech and language development like? How did it compare with siblings' development and with your expectations?**
   The first appearance of stuttering may be influenced by the "processing load" that language acquisition has on a child's speech production, as described in the sections on speech and language development in Chapter 4. Thus, it is important to understand the course of a child's overall speech and language development. I explore the possibility that a child's language acquisition is proceeding so rapidly that his developing motor system cannot keep up. I also examine the possibility that a child's speech and language development are delayed, making her frustrated with finding it hard to talk. As mentioned in Chapter 3 and 4, there is some evidence that poorer speech and language skills may predict persistent stuttering (Yairi et al., 1996).
3. **Describe the child's motor development compared with that of her brothers, sisters, or with other children.**
   I am interested in parents' general impressions. Does their child seem to be developing motor skills like other children her age, or do they think she may be delayed? Some indicators of the normal range of children's gross and fine motor development, as well as their personal-social and speech-language development, can be found in the Denver Developmental Screening Test (Frankenburg & Dodds, 1967) and is shown in Figure 4.2 (child development in the first 5 years).

In my experience, many children who stutter appear to be slightly advanced in their language and, less often, slightly delayed in their motor skills. Or, they may be well advanced in language but have completely normal motor skills. In either case, these children seem to benefit from models of speech produced at a slow rate (Guitar, Kopff-Schaefer, Donahue-Kilburg, & Bond, 1992; also, see the section in Chapter 11 on indirect treatment). Other children who stutter may be delayed in several areas and may need treatment for language and phonology that is integrated with therapy for stuttering (see the section of Chapter 12, "Treatment of Concomitant Speech and Language Problems").

4. **Have any members of your family had speech or language disorders?**
I ask this general question and then ask more specifically whether family members or other relatives have ever had problems related to stuttering, cluttering, speech sound development, or language disorders (see Chapter 15 for a description of cluttering). To confirm that a problem was considered significant (and was perhaps diagnosed), I ask if the person ever received treatment. I use this information when we discuss stuttering as a disorder that may have predisposing factors. Handled tactfully, a discussion of predisposing factors may help parents realize that their child's stuttering was not something they caused, which in turn may reduce their anxiety or guilt, making them more effective in facilitating the child's fluency.

If a parent stutters or formerly stuttered, the parent may have strong negative feelings about the disorder, including guilt that the parent has passed it on to the child. Such feelings should be discussed in the initial interview and throughout any treatment the child receives. The way in which a parent who stutters handles her or her stuttering is also important, because these behaviors serve as a model for the child. It is my observation that a parent who avoids words or otherwise tries to hide stuttering is communicating an attitude that may move the child to the intermediate level faster than if the parent accepts the stuttering, comments neutrally about it in front of the child, and uses facilitating techniques to handle it.

If any of the child's relatives stutter, it is important to find out whether they recovered. Research cited earlier found that among children who were identified within 6 months of the onset of stuttering, those with relatives who did not recover from stuttering were more likely to have persistent stuttering than those with relatives who did recover (Yairi et al., 1996). It is not necessary to tell the parents that unrecovered stuttering relatives may predict persistence, because many of the studied individuals did not have treatment. Instead, I let parents know that treatment would be important if relatives did not recover from stuttering. In my experience, treatment can overcome factors that suggest persistence. After obtaining this background information about family history, I turn to the onset and development of the child's stuttering.

5. **When did you first notice the child's disfluency?**
I have found that if treatment begins relatively soon after a child starts to stutter (within 18 months, rather than after several years), we have a better chance of preventing negative feelings from building up for both the parents and the child. Therefore, I praise parents for bringing a child in promptly for an evaluation if they did so relatively soon after they first realized there may be a problem. Another reason I want to know how much time has passed since onset is that most of the predictive information on chronicity of stuttering is based on children identified within 6 months of onset. For example, Yairi et al. (1996) found that children who naturally recovered began to show a steady decline in their stuttering during the first 12 months after stuttering onset, whereas children whose stuttering persisted for at least 3 years did not show such a decline. Therefore, knowing how long a child has been stuttering helps me make treatment decisions based on findings that some children are likely to recover without therapy.

6. **Was anything special going on in the child's life when the stuttering started?**
This may provide some leads about the kinds of pressures to which a child may be vulnerable, which can help clinicians determine what changes parents can make to reduce stuttering. Events that may precipitate the onset of stuttering include the birth of a sibling, moving to a new home, family travel, prolonged periods of anxiety or excitement, and growth spurts in a child's language or cognition (see Chapter 4). Many times, no special circumstances have occurred at the onset of stuttering. Events surrounding the onset of stuttering should be discussed in a way that helps parents feel they are not to blame for the stuttering. For example, if parents tell me that their child first began to stutter during a busy holiday season or when they were away on a trip, I let them know that this situation at onset is not uncommon in children who stutter. I also indicate that the stuttering would probably have appeared whenever the child felt any of the kinds of stresses that are in a typical home.

7. **What was the disfluency like when it was first noticed?**
Most stuttering begins with easy repetitions, although some children exhibit prolongations and blocks, as well. Some preliminary information suggests that when repetitions sound quite rapid (i.e., when the pause between repetition units is brief), a child is more likely to be stuttering rather than normally disfluent (Allen, 1988; Throneburg & Yairi, 1994). In addition, rapid-sounding repetitions may be predictive of persistent stuttering (Yairi et al., 1996). However, the length of pauses between repetition units cannot be determined accurately without

instrumentation, even though a practiced ear can help clinicians perceive the brevity of pauses between repetition units. This information should be used only to support an overall pattern of findings that will help the clinician decide whether or not to recommend treatment.

8. What changes, if any, have been observed in the child's speech since stuttering was first noticed?
The most interesting changes include the frequency and types of disfluencies and whether and for how long the stuttering diminished greatly or disappeared altogether. As indicated in the discussion of Question 5, children whose frequency of core stuttering behaviors (i.e., part-word and single-syllable whole-word repetitions, prolongations, and blocks) does not decrease during the 12 months after onset are at risk for becoming persistent stutterers. In my clinical experience, if a child's physical tension and struggle during stuttering are increasing, or if stuttering is becoming more consistent and less intermittent, the child is not exhibiting a borderline level of stuttering, and direct treatment should be considered.

9. Does the child appear to be aware of her disfluency?
If a child appears to have no awareness of her disfluencies, I am more likely to categorize her as normally disfluent or as having borderline stuttering than if she notices or seems concerned about her disfluencies. If she shows negative awareness, such as expressing frustration, this may be beginning stuttering. Note that a child may be aware of her stuttering but not particularly bothered by it; some children are even amused by it when it first occurs, though this often quickly changes to frustration. Indicators of a child's awareness include such things as her commenting about her stuttering, either when it occurs or at some other time, responding to the fact that people have brought it to her attention. Awareness is also indicated if a child stops when she is disfluent and starts again or laughs, cries, or hits herself when she stutters. Even without any of these signs, a child may still be quite aware of her stuttering. In a study of 1,096 stuttering children between the ages of 2 and 7, the most frequent response suggesting awareness was asking for help (Boey et al., 2009).

In some cases, preschool children may show more than just signs of frustration. They may show negative feelings about talking and may fear using certain words. They may even comment that they wish they could speak like someone else. These signs of awareness are indications that treatment is warranted.

10. Does the child sometimes appear to change a word because she expects to be disfluent on it?
Parents are usually able to perceive that this is happening because they can sense the child's apprehension about saying a word. I also may ask them if the child changes words in midstream; that is, does she start a word, get stuck on it, and then change it or stop talking? Such behaviors are warning signs. They suggest that the child is avoiding a possible stutter because stuttering is so distressing to him. She may be moving toward a more serious problem, indicating the importance of treatment.

11. Does the child seem to avoid talking in some situations when she expects to be disfluent?
Again, this is something that most parents know because they sense the child's fear of talking, and like the word avoidances discussed in Question 10, this behavior may indicate a need for treatment.

12. What do the parents believe caused the problem?
In some cases, parents may express ideas about the possible causes of their child's stuttering that I believe are appropriate and accurate. In other cases, parents' beliefs about causal factors appear to be incorrect, and I respond by providing more accurate information. I am particularly sensitive to whether or not parents blame themselves or each other for their child's stuttering. This is usually a good time to let parents know that they are not to blame. I tell them that some children may have slight differences in their neurological organization for speech, which may emerge as stuttering during the normal stresses and strains of growing up and learning to talk (see Chapters 2, 3, and 4).

Sometimes, parents are deeply convinced that they caused the child's stuttering. For example, the stress a child feels when their parents divorce can sometimes trigger stuttering. I try to be honest, letting the parents know that this stress may have been related to the onset of the child's stuttering, but that the stuttering was probably dormant and would have probably appeared under other stresses. The parents and I then brainstorm how the child can be reassured of their love, and we discuss ways in which they can play a key role in their child's learning to deal with it appropriately.

13. How do the parents feel about the child's disfluency problem?
The kinds of feelings and attitudes we are looking for are: do they feel concern? Guilt? Do they assume the child will outgrow it? Parental emotions and attitudes are contagious and may influence the child to fear stuttering, particularly a sensitive child. If parents feel guilty or highly anxious, it is important to engage them in positive treatment activities as soon as possible. You will find some activities families can begin with in the section titled The Closing Interview.

14. What, if anything, have the parents done about the child's disfluency?
This question is aimed at finding out how the parents have responded to the child's disfluencies. For example, have they asked the child to slow down or stop and say the word again? Knowing this will help me to decide what to do in counseling them. If parents are correcting the child, I may get them involved in therapeutic activities immediately so that they can develop more appropriate ways of responding. Either in the initial parent

interview or at the end of the evaluation, I let parents know that direct suggestions to children about changing their speech are usually not effective in the long run. I always give them suggestions for specific things they can do instead, such as slowing their own speech without asking the child to slow their speech.

15. Has the child been seen elsewhere for the problem? If so, what were the outcomes?

This information can be important in planning therapy and counseling parents. For example, if their family doctor told them several years ago that the child will outgrow stuttering, this needs to be addressed because they may now be convinced she will not outgrow it. It is wise to comment positively or neutrally on what other professionals may have said or done. So, many children appear to overcome stuttering without treatment that most doctors and nurses believe that their advice to parents to ignore the stuttering will have a good outcome. Some doctors and nurses, however, are learning to distinguish between children who are likely to recover without treatment and those who are not and will advise parents accordingly. By establishing relationships with pediatricians in the community, speech-language pathologists (SLPs) can help facilitate that process.

If the child has been in other treatment previously, knowing what advice the parents were given can be important. Sometimes, parents have been given excellent advice but were not able to follow it. If so, we need to find out why and help them overcome obstacles to helping their child. Sometimes, parents have had their child in successful therapy but have moved away and sought me out to continue the same kind of treatment. In these cases, I try to contact the previous therapist as well as explore with the parents what was done so that we can continue to work in the same direction as before. In some cases, parents come to me seeking a second opinion, and I am able to reinforce what others have said if I agree. In other cases, they may have been advised to ignore the child's stuttering, which may lead me to tactfully discuss the possibility of taking an entirely different direction now that more time has passed or indicators suggest that there may be more helpful alternatives.

16. When and in which situations does the child exhibit the most disfluency? The least disfluency?

This information helps to identify fluency disrupters and fluency facilitators that I will use to help parents facilitate their child's fluency. I have also found it effective to point out whenever possible all of the helpful things the parents are already doing. Just the awareness that their child's stuttering responds to environmental cues and thereby has some logic to it helps most parents feel more able to manage it.

17. How does the child get along with her brothers and sisters and other children?

Although I usually find that children who stutter relate fairly well to others, I want to determine whether a child's stuttering may be interfering with her relationships. Sometimes, when asking this question, I learn about pressure and competition from siblings or teasing by a child who is acting as a bully in the neighborhood or even among her siblings.

18. What is the child's temperament like?

Some children who stutter may be more emotionally reactive than other children, and they may have less capacity for self-regulation (i.e., dealing with that reactivity). The Short Behavioral Inhibition Scale described in Chapter 8 will help assess how sensitive a child is. More emotionally reactive children and those with less ability to self-regulate would be more likely to respond negatively to parents' anxieties about their speech. A child with this temperament may benefit from extra help in learning to cope with arousing stimuli. There is good evidence that families can help a child develop a more resilient temperament (Calkins & Fox, 1994; Zolkoski & Bullock, 2012).

19. What is a typical day like for your child?

It can be helpful to get an idea of how busy and rushed a family is. For one thing, it has been my experience that many children who stutter and their families benefit from having less hectic schedules, particularly if the child seems happier when the home is more tranquil. You can add this information to what the parents told you about when their child stutters most to develop a hypothesis about how much the family's schedule may be affecting the child's fluency. If the child stutters more when things are busy, frantic, and stressed, it may be appropriate to brainstorm with the parents about how everyone can have a little more "downtime." Knowledge of the family's schedule will also help you begin to consider treatment recommendations. Some treatments are demanding of parents' time and attention, and their schedule must be considered in working with them to determine the most appropriate treatment approach for their child.

20. Is there anything else you can think of to tell me that will help me better understand your child's stuttering and your concerns?

Sometimes, it is not possible to direct questions to all areas of concern, and this question provides parents an opportunity to provide information that I have not thought of asking about.

To see an actual parent interview, go to *thePoint* and watch the video "Chapter 9: Assessment and Diagnosis: Parent Interview." Observe how the clinicians learn from the mother about the onset and development of the child's stuttering up to its current status. How do the clinicians facilitate the mother's being able to talk not only about the child's stuttering but also her own reaction to her child's stuttering? What do you think about the clinician using the Stuttering Severity Scale to find out about the range of the child's severity? What do you think about having the child present during the parent interview? How might this change what goes on in the interview?

Clinician-Child Interaction

One of the most important parts of a preschool child's evaluation is the **clinician-child interaction**. Here, the clinician can see "up close" what the child's speech is like, how she responds to various cues, and how well she can modify her disfluency. I always record this interaction for later analysis because it is difficult to make notes as we interact. Video recording is preferable because visual cues are often critical in determining a child's developmental and treatment level. If audio recording must be used, the clinician should make notes on visual aspects of the child's disfluencies.

I focus my interactions on toys or games that are suitable to the child's age. For preschoolers, the Playskool® farm or airport is a good example. I play alongside the child, letting her direct the action, commenting on what she's doing or playing with. I refrain from questions as we begin and talk in an easy, relaxed manner, much as I advise parents to do.

If a child's stuttering is like that described by the parent, I maintain the same speech style throughout the interaction. However, if a child is entirely fluent or normally disfluent and the parents have described behaviors typical of stuttering, I speak more rapidly and ask many questions. Occasionally, I interrupt the child to elicit disfluent speech, which may be more characteristic. I do this to avoid misdiagnosing a child who is stuttering as a typically fluent speaker.

An adult client of mine described an experience that illustrates my concern. When she was 5 years old, she stuttered quite severely, and her parents were understandably concerned. Seeking the best help, her mother took her to a famous university speech clinic for an evaluation. For reasons she never understood, she was relatively fluent throughout the entire evaluation. The clinicians observed her temporary fluency and despite her mother's protestations that her daughter stuttered at home did not diagnose her stuttering and advised her mother to ignore any disfluency. Her disfluency gradually worsened, and she developed severe, chronic stuttering. Nonetheless, I realize that, even by putting pressure on the child, I may not elicit stuttering that the child displays in other settings. Thus, the parents' report and the recording they made before the evaluation are of vital importance for a full understanding of a child's speech.

Talking about Stuttering

Before interacting with a child, I try to determine from talking with a child's parents whether the child is aware of her stuttering. If I think she isn't, I simply observe the child's speech while she and I play. If it seems clear that she is aware of her stuttering, I then try to determine how comfortable the child is in talking about her stuttering. Sometimes, if the child is old enough to understand, I ask her if she knows why she has come to see me. Most children answer noncommittally, but some say something like, "Because I don't talk right." This gives me an opening to discuss the stuttering. I would respond to such a comment by saying something like "It sounds like words sometimes get stuck" or another statement that acknowledges her expression of difficulty with speech. I might also say "Lots of kids that we see here have trouble getting words out. It's OK, if words get stuck sometimes, but we can usually help kids and make it easier for them to talk."

Some clinicians help a child talk about her stuttering by first talking about another child who stutters (Bloodstein, personal communication, 1990). In discussing stuttering with a child, I usually try to use their vocabulary, such as "getting stuck" or "having trouble on words." If a child seems reluctant to talk about stuttering, I drop the issue for the moment and return to playing. Then, later, I will insert a few natural-sounding disfluencies in my speech and comment that I sometimes have trouble getting words out.[2] I might play some more and then insert a few more disfluencies and ask the child if she ever has trouble like this. As before, the child's response will indicate that either she remains unwilling to discuss stuttering or she will give the clinician an opening to discuss, little by little, her disfluency problem. In summary, the goals of these attempts to discuss a child's disfluency are (1) to see if she is willing to talk about her disfluencies and (2) to assure her that she is not alone with the problem and that her parents and I can help her.

A Child Who Won't Talk

At times, I encounter a preschooler who is reluctant to separate from her parents. A shy child may start to cry and cling to her parents. I don't force the child to separate, of course. It is more important to have her positively inclined toward therapy (which she will probably equate with me) than to try to elicit a few stutters. In this situation, I sit quietly while the parent and child play together. After a few minutes, I join in the play, without focusing on the child, and after a few more minutes, I'll comment on what the parent and child are doing or what I'm doing with a tractor or a farm animal or whatever I'm playing with. In most cases, the child will soon say something to me or include me in the play. This interaction, leading to at least a little speech from the child, gives me an opportunity to observe at close range any stuttering the child may have. Only after a child gets comfortable with me do I attempt to discuss her trouble talking and only if I'm sure she is aware of her stuttering.

With some children, I do not attempt to discuss stuttering at all during our initial interactions, and I always take my cue from the child and go slowly in this area. A very shy child, who becomes even shyer if I produce a few easy disfluencies, may be quite turned off to therapy if I invade her space by asking about her stuttering at this point. You can infer many things about a child's feelings from observations rather than from their responses to direct questions.

[2]I believe that it is appropriate for fluent clinicians to put a few disfluencies in their speech and refer to them as they talk with a child about stuttering. Everyone—even the most fluent speakers—has some disfluencies and at times they can be frustrating.

A Child Who Is Entirely Fluent

Some preschool children who stutter may be entirely fluent during an evaluation. In such cases, there are several options. First, the recording I asked the parent to send me may include enough stuttering to provide a good sample for analysis. Second, if a child is in a particularly fluent period, I may reschedule her evaluation for a later time. If my recommendations to the parents enable them to change the home environment enough in the meantime so that the child remains fluent, the parents may wish to postpone the evaluation until and if the child's stuttering returns.

Speech Sample

The following sections describe how to analyze samples of a preschool child's speech. You should have more than one **speech sample** to analyze from the recordings that the parents sent in, the parent-child interaction, and the clinician-child interaction. Because you may want to use the SSI-4 (Riley, 2009) as part of your assessment, you need to follow the procedures it recommends for this analysis. Thus, the sample obtained from the clinician-child interaction should include conversation using the pictures in the SSI-4. Riley recommends that as the child talks, the clinician should "interject questions, interruptions, and mild disagreements to simulate the pressures of normal conversation at home and elsewhere" (Riley, 2009, p. 4). The samples should include at least 200 syllables; samples this long or longer make it more likely that you will have an accurate picture of the child's speech. By making orthographic transcripts of the samples, you can more easily quantify the variables described in the following section on **pattern of disfluencies**. I explain how below.

Pattern of Disfluencies

By analyzing the child's speech sample, I can determine whether or not the child truly stutters and, if so, her developmental/treatment level. I analyze the following six variables to begin this determination. The choice of variables owes much to six individuals who have written about the differential diagnosis of preschool stuttering (Adams, 1977; Curlee, 1984, 1993; Riley & Riley, 1979; Yairi & Ambrose, 1999).

1. *Frequency of disfluencies.* This is calculated from the entire sample and is expressed as the number of disfluencies per 100 words. Both normal disfluencies and those associated with stuttering are included in this count. Normally disfluent children have fewer than 10 disfluencies per 100 words. Frequency is also commonly assessed by calculating the percentage of stuttered syllables (rather than words), by dividing the number of syllables stuttered by the total number of syllable spoken. Details for using both syllables and words are given in "Assessing Frequency" section of Chapter 8.
2. *Types of disfluencies.* I described the following eight types of disfluencies in Chapter 7: part-word repetitions, single-syllable word repetitions, multisyllabic word repetitions, phrase repetitions, interjections, revisions-incomplete phrases, prolongations, and tense pauses. Children who are typically disfluent are likely to have more revisions and multisyllabic word repetitions, as well as many interjections when they are younger than 3.5 years old. Part-word repetitions, single-syllable word repetitions, prolongations, and tense pauses occur more frequently in stuttering children. Another distinguishing measure is the proportion of total disfluencies that are stutter-like disfluencies (SLDs) (i.e., part-word repetitions and single-syllable repetitions, prolongations, and blocks). Fewer than half of the disfluencies of normally disfluent children are SLDs, but about two-thirds of the disfluencies of children who stutter will be SLDs (Ambrose & Yairi, 1999; Yairi, 1997a).
3. *Nature of repetitions and prolongations.* This variable has several dimensions. First, normally disfluent children usually have only one extra unit in their repetitions, li-like this, but sometimes they may have two. As the number of repetition units increases, however, so does the likelihood that the child is stuttering. Second, I listen to the tempo of repetitions. If they are slow and regular, a child is more likely to be categorized appropriately as a typically disfluent speaker. If they are rapid or irregular, it is more likely that the child is stuttering. Third, I look for signs of tension in both repetitions and prolongations. Both visual and auditory cues can help here; tension can be seen in the child's facial expression and heard in her increased pitch or loudness and more staccato voice quality. Children whom I would consider typically disfluent seldom exhibit tension in their disfluencies.
4. *Starting and sustaining airflow and phonation.* The child who we usually consider as stuttering often has difficulty here. You may observe abrupt onsets and offsets of words, especially repeated words, or momentary pauses with fixed articulator positions at the onset of words. Moreover, transitions between words may seem abrupt, jerky, or broken much of the time.
5. *Physical concomitants.* I look for physical gestures that accompany a child's disfluencies, such as head nods, eyeblinks, and hand or finger movements, especially gestures that coincide with the release of a disfluent sound. I also include such extra noises as a child gritting her teeth or clicking her tongue during disfluencies.
6. *Word avoidance.* Another sign I sometimes see in a disfluent preschool child, which suggests that she stutters, is word avoidance. This can be blatant, as when a child starts a word and then changes it, as in "pu-pu-pu...dog," or it may be more subtle, as when she says, "I don't know," when it's clear that she does know. I also ask about word avoidances when I interview a child's parents. When a clinician interacts with a child, she may sometimes miss avoidances in a live interaction, and it may take a viewing of the videotape to pick them up. For example, a few years

ago, I noted on the videotape I watched after an evaluation a very subtle avoidance that I had completely missed during the face-to-face interaction. I had asked the child what he was going to dress as for Halloween. He pursed her lips for a "B," but when he couldn't say the word, he used an avoidance by singing the Batman theme, "Na-na-na-na-na-na-na-nah! Batman!"

In my experience, if a child shows any of the characteristics of stuttering just described, she should be considered at least a borderline stutterer. The presence of tension, stoppage of airflow or phonation, physical concomitants, or word avoidances would place her on a level above borderline. Further details on this placement are given in the sections on diagnosis that follow.

Stuttering Severity Instrument (SSI-4)

Using the 200-syllable or longer samples gathered earlier, you should carefully follow the guidelines in the examiner's manual of the SSI-4 to determine a child's stuttering frequency, duration, and physical concomitant scores. These three scores combined result in a total score which can be used—with the "Percentile Ranks and Severity Equivalents" tables in the manual—to derive a percentile ranking for the child, which compares him or her to the norms for children who stutter. Severity Equivalents that range from very mild to very severe can also be derived from the total overall score. Sometimes, typically disfluent children may be rated as stuttering at the very mild level on the SSI-4. Thus, clinical judgment, informed by your analyses of the types and frequencies of disfluencies, must be used to decide which children are actually stuttering and which are not. Remember that the SSI-4 is not a tool for differentiating stuttering from normal disfluency but for assessing a child's severity.

Test of Childhood Stuttering

As described in Chapter 8, the Test of Childhood Stuttering (TOCS; Gillam & Logan, 2009) can be used for children ages 4 to 12 and is thus appropriate for older preschool children. This instrument evaluates the child's stuttering in a variety of speaking situations and provides a more in-depth analysis of the child's stuttering, but takes more time to administer than the SSI-4. Although I have not used it often, I am aware that it provides additional information about stuttering types, speech rate and naturalness, and effect of time stress on picture naming.

Speech Rate

I assess preschool children's speech rate using the speech sample obtained for the SSI-4. Counting and timing procedures were described in the section on assessment of speech rate in Chapter 8. One sample of speech rates for preschool children is given in Table 8.5. If a child is stuttering and her speech rate is substantially below the range for her age, the extent to which stuttering slows her rate of speech may be a problem for both listeners and the child. Children whose rates are substantially above the norms—or who sound like they are talking too fast—may have the disorder of cluttering, which is described in more detail in Chapter 15.

Feelings and Attitudes

If I am evaluating a preschooler, I begin by asking the parents if they think the child is aware of her stuttering, and I explore observations they have made of her reactions to her disfluencies. If they are convinced that the child is oblivious to her disfluencies and I observe those disfluencies to be without much tension and struggle, I don't talk directly to the child about her stuttering. Instead, I rely on what the parents can tell me during the parent interview about their child's feelings. I am also beginning to use the Impact of Stuttering on Preschoolers and Parents questionnaire (Langevin, Packman, & Onslow, 2010; see Chapter 8) to gather initial information about the child's (and parents') feelings and attitudes about stuttering. However, if the child shows signs of struggle and tension when she stutters, or if the parents indicate that the child is aware through various examples of her frustration with her stuttering, I explore with the child her feelings about getting stuck on words.

In the section on "Talking About Stuttering" when I discussed the child-clinician interaction, I touched upon asking the child about why her mother or father or another caregiver has brought him to our clinic. I will revisit that topic now. Before bringing up the topic of stuttering, I get to know the child by talking with her during various play activities. Then, as we play, I insert a question about her speech, such as "Do you sometimes get stuck on words?" Both the child's verbal and nonverbal responses to a gently asked question about stuttering tell me a lot. Even beyond what I notice when we are talking, I am often able to learn a great deal by watching the video of my interaction with a child. I find that by playing a video recording of my interaction, I am able to devote my undivided attention to observing key segments of the interaction. The recording often provides a rich payload of information about a child's feelings that may not have been apparent to me in the face-to-face meeting. Some children may be quite comfortable answering my question about getting stuck on words, while others are embarrassed, look away, and don't make clear responses. Still others emphatically deny they have any problem talking. If the stuttering is very mild and the child matter-of-factly says she doesn't get stuck, I may tentatively conclude that she really isn't aware.

Assessment of the feelings and attitudes of a preschooler leads me to conclude tentatively whether a child (1) is unaware of her disfluencies, (2) is occasionally aware of them and, even then, is seldom and only transiently bothered by them, (3) is aware and frustrated by them, or (4) is highly aware, frustrated, and afraid of them. The levels of awareness and emotion that a child has about her stuttering are an important consideration in planning treatment, as we shall see.

In addition, the questionnaire for parents described in Chapter 8—Short Behavioral Inhibition Scale (Ntourou et al., in review)—can be used to learn about how sensitive the child is. Children who are very sensitive will often be reluctant to talk about stuttering and the approach to this topic should be gradual.

Other Speech and Language Behaviors

When I evaluate a preschool child's speech for stuttering, I also screen for possible speech sound, language, and voice problems. In addition, I make sure that her hearing has been checked recently and if not, arrange to have a hearing screening.

A child's language and articulation problems can usually be detected in the recorded parent-child or clinician-child interactions. When I suspect problems in these areas, I administer formal tests. You may wish to consult Bernthal, Bankson, and Flipsen (2017) and Velleman (2015) for testing articulatory and phonological disorders and Paul and Norbury (2012) for assessing language disorders. I will discuss the management of concomitant articulation and language disorders in Chapter 12, which deals with treatment of beginning stuttering.

My view of the relationship between language and stuttering, which I described in Chapters 3 and 4, is that one of the pressures on a child who stutters may result from language development that is much more advanced than motor development. Thus, in evaluating a child's language and articulation, I explore the possibility that her language exceeds age expectations. In addition, I observe her language usage and motor abilities and question parents about her general motor development and the intelligibility of her speech.

When language development outstrips motor development, there may be a risk that a child will try to produce long sentences at a relatively fast pace with a speech system that, at this age, is better suited to a slower rate. A child's motivation to speak quickly may come from her own eagerness to express complex thoughts, from her parents' pleasure at her adult-like speech, or just from the fact that adult speech rate models affect the child. We have demonstrated this with typically developing children—typical in both language and fluency (Guitar & Marchinkowski, 2001). We demonstrated that if a mother talks at her typical rate and then slows down her rate, and then repeats that sequence, the child will change her speech to match the mother's.

For a child who stutters and who also has advanced expressive language abilities for her age, rate of speech production may be an important factor to target in treatment. How rate is targeted in intervention depends on the child's level of stuttering. If the child is relatively unaware of her stuttering and does not seem to be reacting to it with escape or avoidance behaviors, and her frequency of stuttering is relatively low, I am likely to use an indirect treatment approach. I would train parents to use a slower speech rate when speaking to the child as part of the treatment, with the expectation that their model of a slower speaking rate will influence the child to speak more slowly, thereby putting fluency within her reach. In such cases, I also explore ways in which the family may be putting pressure inadvertently on the child's language skills by expecting a higher level of language development than the child can achieve.

Verbal activities that some parents may particularly enjoy with their children, such as puns, wordplay, and teaching the child multisyllabic words, may convey to a child that the parents place high value on verbal ability. For most children, this would be an incentive to develop their verbal skills. But, for children vulnerable to fluency breakdowns, their parents' pride in their verbal proficiency may stress their ability to perform, resulting in increased disfluency. For those children who are really struggling with stuttering, parents' focus on verbal performance may create in the children feelings of shame at their verbal ineptitude.

It is useful to compare a child's language (syntax) scores with her vocabulary scores. Researchers (e.g., Anderson & Conture, 2000; Choo et al., 2016; Conture, 2001) have shown that many children who stutter have a disparity between syntax and vocabulary scores that is greater than that for peers who are typically developing. Interestingly, it has also been shown that children who have lower language abilities, relative to peers, at the beginning of treatment show greater long-term decrease in stuttering as a result of treatment (Richels & Conture, 2010).

As I review my observations of a child's speech and language, I consider not only the possibility that a child's language is advanced relative to her speech-motor abilities but also the possibility that her motor abilities are markedly delayed. A few children have motor problems that impair their coordination of respiration, phonation, and articulation with language production. Many are aware that speech is difficult for them and have already felt frustration and shame, not just about stuttering, but about the way they speak and how they perform other fine motor tasks. Therefore, to help these children improve their feelings about themselves as talkers, the parents and I work on their speech-motor skills. These children seem to benefit especially from models of slow speech as well as activities that teach them to speak more slowly.

In addition to exploring the possibility of language and articulation difficulties, I also assess a child's voice. A hoarse voice may be especially significant in a preschool child who stutters because it may be a sign that the child has increased tension in her laryngeal muscles, perhaps in an effort to cope with stuttering. I look closely at how the child is handling her blocks and listen for signs of excess laryngeal tension, such as pitch rises, increases in loudness, and hard glottal attacks. Because many of the techniques I use in treatment of stuttering result in a more relaxed style of speaking, I usually don't treat voice separately from stuttering. However, if a child has voice problems other than hoarseness, or if hoarseness does not diminish with stuttering therapy, I refer the child to an otolaryngologist for assessment and then follow treatment approaches such as those suggested by Boone, McFarlane, Von Berg, and Zraick (2014) that are appropriate given the child's underlying pathology.

Other Factors

In Chapter 4, I described a number of possible developmental influences on stuttering. In this section, I review them briefly so that they may be recognized if they are important in a particular preschool child's stuttering. Because much of this information can be obtained from a parent interview, you may wish to consult Chapter 4 for further details on developmental influences before conducting a parent interview.

Physical Development

I like to ascertain whether a child has age-appropriate gross motor skills and whether her oral motor development is typical. Figure 4.2 in Chapter 4 presents information about motor development. Most children learn to walk at about age 1 but usually do not learn to walk and talk at the same time. If a child I am evaluating was delayed in walking but average or advanced in talking, I may explore the possibility that the onset and evolution of her stuttering were associated with her delayed motor development.

Cognitive Development

When I consider a child's cognitive development, I want to learn whether there is cognitive delay, which can be associated with increased disfluency. I also want to know if a child may be going through a period of rapid cognitive growth that might, hypothetically, take a temporary toll on fluency. This information is likely to come to me as part of the child's case history. However, if I suspect cognitive delay and cognitive testing has not been done, I may recommend a referral to the early childhood special educator or school psychologist.

Social-Emotional Development

As a child grows, various tensions develop between her, her parents, and her siblings. Between ages 2 and 5, many children may display negativity in ways that are felt throughout the family (Dowling, 2014). When I ask a child's parents about conditions surrounding the onset or worsening of a child's stuttering, I explore social-emotional factors as well as environmental and developmental factors.

In Chapter 4, I described various life events that may affect a child's stuttering. In the parent interview, I examine life events surrounding the onset of stuttering to see if upsetting events or ongoing situations may be linked to the child's stuttering. Some events, like the birth of a sibling, may be happy ones, but they can create disturbances in the psychological balance of a family.

Speech and Language Environment

I have referred to the child's communication environment before, but here I will be more explicit. Many children have their hands full trying to compete verbally with fast-talking, articulate adults. Children who stutter may find this particularly hard. If the family has sent, as requested, a video or even audio recording of the parents and child talking, I observe the parent-child interactions carefully for indications of a complicated verbal environment, such as rapid speech models without many pauses, which may be like rough water to a beginning swimmer.

Diagnosis

Now, I will turn to the task of pulling together the information gathered in an assessment and making a diagnosis of a young client's problems. One of the clinical questions that must be answered is whether the child is truly stuttering. Once you have (tentatively) answered that, you can answer the other clinical questions and describe the child's stuttering, her reactions to it, and an appropriate treatment choice.

Determining Developmental and Treatment Level

In determining an appropriate treatment for the child, I begin by trying to figure out if a preschool child is normally disfluent and, if not, her level of stuttering: borderline or beginning stuttering. In the following paragraphs, I briefly review these levels.

Typical Disfluency

All of the following characteristics must be met for a child to be considered normally or typically disfluent. The child has fewer than 10 disfluencies per 100 words; these disfluencies consist mostly of multisyllable word and phrase repetitions, revisions, and interjections. When disfluencies are repetitions, they will have two or fewer repeated units per repetition that are slow and regular in tempo. The ratio of stuttering-like disfluencies to total disfluencies will be less than 50 percent. All disfluencies will be relatively relaxed, and the child will seem to be hardly aware of them and certainly will not be upset when she is aware.

A child may be considered to have borderline or beginning stuttering if she has any of the characteristics described in the following paragraphs. Place her at the level—borderline or beginning—that includes the child's most salient characteristics.

Borderline Stuttering

The child I place in this category has more than 10 disfluencies per 100 words, but they are loose and relaxed. They may be part-word repetitions and single-syllable word repetitions, as well as prolongations, and the repetitions may have more than two repeated units per instance. Stuttering-like disfluencies will be above 50 percent (Yairi, 1997a), and the disfluencies may cluster on adjacent sounds (LaSalle & Conture, 1995).

Beginning Stuttering

Beginning stuttering usually occurs in children between 3.5 and 6 years old. The key features at this level are the presence of tension and hurry in the child's stuttering. Disfluencies may have some of these characteristics: rapid, abrupt repetitions, pitch rises during repetitions and prolongations, difficulty starting airflow or phonation, and signs of facial tension. Just the occasional appearance of these signs would make me believe the child is a beginning stutterer. A beginning stutterer also shows that she is aware of her stuttering (in some, this may be subtle) and may be frustrated by it. She *may* use a variety of escape behaviors, such as head nods or eyeblinks, in terminating blocks. Occasional avoidance may occur. For example, a child who has developed language to the point of using "I" instead of "me" but begins to stutter on "I" at the beginnings of sentences may begin substituting "Me" for "I" to avoid the frustration of stuttering on "I."

Some children are relatively advanced for beginning stutterers. These are children who avoid words and situations, and their behavior and demeanor clearly suggest some fear and shame about stuttering. For example, they may use a variety of starters to begin sentences and look away or appear embarrassed when they stutter.

Although I use information from all sources to determine a child's developmental and treatment level, I have found that my own observations of parent-child and clinician-child interactions are most useful in making this (tentative) decision. Parents are helpful in describing long-term changes in their child's stuttering, but they frequently miss avoidance behaviors, such as starters, circumlocutions, and postponements, which are critical indicators of this more advanced level of stuttering. Parents' reports do provide, however, as much information about a child's feelings and attitudes as I usually gather in observing interactions in the clinic. Thus, parent reports plus my own observations provide valuable, complementary data. A vital adjunct to direct observations is video recordings of parent-child and clinician-child interactions. I sometimes revise my initial placement of a child in a developmental/treatment level after viewing video of the interactions I have already directly observed.

Risk Factors for Persistent Stuttering

Risk factors are those elements within a child or in her environment that make it more or less likely that she will persist in her stuttering (Guitar & Guitar, 2003) or take longer in treatment. Table 9.1 describes several of these factors. For some **risk factors for persistent stuttering**, you'll be able to

TABLE 9.1 Risk Factors for Persistent Stuttering or Extended Treatment

Factors within Child	Factors within Environment
Family history. If child's family history indicates that one or more relatives had persistent stuttering and did not recover without treatment, the child is more likely to have persistent stuttering (Ambrose, Cox, & Yairi, 1997).	**Others' reactions to stuttering.** Clinical observations suggest that if family is critical or impatient with child's stuttering, persistence is likely. More sensitive children are probably more affected by family's reactions to their stuttering.
Gender. If child is a boy, persistent stuttering is more likely (Ambrose, Cox, & Yairi, 1997).	**Family communication style.** Studies suggest that when parents' language is more complex, stuttering is more likely to persist (Kloth, Janssen, Kraaimaat, & Brutten, 1998; Rommel, Hage, Kalehne, & Johannsen, 2000).
Speech and language skills. If child's language, phonological skills, or nonverbal intelligence is below normal, he is likely to persist in stuttering (Yairi et al., 1996). However, some studies question whether language skills are predictive of persistence (Watkins, Yairi, & Ambrose, 1999). Also, if there is a disparity between child's vocabulary and syntax, child may be at risk for continued stuttering or extended treatment (Conture, 2001).	**Family expectations.** Clinical observations suggest that high expectations for academic, athletic, and social or verbal performance can stress children who stutter, making the stuttering more likely to be persistent.
Sensitivity/temperament. Some evidence shows that children with inhibited or sensitive temperament may take longer in treatment or not reduce stuttering as much in treatment (Richels & Conture, 2010).	**Life events.** Many writers (e.g., Van Riper) have suggested that stressful events may precipitate or perpetuate stuttering. These may include birth of a sibling, death of a relative, or emotional or physical conflicts in the home or in the environment.
Reactions to stuttering. If child reacts to stuttering with emotion and secondary behaviors, treatment may take longer. It may be related to temperament because emotional reactivity may cause more learned reactions (see Chapter 6).	**Family's schedule.** Clinical observations suggest that very busy homes in which children are overscheduled can put stress on a child who stutters. However, if child is successful in hobbies, sports, and other activities, this can bolster self-confidence.

get the information you need to determine a child's risk of persistent stuttering from the case history form, questionnaires, parent interviews, and observations of the child.

Drawing the Information Together

After I have completed the assessment tasks, I consolidate the information I have gathered, develop a tentative diagnosis, and meet with the family in a **closing interview** to discuss my findings and their desires and expectations. If I had been able to get a recording from the parents beforehand, ideally, I would have carefully analyzed it before the assessment and would present the results of my analysis in the closing interview. The same is obviously true for the other information I obtained before the assessment, such as the Behavioral Style Questionnaire (McDevitt & Carey, 1995) that I described in Chapter 8. Some data, like my analysis of the recordings of parent-child and clinician-child interactions, may not be completed by the time of the evaluation, but results will be included in my assessment report. Thus, for the closing interview, I rely on a combination of previously acquired quantitative data, some of the quantitative data I acquired as I talked with the child, such as frequency of stuttering, and the qualitative data gleaned from my observations and interview questions.

Before the closing interview, I spend a few minutes studying my findings or discussing them with students or colleagues if I have been working with a team. I try to make sure that I have obtained enough information to answer two key questions: what is this child's developmental/treatment level of stuttering, and what is the appropriate treatment? Working with the family, we can decide where to go from here. A few years ago, I began a practice of writing up (often by hand) a brief, one-page summary of our findings and recommendations prior to the closing interview. I share a copy of this recommendation sheet with the family so that we will have a common reference as we discuss the evaluation and where to go from here. They can share this with other family members, and if appropriate, the family can begin to make some changes immediately, without having to wait for the formal written report, which may take several days to prepare. A sample is shown in Figure 9.4.

Dear Katy and Charlie,

It has been such a pleasure meeting you and Susie today. Susie is obviously very bright and talented, and her language skills are impressive. She was also a delight to play with, showing enthusiasm and creativity.

During Katy and Susie's play together, Katy's warmth and attentiveness were very evident. We think it was particularly helpful that Katy kept the focus of play on what Susie was interested in, letting her take the lead.

Susie has great potential for improving her speech because of your good work with her. Children her age sometimes recover without formal treatment, but we are available should formal treatment be required. We will keep in contact with you about Susie's progress toward greater fluency.

To speed her recovery, we have a few recommendations:

1) Continue your facilitating manner of interacting with Susie. This includes using a slow and relaxed speaking style when you are talking and playing with her. Also, allowing plenty of pauses in your speech will assure her that she has plenty of time to talk. If others can do this as well when talking with Susie, she will benefit.

2) When possible, reduce the number of questions you ask Susie. Instead, try to make comments such as "I wonder if this hat goes on your doll," rather than "Where does this hat go?"

3) If Susie expresses frustration with her occasional disfluencies, respond in a reassuring manner, empathizing with her and letting her know that lots of kids get hung up on words sometimes, and that talking will get easier.

Again, we want to say how much we enjoyed having you visit today. As questions and concerns arise, please contact us by phone or email.

All the best,

Alyssa Jones, Alexandra Patch, and Barry Guitar

Figure 9.4 Sample brief comments given to family at the end of meeting.

Closing Interview: Recommendations and Follow-Up

Before I begin, I remind myself to take the necessary time to listen to the family's questions that may arise at any time during the closing interview. When I begin, I always make some positive comments about the child and the family and then describe to the family characteristics of the child's stuttering that I observed in parent-child and clinician-child interactions and the preassessment recording, if I obtained one. I stay away from jargon and strive to be as clear and straightforward as possible. I briefly describe the child's stuttering behaviors, such as easy, tension-free repetitions that may be typical disfluencies, or struggle behavior accompanied by avoidances that may indicate unambiguous stuttering. I refer to the important information that the parents provided in the case history and our interview, such as the child's expressions of frustration or requests for help. Some children will not need referral for treatment, such as when the child has only a relatively few typical, tension-free repetitions (both during the evaluation and as reported at home). Others will show these typical disfluencies quite frequently and may have several iterations of each repeated sound or syllable, li-li-li-li-li-like this. These children may have borderline stuttering. If a preschool child has signs of tension, fixed articulatory postures (blocks), and/or clear evidence of awareness and frustration and/or escape behaviors as they try to free themselves from their stuttering, I would classify the behavior as beginning stuttering. Treatment options for these children are described in the next few paragraphs. More details about treatment approaches for preschool children are given in Chapters 11 and 12.

If stuttering is a serious concern, I say so, and if the parents have expressed feelings of guilt about their child's stuttering, I again reassure them that they are not to blame but that they will be crucial in helping to resolve it. Next, after answering questions, I describe appropriate treatment approaches, such as environmental changes, indirect treatment, and direct treatment, which will differ depending on the developmental/treatment level of the child's problem.

In the video clip of the child on *thePoint* (as "Chapter 9: Assessment and Diagnosis: Preschool Child-Closing Interview"), you will see at the end an example of the way we conduct the closing interview. On the right in the video is the mom with the child and then you see two graduate students, one with her back to the camera. On the far right is the supervisor, Dr. Danra Kazenski, ready to help out when needed. The clinicians make several comments about the child's positive traits and existing influences that may help lead to recovery. They also note that the child has been stuttering more than a year and, if anything, her stuttering is increasing. These observations lead them to their recommendation that treatment should begin immediately. Then, the clinicians recommend that the mom fill in the Severity Rating chart daily and share it with Dr. Kazenski weekly. Finally, therapy scheduling is discussed.

Recommendations for Children with Typical Disfluency

If I believe that a child's speech is typically disfluent, I deal with the family's concerns rather than the child's disfluencies. Most families benefit from knowing how I reached my tentative conclusion, so I provide them with information about normal disfluency, such as the following: "During their preschool years, many normal children pass through periods of disfluency. Interjections, revisions, pauses, repetitions, and prolongations are common during these periods, but they usually occur in fewer than 10 of every 100 words. Interjections and revisions are more common than part-word repetitions, and part-word repetitions usually have only one or two repeated units per disfluency. Children who are normally disfluent are largely unaware of their disfluencies, do not react negatively to them, and gradually 'outgrow' them."

In most cases, I use analogies to help the family understand their child's disfluent speech. For example, I may point out that learning to speak is like learning many other skills, such as riding a tricycle or learning to skate, and that a learner falls down a lot in the early stages. I look for analogies that will fit the family's experiences to help them understand why their child is disfluent and how valuable an accepting environment can be for a child's self-esteem. Parents who are concerned about their child's typical disfluencies usually feel reassured when they find out that this is not uncommon. In those rare cases when parents are still not convinced that their child's speech disfluencies are not stuttering, I teach them how to slow their speaking rates and increase pausing. I sometimes use a video from YouTube of a slow and relaxed speaker (such as "Fred Rogers' 2002 Dartmouth College Commencement Address") to illustrate how it sounds. Then, I set up another appointment to discuss their progress and the child's speech. If parents really are concerned and seem likely to continue worrying and perhaps correcting their child's speech, a few sessions focused on the normalcy of their child's speech and the changes they have made in the family's environment can be helpful to feelings of well-being may also be an ounce of prevention.

Finally, I always keep the door wide open for all parents of normally disfluent children. I reassure them that I am available to talk with them if they become concerned again and will be ready to work with them if their child does begin to stutter.

Recommendations for Children with Borderline or Beginning Stuttering

My theoretical perspective on stuttering provides guidelines for the treatment of preschool children (e.g., see Chapter 6). First, the child's fluency should be enhanced. This can be done using an indirect approach in which the family uses a slower speech rate with pauses, in addition to other possible changes that make it more likely the child will find it easier and more rewarding to talk. For older preschool children, I often (but not always) use a direct approach that is focused on rewarding fluency. Second, the child should be helped to decrease or eliminate defensive responses to her stuttering. This may be done by increasing the child's fluency and responding matter-of-factly to stuttering, as in the Lidcombe Program (see Chapter 12). It can also be a part of an indirect treatment approach in which both the family and the child are guided to accept the present level of stuttering as fluency is increased, as in the parent-child interaction therapy (see Chapter 11).

For those preschool children evaluated fewer than 12 months after the onset of stuttering, there are guidelines to help decide which children should begin treatment and which can be followed for a period of time without treatment. First, children whose stuttering-like disfluencies (part-word and single-syllable word repetitions, prolongations, or blocks) steadily decrease during the first 12 months after onset are more likely to recover without formal treatment. Turn to Table 9.2 for a more complete list of factors suggesting natural recovery is likely.

I believe that any preschool child who has borderline or beginning stuttering should be treated or followed carefully for several months because if treatment is warranted, it should begin early. I stay in telephone or e-mail contact with families of children who are close to onset whose stuttering is diminishing, who have other indicators suggesting recovery without treatment is likely, and whose families are not overly concerned. However, if families are highly concerned or the child's stuttering is not decreasing and there are only few indicators of recovery, I begin treatment as soon as possible.

When I recommend therapy, my closing interview with parents is usually the first of many sessions we will spend together. Consequently, I don't need to accomplish everything in this meeting. Because treatment of any preschool

TABLE 9.2 Factors That May Be Associated with Increased Likelihood of Recovery from Stuttering without Treatment*

Factor	Comment
1. Decrease in stuttering-like disfluencies during the 12 months after onset	This is an important predictor of recovery. Thus, it is important to follow preschool children and continue to assess their disfluencies.
2. Female sex	Evidence suggests females are more likely to recover.
3. No relatives who stutter, or relatives have recovered from stuttering	Preliminary evidence suggests that persistent stuttering may run in families.
4. Good language and articulation skills	Both receptive and expressive language skills should be considered. Evidence of early phonological problems may predict persistent stuttering.
5. Good nonverbal intelligence scores	Children with persistent stuttering had normal but slightly lower nonverbal skills.
6. Outgoing, carefree temperament	Our clinical experience suggests these children who begin to stutter often outgrow it.

*When a young preschool child is assessed within 1 year of stuttering onset.
Factors 1 to 5 are based on evidence cited in Andrews et al. (1983), Yairi and Ambrose (1992a, 1992b), and Yairi et al. (1996).

child who stutters is often focused on the home environment, we frequently begin our discussion with things the parents can do at home. The chapters on treating preschool children (Chapters 11 and 12) contain more extensive discussions and guidelines for involving the family in treatment, but I will make some initial suggestions here.

In my experience, parents who are active in the ongoing assessment process from the beginning feel more hopeful, less guilty, and more motivated to be involved in treatment (see also Zebrowski & Kelly, 2002). Therefore, in the closing interview, I ask parents of preschool children who will soon start treatment to begin observing and recording the day-to-day variations in their child's fluency. Having them assess fluency in the home environment also gives me a more valid indication of changes in stuttering than if assessments are done only in the clinic.

I teach parents to use the Severity Rating Scale (Fig. 8.4) (Onslow, Andrews, & Costa, 1990; Onslow, Packman, & Harrison, 2003; Onslow et al., 2018)—a form they use at the end of each day to record a number from 0 (no stuttering) to 9 (extremely severe stuttering), which is their estimate of the severity of their child's stuttering condensed from observations over the course of the day. Parents begin by rating the severity of the child's stuttering during the parent-child interaction that has just taken place in this evaluation session. The clinician also rates the severity of this sample. If the parents' and clinician's ratings differ by more than one point, the parents and clinician discuss the ratings and watch the recording of the interaction to help them come to a consensus. If more than one parent or another family member will be using the Severity Rating Scale, each person should be trained until her or her ratings are within one point of the clinician's rating of each sample. In addition to rating the child's severity every day, parents can use this form to record comments and questions they would like to discuss when we meet at the next session.

If a child with borderline stuttering is being followed but not formally treated, severity ratings remain an important part of the monitoring process. Clinicians can obtain information about the child's stuttering via phone calls or e-mail on a regular basis, and parents can report their severity ratings for each day as well as discuss issues of concern and ask questions. In addition to monitoring the severity of a child's stuttering, it is often helpful to brainstorm with the parents about ways in which the environment might be made as facilitating as possible for their child's speech. I will discuss this in more detail in the following paragraphs.

For the younger preschool child with borderline stuttering who is being treated (i.e., a child whose parents are very concerned or who has multiple risk factors for persistent stuttering), the closing interview is a time when further appointments may be set up and changes in the family environment can be initiated. Such changes will be determined by the clinician's observations of parent-child interactions, the parent interview, and ideas that parents may have about what they would like to change. In my experience, one of the most powerful ways that parents can facilitate fluency is to set aside 10 to 15 minutes each day, preferably in the morning, for child-directed interactions. This is a one-on-one interaction without other children interrupting. In two-parent homes, parents may need to alternate which one does the one-on-one activity so that the other parent can watch the other children. Or a parent may conduct the session when the siblings are at school or napping. During these interactions, the parent primarily listens to the child and plays whatever games the child chooses. When the parent speaks, he or she should use a slow rate with frequent pauses, somewhat like television's Mr. Rogers. I have found this works best if the clinician models this interaction style and then watches the parent carry it out. More information about changing the family environment is given in the chapter on treatment of the young preschool child with borderline stuttering (Chapter 11).

I also give parents of these children reading material or a video recording to help them better understand stuttering and what they can do to help their child. The book *Stuttering and Your Child—Questions and Answers* (Conture, 2002) gives many good suggestions and is available from the Stuttering Foundation (www.stutteringhelp.org) for very little money. The video, *Stuttering and Your Child: Help for Parents* (Guitar & Guitar, 2003, SFA publication no. 70), is also available from the Foundation, both inexpensively through the online store and free as a streaming video on www.stutteringhelp.org. Another video, *Preventing Stuttering in the Preschool Child: A Video Program for Parents* (Skinner & McKeehan, 1996; Communication Skill Builders), is highly instructive.

For older preschool children with beginning-level stuttering, I recommend (1) starting treatment as soon as possible (2) with a direct approach. These and other options for therapy should be described to the parents, and with the clinician's guidance, they should make an informed choice about whether to choose this option. In some cases, the family will be able to make their decision immediately. In other cases, they may need time to consider the possibilities. If they choose to begin treatment immediately, one or more family members should be trained in recording daily severity ratings before they leave, and the next session should be scheduled. If the session can be scheduled within a week or two, they should be asked to bring in their severity ratings with them. If it has to be delayed, the clinician should be in contact with the family through e-mail or telephone each week to discuss their severity ratings until formal treatment can begin. During therapy, parents will bring in their severity ratings each week to discuss them with the clinician.

If treatment cannot begin for several weeks, I ask a parent or another family member to conduct one-on-one interactions with the child like those described above for the child with borderline stuttering. If the family is able to begin treatment immediately, the clinician can start the parents on appropriate activities. Clinicians who carry out therapy themselves with the child will probably have a parent watch the first few sessions before beginning direct activities at home. My own preference is to use the Lidcombe Program (Harrison & Onslow, 2010), which is a parent-delivered treatment described, along with others, in some detail in Chapter 12. When the parents agree with use of the Lidcombe, I describe the first phase of this treatment program—a daily parent-child session conducted at home—to the parents. In these sessions, parents engage the child in an activity at an appropriate linguistic level to elicit fluent speech and reinforce fluent utterances, where appropriate means at a level that is easy enough to almost assure fluent speech. After explaining this to the parent, I model this type of interaction and then observe the parent as she or he tries it.

The closing interview should end when the family seems to have a good understanding of the clinician's findings, and they and the clinician agree what the next steps should be. Because a family may come up with new questions and concerns in the days following the evaluation, it is important to conclude the interview with information about how they can contact the clinician.

SCHOOL-AGE CHILD

Preassessment

Evaluation of the school-age child is different from evaluation of the preschool-age child because the child's stuttering will by this point probably be more severe. A child in this age group commonly stutters with tension and struggle, and he will be frustrated and embarrassed by it. The reactions of the child's peers are important as well.

Clinical Questions

As with preschool-age children, it is important to begin an evaluation with certain questions in mind. What is the child's stuttering like? More specifically, what is this child's frequency of stuttering? What types of disfluencies does he display, and what is the percentage of SLDs? What is the child's severity? What is his speech rate? With rare exceptions, the question of whether the youngster is normally disfluent or stuttering is not an issue. By age 6, most children who stutter do so in ways that are quite different from the normal disfluencies typical for their age.

Another question is what emotions and attitudes does the child have about stuttering and about speaking? Schoolchildren with notable fear and avoidance may need special attention to these feelings and behaviors. Information about risk factors (e.g., gender, family history) is important but not as critical as they are for a preschool child. By the time a child is in school, natural recovery is less likely than in the preschool years; thus, an absence of risk factors doesn't warrant withholding or delaying treatment.

Information from the child's teachers, the clinician's observations of his speech in class and in the treatment room, and information from his family are all required to assign the child a developmental/treatment level. Questions about treatment of children in the public schools can be answered only in the context of federal and state laws, which are considered in the next section. With any school-age child, it is vital to determine the child's school performance and whether stuttering interferes with it.

Public School Considerations

The **Individuals with Disabilities Education Act** (IDEA 1997 and changes made in 2004) and individual state laws mandate the procedures that public school clinicians must use for gathering information about a child's disability and deciding on treatment. Every state will have their own guidelines so what I write here may not be exactly what is expected in the state you practice in. Check your state's guidelines. Many states use a concept called Multi-Tiered System of Supports (MTSS) to make sure that all students are getting the educational input and support they need. The tiers of support are in a hierarchy from less intense to more intense extra support.

Tier 1 is support provided by changing the educational environment for a student. Speech-language pathologists are usually members of a team that consults with the teacher and parents to determine if a child's difficulty can be resolved by making changes in the educational setting. An example of such modifications might be discussions between the child and teacher about how the teacher can facilitate the child's class participation. If stuttering continues to be a problem in the classroom after the modifications have been in place for a designated time period or if the child's stuttering is quite severe, the SLP can provide some therapy outside the classroom under a Tier 2 plan. If this seems to work for the child, it can be continued, but at some point when therapy is ongoing, the child should be placed on an Education Support Team (EST) Plan. At the same time, the SLP should document changes that are occurring in response to the treatment (changes are sometimes called "response to intervention" or RTI). The support team may consist of the SLP, administrators, special educators, and others. In some schools and with some children, Tier 2 therapy may be the best approach.

Tier 3 is more serious and requires—in most states—that the child's stuttering (and/or related issues) meets the state's eligibility standards and that the child's stuttering has an adverse effect on his education. The child then could be placed on Individualized Education Plan (IEP) and receive direct services. The step to reach Tier 3 would be a formal evaluation by the multidisciplinary team to determine if the child meets all the requirements. As part of this evaluation, the clinician discreetly observes the child in the classroom and confirms (or disconfirms) that the child is stuttering. The clinician then discusses the child's problem with the teacher and the school's special education administrator. Next, the clinician, teacher, or administrator contacts the child's parents to ask permission to do a formal evaluation of the child. If permission is given, the clinician gathers information on as many dimensions of the child's stuttering as possible. Typically, this will include the frequency, severity, and types of stuttering observed in two or more situations, the child's feelings and attitudes about stuttering and speaking, concomitant speech or language problems, and overall communicative performance. The clinician uses standardized tests such as the SSI-4, observations, and interviews with the child and his family as well as with his teachers and others at school who know him. After this information is gathered, a team composed of the clinician, teacher, special education administrator, and the parents meets to decide two issues. The first is whether the child's stuttering problems meet the state's criteria for eligibility, and the second is whether the child's stuttering adversely affects his educational performance. These two issues are discussed in detail later in this chapter, after the sections on the parent, teacher, and child interview.

Initial Contact with Parents

Whether contact is made because the child has been referred to the school clinician or because the parents have made an appointment at a private or university clinic, the clinician's most important task is to listen and try to understand the parents' point of view. If the school clinician is telephoning the parents for permission to evaluate their child, she should describe the process by which the child was identified and convey her and the school's desire to help the child achieve his potential as an effective communicator. It will be helpful to briefly describe the disfluencies that identified the child as stuttering and to find out if the parents have also noticed them. The clinician should calmly convey her interest in the child and his stuttering in an accepting tone of voice, particularly because parents may fear that they are being blamed for the child's stuttering. It may help also to comment that current views suggest that stuttering may be the result of how the child's brain is organized, although its exact cause is unknown. The evaluation process should be described and permission sought. If the parents agree to an evaluation, this is a good time to ask them to fill out a case history form and, if possible, send a video recording of the child's speech. It may be beneficial for the clinician to talk to the child as well and ask his permission to have his parents video record his speech at home. In some cases, the home video is easier to obtain once the clinician has gotten to know the child and has conveyed her acceptance and interest in the child and his stuttering.

When the evaluation will take place in a clinic rather than school, the clinician should call the parents and let them know what will take place in the evaluation, get some preliminary information about the child and his stuttering, let them know they will receive a case history form to complete and return, and request a video from home prior to the evaluation. As with the school clinician's telephone call, the parents' point of view about stuttering must be understood. Even though they will have a chance to talk over their concerns in person, they may also want to talk and ask questions in this preliminary telephone call.

Case History Form

The form used for this age group is the same one used for preschool children (Fig. 9.3). Some of the questions about speech and language development may be difficult for parents to recall. This is not critical for evaluating a school-age child, but it is important to probe for other speech and language problems that may be contributing factors in the school-age child's stuttering. An important section on this form deals with how the problem has changed since it was first noticed, what has been done about it, and how others have reacted to it. In addition, the section on educational history lets us know if the child is having problems in school.

Audio/Video Recording

Obtaining a recording (preferably a video recording) of the child speaking at home or elsewhere will help clinicians prepare for the evaluation because they can get a preview of the child's pattern of stuttering, analyze the sample ahead of time, and plan the assessment more carefully. For example, if a sample from home has little or no stuttering, the clinician may want to obtain another sample in a more difficult speaking situation. Up to a point, more varied samples of a child's speech lead to a more valid assessment. If a pre-evaluation sample has lots of avoidance behaviors on it, clinicians can prepare questions to ask the child about what he does when he expects to stutter.

Assessment

Parent-Child Interaction

When I conduct an evaluation in a clinic, I usually first observe the child's speech with his parents while they are involved in an activity that promotes speech, such as how their favorite sports team is doing or describing a book or movie that they liked. I video record this with the participants' permission for later analyses and then pay close attention to both the child's stuttering behaviors and the parents' responses and interaction style.

Parent Interview

This description of the parent interview assumes that the parents have brought their child to a clinic for the evaluation. When the evaluation is school-based, the clinician can get much of this information by telephone and follow-up with a face-to-face meeting at school.

Begin a clinic-based interview by sharing some positive observations about the child and his family and then describe the course of the evaluation. Before obtaining more background information to fill in gaps left by the case history, ask parents an open-ended question, such as requesting them to describe their concerns about their child's speech. Only after the parents or caregivers have had a chance to express their worries and observations do I ask follow-up questions. As I do with parents of preschool children, I explore the onset and development of the child's stuttering, his reactions to it, family members' reactions, and any gaps in the case history. I also ask parents of a school-age child about his school experiences. Does he like school? Does his speech seem to bother him there? Do you think he participates less in school because of his stuttering? Is he teased or bullied about his stuttering? Do you think he stutters more at school than at home? Has he gotten therapy at school? Has that helped? Has he liked it?

As I ask parents questions about the child's stuttering at home and school, I listen for responses that may help me understand factors explaining why the child's stuttering has persisted into elementary school. Here are some of the questions I think about as I try to assimilate the information I am getting from the parent: is the child sensitive about his stuttering? Are the family and child comfortable talking about stuttering? Is the family supportive of the child and his ways of coping with his stuttering? Is the family motivated to participate in therapy?

Teacher Interview

The more assistance we can get from a child's teachers, the more we can help the child. We need to approach teachers respecting their heavy responsibilities and their concern for all of their students, including the one with whom we are working. But, we also should anticipate that they may neither understand nor know what we do to help a child who stutters. As I conduct a **teacher interview**, I try to sense what they would like to know about stuttering and my treatment approach. The following questions serve as guidelines for the types of things I want to find out.

1. **Does the child talk in class? Does he stutter? What is his stuttering like? How does he seem to feel about his stuttering and about himself as a communicator?**
   Here, I am trying to determine how much the child stutters in class and whether his stuttering keeps him from talking as much as he might otherwise if he did not stutter. I may also get a flavor of how the teacher feels about the child, his communication abilities, and his stuttering.
2. **Does stuttering interfere with the child's performance in school?**
   This question is obviously related to the previous one about the child's stuttering in class. But, it also may give us some information about how much the child may avoid speaking, especially volunteering in class. I ask about disparities between his oral and written performance; a large disparity may indicate that he declines to talk or says "I don't know" even when he knows the answers.
3. **Do other children tease him about stuttering?**
   Most school-age children who stutter are teased, at least a little, and I want to get more information about how much he is teased (or bullied) and how it affects him.

I also want to find out about any school policies that relate to bullying since teasing may be just the tip of the iceberg, and many schools are developing strategies for addressing both problems.

4. **How does the teacher feel about stuttering, and how does he or she react to it?**
I am often able to get this information indirectly, from what he or she said before, but if not, I ask directly. Teachers are also likely to ask how they *should* respond to a child's stuttering, which is an important issue because a teacher's response often influences how the class responds. This and other issues related to the child's speech in the classroom are discussed in the chapter on intermediate stuttering (Chapter 13).

Classroom Observation

In addition to the information obtained from teacher and parent interviews, direct **classroom observation** can help clinicians understand the severity of a child's stuttering and the degree to which it interferes with his academic adjustment. If a child is to receive services in the school, the clinician must establish that the child's stuttering is interfering with his education. One way to verify this is by firsthand observation of a child in the classroom.

You should arrange with the teacher to come to the classroom at a time when the child will have opportunities to participate in class and observe the class as unobtrusively as you can. By observing the class when many students are participating, not just when the child you are evaluating is talking, you will not call as much attention to him. Most school-age children want to be like their peers and dread being singled out. I let the child know beforehand that I will not be interacting with him so no one will know I am there to observe him. I let him know that I only want to hear his speech in class. Notice whether the child participates in class discussion. If called on, does he speak in a straightforward manner or does he hesitate or deploy any postponement devices, such as repeating "uh" several times? Does he answer "I don't know?" This is a reply many children who stutter (including me, when I was in school) use to avoid speaking and thus risk stuttering—even when they know the answer. If the child does talk in class and happens to stutter, notice how other children react to his stuttering. Do they giggle and look at each other and make comments under their breaths, or do they seem normally attentive? Because the classroom is the arena where children learn, socialize, and develop communication skills, it should be a target of assessment and treatment.

Child/Student Interview

After I obtain parents' consent to evaluate a child, I arrange for the child to come to the treatment room. Here, I set about to make him feel that my room is an **accepting environment** where he can have fun and also discover how he can make his speech much easier. School-age clients sometimes tell me that it helps just to have someone to talk to about stuttering and other things that are bothering them. This can occur only after a trusting relationship is established, and the initial interview is the beginning of building that relationship.

During our first encounter, it is important for a child to feel that I am genuinely interested in him as well as his stuttering. I usually begin by asking what he likes to do, who his friends are, and who is in his family. Then, I tell him a little about myself and how I work with other kids who sometimes get stuck on words. As the child talks, I note whether he stutters or not and how he stutters. When a child's body language and behavior tell me he's comfortable in the session, I talk to him about his speech. The following questions are not asked one right after another but over a session or two. Often, it is more effective to make the question a comment, such as phrasing the first question below as "Sometimes kids have trouble getting words out. Their words just seem to stick a little bit." Then, leave some silence to see if the youngster will talk about his own speech. Whatever you do, don't ask the questions "bang-bang-bang," one right after the other. The questions I list below are just to give you ideas for talking to the child about his experiences and feelings. For most children, talking about their stuttering will make them anxious so you need to do things that relieve their feelings as they talk. Playing a game while you talk is helpful as long as it isn't so engrossing that talking about his speech annoys him because it distracts him from the game.

1. **Do you ever think that you have any trouble talking?**
I rarely see school-age stutterers who are unaware of their difficulty. However, if a child regards his problem as minor or seems genuinely unaware of the problem, I avoid giving it undue emphasis or creating an unfavorable attitude about it. Thus, my first talk with a child is usually low-key, and if he truly doesn't seem to be bothered by his stuttering, although his parents and teachers are, I respect his perception and try to treat it as a relatively minor problem, but I remain aware that the child may be bothered by his stuttering much more than he wishes to let on at first.
2. **What happens when you get stuck on a word? When does it happen? Is it different at different times?**
I am looking for several things here. One is to learn the words the child uses to describe his stuttering so that I can use them when talking with him about it. I also want to find out if the child is unaware of some of his stuttering behaviors, if they seem to be too painful for him to face, or if he just doesn't like talking about them. Even more important, these questions let a child know that the clinician really wants to understand his problem.
3. **Have you learned to use any helpers or "tricks" to get words out? Do you sometimes avoid certain words?**
With this question, I can convey that I understand what some people do when they stutter. I can also let a child know that I am nonjudgmental about the "tricks" he

uses by conveying my acceptance and interest in his descriptions. In addition, I am also exploring which level the child's stuttering has reached by determining if he is using escape and avoidance behaviors.

4. **Are certain speaking situations more difficult?**
   This is another question that helps me understand what a child is experiencing while conveying my understanding.
5. **Most kids who stutter get teased or picked on about their speech. Do you ever get teased about your stuttering? What do you do when that happens? How does it affect you?**
   Many children who stutter are teased about their speech but are not willing to talk about it straightaway with someone they don't know well. So, this question is a "feeler," and if the child denies being teased, the clinician should not dwell on it now.
6. **How do you feel about your speech?**
   To help a child express feelings about stuttering, I can suggest some possibilities by asking, "Does it make you mad sometimes?" or "Do you wish you didn't get stuck?" Don't be surprised, however, if a child says it doesn't bother him because his feelings may have been rejected, perhaps unintentionally, by adults. Adults may say, for instance, "You shouldn't feel that way," or "Why do you let it bother you?" An effective clinician will show the child that whatever feelings he has are OK and that the clinician is really trying to understand. Real discussions of feelings probably won't begin until a child has learned to trust the clinician deeply. However, in this first interview, I may be able to infer what some of the child's feelings are and, from that, understand how far his stuttering has advanced.

   Another avenue to elicit feelings is through drawing pictures. For some children, drawing makes it easier to talk about feelings. The child doesn't have to look directly at the clinician, and his self-consciousness may be decreased by his focus on drawing. I usually suggest to a child that both of us draw whatever we would like, and as we are drawing, I talk about feelings. If this goes well, I bridge the gap between the drawing and talking by suggesting that the child might want to draw a picture of what stuttering is like or what he feels like when he stutters. I have found that this technique can make extensive discussion of feelings much easier for some children. In some cases, children have used their drawings when they talked about stuttering with their class once therapy has helped them feel more comfortable with themselves and their speech.

   Some of the activities in the workbook titled *The School-Age Child Who Stutters: Working Effectively with Attitudes and Emotions* (Chmela & Reardon, 2001) are helpful in exploring a child's emotions in both the evaluation and treatment. I will discuss some of these a little later.
7. **How do your parents feel about your speech? Do they ever say anything or give you advice?**
   This helps me determine what sorts of experiences the child may have been going through at home. One parent may be much less accepting of a child's stuttering than the other. Whatever I find out may help me enlist the parents' participation in treatment.
8. **Can you think of anything else important for me to know about you or about the trouble you sometimes have when you talk?**
   This lets the child know that I am interested in him and that his ideas are important to me.

Speech Samples

Preliminaries

With a school-age child, I video record him talking for 10 minutes about school and other activities in the therapy room. I prefer not to turn on the recorder the moment the child walks into the room. Instead, after talking for a few minutes, I ask the child if he would mind my recording our conversation as we talk. If it's OK with the child, I record a sample that optimally includes 300 to 400 syllables of his speech. For those few children who are reluctant at first, I explain that I need a recording of their speech to understand their stuttering better. In rare cases, I might need to postpone recording until the child is more comfortable with me. After recording the speech sample, I ask the child to read approximately 200 syllables of age-appropriate material. I often use the SSI-4 examiner's manual, which has 200-syllable reading passages at the third, fifth, and seventh grade levels.

If possible, I also obtain a video recording from home for a second sample. In some instances, you may not be able to get a second recorded sample from home or elsewhere. Even if you are not able to record a second sample, write down your impressions of the child's stuttering, including the amount of stuttering and the core and secondary behaviors you observed.

Pattern of Disfluencies

A school-age child is likely to show beginning or intermediate stuttering, so you want to know as much as possible about the amount of tension in the child's stuttering, the escape behaviors he uses, and the extent to which he avoids words and situations. You can obtain this information directly by observation or indirectly through parent and teacher interviews. As with adults or adolescents who stutter, I use this information not only to decide at which developmental/treatment level to place the child but also, when appropriate, to plan the process of unlearning conditioned responses, which, once created, now maintain the child's pattern of stuttering.

Stuttering Severity Instrument (SSI-4)

Samples of conversational speech and reading are needed to calculate scores on the SSI-4. Administration and scoring of the SSI-4 were described in Chapter 8.

Speech Rate

The samples you collect for rating severity with the SSI-4 can also be used to assess the child's speaking rate. The purpose of assessing speech rate is to get some idea of how much the child's stuttering interferes with the rate of speech he normally uses. As I help the child manage his stuttering, I expect a steady increase in his speech rate toward normal levels.

Normal speech rates for schoolchildren measured in syllables per minute are given in Table 8.5. These rates were obtained from children's conversations with a clinician about holidays, hobbies, school, and home activities. They were calculated by including normal pauses in their conversation but excluding pauses longer than 2 seconds for thought. It is reasonable to expect that children's speech rates in other states will be similar.

Trial Therapy

Trial therapy with a school-age child will help me understand how easily a child can talk about his stuttering, including about his feelings. If the child is able to make even small changes in his stuttering, though they will be only temporary in this trial therapy, he will gain hope and motivation for our work together.

I usually begin by asking the child to identify moments of voluntary stuttering in my own speech. I explain that I will be putting stutters in my speech and want to see if he can catch me. It's more fun if I can use a small reward for his successes. For example, I might give him tokens to be cashed in later for an activity that he would find really cool, like throwing a ball to knock down a pyramid of cans. I then tell him about my favorite recent movie or television show (something he can later talk about himself) and put in a variety of stutters in my speech. As I talk and encourage him to catch my stutters, I let him know how good he is when he catches one of my stutters without my help and hand him a token, a piece of candy or a sip of soda. After a few successful catches, we switch roles and I ask him put in some stutters—pretend or real—as he talks about a movie, TV show, or any other handy topic, and I try to "catch him." Each time I catch a stutter of his (with his permission), I make a positive comment about his stutter and give him a reward. Rewarding stutters of school-age children causes no harm; in fact, it reduces negative emotion, which is a very positive step in treatment.

As the child becomes tuned in to his stutters by my catching them and commenting interestedly on them, I begin to explore with him both what he does when he stutters and how he feels. For example, after I have commented on a stutter, I might say, "OK, let's see what was going on there. Seems like you were squeezing pretty hard with your lips," if that was what he seemed to be doing. "Did you feel that? Let me try it." Then, I would try to emulate what he had done on the sound he had stuttered on. "Did I have that right? Can you make it happen again? Can you stutter on the same word?" I encourage him to pretend to stutter if he doesn't have a real one when he tries again. If he does stutter on it again or pretend to, I say, "Wow. That was great. You really did that stutter well!" If he doesn't want to stutter again, I let it go and try again later, after we do something more fun for him.

Take a look at the video clip of me working with a child when we both practice stuttering on the word "apple." It's in the Trial Therapy segment of the series of Chapter 9 video clips on *thePoint* on evaluation of school-age children. Note how I coach the student to try to stay in the moment of stuttering and finish the stutter with less tension. After a few tries, this child does a pretty good job of staying in the beginning sound and easing off on his tension before finishing the words. Throughout, I praise his stuttering, letting counterconditioning (associating something positive—my praise—with something that has been frustrating and even fearful for years) reduce his negative emotions.

Because emotions are such a large part of stuttering, it is important to explore how the child feels about his stuttering as well as what he does. The child and I have been talking about his moments of stuttering and so I begin to ask him about how one of those stutters feels. After he has stuttered, I show my interest and curiosity and then ask him, "How did it feel when you stuttered that time? I mean, how did it feel inside of you?" If he seems not to quite understand, I might suggest, "Lots of kids tell me that stutters feel bad, like they wish they didn't stutter. Is that about how it feels to you?" After a little bit of talking about how his stutter feels to him, I might ask him to draw his stutter. With some encouragement, and with me offering to draw something of mine I don't like, a child will usually draw a picture that we can then discuss.

For some children, you can sense when they've done enough. That's a time to stop and do something different. If the child seems like he can deal with a little more, I might see if he can make a little change in his stuttering by not just blasting through it but instead staying in the stutter and letting some of the tension go. As always, I first demonstrate what I'm asking the child to do. I have the child signal me by pointing to me when he wants me to stutter and make me hold on to the stutter for several seconds by continuing to keep his finger pointing at me. Then, we reverse roles and I coach him to hold onto either voluntary or real stutters. Coaching is essential because it will be unnatural for him to hold onto a stutter and he may need some practice until he can do it. I also coach him, while he's holding on to the stutter, to let it go slowly and loosely when he's ready to move on. Typically, my models of holding onto a stutter, my enthusiasm, and the reinforcements I use enable most children to be able to carry out these activities. Note that if the child cannot do these activities, it suggests a higher level of fear or an inability to focus on the task. These possibilities usually mean that a child needs a slower approach, and I will consider helping him reduce fear of stuttering before attempting to hold onto stutters.

In the rare case that the child doesn't seem to have much or any negative emotion associated with his stuttering, I might try teaching the child a few fluency skills such as those described in Chapter 13 on treatment of stuttering in school-age children. This approach doesn't deal directly with any tension or fear about stuttering. It simply teaches the child to talk in a way that is likely to engender fluency. I use a word list and give the child an example by producing each word myself before he tries it, using a slow rate and gentle onset of voicing. The severity of the child's stuttering will determine how slowly I begin the word; my aim is to use modeling of slow rate and easy onset to produce fluency in the child. Once he can say words after me in that slow fashion, I then ask him to say each of several words again, but without my model. If he can do this, I create sentences beginning with those words said slowly and with an easy onset (but with the remainder of the sentence produced at a near-normal rate) and again assess whether he can repeat them fluently with my model and then without.

These exercises help me determine how well the child can make changes in his speech and his stutters. By using a large amount of modeling and appropriate reinforcement, I can often take the child quite far along in the time I have.

Feelings and Attitudes

One of the best assessments of a child's feelings and attitudes about his stuttering is the clinician's judgment. In the trial therapy and just by observing the child's stuttering, the astute clinician can usually tell if the child has mild, moderate, or severe negative feelings and attitudes about his stuttering. Watch how the child responds when asked about his stuttering, and note how much he avoids stuttering. When the child does stutter, observe how calm he is and how consistent his eye contact is.

After the clinician has gotten to know the child a bit, she may want to administer a paper-and-pencil assessment of attitude. Figure 8.7 in the previous chapter depicts the A-19 scale (Guitar & Grims, 1977), a measure developed to assess children's communication attitudes. This scale consists of questions that were found to distinguish children who stutter from those who do not, but the differences were not great. Hence, if treatment is effective, a child's attitude about communication may change, although this has not been established by research. One of the best uses of such measures is as a starting place for discussions about how a child's stuttering is affecting him.

In addition to the A-19, the Communication Attitude Test has been tested on nonstuttering children (Brutten & Dunham, 1989) and shown to differentiate them from stuttering children (De Nil & Brutten, 1991; Vanryckeghem, Brutten, & Hernandez, 2005). It has also been found to have good test-retest reliability for this purpose (Vanryckeghem & Brutten, 1993; Vanryckegham, Vanrobayes, & De Niels, 2015).

Many informal methods of assessing feelings and attitudes are given in the workbook, *The School-Age Child Who Stutters: Working Effectively with Attitudes and Emotions* (Chmela & Reardon, 2001). These include such activities as a "Worry Ladder," in which a child lists his worries in a hierarchy, and "Hands Down," which elicits things the child likes and does not like about himself. Although the reliability and validity of these tools have not been determined, they provide useful starting points for communication about feelings and attitudes.

With some children, both formal and informal methods of assessing feelings will be productive during the evaluation. But, others will hold back until they have developed a trusting relationship with the clinician. Thus, clinicians should be mindful that information about a child's feelings and attitudes obtained in a first meeting may not be complete or accurate.

Other Speech and Language Disorders

In my discussion of the preschool child, I described the importance of screening speech sound production and language. The same abilities should be screened in the school-age child. You can use the Goldman-Fristoe Test of Articulation-3 (Goldman & Fristoe, 2015) and the Hodson Assessment of Phonological Patterns (HAPP-3) (3rd ed.) (Hodson, 2004) for speech sound production. For language, I would suggest the Clinical Evaluation of Language Fundamentals-5 Screening Test (Wiig, Secord, & Semel, 2013) and the Peabody Picture Vocabulary Test 5 (Dunn, 2018) and Expressive Vocabulary Test 2 (Williams, 2007) for vocabulary. The child may have a previously diagnosed language or speech sound production problem and may be in therapy. If so, the clinician should seek out details of any current or previous therapy. If a child is receiving or has received therapy for speech sound disorders or language disorders in the past, the clinician should find out details about the type of treatment the child received and how the child responded. Did his articulation or language difficulties improve? Did his stuttering first appear or worsen during treatment? If so, the clinician should pay particular attention to indications that the child may think of himself as a poor speaker and may believe that speaking is difficult. The interviews and questionnaires I suggested in the previous section on feelings and attitudes will help you explore this possibility, and the therapy approaches described for treatment of school-age children (Chapter 13) are designed to help a child regain confidence in his ability to speak easily and well.

Other Factors

Other factors, such as those described in the following sections, can influence the outcome of treatment. We recommend evaluating all factors that may have precipitated or are maintaining a child's stuttering so that they may be included in the child's overall treatment plan.

Physical Development

My main concern in this area is that motor development may be lagging behind language development. A child with speech-motor delays may benefit from therapy that helps him coordinate respiration, phonation, and articulation, thereby reducing stuttering. He may also benefit from procedures that help him learn to stutter easily and openly, rather than becoming tense and frustrated if his fluency breaks down under stress. Such children's treatment should also focus on building self-esteem, which may be low in children who are not well coordinated. One way to help build a child's confidence is to figure out what he is good at or what he would like to improve his mastery of and encourage that. I sometimes make up games, like tossing a ball into a wastebasket at greater and greater distances and have the child practice this during breaks from working on speech. Most children will delight in improving their skill at tasks at which they have some success, especially when they can do better than the clinician.

Cognitive Development

I try to find out whether or not cognitive stresses of school may be increasing the general demands experienced by the child, which I'll discuss further in a following section on academic adjustment. If a child has academic difficulty or a learning disability, we may need to adjust our approach to treatment to make sure that he understands our explanations and examples.

Social-Emotional Development

I am interested in how well a child fits in with his classmates, how comfortable he feels about talking and relating to others, and how often he feels a need to hide his stuttering. Some children are friendly and outgoing even though they stutter and are supported by their classmates. These social skills are a positive factor in their prognoses for recovery from stuttering. Other children may be very sensitive or self-conscious, and stuttering compounds their self-concern and keeps them from relating easily to others. Such children need help in relating more easily to their classmates. Evaluation of this component can be accomplished through teacher, parent, and child interviews; classroom observation may be helpful, too.

I am also concerned with the extent to which a child's home environment provides support and security. This information comes primarily from parent/family and child interviews. Parents often provide insight into conditions surrounding the onset of stuttering and conditions under which it gets better or worse. I sift through this information and, with the parents' help, determine whether something can be done to improve the child's self-esteem. For some children, school psychologists and private psychotherapy have been helpful in building self-esteem and helping them improve their social adjustment.

Academic Adjustment

Parent, child, and teacher interviews allow me to find out how well the child is doing in school and how much he likes it. Stuttering may appear for the first time or worsen when a child is under the stress of learning many new things. For example, reading aloud in class when just learning to read is likely to put substantial demands on a child's resources for language formulation and speech production. The child must make "second-order mappings of meanings and lexical units from speech" (Gibson, 1972) while simultaneously translating the written representation into units appropriate for speech production. Thus, some academic challenges may be more demanding for a child who stutters, and his stuttering in school should be understood in relation to this. In practical terms, clinicians can determine if a child needs extra help in certain academic areas through discussions with his teachers about which speaking situations in school are most difficult for him. If the child has more difficulty in certain academic situations, these should be given extra attention in treatment when planning generalization of more fluent speech.

Diagnosis

At this point in a clinic-based evaluation, the clinician pulls together the information collected from (1) the case history; (2) parent, teacher, and child interviews; (3) speech samples; and (4) classroom observations. This information helps the clinician determine the developmental/treatment level of the child's stuttering, which will give direction for selecting a treatment approach.

Occasionally, a school-age child is referred for stuttering, but it may not be at all clear whether he or she stutters or only has a high level of typical disfluency. You probably know some adults who are quite disfluent but don't consider themselves as stuttering and are not inhibited about talking. When a school-age child seems genuinely unbothered by his disfluency and does not avoid speaking or show excess tension or other escape behaviors, he should be given the option of therapy, but he should not be forced to accept it. I have talked with several adults who felt they were unfairly badgered about their speech and think they would have coped quite well and probably outgrown the disfluency except for the pressure on them to "do something about it." Instead, they became quite self-conscious of it and developed a serious stuttering problem. These may be real examples of the "diagnosogenic" theory of stuttering discussed in Chapter 6.

Despite the rare exceptions just described, most schoolchildren are at beginning or intermediate levels of stuttering. Beginning-level stuttering is most likely to occur in younger school-age children and is characterized by physical tension, hurry, escape behaviors, awareness of difficulty, and feelings of frustration, but lack of avoidance. The intermediate level also involves tension, hurry, escape behaviors, and frustration, but also includes notable avoidance behaviors as a result of fear and anticipation of stuttering. It is important that we understand whether the key stimuli for a child are only in his experience of being stuck in a stutter (escape behaviors) or are *also* in the anticipation of stuttering (avoidance behaviors). As I'll discuss in future chapters, treatment for these two levels of stuttering should be different because we need to decondition the link between anticipated stuttering and the preparatory tension that occurs when a child (or an adult) fears a stutter coming up and tries to fight it.

In addition to a child's stuttering behaviors and feelings, developmental and environmental pressures currently affecting the child must be considered in planning treatment. Such pressures can be uncovered from parent, teacher, and child interviews and the speech sample. Some pressures may result from other speech and language disorders, motor problems, or pressures in the child's home. Goals can be formulated with the parents' input for alleviating those pressures that can be changed and helping the child cope with those that can't be changed. Some pressures can be dealt with in treatment, but others may require parent counseling or referral to other professionals.

Closing Interview

When parents have been able to be involved in my evaluation of the child, the closing interview provides an opportunity to summarize my immediate impressions for the parents and make recommendations about treatment. It also provides an opportunity to discuss the crucial role parents can play in reducing environmental pressures. I point out the many beneficial things they have done about their child's speech and assure them that stuttering was not caused by anything they have done. Although some parents may have created conditions in which a child's predisposition to stutter has been transformed into a serious problem, it does not help to make an issue of this. Rather, we want to convince them that they are in a key position to help.

After describing clearly and simply what I observed about the child's stuttering, I summarize my thinking about appropriate treatment. I do this in only general terms because parents' main concerns at this time are not the details of treatment but the prospects for their child's future. Therefore, I rely on my experience to describe likely outcomes. For example, I might say that a combination of many factors will determine the child's outcome. These include the natural increases in fluency that occur as a child matures, feelings of self-acceptance that a child develops when he finds that people accept him whether or not he has trouble with his speech, and his learning ways to speak more fluently. When I talk about the child's prognosis, I always include some aspect of the parents' role, such as their acceptance of the child's speech or their participation in treatment, as part of the formula for recovery. Sometimes, a key aspect of the parents' acceptance of stuttering is realizing they are not responsible for curing it. If I feel that there is a good chance the child will have some stuttering remaining after therapy, I talk with the parents about this possibility, indicating that many people who have some stuttering remaining lead highly successful lives. A few who come to mind are Malcolm Fraser, a very successful businessman who founded the Stuttering Foundation, Billionaire Walter Annenberg who was ambassador to Great Britain, singer Ed Sheeran, and, if they are Democrats, Vice President Joe Biden.

After summarizing my impressions and describing some of the ingredients for recovery, I discuss some of the things the parents can do to promote recovery. Specific suggestions depend on findings from our interviews, but the sections on parent counseling in the chapter on treatment of stuttering in school-age children present general ideas for parents' involvement. Discussion of the family's involvement in therapy is the most important part of the closing interview and in fact may continue for several more meetings. If I treat the child directly and in a clinic rather than in a school setting, I meet with parents weekly as part of treatment. In these meetings, I continue to help them explore how various changes in the home environment can facilitate their child's fluency.

Public School Setting

The sequence indicated by Multi-Tiered System of Supports (MTSS—see the section on "Public School Considerations" earlier in this chapter) is that after a referral for stuttering is made, the SLP may start by informally assessing the child's speech by talking with him, visiting his classroom, and talking to his teacher. But first, before assessing the child's speech, the SLP should contact the child's family to ask permission to do so. This contact would require that the parents be told what the school's concerns are—in a general way—and it is an opportunity to find out if they have noticed the child's stuttering also and if they have their own concerns. Once permission is obtained and the child is assessed, the SLP may then start to meet the child's needs at a Tier 1 level by having the teacher try to give the child opportunities to talk in low-stress situations like in small groups. The teacher should also monitor the child's speech in class to further assess how much, if any, it interferes with his classroom participation. She can also become aware of how other children are responding to the child: are other children reacting to the child's speech? Interrupting? Teasing?

It is usually important to involve the child's parents/family in treatment if possible. The SLP can meet with them and, if appropriate, include the child so that suggestions can be explored about how the family can help the child's speech. Specific ideas are given in more detail in Chapter 13, on the treatment of school-age children.

Returning to the SLP's work with the child in school, after 4 to 6 weeks of Tier 1 classroom environment modification, the child's stuttering is not improving; the SLP can move to Tier 2, which involves trial "pullout" therapy (in the SLP's room) for 4 to 6 weeks, to see if that is meeting the child's needs. If the child needs further pullout therapy, the SLP may want to involve an Education Support Team (EST) (SLP, administrator, special educator, and appropriate others). The EST can develop a plan that includes goals and objectives and could continue for some time.

If the child has other challenges, such as reading problems, or if the child is quite severe, it may require a special education assessment and eventually an Individualized Education Plan (often referred to as an IEP). If this were the case, the formal evaluation by the team would be comprised of parent input, a detailed assessment of the child's stuttering using standardized measures such as the SSI and assessment of the child's attitudes and feelings, and demonstration that the child's speech (and/or other challenges) prevents him from obtaining an adequate education. In other words, the team needs to show that the child meets eligibility standards (severe enough challenges) and that the challenges (stuttering alone or combined with other handicapping conditions) are having an adverse effect on his education. Evidence of adverse effect can be obtained from measures of communicative functioning in school, such as the *Teacher's Assessment of Student Communication Competency* (Fig. 8.8) (Smith, McCauley, & Guitar, 2000), observations of the child in the school, and interviews with teachers and parents. Lisa Scott Trautman (personal communication, July 30, 2003) noted that adverse effects can be shown by demonstrating that the child cannot meet the school district's curriculum objectives because of his stuttering. Examples of such objectives might be that students will be active in class discussions or that students must be able to speak effectively in front of a group.

If the evaluation determines that the student is eligible for services, an IEP team, often headed by the SLP, develops measurable goals and short-term objectives (also called "benchmarks") as well as services to be provided that will help the student improve his performance in all aspects of the educational setting. These goals and objectives are considered in detail in the chapters on treatment of beginning and intermediate stuttering.

I have made available a series of video clips of our evaluation of a school-age child. You can find them on *thePoint*. The evaluation of this school-age child begins with an interview of his parents. The child, whose name is Cameron (Cam for short), is 7 years old and, as you will see, his stuttering has been getting worse. Cam had been more fluent as the result of treatment administered by a school clinician. Recently, however, the effects of the former treatment have worn off and Cam became increasingly upset by his stuttering. We began the interview by asking an open-ended question: "Why don't you tell me about Cam's speech?" The parents then describe Cam's stuttering and their empathetic concern about it. Interestingly, they mention that he felt better after watching the Stuttering Foundation video "For Kids by Kids." Cam refers to this video in the later clip about trial therapy. The parents also relate that Cam talked to his class about his stuttering, letting them know about it and asking them not to tease him. (Such openness about stuttering is rare in a child this age.)

In the second clip of Cam, notice the things he does when he stutters. For example, when he stutters on "ink," he simply prolongs the vowel, without a great deal of struggle and no avoidance. He doesn't shut off his voicing. This suggests that for him—at this point—being stuck in a stutter is not a terrifying experience requiring a big reaction. Later in this clip, he talks openly about his accessory behaviors, such as looking up at his hair when he stutters. This openness to discuss aspects of his stuttering so matter-of-factly is a very positive prognostic sign.

In the next clip, we experiment with trial therapy to see if Cam can tolerate staying in his stutter. As he talks about holding in his stutters rather than letting them out, he is unusually candid. Not many school-age children will be this open, and it usually takes some time to get them comfortable talking about their stuttering. In the trial therapy, I ask Cam to stay in the stutter and feel it loosen up. We talk about practicing in the therapy sessions and not having to do anything embarrassing with his speech in public.

The last clip is a wrap-up of the evaluation. This does not show everything we said and did, but you can get an idea of how we praise Cam and his family for the openness they are all showing about the stuttering. In the last few minutes, we discuss his coming to our clinic to work on his stuttering. That therapy, which Cam needed intermittently for several years, is discussed and shown in Chapter 13 on the treatment of stuttering in school-age children.

ADOLESCENT/ADULT

The assessment of an adolescent or adult can be very rewarding. Although some clients may be discouraged because they have been stuttering for years and are understandably skeptical that you can really help them, many are highly motivated to work on their speech and ready to begin this work during the evaluation. Your challenge is to take advantage of this motivation, get them working immediately, and give them realistic hope that hard work and resolve can change their speech and maybe their lives. Many aspects of my recommendations for assessment of an adult are adopted from Van Riper. Some of these I learned from his book, *The Treatment of Stuttering* (1973). But, other components came from my experience of being assessed by Van Riper himself, when I was 20 years old.

Preassessment

Clinic versus School Assessment

This section is written as though the evaluation is being carried out in a clinic rather than a school. When the setting is a public school, the evaluation process is determined by the Individuals with Disabilities Education Act (IDEA, 1997) and the laws of each state. The guidelines for this process were described in the previous section on evaluating a school-age child. For the adolescent, an additional consideration is his participation in the IEP process and his transition beyond high school. When a student reaches age 14, his input is sought by the IEP team, and he gradually becomes an active member of the team, not only with regard to his present situation but also in terms of his aspirations beyond secondary school. When a student reaches age 16, transition plans are a mandated part of the IEP. At age 18, students take over responsibility from their parents for signing off on documentation.

Case History Form

A case history form is sent to adolescent and adult clients several weeks before their appointment. A copy of this form is shown in Figure 9.5. Adolescents and their parents should be told that a collaborative effort to fill it out is permissible. This form allows the clinician to learn ahead of time whether the client referred for stuttering may have a different or additional disorder. The form, along with the OASES, gives the clinician information about the extent to which stuttering, if that is the problem, affects a client's life.

STUTTERING CASE HISTORY FORM – ADULT

Instructions: Please fill out this form in as much detail as possible. You can be assured that this information will be treated as confidential. If information is not available, please specify the reason so that we will know that the question has been considered. **Please return this form prior to your appointment.** Thank you.

Date: ______________________

Name: ______________________ Gender: M F

Address: ______________________ Telephone: (home) ______________

______________________ (work) ______________

E-Mail Address: ______________________ Cell Phone: ______________

Date of Birth: ______________________ Place of Birth: ______________

Referring Physician: ______________________

Marital Status: ______________________

Education Level: ______________________ Occupation: ______________

Employed by: ______________________

Referred to this Center by: ______________________

Name of spouse/nearest relative: ______________________

Address: ______________________ Telephone: ______________

HISTORY OF STUTTERING

Are there other individuals in your family background or immediate family who stutter?

____

Give approximate age at which your stuttering was first noticed: ______________________

Who first noticed or mentioned the stuttering? ______________________

In what situation did this occur? ______________________

Describe any situations or conditions that you associate with the onset of stuttering:

____

____

____

What were the first signs of your stuttering? (If you don't remember, you might ask your parents or siblings.) ______________________

____

Was the stuttering always the same or did it occur in several different ways? ______________________

____

If they occurred in different ways, how were they different from one another? ______________________

____

Figure 9.5 Case history form for adults and adolescents.

Did the first blocks seem to be located in the tongue? lips? chest? diaphragm? or throat?

____

Approximately how long did each block (on one word) seem to last? ______________________

____

Was the stuttering easy or was there force at the time when the stuttering was first noticed?

____

Were the words that were stuttered at the beginning of sentences, or were they scattered throughout the sentence being said? ____

____

When stuttering first began, was there any avoidance of speaking because of it? Give examples, if any. ____

____

At the time when stuttering was first noticed, what was your reaction?

Awareness that speech was different? __________ Indifference to it? __________

Surprise? __________ Anger or frustration? __________ Shame? __________

Fear of stuttering again? __________ Other? __________

What attempts have been made to treat the stuttering problem? ______________________

____

DEVELOPMENT OF STUTTERING

Since the onset, have there been any changes in stuttering symptoms? Check those that are appropriate.

Increase in number of repetitions per word __________

Change in amount of force used (increased? decreased?) __________

Increase in amount of stuttering __________

Increase in length of block __________

Periods of no stuttering __________

More precise in speech attempts __________

Lowered voice loudness __________

Slower rate of speech __________

Change in location of force when stuttering, if force is present __________

Looking away from listener __________

Describe any of the above that apply ____

____

____

Figure 9.5 *(Continued)*

Were there any periods (weeks/months) when the stuttering disappeared? ____________________

____

Were there any periods (weeks/months) when the stuttering increased? ____________________

____

Can you give an explanation for these "worse" periods? ______________________________

____

CURRENT STUTTERING

Are there any situations that are particularly difficult? If so, please describe. ______________

____

List any situations that never cause difficulty. ______________________________________

____

Answer the following "yes" or "no" as they apply to your stuttering. Do you stutter when you

Talk to young children? __________ Say your name? __________

Answer direct questions? __________ Talk to adults, superiors at work, teachers? __________

Use new words that are unfamiliar? __________ Use the telephone? __________

Read aloud? __________ Recite memorized material? __________

Ask questions? __________ Talk to strangers? __________ Speak when tired? __________

Speak when excited? __________ Talk to family members? __________

Talk to friends? __________

Do you know any stutterers? __________ Describe your relationship with them. ______________

____

Do you feel that stuttering interferes with your career? __________ Social relationships? __________

Success in school? __________ Success on the job? __________ Daily life? __________

Describe what your stuttering currently looks and sounds like. ________________________

____

____

MEDICAL, DEVELPMENTAL AND FAMILY HISTORY

If possible, describe mother's health during pregnancy and/or your birth history (i.e., complications). ____

____

____

Describe any development problems during infancy or early childhood (i.e., late to walk, feeding problems, food allergies, late to talk). ____

____

Figure 9.5 *(Continued)*

Are you: Right-handed? __________ Left-handed? __________ Both? __________ Is there any evidence of visual, artistic abilities in your family? ______________________________

Were you sensitive as a child? ______________________________

Would you describe yourself as sensitive now? ______________________________

List your history of any significant illnesses, injuries, and/or operations:

Date	Fever	Complications	Treatment	Physician

List all present physical disabilities. ______________________________

____

Any chronic illnesses, allergies, or physical conditions? ______________________________

____

Vision normal? __________ Hearing normal? __________ List any medication you take regularly or are taking currently. ______________________________

Describe any learning or reading problems you experienced as a child or are currently experiencing. ______________________________

____

Do any members of your family have speech or language problems or learning disabilities? If so, describe. ______________________________

____

SOCIAL HISTORY

Hobbies ______________________________

Leisure time activities ______________________________

Describe any previous therapy you have participated in to aid your fluency. When? Where? With whom? Length of time? The outcome? ______________________________

____

____

Add anything else you would like to include and think might be important: ______________________________

____

____

In addition, what goals would you like to see accomplished as a result of this evaluation? __________

____

____

Signature: ______________________________ Date: __________

Figure 9.5 *(Continued)*

Attitude Questionnaires

I assess clients' communication attitudes through observations, interview questions, and questionnaires. Because I want to be able to analyze completed questionnaires before the diagnostic interview, I prefer to send them to clients and ask them to complete and return the questionnaires before the interview. If this is not possible, clients can complete them when they arrive for an evaluation before the initial interview or, as a less desirable alternative, after the initial interview. Prior to the interview, follow-up questions based on information from the case history and questionnaires, which are described in the section on feelings and attitudes, can be prepared to further explore a client's attitudes.

Audio/Video Recording

It is important to sample a client's speech in several situations to get an adequate picture of his stuttering. I ask clients to video or audio record themselves talking in one or two different situations outside the clinic and get the recording to me prior to the evaluation. It is usually easy for clients to record themselves talking to someone on the phone, recording only their own voices and not the person on the other end of the line, therefore not violating the other person's privacy. Some clients can also record themselves talking face-to-face with a friend or family member, obtaining their permission to record. If I listen to the recording(s) before an evaluation, I am better prepared to understand the client's stuttering and to plan various trial-therapy strategies.

Assessment

Interview

I begin by welcoming the client and reviewing the procedures I will use to evaluate his stuttering, such as interviewing him about his stuttering and his feelings and attitudes, video recording his speaking and reading, examining what he does when he stutters, and trying to determine if he can change it. I let him know that after the initial part of his evaluation, I will ask him to wait while I analyze the information I've obtained before meeting with him to share my findings and recommendations. If there are any forms or questionnaires I haven't already obtained from him, I'll have him complete those while I analyze the other data. I video record the interview, and even though I have indicated that video recording will be part of the evaluation, I ask the client again, just prior to turning on a video recorder, whether he minds if I record our conversation.

I begin our interview with an open-ended question such as "Tell me about the problem that brings you here today," or "Why don't you tell me about your stuttering?" The first question might be used if I don't know what is motivating the client to come for an evaluation at this time; the second question I use when I already know from prior information why the client has come right now.

Once a client has had a chance to describe his speech problem, I ask further questions to try to get a deeper understanding. The following are typical questions that I ask with a brief commentary about why I'm asking them. Sometimes, I group several questions together (e.g., a question to start the client talking about a particular topic and follow-up questions that I ask if the first question doesn't elicit all of the desired information). I ask only one question at a time, listen carefully to the client's response, and try to understand the client's underlying feelings.

1. **When did you begin to stutter? How has the way you stutter changed over the years?**
   I realize that in answering the first part of this question, a client may just be reporting what parents told him about his stuttering. The accuracy of his response may be questionable, but at least I'll learn his perception of the onset. The second part of the question—about changes over the years—may reveal what kinds of things affect the way the client stutters. Does he stutter more severely because of a recent job change or a threat to his self-esteem, such as a divorce or loss of employment? Less frequently, I may find out that a client began to stutter in late adolescence or as an adult. If so, I would want to consider the possibility of neurogenic or psychogenic stuttering, which is discussed briefly in the upcoming section on "Diagnosis" and more fully in Chapter 15, on other fluency disorders.
2. **What do you believe caused you to stutter?**
   This may give some insights about a client's motivation. For example, a woman whose speech I once evaluated reported that her mother and several brothers stuttered and that her stuttering was therefore a genetic problem that could not be helped. This led us to confront the issue of whether or not she was likely to change. (Yes, change is quite possible no matter what a client's genetic history.)

   In addition, I sometimes find that clients have misinformation about possible causes of their stuttering. If I can give them more appropriate information, their attitudes about the problem may change, and their motivation may increase. I have met individuals who come to the evaluation believing that their problem is entirely psychological. After I discuss current views of stuttering, they are relieved to know that they are likely able to modify their speech without long-term psychotherapy.
3. **Does anyone else in your family stutter?**
   I might find that a parent stutters, which can be significant because a parent's attitudes about his or her own stuttering may have had a profound effect on the client. Moreover, knowing about other family members who stutter and how they have responded to it may provide

a better understanding of the factors related to this client's stuttering, which may be useful in treatment. For example, someone I am interviewing may have had a parent who stuttered but who never talked about it. I might then want to explore whether the individual I am working with feels especially ashamed of his stuttering or, on the other hand, whether it gives him an important bond with the parent, or both.

4. **Have you ever had therapy for your stuttering? What did the therapy consist of? How effective do you think it was?**
This information is important in planning therapy. For example, if a client had received a type of therapy that he felt did not help, it would be unwise to use that type of therapy with this client. But, if a client has had success with therapy but has regressed slightly or moved away before treatment was finished, using this type of therapy again may be most appropriate. It is important that clinicians be familiar with various types of therapy that clients may have undergone. Most current therapies emphasize either modifying stuttering behaviors (**stuttering modification**) or learning to talk in ways that eliminate stuttering (**fluency shaping**).
5. **Has your stuttering changed or caused you more problems recently? Why did you come in for help at the present time?**
Responses to these questions allow clinicians to see the current problems faced by the client and also obtain some inkling of the client's motivation. For example, a client may have been offered a promotion if he can improve his speech or may have recently learned of the clinic's treatment program and is hoping for some relief from a long-standing problem. The following four questions about the client's pattern of stuttering are closely related to one another:
6. **Are there times or situations when you stutter more? Less? What are they?**
7. **Do you avoid certain speaking situations in which you expect to stutter? If so, which ones?**
8. **Do you avoid certain words on which you expect to stutter? Do you substitute one word for another if you expect to stutter? Do you talk around words or topics so you won't stutter?**
9. **Do you use any special movements or extra sounds to get words out? Escape behaviors?**
These four questions will provide information that is useful in planning therapy because they tell us something about the client's most difficult situations, how he feels about them, and how he deals with them. This information may also corroborate what has been learned from the questionnaires that the client completed and will also reveal how aware he is of his stuttering behaviors.
10. **Have your academic or vocational choices or performance been affected because you stutter? How?**
The client's answers can be used to help plan later stages of treatment in which new behaviors and new challenges are attempted. They may also prompt the clinician to refer clients in later stages of treatment to an academic or vocational counselor to help them make more appropriate choices for themselves.
11. **Have your relationships with people been affected because you stutter? How?**
As with Question 10, I can use this information to plan a client's hierarchy of generalization, moving from easy to difficult social situations gradually if the client finds social interactions difficult. I also need to know how much a client blames his stuttering for any of the difficulties he has in social interactions. A client may be socially inhibited because he is sensitive and vulnerable to expected listener reactions. Such sensitivity can be assessed by observing his facial expressions and body movements while stuttering as indicators of affect. If he appears to be relatively unaffected emotionally by his stuttering but professes to have difficulty relating to people, he may benefit from counseling or psychotherapy that focuses on resolving this interpersonal difficulty.
The decision to refer an individual for psychotherapy as an adjunct to stuttering therapy can seldom be made in the evaluation session. It may be that a few therapy sessions are needed to learn more about a person and to develop the client's trust before a successful referral can be made. If psychotherapy is recommended too hastily, a client may believe that I think his stuttering is too great a problem for me to handle, perhaps an insurmountable problem or one that I secretly believe is due to a psychological disorder. However, if I work with him and he starts making some progress before I refer, he will likely feel supported and may be more likely to benefit from psychotherapy.
12. **What are your feelings or attitudes toward your stuttering? What do you think other people think about your stuttering?**
A client's responses will be used to help determine some of the foci of treatment, such as desensitization procedures to decrease fear as well as shame or guilt about stuttering. Perceptions about others' views of his stuttering may need to be confronted with various "reality-testing" tasks to find out what people really think.
13. **What are your family's (parents', spouse's, children's) feelings, attitudes, and reactions toward your stuttering and toward the prospect of your being in therapy?**
This information can identify sources that may positively or negatively affect a client's motivation and may be an important consideration in planning therapy.
14. **Is there anything else that you think we ought to know about your stuttering?**
This gives the client a chance to get anything off his chest that he may be holding back or an opportunity to discuss issues that occurred to him only after other questions were asked.

15. Do you have any questions you'd like to ask me? Sometimes, an adolescent or adult has questions about stuttering that he has been reluctant to ask, and this may give the clinician an opportunity to answer them. On the other hand, a client may want to ask about the length and type of treatment or other issues that are best dealt with after his assessment is completed. In this case, the clinician explains why he needs to delay responding but will keep the questions in mind to answer during the closing interview.

Speech Sample

In this part of the evaluation, the client's overt stuttering behaviors are assessed. Although I always video record the entire evaluation, if the client has given permission, I pay particular attention to the recording of this section because I will need to analyze it carefully afterward. In the first 5 or 10 minutes of the interview, I try to let the client talk as much as possible without my interrupting or asking too many questions. This is a conversation, but one in which the client does most of the talking—at first. Clinicians use a variety of procedures for assessing overt stuttering. Next, I shall describe in detail the tool I currently use and then note other available options.

Stuttering Severity

As indicated in the previous chapter, stuttering severity is usually measured using the Stuttering Severity Instrument (currently, SSI-4; Riley, 2009), a moderately reliable tool that is commonly used to assess the severity of stuttering. To obtain appropriate samples, I have the client talk about a familiar topic, such as his work, school, hobbies, vacations, sports, or entertainment. It is important to get about at least 300 syllables of the client's talking, so 5 or 10 minutes is usually enough, depending on the client's fluency. Then, I provide the client material at an appropriate reading level, such as the passages in the SSI examiner's manual, and ask him to read aloud for about 3 minutes to get 200 or more syllables of reading.

As I noted earlier, we often gather more than one sample of spontaneous speech from adults and adolescents. A sample of speech during a telephone conversation in the clinic can be video recorded and scored using the SSI. In addition, I use samples the client has brought or sent in. If the sample from another environment is audio recorded rather than video recorded, I score it for both frequency of stuttering and speech rate, as described below.

Other Measures of Stuttering

If I am assessing stuttering many times throughout the course of treatment or assessing samples that I cannot visually analyze, such as those audio recorded by a client in his natural environment, I use a combination of frequency of stuttering (percentage of syllables stuttered) and speech rate (syllables spoken per minute). These measures, which were first described in Andrews and Ingham (1971), together require much less time than the SSI.

Starkweather (1991) has presented a case for capturing the amount of time that stuttering takes. This is done by totaling the duration of all disfluencies and pauses in a sample and dividing this total by the overall time spent in speaking, thereby giving the clinician a measure of how much an individual's stuttering interferes with the rate with which he can communicate information.

As part of a determined effort to improve the reliability of stuttering measures, Ingham and his colleagues (Cordes & Ingham, 1999; Ingham, Cordes, & Finn, 1993; Ingham, Cordes, & Gow, 1993) developed a time interval system of assessment. They have shown that when judges determine whether or not 4-second intervals of continuous speech contain one or more stutters, interjudge reliability is higher than when moments of stuttering are counted; however, the clinical usefulness of this procedure has not been determined.

Speech Rate

In addition to measuring stuttering severity using the SSI, I also assess a client's speech rate. I believe, as many other clinicians do, that speaking rate often reflects the severity of stuttering, as well as its effect on communication. If a client's speech rate is markedly slower than normal, communication may be difficult for him. A description of the procedure for measuring speech rate was given in Chapter 8, "Preliminaries to Assessment."

Normal speaking rates of adults range from around 115 to 165 words per minute, or about 162 to 230 syllables per minute, with a mean of 196 syllables per minute (Andrews & Ingham, 1971). Adults' normal rates for reading aloud are faster, ranging from about 150 to 190 words per minute (Darley & Spriestersbach, 1978), or about 210 to 265 syllables per minute (Andrews & Ingham, 1971).

Pattern of Disfluencies

Throughout my evaluation of adult or adolescent stutterers, I observe the client's patterns of stuttering. For example, I try to roughly determine the proportions of core behaviors that are repetitions, prolongations, or blocks and ask myself a number of questions about the client's stuttering. During blocks, where and how does he shut off airflow or voicing? What are his escape and avoidance behaviors? Does he end the stutters quickly with pushing and tension? Is he able to tolerate being in blocks, or does he speak in unusual or vague ways to avoid stuttering? More details on various escape and avoidance patterns can be found in Chapter 7 on the development of stuttering. My aim, as I study the client's stuttering, is to figure out how much fear of stuttering there is. If there are a lot of avoidances and urgent escape behaviors, I would hypothesize that the client has a fair bit of fear of stuttering, and I need to focus on that, first.

As I explore the behaviors that constitute a client's stuttering, I comment on them, question him about how typical this sample of his stuttering is, and ask about the escape and avoidance behaviors we've observed. If a client doesn't seem too uncomfortable confronting his stuttering, I ask him to teach me how to stutter like he does, and we work together, with both the client and myself emulating his various types of stuttering. This does not need to be an exhaustive exploration, because I will do much more in treatment. Here, I am trying to accomplish three tasks: (1) begin to decrease fear a little, by modeling an "approach" rather than "avoidance" attitude toward stuttering, showing calmness and objectivity about behaviors that the client may feel are shameful and perhaps even terrifying, (2) study the client's emotional reaction when he comes face-to-face with his stuttering and perhaps reduce some of his fear, and (3) teach both of us about what the client does when he stutters so that he can begin to become less emotional about it and thus, eventually, stutter in a way that is close to typical speech.

Trial Therapy

I try therapy techniques with clients during their assessment sessions for several reasons. First, I try to get an idea of how a client responds to different therapy approaches, which provides me with information I may use in talking with him about possible treatments. Second, trial therapy can help me to make a differential diagnosis between developmental stuttering and stuttering with a neurological or psychological etiology. Third, it gives clients a preview of things to come and provides them with motivation to follow through on treatment. There is a fourth reason: to give the client hope that he can change.

I begin by asking a client to modify his stuttering, which can be done easily in the context of studying his patterns of disfluency, as described in the preceding section. In fact, this exploration of stuttering with a client is a condensed version of the first stage of treatment that aims to change stuttering to an easier pattern. Once a client is able to emulate his stuttering to a small degree, I carry out trial therapy by coaching him through the following sequence:

1. First, I encourage him to stutter, telling him we must have a sample of the behavior we are trying to change. Then, I ask him to "freeze" during a moment of stuttering but maintain the level of physical tension and posture of his stuttering as I encourage him to stay in the moment of stuttering. In other words, I ask him to catch a stutter and prolong it. This may require a little or a lot of modeling of how to hold a moment of stuttering right on the sound that's being stuttered. This is easier with a continuant sound, like /m/, but will be harder and need more coaching for plosives, such as /b/. You will probably have to model for the client how to prolong the posture required for holding a stutter on a plosive. It is key that you and he identify the exact posture that is associated with the moment of stuttering and hold onto it. When I model this for the client, after I demonstrate staying in the moment of stuttering, I always finish the word slowly and easily, which I will ask him to do, later. It is important that during this activity, the clinician praises the client enthusiastically for catching and holding onto a moment of stuttering. This helps the counterconditioning process—pairing a positive stimulus with a behavior about which the client feels negative. Also, anything you can do to inject humor into this process will help the counterconditioning.
2. Have the client become aware of what he is doing right when he gets into the stutter. For example, where is he holding back sound or airflow? Lips? Tongue? Larynx? All three? As you are helping him explore what he's doing when he stutters, use plenty of praise for being able to stay in the stutter. This is an experience charged with fear and frustration for most adolescent and adults who stutter. Try to create something very different—a satisfying experience that you provide by rewarding their maintaining of this stuttering moment. It's similar to treatment for a phobia: staying in contact with a feared object (a spider or even, in some cases, a rabbit) reduces fear if there is reward provided by another person. It has been said that an individual's physical awareness of what he is doing with his body as he stutters can be an antidote to the fear he might otherwise be feeling (Zebrowski, personal communication, October 18, 2011, channeling the famous clinician Dean Williams). This may be related to the use of proprioceptive awareness to manage stuttering, which may be effective because it bypasses a faulty auditory monitoring system (Van Riper, 1973).
3. Have the client change his behaviors that are maintaining stutters by (1) releasing excess physical tension wherever he can feel it, (2) starting to move structures that are being rigidly held, (3) getting voicing or airflow going, and/or (4) allowing himself to breathe. I may stop a client's trial therapy here if he is unable to release the physical tension or does it only with obvious difficulty and frustration.

If a client seems able to make these changes easily, I go one step further. I ask him to hold onto the stutter, which has become voluntary by now, and to prolong the airflow or voicing for several seconds (while I tell him how great it is that he can do this!) and then produce the remainder of the word slowly. (Some of my clients call this "catch and release.") If a client is able to do this with coaching, I ask him to do it while reading without my coaching. This is enough. No matter how much or how little our client is able to do, I want to stop when he is feeling successful.

Another approach to trial therapy—one that I would only use for a client who seems to have little or no fear of stuttering—is to change the client's habitual way of talking so that stuttering is decreased substantially or prevented. Adolescents and adults who fear stuttering, especially those with avoidance behaviors, will probably continue to have fear even if they learn a new way of talking to (temporarily) replace stuttering. The fear will often create a relapse in the new fluency. However, with those few clients who are unafraid of stuttering, I experiment with a slow way of talking that produces fluency. I begin by reducing my own speech rate as I describe the aim of this exercise to the client, which is to produce words very, very slowly. I use a written sentence that begins with a vowel or a glide, going over it word by word, teaching the client to use gradual and gentle onsets of voicing and to stretch each sound, whether vowel or consonant. This is essentially the "prolonged speech" or "fluency-facilitating targets" used by some fluency-shaping approaches, such as the Camperdown Program (O'Brian et al., 2017) and the Fluency Plus Program (Kroll & Scott-Sulsky, 2010). The clinician needs to provide a good model for each word and to give feedback frequently. When words are produced slowly enough with each part of the speech production system (respiration, phonation, and articulation) moving in slow motion and without excess tension, then fluency results. After a client is able to produce each word of the sentence in this way, he is then coached to produce the entire sentence, linking each word to the next. Breath supply should be monitored closely, so that pauses for breath are taken whenever the client would take a breath naturally. Again, accurate modeling and frequent feedback are crucial at earlier stages of treatment.

As an example, the sentence, "Apples are a red fruit," should take from 15 to 20 seconds to produce, with a pause for a new breath after the word "a." The /p/ in "Apples," the /d/ in "red," and the /t/ in "fruit" each should be produced without stopping airflow, making these plosives sound like fricatives. If clients are particularly adept at this, they can be taken all the way to saying short sentences in conversational speech that are produced in this slow, fluent manner. However, clients who have difficulty should be coached only through the production of the short, written sentence, and care should be taken to stop this activity before they experience failure.

This therapeutic approach—fluency shaping—I would only use with the rare client who shows little fear of stuttering and who appears to have a relatively robust (nonsensitive) temperament.

Feelings and Attitudes

A variety of questionnaires can be used to assess various aspects of a stutterer's feelings and attitudes about communication and stuttering. In Chapter 8, I described those questionnaires that I use regularly. These include the OASES (Yaruss & Quesal, 2006), the Modified Erickson Scale of Communication Attitudes (S-24) (Andrews & Cutler, 1974), the Stutterer's Self-Rating of Reactions to Speech Situations (Johnson, Darley, & Spriestersbach, 1952), the Perceptions of Stuttering Inventory (Woolf, 1967), and the Locus of Control of Behavior Scale (Craig, Franklin, & Andrews, 1984). Any of these (I might use only the first three) can be sent to the client before the evaluation and returned so that the clinician can score them ahead of time and have a preliminary idea about the client's emotions related to his stuttering.

Much of the exploration of emotions, however, is done informally, rather than through the questionnaires cited in the last paragraph. This work goes throughout the treatment, but is started in the initial evaluation interview. As feelings are being expressed and the clinician creates an atmosphere of calmness and tolerance, the client-clinician relationship is begun. As they converse, the clinician tries to understand the client's feelings, sometimes asking questions to elicit them and sometimes restating the expressed feelings in a way that demonstrates she is interested in them and accepts them. This approach is therapeutic. It is described by Carl Rogers in his book *Counseling and Psychotherapy* (1942). In this book, Rogers not only describes how the clinician works but also provides a detailed transcript of his work with a client who stutters (and has other issues) in his chapter "The Case of Herbert Bryan." We will revisit the counseling relationship in the next chapter, but for now, I will make a few comments about eliciting feelings in the evaluation interview.

In the assessment interview, described earlier, I wait until I have recorded about 5 to 10 minutes of the client's relatively uninterrupted speech to use for assessment of stuttering, and then I begin to explore the client's stuttering and his feelings about it. As I suggested in the section on "The Pattern of Disfluencies," I often stop the client and ask about the stutters that he has and we study them together. As I do this, I also probe the client's feeling with such comments as "When you get stuck like that, how does it feel?" or "If you get in a block like that when you are talking to someone what are the feelings that go with it?" Before the assessment interview begins, I try to read the client's intake questionnaires, such as the OASES or Erickson S-24, to get some ideas about what are some of the emotional issues related to his stuttering. I use that information to explore the client's feelings—both those about being a person who stutters (such as shame) and those that rise up when the client is (1) anticipating a stutter, (2) is trapped in a stutter, and (3) has just stuttered. It may also help to have the client try to get in touch with sensations within his body that are associated with these feelings.

Other Speech and Language Behaviors

As I interact with a client during the interview, I informally assess his comprehension and production of language, his articulation, and his voice. I also screen his hearing. If I suspect that there may be an articulation, language, voice, or hearing problem, I follow up with further evaluations. Adolescent language assessment procedures can be found in Nippold (2016), Nelson (2010), and the Screening Test of Adolescent Language (Prather, Breecher, Stafford, & Wallace,

1980), although dated is still useful. Procedures for assessment of speech sound production can be found in Bernthal, Bankson, and Flipsen (2017) and in Velleman (2015). I let a client's concern about other disorders guide us in treatment. If, as I have found occasionally, a stuttering client also produces distorted /s/ or /r/ sounds, I discuss it with him. If he is not concerned, I don't believe it is necessary to treat that problem. However, if I believe that an articulation, language, or other problem handicaps a client communicatively, I advise treatment for that problem also. Sometimes, I deal with voice problems differently. I have found that some stutterers may be hoarse, but I suspect this may be the result of laryngeal tension related to stuttering. If stuttering treatment is successful, hoarseness may disappear. Again, I take my cue from the client. If the problem bothers him and isn't remediated by treatment, I address it. If hoarseness is of recent origin and not associated with a cold, I may refer him for an otolaryngological examination to rule out serious laryngeal pathology.

Other Factors

In this section, I will discuss the evaluation of the following factors: intelligence, academic adjustment, psychological adjustment, and vocational adjustment. Each of these factors can affect the treatment of an adult or adolescent stutterer and therefore must be considered in planning therapy. The factors are considered briefly here, but some are covered in depth in the chapter on other fluency disorders (Chapter 15).

If a client has below-normal intelligence, he may have difficulty following the regimen of a typical therapy program. Usually, clinicians know beforehand if a client scheduled for an evaluation has Down syndrome or some other condition often associated with significantly below-average intelligence. An adolescent who stutters who has been identified as developmentally delayed will likely already be receiving special education. Adults, too, are usually identified as developmentally delayed if this is the case, and either the referral source will report this or a guardian will have filled out the case history form. I have been recently been working with an adult who stutters and has Down syndrome. He has been able to benefit from a treatment program focused on reducing avoidance behaviors and learning to stutter in an easier way.

Problems of academic adjustment in an adolescent who stutters usually become apparent from either the original referral or interviews with the child's teachers as part of the evaluation process. These interviews are described in more detail in the section on the school-age child. An example of poor academic adjustment relevant to stuttering could be a student's conflict with a teacher who insists on oral presentations that the student is unwilling to do. The IDEA 1997 process mandates a team approach to solving such problems. This process (e.g., MTSS) was described earlier and will be given more attention in the chapters on treatment.

The research reviewed in Chapters 2 and 3 suggests that there are no group differences in the psychological health of stutterers and nonstutterers. However, we sometimes see individuals who stutter who do not function well in their environment. They may be unable to achieve a satisfying marriage, may be unable to hold a job, or are socially withdrawn. Clinicians need to be alert to the effects that adjustment problems may have on treatment. If psychological problems are suspected of interfering with treatment progress, the clinician may wish to refer the client for a psychological evaluation. In such cases, the clinician should take care to ask professional colleagues for recommendations regarding the most effective psychotherapists in the area.

Psychological problems that are relevant to stuttering also may become apparent during the interview when the onset of stuttering is explored. Sudden onset after a psychological trauma, particularly if onset is in late adolescence or adulthood, may indicate a more psychologically based stuttering. I have found that if the psychological effects of the trauma have subsided, an adolescent or adult client may respond well to the integrated approach to treatment described in Chapter 14. If it is clear that psychological factors are still affecting the client's speech and behavior or if there is doubt, I refer the client for a psychological evaluation. Unless the disorder is a psychosis, in which case stuttering therapy may not be recommended until that problem is being well managed, clients with psychological problems may respond well to a combination of psychotherapy and stuttering therapy.

Interview with Parents of an Adolescent

Adolescents strive to become more and more independent of their parents, and I have found that therapy works best if an adolescent is treated as an adult. I begin fostering independence by talking first to teenage clients separately from their parents so that they can give me their own views of the situation and how they view the prospect of treatment. I ask them if they would like to be present when I talk with their parents and if there's anything the adolescent client has said to me that he would not like me to share with his parents. In the next paragraph, I'll describe an interview with the teen's parents when he has requested not to be present in the interview.

I begin the interview by asking the parents to describe the problem as they see it and encourage them to express their fears, concerns, and frustrations, as I listen carefully. I try to get an understanding of how their child functions within the family and usually ask such questions as "What is his stuttering like at home?" "How does he seem to feel about it—is he embarrassed or does he show fear of talking or anger about his speech?" "How do you feel about it?" "What are your and other family members' reactions to it?" "What do you do when he stutters?" "Has he been seen anywhere else for therapy?" "If so, what were the results?" Even though I am putting some of these questions in groups, I am careful to ask one question at a time and listen carefully to the answer before I ask another question. Although parents, in an interview without the teen, may ask what can be done to help their child and what they should do, I prefer to wait until I am meeting with both the parents and the teen before answering these questions.

If I am meeting with the parents and the teen together, at some point, I let the parents know that I will respect the teen's confidentiality in terms of what he shares with me when we are working together. In a joint meeting with parents and teen, I also try to begin with a discussion of all the good things the teen has going for him—such as his participation in sports, achievements in school, friendships, or abilities with electronic devices. Remember we will be talking about the teen's stuttering—something he probably feels at least a little ashamed about. Thus, the atmosphere needs to be leavened with talk of the teen's good qualities so that both parents and teen feel hope about the future. Previously when I interviewed the teen, I have probably done some trial therapy, and, if the teen has given me permission, he and I share how well he is able to confront his stuttering (if that is the case). We might then let the parents know what sort of things the teen will be doing with his stutters so the parents can appreciate that if stutters appear worse or more evident or longer at times, it is all part of the plan.

I meet with the parents and teenage clients together to seek mutual agreement about their respective roles in treatment. This is often an important time. It serves to let teens know that I respect their ability to work independently from the parents, and it serves to let the parents know that they can be most helpful by being supportive but not directive.

Diagnosis

After I gather the information just described, I need to determine whether the client stutters and, if so, what treatment level is appropriate. Typically, teenage clients are more likely to have advanced rather than intermediate-level stuttering; however, some are still in the intermediate stage. But first, let us consider the possibility that a teenager turns out *not* to have a problem with stuttering.

In rare cases, teens who are normally but highly disfluent may be referred by teachers, employers, or friends. Most have phrase repetitions, circumlocutions, revisions, and hesitations, which are the types of disfluencies described in Chapter 7 as normal. Such disfluencies are observed relatively infrequently after children's elementary school years; however, some adolescents and adults may simply be at the disfluent end of the continuum of normal fluency. In addition to the differences in type and number of disfluencies, secondary behaviors and negative feelings and attitudes will be absent. Our role in such cases is to explain to the individual and to the referring person (if this is a referral) that this kind of speech is not abnormal and need not be of concern. It may also be emphasized to the referring source that excessive attention to these disfluencies may be more harmful than helpful. If the client or referring person feels strongly that the disfluent speech interferes with communication, a fluency-oriented treatment described in the chapters on treating intermediate and advanced stuttering may be offered to the client.

Another need for differential diagnosis, in addition to identifying cases of normal disfluency, is ensuring that cluttering, neurogenic disfluency, and psychogenic disfluency be identified and distinguished from "typical" or "developmental" stuttering. Moreover, it is also necessary to rule out disfluencies caused by word-finding difficulties that we might find in a person with a learning disability.

Some of the salient features of cluttering in adults and adolescents are rapid, sometimes unintelligible speech; frequent repetitions of syllables, words, or phrases; lack of awareness or concern about their speech; disorganized thought processes; and language problems. Cluttering often coexists with stuttering, and both disorders may respond to a highly structured, fluency-shaping approach for treatment. Evaluation and treatment procedures for cluttering are described in Chapter 15.

Neurogenic disfluency in adolescents or adults is usually the result of stroke, head trauma, or neurological disease. Symptoms are likely to be repetitive disfluencies but may include blockages as well. Because stuttering commonly begins in childhood, if a client reports onset of stuttering after age 12, a neurogenic-based disorder is a possibility. In almost all such cases, onsets of neurogenic-based fluency problems are clearly linked to a well-defined episode of neurological damage. A section of Chapter 15 is devoted to evaluation and treatment of neurogenic stuttering.

Disfluency that begins in adolescence or adulthood can also result from psychological trauma. When late-onset disfluencies are seen that are associated with psychological stress and conflict or the onset of a psychiatric condition, psychogenic disfluency should be suspected. Traditional treatments, such as those described in the chapters on treatment of intermediate and advanced stuttering, may or may not be helpful. The patient should be referred for both psychological and neurological assessments, so that treatment needed in these areas will be identified and provided. See Chapter 15 for more information.

When a clinician determines that stuttering treatment would be appropriate for a client, whether the stuttering had a typical onset during early childhood or has another etiology, the focus turns to a consideration of what level of treatment to select for the client. As I indicated earlier, adult and adolescents are most likely to be at advanced developmental and treatment levels. Signs of this level include the core behaviors of repetitions, prolongations, and blocks, all with tension; the secondary behaviors of escape and especially *avoidance*; and strong negative feelings and attitudes about communication in general and stuttering in particular.

Determining Developmental and Treatment Level

The determination of a developmental/treatment level for an adolescent or adult stutterer is based largely on the client's age. Intermediate and advanced treatment approaches are well suited for clients whose core behaviors are blocks, who have escape and avoidance behaviors as secondary symptoms, and whose attitudes about speech are relatively negative. A client suited to the advanced-level treatment will usually have more entrenched negative attitudes about speech and himself as a speaker simply because he has been stuttering longer. It's possible that someone who is at the advanced level will have developed an extensive repertoire of avoidance behaviors so that actual stuttering behaviors are rare, but the individual's life is highly constrained by his efforts to avoid and hide his stuttering. The major difference between intermediate and advanced treatment levels is that more independence and responsibility are required of clients for treatment at the advanced level. Consequently, clinicians ordinarily place adult clients at the advanced level but determine an adolescent's placement based on how much responsibility he can take for self-therapy.

Intermediate Stuttering

A client whose stuttering is at the intermediate level will probably be younger than midteens. His stuttering pattern will be characterized by escape and avoidance behaviors and considerable tension on blocks, prolongations, and repetitions. He will also be avoiding some speaking situations. Moreover, his feelings and attitudes, as revealed in questionnaires and interviews with him and with his parents and teachers, will suggest many negative speech attitudes.

Advanced Stuttering

Individuals who fit into the advanced developmental/treatment level are well into their teens and sufficiently mature to handle the assignments used in advanced treatment. Their stuttering pattern is similar to intermediate stuttering, but their patterns of avoidance and escape may be more habituated (i.e., patterns appear to be highly automatized and rapidly performed). They will probably avoid difficult speaking situations whenever possible, and I often find strong negative self-concepts and negative anticipations of listener reactions as well. An individual with advanced stuttering may feel, for example, "I must be awfully incompetent to talk like this," or "People think I'm dumb because I stutter."

Closing Interview

I will assume here that the client is a person with developmental stuttering rather than another type of fluency disorder. By this point in the evaluation, I have a pretty good picture of his stuttering and how I will start therapy. I begin by summarizing my impression of his stuttering pattern (i.e., core and secondary behaviors) and his attitudes and feelings. One of my aims is to let him know I have some understanding of his stuttering and why he does what he does when he stutters. I feel it is important to let him know that, given his level of stuttering, it is no surprise that he would use the various secondary behaviors and avoidance tactics that he does. I accept these behaviors rather than criticize them and let him know that I feel I can work with him and help him discover other ways to respond. I try to ensure that he feels he will not be alone, that I will be working alongside him, and that I will gradually give him more and more responsibility to work on his own.

Then, I briefly describe some therapy options and discuss the possibilities with him. With my guidance, the client and I decide on a treatment approach. Afterward, I give him some written suggestions to begin the process of his taking responsibility for part of his treatment. This will also take advantage of the fact that, as indicated earlier, many clients are highly motivated to change at the time they come for an evaluation. I may not do this with adolescents, but there are exceptions. Some adolescent clients are reluctant to participate in therapy rather than being highly motivated because of their desire to close ranks with their peers and distance themselves from adults. With adolescents, I often end our evaluation session by striking a bargain to try at least four sessions of therapy before they make a decision about treatment. I may also recommend the website for the Stuttering Foundation (www.stutteringhelp.org) where they can click on the "Teens" link on the bar at the top of the page. This leads them to streaming videos for teens as well as a good deal of written material for free and links to other Internet sites with resources for teens. These items will help them learn about therapy and develop realistic and motivating expectations about its potential outcome. Sometimes, it helps to have a teen who stutters talk with a former or current teenage client who also stutters. This can provide substantial hope.

If the client has few avoidances and relatively mild stuttering, I am likely to start treatment with fluency shaping. If the client's stuttering is moderate to severe and/or he has relatively many avoidances and fears, I am likely to start with stuttering modification treatment. See the next chapter for an overview of both approaches. An exception that I may make is when a client has many fears and avoidances, but seems unwilling to confront them. I may begin working with this client using fluency shaping. Some clients who are at first unwilling to "touch the hot stove" of stuttering will be able to confront and change their stuttering if they first get some fluency through fluency shaping.

At the end of the closing interview, I ask a client if he has any questions about the evaluation. I also try to answer the questions asked in the initial interview that I postponed for response until after the evaluation. Adults and adolescents sometimes ask how long treatment will take. This is a reasonable question, given that they need to budget time and money to undertake treatment, but I have no easy answer for this difficult question. With appropriate cautions about individual differences and unexpected issues, I reply that with hard work and a willingness to tackle difficult situations and to confront fears with my help, I believe that considerable progress can be made within a year of the onset of treatment.

A video recording of an evaluation of an adult with advanced stuttering is available on the website. Although the recording omits discussion of the questionnaires usually given, it does capture the gathering of the speech sample, at the same time that the clinicians explore the onset and development of the client's stuttering. The client is questioned about his motivation for treatment, trial therapy is administered, and the client and clinicians develop an assignment for him to begin to work on immediately. At the end of the session, the client leaves with a positive feeling that he can change his stuttering and meet his goals. Aspects of the evaluation that you should pay particular attention to are described below.

On *thePoint*, you will find video clips of a young adult—Ben Barnet—that illustrate key aspects of an evaluation of an individual with advanced stuttering. You will find the first clip under Chapter 9: Assessment and Diagnosis, "Video 9-1: Diagnostic Evaluation: Introduction." In this clip, the clinicians obtain a sample of his speech when they ask him to tell them about the onset of his stuttering and his previous therapy. As you listen to his speech, notice his occasional repetitive stutters, a few blocks, and some avoidance behaviors (e.g., starters). Compare his fluency when speaking compared to his fluency when reading.

In the second clip, "Exploring Ben's Stuttering," the graduate student clinicians find out about his motivation for therapy and explore with him what his stuttering is like. What do you observe about (1) the types of stutters he has, (2) his avoidances, and (3) how aware he is of what he's doing when he stutters?

The third clip, "Exploring Ben's Avoidance Behaviors," focuses again on his motivation for therapy. It is clear that Ben feels his stuttering holds him back from fully participating in life. Underlying this, I think, is his being unwilling to say exactly what he wants to say because he's reluctant to stutter.

The clinicians carry out some trial therapy (in the clip with that name) that helps Ben go ahead get into his stutters, rather than avoiding them. They see if he can stay in his stutters and hold onto them and discover that when he doesn't fight them, the stutters gradually release themselves.

Because Ben understands what he must do to reduce his stuttering, the clinicians end the session in the "wrap-up" helping Ben develop an assignment to "get into the stutter." The clinicians help Ben understand that the more he confronts his fear of getting stuck, the more he will learn that the stutters will release themselves if he courageously stays in his moments of stuttering and accepts them. This will give him a feeling that he can control what he once feared.

Ben returned to our clinic 5 years later after carrying out this assignment day after day, month after month. In the video clips titled "Commentary," he reviews the recording of his initial evaluation and provides insights into what he was feeling and doing at that time as well as revealing how much his stuttering has changed. We will discuss the Commentary video clips later in the book when we discuss treatment of stuttering in adolescents and adults.

SUMMARY

- In evaluating a client who may stutter, your task is to decide:
  1. Whether his disfluencies warrant treatment
  2. If they do, you should also find out more about his history, current environment, speech behaviors, and reactions.
  3. What treatment seems reasonable given these findings
- In assessing a preschool child, the important questions to answer are:
  1. Whether the child is stuttering or is normally disfluent
  2. What the probabilities are that he will recover without treatment
  3. If treatment is warranted, whether indirect (for borderline stuttering) or direct (for beginning stuttering) is best
- It is important to obtain some information prior to the formal assessment. This includes a recording of the child's speech at home and a completed case history.
- Key elements of the assessment for a preschool child are:
  1. Observation of parent-child interaction
  2. Parent interview
  3. Clinician-child interaction
  4. Analysis of child's speech
  5. Screening of language, articulation, voice, and hearing
  6. Determining risk factors
  7. Deciding on the child's need for treatment
  8. Making follow-up recommendations to family
- In assessing a school-age child, the important questions are:
  1. How the stuttering is affecting the child's performance in school
  2. How the child feels about his stuttering
  3. How motivated he is to work on it
  4. How supportive the parents are of the child's problem
  5. How supportive the child's teachers are
- The assessment of the school-age child may proceed differently if he is being seen in a clinic or at school. If seen at school, the IDEA affects the process and mandates how assessment is carried out. If seen in a clinic, the clinician will have more contact with the family but needs to reach out to the school setting.

- Key elements of the assessment for a school-age child are:
  1. Initial contact and formal interview with the child's parents
  2. Interview with the child's teachers
  3. Interview with the child
  4. Analysis of speech
  5. Trial therapy
  6. Assessment of other factors, including academic adjustment
  7. Determination of appropriate treatment
- In assessing an adolescent or adult, the important questions are the client's level of motivation and ability to carry out assignments independently; the severity of stuttering and degree of avoidance; the client's feelings and attitudes about his stuttering; whether the problem is typical "developmental" stuttering or is cluttering, psychogenic, or neurogenic stuttering; and the appropriate type of treatment.
- Key elements of the assessment of an adolescent or adult are:
  1. Obtaining preliminary case history, attitude questionnaires, and recordings made outside of the clinic
  2. Interviewing the client
  3. Analyzing the client's speech
  4. Conducting trial therapy
  5. Interviewing parents if client is an adolescent
  6. Determining appropriate treatment
  7. Summarizing findings and making recommendations in closing interview with client
- Whether the person is to be treated as a normally disfluent speaker or as someone who stutters depends on your interpretation rather than a score. You must weigh what you see and hear to determine whether they indicate stuttering, normal disfluency, or even another disorder. From the flood of information you have gathered, you must extract the essential characteristics that support your choice of treatment.
- To hone your judgment, make evaluations a continuing process. The procedures I have suggested for assessment and diagnosis in this chapter will give you a good start, but stuttering is highly variable, and no individual can be completely evaluated in just an hour or two. Consequently, you will overlook an important element at times, and sometimes a vital clue will not be present in the samples of behavior you see during an initial evaluation. With good ongoing evaluation of a client, you will be able to change decisions and redirect therapy as additional information and understanding become available. You will also be able to evaluate the effectiveness of your treatment and improve it when needed.

STUDY QUESTIONS

1. How do you determine whether a preschool child is stuttering or is normally disfluent?
2. Why is it useful to obtain audio/video recordings of a preschool child's stuttering before the evaluation?
3. What are some indications that a parent of a preschool child who stutters feels she or he is to blame? How can you help the parent deal with those feelings?
4. What do you tell the parent of a preschool or school-age child who asks you what causes stuttering?
5. What are the variables assessed in the speech of a preschooler to determine his developmental/treatment level?
6. What are the advantages and disadvantages of talking to a child about his stuttering?
7. Compare the involvement of the parent and the teacher in the evaluation of a school-age child.
8. In what various ways do we assess the impact of the school environment on the school-age child who stutters?
9. What are the benefits of obtaining both a reading and a conversation sample with schoolchildren and adults?
10. In the section on evaluation of the adult and adolescent, what different pieces of information that you may gather from the interview questions help you to assess the client's motivation?
11. What are two reasons we suggest continuing evaluation after the initial assessment of clients who stutter?
12. Compare the assessment of the feelings and attitudes of a school-age child with the assessment in an adult.
13. What are the stages of management (from less to more formal treatment by the SLP) for a school-age child who stutters?
14. What are the goals of trial therapy?
15. What are the major questions to be answered in the evaluation of an adult?

SUGGESTED PROJECTS

1. Role-play the part of a clinician in a parent interview, having a friend or classmate play the part of a parent. Practice your listening skills by only listening and asking no questions as the "parent" describes in detail his or her child's stuttering problem. Switch roles, and then compare your impressions of the experience both as the parent and as the clinician.
2. Pair up with a friend or classmate who could pretend to stutter or with a person who stutters, and practice trial therapy (including exploring feelings) that is appropriate for a school-age child and then appropriate for an adult. Try both approaches, modifying stutters to make them less severe and modifying speech to produce fluency.
3. Pair up with a friend or classmate who doesn't stutter, and have them talk rapidly about a complex topic so he or she produces normal disfluencies. See if they are able to "catch" their normal disfluencies and hold onto them (e.g., turn single repetitions into multiple repetitions or make prolongations longer). Can this be done with normal disfluencies? With only certain types of normal disfluencies?
4. Find websites on the Internet that contain helpful information for (1) parents of children who stutter, (2) school-age children who stutter, (3) teens who stutter, and (4) adults who stutter.
5. One of the challenges for clinicians is to get a good speech sample from a child who may be somewhat shy or reluctant to talk to someone she doesn't know well. Experiment with different ways of interacting with a child until you find a "best" method. For example, try asking lots of questions, try just playing quietly alongside a child, and try playing with a child and making comments about things you are playing with together.

SUGGESTED READINGS

Conture, E. (2001). Assessment and evaluation. In *Stuttering: Its nature, diagnosis, and treatment*. Boston, MA: Allyn & Bacon.

In this chapter, Conture covers many details of the assessment not dealt with in the chapter that you have just read. Among these are finer points of audio and video recording, general interview procedures, and analysis of the speech sample. Conture also discusses concomitant problems like attention deficit hyperactivity disorder, Tourette's syndrome, neuromotor problems, and word-finding problems.

Guitar, B. (2010). Stuttering. In M. Augustyn, B. Zuckerman, & E. Coronna (Eds.), *The Zuckerman Parker handbook of developmental and behavioral pediatrics for primary care*. Baltimore, MD: Lippincott Williams & Wilkins.

This brief chapter for pediatricians summarizes key questions and important information for parents, criteria for referral, and initial treatment strategies.

Logan, K. (2014). *Fluency disorders*. San Diego, CA: Plural Publishing.

Logan, who himself is a person who stutters, provides excellent guidance in doing clinical assessments, including how to obtain valid speech samples, make detailed analyses of them, and come up with treatment recommendations.

Manning, W., & DiLollo, A. (2017). *Clinical decision making in fluency disorders* (4th ed.). San Diego, CA: Plural Publishing.

These authors have had a great deal of experience in the field of stuttering and present excellent ideas about diagnosis and evaluation.

Richels, C., & Conture, E. (2010). Indirect treatment of childhood stuttering: Diagnostic predictors of treatment outcome. In B. Guitar, & R. McCauley (Eds.), *Treatment of stuttering: Established and emerging interventions*. Baltimore, MD: Lippincott Williams & Wilkins.

This unique chapter uses the authors' Communication-Emotion Model of Childhood Stuttering as a rationale for their thorough evaluation of a child's speech and language, as well as emotional factors in the child's life. Variables measured before treatment predict short- and long-term outcomes.

Shafir, R. Z. (2000). *The zen of listening: Mindful communication in the age of distraction*. Wheaton, IL: The Theosophical Publishing House.

This is an excellent introduction to the practice of careful listening. Shafir is a speech-language pathologist who has developed her ability to listen to clients and writes eloquently about the healing powers of mindful listening.

Shapiro, D. (2011). *Stuttering intervention: A collaborative journey to fluency freedom*. Austin, TX: Pro-Ed.

This is a very fine textbook on many aspects of stuttering—its nature, assessment, and treatment, written by someone who has coped successfully with his own stuttering for many years. The chapters on (1) preschool children, (2) school-age children, and (3) adolescents, adults, and seniors who stutter have insightful sections on assessment and diagnosis, as well as treatment.

Van Riper, C. (1973). *The treatment of stuttering*. Englewood Cliffs, NJ: Prentice-Hall, Inc.

In his text, on pages 215–219, Van Riper gives a step-by-step description of his process of assessing an adult's stuttering. Not surprisingly, Van Riper's approach takes into consideration that each client will be unique and his individual needs for therapy must be understood.

Yairi, E., & Ambrose, N. (2005). Assessment of early stuttering. In E. Yairi, & N. Ambrose (Eds.), *Early childhood stuttering*. Austin, TX: Pro-Ed.

This chapter gives a thorough description, based on assessment experience with hundreds of children, of how to obtain samples and analyze speech of preschool children who stutter. Information regarding prognosis is given by the experts.

Yaruss, S. (2002). Facing the challenge of treating stuttering in the schools: Part 1. Selecting goals and strategies for success. *Seminars in Speech and Language*, *23*, 153–159.

This volume of "Seminars" is a rich source of information for school clinicians. Experienced clinicians, many of whom work in the schools, have written chapters on a wide variety of topics, including interpreting IDEA 1997, doing an evaluation in a school setting, and planning therapy for school-age children.

10

Preliminaries to Treatment

Chapter Objectives

After studying this chapter, readers should be able to:

- Understand the most important attributes of an effective stuttering clinician
- Understand how the clinician's beliefs about the nature and development of stuttering affect her choices about treatment procedures at different ages
- Understand what important goals are for stuttering therapy and how they may vary depending on the client's age
- Understand the therapy procedures used to meet the goals selected for a client's treatment

Key Terms

Abnormality of stuttering: Characteristics of an individual's stuttering that make it stand out or be distracting to the listener. Examples are facial tension and facial grimacing, body movements used to release stutters, and avoidances that make it difficult for the listener to follow what the individual is saying, such as "well, um, you see, that is....."

Clinician's beliefs: The perspective a clinician takes on the nature and development of stuttering that leads to her choices of assessment and treatment strategies

Cognitive behavior therapy (CBT): Treatment based on the notion that persons' perceptions of and thoughts about situations and themselves determine their feelings and behavior. CBT aims to help the persons see situations and themselves more realistically and more compassionately.

Critical thinking: An attitude of mind that encourages questioning; in the current context, the questioning is about whether a treatment will be effective for a particular client

Emotions related to stuttering: Physiological responses and conscious feelings that arise in a person who stutters, in regard to the act of stuttering or the fact of being someone who stutters

Empathy: Ability to put oneself in another's place and to identify with the feelings that the other person has

Evidence-based practice: A commitment to use research evidence, client goals, and clinician expertise when choosing assessment and treatment goals and tools

Fluency-facilitating environment: A climate in one or more situations that makes it easier for an individual who stutters to speak more fluently. For example, when parents speak more slowly than usual and increase pausing. Another example would be when family members are accepting of stuttering.

Genuineness: Honesty about life, oneself, and other people; a sense that the genuine individual is comfortable with herself, speaks straightforwardly, and takes actions that are congruent with her thoughts, beliefs, and attitudes

Therapy protocol: A detailed plan for carrying out treatment

Warmth: A feeling of positive regard for another person, often conveyed by tone of voice or body language

Before presenting the details of treatment in the next four chapters, I want to provide some background for the **therapy protocols** you can use, as well as how and why you use them. First, I'll describe important attributes of the clinician who works with people who stutter and how his or her beliefs about the nature of stuttering influence treatment decisions. Then I'll discuss commonly held goals for stuttering therapy and finally the procedures to meet them.

CLINICIAN'S ATTRIBUTES

The clinician is probably the most important ingredient in stuttering therapy other than the client. A clinician's knowledge, skills, and personality have a major influence on outcome. This is true whether therapy's major focus is to change behaviors, thoughts, or feelings—or some combination of these. In this section, I discuss some of the attributes that I think make a clinician effective, and I suggest how these can be developed. Unfortunately, there are no data that I'm aware of to support the importance of these attributes for stuttering therapy. In the field of psychotherapy, Carl Rogers (1961) and others have spent a considerable amount of time and effort measuring the effects of some of these clinician attributes on treatment success. In the field of stuttering treatment, Manning and DiLollo (2018), Shapiro (2011), and Zebrowski (2007) have excellent chapters on the role of the clinician and the importance of the clinical relationship.

Much of my thinking about the treatment process has been influenced by my experiences as a client and later as a student of Charles Van Riper. He was a master clinician of stuttering therapy. Let us begin then with Van Riper's (1975a) description of three important clinician characteristics: empathy, warmth, and genuineness.

Empathy

Empathy, in this context, is the ability to understand the feelings, thoughts, and behaviors of someone who stutters. You might think that this is much easier for clinicians who stutter. However, Van Riper's own clinician, Bryng Bryngleson, was a fluent speaker who showed an impressive understanding of individuals who stutter. Once, Bryngleson assigned

Van Riper the task of voluntarily stuttering to 10 strangers, but Van Riper was unable to carry it out. Exhausted from trying again and again and failing over and over, Van Riper sought out Bryngleson in his office. Bryng, as he was called, jumped up from his chair and headed for the door, saying, "It's OK, Van, just follow me and watch." Bryng then went into a nearby tobacco store, walked up to the clerk, and pretended to stutter—with the longest, loudest stutter that Van Riper had ever heard, causing the clerk to cower behind the counter. Van Riper was astounded. That single demonstration by his clinician had a huge impact on Van Riper. He felt deeply supported by Bryngleson's acceptance of his failure and Bryngleson's willingness to risk ridicule to help him. Remember this when you wonder how to show your clients empathy for their stuttering.

You can also get some idea of what clients experience by going out in public like Bryngleson did and stuttering voluntarily, though you don't have to stutter as long or as loud as Bryng did. My students are required, over the course of the semester, to carry out 15 pseudo stutters—to friends, family, and especially to strangers—and to keep a journal of their own emotions about their experience. Every year they tell me that this assignment—which they hated me for at the time—opened their eyes to the challenges of stuttering. They find out not only how embarrassing it is to stutter but also how listener reactions can make them feel—both good, if a listener is accepting, and bad, if she is rude.

You can also develop empathy with all your clients by working on your ability to listen deeply and acceptingly. It will also help to observe your clients' body language, posture, and the words they use. Van Riper said that he could improve his understanding of a client's feelings if he assumed the same body posture that the client had (C. G. Van Riper, personal communication, April 1965). Levine (2010), a psychotherapist working with patients who have experienced emotional trauma, writes eloquently about how a client's posture will often convey his or her emotional state. The clinician may detect those emotions because his own body nonconsciously imitates the client's posture and thus communicates the emotions to the clinician himself. He notes, "Therapists working with traumatized individuals frequently pick up and mirror the postures of their clients and hence their emotions of fear, terror, anger, rage and helplessness" (Levine, 2010, p. 46). Even if many of our clients who stutter cannot be described as traumatized by their stuttering, still they will have strong emotions relating to their speaking difficulty, even if they themselves do not recognize it. By noticing these, the clinician can, over the course of therapy, help the client to deal with them.

Reading stories written by people who stutter and parents of children who stutter will also help you better understand the experiences that have shaped their feelings. Good examples of such writings are *V-V-Voice: A Stutterer's Odyssey (Damian, 2014), Living with Stuttering* (St. Louis, 2001), and *Forty Years after Therapy: One Man's Story* (Helliesen, 2002). I will describe these books and others in the suggested readings at the end of this chapter.

Warmth

This attribute has also been referred to as "unconditional positive regard" (Rogers, 1957). Much of it is conveyed in the tone of voice, facial expression, and body language of the clinician. Genuine caring comes from the heart and is conveyed automatically when it is present in the clinician. Clients whose clinicians demonstrate **warmth** feel accepted, liked, and nurtured. Warmth creates an environment that supports learning and helps clients respond to the challenges involved in making difficult changes, such as being open about their stuttering. Warmth is also expressed in the comments the clinician makes when a client has done something well. This is sometimes harder than you think. It surprises me when I watch a video recording of one of my therapy sessions, how many opportunities I miss reinforcing the client with a "Good!" or "Well done!" Therefore, I try to watch videos of myself working with a client to discover things that I need to work on. Although it is initially painful for all of us to watch video recordings of ourselves, this is one of the best ways we can improve. Clinicians should become aware of how much or how little enthusiasm they show and how much warm encouragement they give to their clients. These are important tools of therapy.

Genuineness

Van Riper (1975a) described a third characteristic of good clinicians: "**genuineness**," which he equated with Rogers' (1961) "congruence." Both terms refer to a clinician's honesty and self-acceptance. The clinician just tries to be who she is, "roughness, pimples, warts, and everything" as Oliver Cromwell said on having his portrait painted (http://www.thehistoryblog.com/archives/1773). Genuineness allows clinicians to be honest with their clients, not sugarcoating the hard lumps of reality that must be swallowed if real progress is to be made.

In his video "Adult Stuttering Therapy," Van Riper said to his client with his characteristic bluntness, "Why do you have to have all that junk in your speech? Can't you just go ahead and say the word, starting with the first sound and working your way through it slowly, syllable by syllable?" (Van Riper, 1975b). My students always thought this side of Van Riper was cruel and couldn't understand why he would be so blunt. But I think Van Riper is just doing something vital in his therapy. He is showing the client that he can be hard. This means that the client would feel that Van Riper is tough enough for the client to hate him, to be angry with him, even to be able to express his rage toward him at times. All these things—as well as the opposite—feelings of love and caring toward the clinician are components of deep and effective therapy when we work with older children and adults. When a client senses the clinician's genuineness, he gains trust and begins to believe that his clinician means it when she asks about his thoughts and feelings so that he can let go and honestly express those feelings, convinced that the clinician will understand and accept him and his feelings, and be strong enough to be unhurt by them. Clinicians can cultivate their genuineness and strength by being open about their abilities and their limitations and learning self-acceptance through psychotherapy, meditation, spiritual practice, or other experiences that help them accept both their weaknesses and their strengths. This "groundedness" in the clinician will allow her to feel frustration and anger toward the client (and not have to express it) when the client shows resistance in treatment.

A Preference for Evidence-Based Practice

There are more traits than those three listed above that characterize good clinicians. One is a clinician's desire and ability to base her clinical practice on evidence of its effectiveness, called **evidence-based practice**. In choosing tools and approaches for evaluating and treating someone who stutters, a clinician who wishes to grow looks for evidence of the effectiveness and appropriateness of treatment approaches she is using or considering. She works together with the client or family in the diagnostic evaluation to determine which treatment approach is likely to meet the client's or family's goals most effectively. She measures the client's progress during treatment to assess whether this approach is working with this person. She is flexible, creative, and insightful enough to find ways of altering treatment if it is not working.

Many treatments, including some described in this text, have relatively little published data that support their effectiveness. For example, my approaches to school-age children and adolescents/adults have been derived from years of experimenting in a more casual way, and only now have I developed enough consistency to start collecting data to be disseminated. This does not preclude their being used. However, when my or any other treatment not supported by strong research evidence is used, the clinician should be particularly careful to assess how well particular treatment procedures work for *her* clients with measures made before, during, and after treatment. In addition, for those clinicians who find particular treatment protocols very effective, obtaining research evidence on them to share with others would represent a valuable contribution to the field. Ideas and information on evidence-based practice can be found in Bernstein Ratner (2005), Bothe (2004), Frattali (1998), Guitar (2004), Guitar and McCauley (2010), Pietranton (2012), and Sackett, Straus, Richardson, Rosenberg, and Haynes (2000). The American Speech-Language-Hearing Association (ASHA) has provided member access to useful tutorials on evidence-based practice at http://www.asha.org/Members/ebp/web-tutorial/.

An interesting example of an early attempt at evidence-based practice is the data that Van Riper (1958) kept as he experimented with different forms of treatment for stuttering. He attempted to write down in detail what variations he made with his treatment protocols each year and reassessed his clients 5 years after they had finished therapy. Although he admits his methods are not perfect, the chapter in which he presents 20 years of experiments in stuttering treatment is a fine example of evidence-based clinical practice for its time, more than 60 years ago (Van Riper, 1958). In this spirit, in the treatment chapters that follow, I suggest ways in which clinicians today can measure client progress.

A Commitment to Continuing Education

Another important attribute for clinicians is the habit of continually updating knowledge gained in graduate school. New methods of evaluation and treatment are developed every year, and new data on treatment effectiveness become available. It is vital for the clinician to keep up to date with the latest and best practices. Journals are the best source of this information, but recent editions of books that review diagnostic and treatment methods for stuttering can also be helpful. Books are likely to provide more background information than journal articles that may help you think about how well the method will fit with your client and your current level of expertise.

New approaches to treatment often require training. Short courses at the annual ASHA convention and workshops offered through schools, hospitals, state associations, and other institutions are excellent sources of such training. However, before adopting a new approach, a clinician should critically analyze the quality of evidence that supports its claim to effectiveness.

Critical Thinking and Creativity

Clinicians should become discriminating consumers and ask, "Which new diagnostic tools and treatment approaches are effective, and which clients are they appropriate for?" This demonstrates **critical thinking**. Some new approaches are not all they are cracked up to be. For example, many years ago, a well-known psychologist and his colleagues (Azrin & Nunn, 1974) suggested that teaching clients simply to take a breath and relax before speaking was an effective treatment for stuttering. Researchers at another clinic tested the approach and found it to be far less effective in their clinic than its developers had suggested (Andrews & Tanner, 1982). Nevertheless, there may be some aspects of relaxation and breathing that are useful for some clients in the hands of a clinician who becomes skilled at integrating these tools into a broader approach.

Another critical question is "Will this approach work for my clients in my environment?" Often a treatment that works under laboratory conditions with carefully selected participants does not work as well in the real world of a public school, for example. But a clinician may be able to adapt an approach to suit her situation. For instance, an approach developed for very young children in tightly controlled clinical studies with total fluency as its goal may need to be altered so that some degree of easy and open stuttering is an acceptable outcome when used with older children.

CLINICIAN'S BELIEFS

It is important for clinicians to weigh their beliefs about the nature of stuttering against the available data and then develop clinical procedures compatible with the **clinician's beliefs**—procedures supported by data, ideally data collected by others as well as the clinician. My own beliefs about the etiology and development of stuttering that were presented in the first few chapters are reviewed here only in enough detail to illustrate the relationship between beliefs and treatment procedures. My beliefs are that predisposing physiological factors interact with developmental and environmental influences to produce or exacerbate core behaviors that often (but not always) begin as repetitions. When children experience these early disfluencies as feeling out of control or as causing listeners to show alarm, they nonconsciously increase the amount of physical tension and they may speed up their attempts to say the word. The increase in tension makes the disfluencies even more distressing to them, compounding the problem. They then may add escape and avoidance behaviors to their behavioral repertoire as well as negative feelings and attitudes to their repertoire of emotional reactions. They learn escape behaviors through instrumental conditioning, speech fears and other negative emotions through classical conditioning, and word and situation avoidances through avoidance conditioning. All of these factors and how they contribute to stuttering are reflected in the details of how learning influences the development of stuttering in Chapter 5 and in the description of the stages of stuttering development I described in Chapter 7.

How does this point of view about the etiology and development of stuttering affect treatment? Let's use the management of school-age children who stutter to illustrate this point. In my view, a child's treatment plan is determined by his developmental level of stuttering—which reflects the likely behaviors and emotions he has added to his speech and feelings about his speech. Each advance in level requires new components in treatment. A first grader with borderline stuttering who is not embarrassed or afraid to talk and who doesn't avoid talking requires a different treatment than a fifth grader with intermediate-level stuttering who has developed fears and avoidances in response to his stuttering. In my view, the first grader with borderline stuttering may be treated with an approach that focuses on increasing fluency and deals only minimally with negative feelings and avoidance behaviors. On the other hand, the fifth grader needs help to reduce the tension and struggle *and* the fears and avoidances. In contrast to these ideas about treatment, a clinician who doesn't believe that fears and avoidances are crucial in understanding and managing stuttering might treat both children with the same approach.

Another way in which a clinician's beliefs can affect management is in the assessment procedures she uses. Assessment tools should provide clinicians with information that is essential for planning treatment and measuring progress. In evaluating the first- and fifth-grade children described above, I would evaluate each child's feelings and attitudes about his speech, as well as his use of word and situation avoidances, to accurately determine each child's developmental/treatment level and decide which aspects of the problem to focus on first. Another clinician—for example one who is atheoretical or unconcerned about the etiology and development of stuttering—might simply want to measure each child's frequency and severity of stuttering.

A third way in which a clinician's beliefs about the nature, development, and treatment of stuttering can affect clinical behavior relates to how she counsels the parents of her clients. In counseling the parents of these two school-age children, my beliefs would guide me to describe the etiology of stuttering as being related to the way a child's brain processes speech and language. Using terminology appropriate to the parents, I would talk about brain organization and development that may predispose a child to stutter, and I would emphasize that this suggests that parents don't cause stuttering. I would also explain that the child's way of producing speech and language can become more effective, which means that parents can be vital in helping a child overcome or manage his stuttering. I would also discuss with parents the importance of factors in the environment that might be contributing to the child's stuttering problem and discuss ways of modifying these factors. Lastly, I would use my understanding of the development and nature of stuttering to give parents a general idea of the course of therapy and possible outcome. Clinicians with other beliefs might not go into the nature of stuttering because they feel it is not well understood and would instead just counsel the parents about their role in the child's treatment.

TREATMENT GOALS

Treatment goals will vary with a clinician's beliefs, the client's age, and the developmental/treatment level of his stuttering. Nonetheless, it is still possible to describe the likely range of goals that clinicians tend to have for clients who stutter and to suggest which goals are likely to be paramount for which level. Individuals differ in their strengths and weaknesses at the outset of treatment, and these change as treatment proceeds. Thus, a clinician needs to ask herself: "What does this client need? What does he need from me? What does he need from me right now? And why?" (Van Riper, 1975a, p. 477).

As I said earlier, the clinician is not the only one who determines the goals of treatment. Clients and their families have an important role to play in choosing goals that are paramount for them. Ongoing discussions between clinicians and clients about treatment goals strengthen clients' motivation to achieve them and enhance the relationship between clients and clinicians. The following statement by Donald Baer (1990), an eminent behavioral psychologist, expresses this philosophy.

> *It seems only reasonable to learn that when stutterers are given control of the therapeutic consequences that presumably can change their output, some of them choose different targets than would their therapists or, probably, other stutterers, and some of them target not so much their speech output as they do a private response that they describe as sense of "imminent loss of control" (p. 35).*

Perkins, Kent, and Curlee (1991) described the feeling of loss of control as a key element in stuttering, perhaps the heart of it. We will revisit the concept of loss of control when we discuss the goal of reducing negative feelings about stuttering in a following section.

Reduce the Frequency of Stuttering

This can be achieved in a variety of ways, but it is important to reduce the frequency of stuttering without creating other behaviors, such as taking deep breaths before speaking that may be distracting to the listener (and speaker) and may therefore hamper communication. This goal is appropriate for all ages and levels of stuttering. For preschool children, the goal should be to reduce frequency of stuttering to essentially zero.

Reduce the Abnormality of Stuttering

I think much of the **abnormality of stuttering** comes from the conditioned tension and struggle behaviors that occur during moments of stuttering. It shows up as squeezing of facial muscles as the person is trying to say a word that feels blocked. Reducing this tension and struggle is an important goal for school-age, adolescent, and adult clients. In addition, behaviors that occur before the stutter (avoidance) and behaviors that are deployed to terminate the stutter (escape) should be eliminated or at least greatly diminished. These include (1) avoidance behaviors, such as the repetition of the sound "uh" before saying a word, and (2) escape behaviors, such as eye blinks and head nods used to terminate a block. For some school-age children and older clients, it may not be possible to eliminate their stuttering. Instead, the stuttering can be changed so that it is easy and comfortable both for the speaker and the listener and doesn't interfere with communication. Van Riper and other experienced stuttering clinicians have suggested that a person who stutters may not always have a choice *whether* he stutters but he does have a choice about *how* he stutters. This choice includes stuttering in a way that is easier and briefer than his old habitual pattern. This new way of stuttering reduces fear because it feels and sounds more like normal speech and is often unnoticed by the listener. Once the person has confidence in his ability to stutter this easily, he is less likely to increase muscle tension in response to an actual or anticipated stutter.

Reduce Negative Feelings about Stuttering and about Speaking

Many individuals who stutter appear to have a temperament that is sensitive and somewhat perfectionistic. See my theoretical perspective in Chapter 6 for support for this contention. They are thus vulnerable to feelings of embarrassment, fear, shame, and other negative feelings associated with their stuttering. A cycle can develop in which stuttering gives rise to negative feelings, which, in turn, increase tension and other struggle behaviors, which then generate more negative feelings. Classical conditioning plays a major role in this cycle. Therefore, treatment strategies to deal with classically conditioned behaviors, strategies such as deconditioning and counterconditioning, are crucial in treatment. These and related approaches are discussed in the chapters that describe treatment of school-age children (Chapter 13) and treatment of adolescents and adults (Chapter 14). Reducing negative feelings is an important goal for many clients beyond age 6 or 7, although a few school-age children and even older clients may not have strong negative feelings about being someone who stutters. They may, however, have feelings of frustration about their impediment to speaking easily. Most of these feelings can be changed significantly—either directly or indirectly—through treatments that give the client repeated experiences with effective communication and ease of speaking. One major difference among treatment approaches is whether they deal with clients' negative feelings and emotions directly or indirectly.

An example of facilitating changes in negative feelings about stuttering can be seen in the first phase of treatment using stuttering modification, called "identification." The clinician helps the client explore his stuttering and get to know it in an accepting environment. Figure 10.1 shows a clinician showing warmth and curiosity about a client's severe stuttering block. When the person who is stuttering encounters someone who is interested in his stuttering and does not reject it, he feels a little less negative.

Before we leave this section, I would like to discuss a negative feeling we can label "loss of control." In Chapters 5 and 6, I talked about a nonconscious response to feelings of loss of control: increased tension. This tension is a defensive response to relatively loose disfluencies that are often the first sign of stuttering in a preschool child. This experience—feeling loss of control—soon becomes conscious and remains an important part of stuttering as a child grows up. Key components of treatment, such as staying in the stutter, accepting it, and letting it relax are intended to reduce the negative feeling that an individual has that his speech—his stuttering—is out of control.

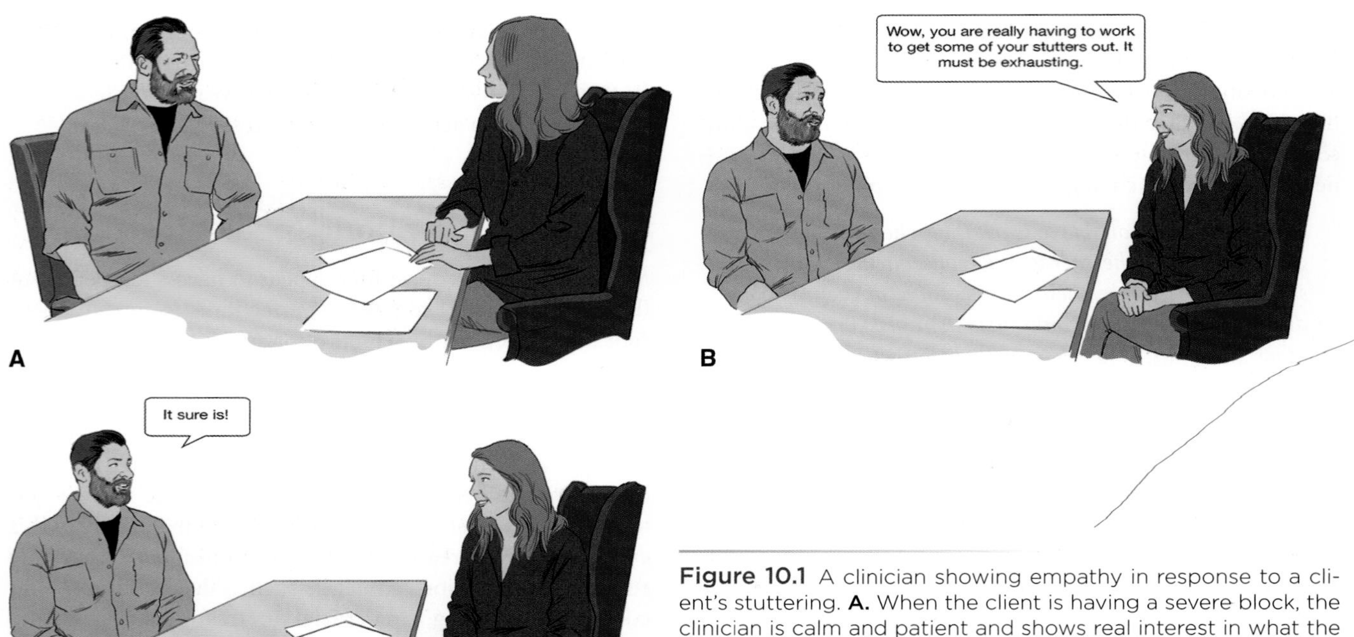

Figure 10.1 A clinician showing empathy in response to a client's stuttering. **A.** When the client is having a severe block, the clinician is calm and patient and shows real interest in what the client is saying. **B.** When the client finishes his stuttered word, the clinician makes an empathic response. **C.** The client, upon hearing the clinician's empathic response, relaxes a little and responds appreciatively.

Reduce Negative Thoughts and Attitudes about Stuttering and about Speaking

In the chapter on the development of stuttering, I described how people who stutter may acquire negative self-concepts through repeated experiences of stuttering and perceiving—sometimes correctly and sometimes incorrectly—that listeners are impatient or disapproving. Over time, a person's negative expectations in speaking situations become more engrained. This can lead to more stuttering. If a person who stutters expects rejection or disapproval, he may try very hard not to let the stuttering occur—not to let the stutter out—by adopting fixed, tense articulatory postures that trigger blockages. These are often devastating to the individual who stutters and make him feel helpless and out of control. This then "snowballs" downhill, gathering speed, from negative thoughts to more stuttering to more negative thoughts, on and on. This avalanche of events is at the heart of much chronic stuttering.

Good treatment can unroll the giant snowball. Clients can be toughened up (desensitized) to the experience of stuttering, decreasing their fears and negative expectations. They can also be shown how to say their feared words without as much struggle. As a result, they will approach speaking opportunities with more relaxed speech muscles and find themselves stuttering more easily or not stuttering at all. This in turn will lead to more positive expectations, which can lead to easier or less stuttering; thus a positive cycle begins to replace the negative one that got them to a place of more severe stuttering and very negative feelings about themselves.

A different approach besides unrolling the snowball and gradually decreasing fear of the experience of stuttering is to give the client repeated experiences of being fluent—in many situations, with increasing linguistic and social demands over a relatively long period of time and with much success and little failure. The aim is to replace expectations of stuttering with expectations of fluency. This seems to work best, in my experience, with younger clients and with adults who have few avoidance behaviors. For those with much avoidance, the strategies described below can help.

Reduce Avoidance

Avoidance behaviors, as you will remember, are evasive maneuvers taken by individuals to keep from stuttering. Sometimes they may occur very close in time to the expected stutter, such as saying "um" or "well" just before attempting to say a feared word (as illustrated in the video of Ben in the adult diagnosis clips). Other times they may be quite separated in time from the expected stuttering, such as *not* volunteering to be in a school play or by driving 20 miles to talk to someone rather than telephoning her. Some individuals who stutter may have an innate predisposition to avoid negative stimuli because of their temperaments, as described in Chapters 2 to 6. Avoidances keep stuttering "hot," because they prevent an individual from learning that it is possible to stutter in an easy fashion and communicate well. Reducing avoidance is usually not the first treatment goal on the list, although it may be one of the most important goals for more advanced levels of stuttering. Usually, before helping clients reduce avoidances, clinicians need to help them reduce negative emotions about stuttering and teach them to stutter more easily. Reducing avoidances is a major goal for older children and adults, but again, some approaches work indirectly by giving them tools to increase fluency, which then, one hopes, reduce fear and thus decrease avoidances.

Increase Overall Communication Abilities

The ability to communicate easily and well varies a great deal from client to client. It may be affected by severity of stuttering, temperament, avoidances, and communication models in the family. For many of us who work with individuals who stutter, effective communication is an important treatment goal. Some clients will become good communicators once the frequency and severity of their stuttering, along with their negative feelings and attitudes about speaking and stuttering, have been reduced. For other clients, guided practice and structured experiences in communication are essential. Once clients feel they can communicate easily, they often begin to seek out talking experiences, their avoidances drop away, and they become comfortable and open about any remaining stuttering that occurs. The goal of effective communication is most needed for older children and adults who have developed avoidances. Many of these clients, especially those with more severe stuttering, have been preoccupied with their stuttering and not spent much time learning to communicate effectively (Curlee, personal communication, March 3, 2004). They may still have hesitancies and a herky-jerky style of speaking that lacks the fluidity of normally fluent speech.

A good example of how stuttering—especially the fear of stuttering—can affect communication is shown in the video of Ben Barnet's initial evaluation on this book's Web site.[1] When asked why he is seeking therapy, he says, in essence, that he doesn't say what he wants to say. His talking is hard for listeners to understand because he has so many avoidances and "work-arounds" when he fears he will stutter that his narrative is hard to follow. Compare his style of talking in the evaluation video with his new way of expressing himself that is evident in the "Commentary" video clips made 5 years later.[2]

Create an Environment that Facilitates Fluency

This goal is paramount for working with young children who can often be treated by helping the family reduce pressures on the child's speech and increase positive aspects of the child's speaking environment in order to create a **fluency-facilitating environment**. For example, family members can spend one-on-one time with the child, using a slow speech rate and careful listening skills, thereby increasing the child's daily opportunities to experience fluency. The child's environment may be made more positive through praise and appreciation of his fluent speech and/or his other accomplishments. This goal of improving the child's speaking environment may also be important for school-age children. However, teachers and aides, as well as family members, need to be enlisted in facilitating the child's fluency. Older clients can make their environments facilitating to both fluency and easy stuttering by being open about their stuttering and sharing with others how listeners can be most helpful to them.

Increase Freedom to Speak

This goal is similar to what Shapiro is referring to in the title of his book *Stuttering Intervention: A Collaborative Journey to Fluency Freedom* (2011). For me, freedom to speak means being able to say what you want to say, when you want to say it. There may be some stuttering, but the individual doesn't hold back from speaking because of it. Moreover, the individual's own reaction to his or her stuttering is not strong and therefore he or she is able to maintain natural eye contact and connect with the listener and communicate effectively. Because the person is free to speak, his or her struggle will be minimal because there is little negative emotion associated with their stuttering and thus the tension and holding back are hardly present.

THERAPY PROCEDURES

The aim of this section is to outline the tools and strategies that clinicians can use to work on each of the treatment goals described above. By understanding which procedures are most likely to be useful in achieving each goal, clinicians can select those procedures that best suit each client and are in accord with their own beliefs. The procedures outlined here are more fully described in the therapy sections on each developmental/treatment level.

My belief about stuttering treatment is that the emotions associated with stuttering must be understood and dealt with if therapy is to be successful. Therefore, I begin talking about procedures with a substantial discussion of how the clinician is involved in the process of helping the individual or his family reduce negative emotions.

Procedures to Help Clients and Families Deal with Their Emotions Associated with Stuttering

In many books, this section might be called "counseling," but I prefer to describe this process as working with **emotions related to stuttering**. The clinician's attributes of empathy, warmth, and genuineness are vital for reducing the negative

[1]See Chapter 9, "Assessment and Diagnosis," videos 9-1 through 9-5.

[2]See Chapter 9, "Assessment and Diagnosis," videos 9-6 through 9-12 Commentary.

emotions that can impede improvement in fluency and communication, as well as for facilitating positive emotions that can foster recovery. Although there are similarities in how the clinician responds to the parents of a child who stutters and how she helps older children and adults, there are enough differences that I will describe them separately.

In the treatment of preschoolers, working with the child's family is paramount. The family must develop faith in the clinician's abilities. They also must feel her understanding and acceptance of their feelings and of the family itself. The clinician must display this even if the family have been trying to stop the child's stuttering in ways the clinician feels are not helpful. In the initial meetings, the family is likely to feel anxious because they have watched their child struggle, for weeks or even months, not knowing how best to help her. The clinician must listen with care to how the parents (or other family members or caregivers) describe the child's stuttering, the child's response to it, and the family's own responses to it. Listening to their feelings throughout the course of treatment will provide support for the family and will convey the all-important idea that they and the clinician form a team working together to help the child. As the clinician listens, she acknowledges their feelings, sometimes restating them to make sure she understands. She refrains from simple reassurance, but instead, brings them hope by showing them evidence that the child is making progress, sharing information about recovery, and helping them realize all the positive things the child has going for him. Particularly important is the clinician's empathy for their expressions of frustration, discouragement, and guilt. It is sometimes hard for new clinicians to realize how much their empathy for a family's negative feelings can provide the family relief even in their moments of despair. In summary, in working with young children and their families, the clinician must be aware that the child's and family's emotions can be a part of the reason that stuttering may worsen after onset and that treatment can reverse this.

In treating clients older than preschoolers, the clinician works more with the client directly, rather than his family. The clinician's role in helping the client deal with emotions is to create an atmosphere in which the client feels more and more comfortable expressing feelings. These feelings may include shame and fear, and sometimes anger toward the stuttering, the clinician, and listeners. The clinician should point out that such feelings are normal when a person has stuttered for a number of years and has experienced listeners' impatience, rejection, or even teasing.

In the early stages of therapy, as the client learns more about his own stuttering, the clinician's genuine interest and curiosity about the stuttering have the potential to counteract the negative feelings the client may have—expressed or unexpressed—toward his stuttering. The goal is for the client to accept his stuttering and take responsibility for changing it. For this to happen, the clinician must show her acceptance of it. Another goal is to help the client build up tolerance to the frustration and the fear of "being stuck" as a means to reducing tension and struggle. Activities to accomplish this include stuttering openly, without avoidances, and stuttering voluntarily on nonfeared words. These activities usually cause an increase in emotion and resistance, giving the clinician an opportunity to help the client explore and accept his feelings. The clinician asks the client how he's feeling about doing these tasks, listens attentively, and doesn't ask the client to work on his stuttering while he talks about feelings.

To learn more about the clinician's skills in listening empathically, I recommend studying the tutorial by Lieberman (2018) that describes in detail the counseling that is so important for speech-language pathologists and audiologists in working with individuals who have communication disorders. Lieberman notes that the helping relationship—in which the clinician creates a safe and supportive environment—is paramount for a client's making progress. At the heart of this relationship is a therapeutic alliance that is gradually formed between the client and clinician. This alliance helps the client feel that they are not doing the work of therapy alone. They feel supported and accepted *as they are*, whether they are leaning forward in progress or slumped in self-pity. It is what Van Riper's therapist, Bryngleson, provided in Van Riper's moment of need when he couldn't complete the assignment of 10 voluntary stutters.

I want to turn to the emotions that arise directly from the confrontation of old stuttering patterns and the learning of new behaviors. An important goal in therapy that seeks to teach the client to stutter more easily is for the client to learn to stop rewarding the old struggle behaviors. This is done by progressively changing the form of stuttering from tense and rapid to loose and slow. To help the client do this, many clinicians, myself included, teach him to stay in the moment of stuttering, accept it, and allow the tension to reduce so that a slow, relaxed ending to the word can be produced. As this goal is being worked on, many emotions and resistances usually arise, as I said earlier, and these are opportunities for the clinician to help the client express them, explore them, and accept them so progress can be made. Previously, the client may have been afraid of listeners' reactions to his stuttering; now he may be afraid of listeners' reactions (real or imagined) to his managing his speech by slowing his speech rate, using easy onsets of phonation, or staying in the stutters even beyond the moment when they can be released. These are things that the client may have to do to reduce tension and struggle, but they are often hard to do with friends, family, or strangers. The clinician can help the client learn that, by and large, listeners respect a person who is openly working on his challenges. And when listeners are impatient, anxious, or rejecting, it is because they have their own issues, and the client can learn to tolerate and transcend these reactions. Seeing those reactions as the other person's problem places the person who stutters in a more powerful position from which they can more easily act (by helping their listener understand) rather than react (by thinking the listener's response is their fault).

There is a rhythm to treatment of older children and adults who stutter. The clinician guides the client to carry out various tasks. Before, during, or after carrying them out, the client feels various emotions that are related to the stuttering and to changing it. The clinician helps the client express these emotions, and together they accept them, then move on to work on the next step together. The clinician's role in this process has been described in this way:

> *[People who stutter] need a permissive figure to whom they can ventilate their anxieties and frustrations. They need a companion who can share their difficulties in communication without becoming punitive or upset. They need someone to point out a possible pathway out of communicative deviancy and who will stay with them even when they fail. They will learn all they need to about themselves by working with their stuttering. Perhaps what we are saying is that the stutterer needs a very good teacher rather than a psychiatrist. (Van Riper, 1958, p. 381)*

Before leaving this section on emotion, I want to describe some of the things I have done to help children express and release emotions in an acceptable way. These activities are included in Chapter 11 on treatment of school-age children and are illustrated in the videos that accompany that chapter.

One way I ease into a discussion of feelings with children is to have them draw a picture of their stuttering. One of my former clients, David, depicted his stuttering as a rock that was stuck in his throat and kept words from coming out. He was able to talk about how uncomfortable it was and how he had to send an army of spear-carrying soldiers down into his throat to try to get the word out. As we looked at his drawing together, he was easily able to express his frustration and embarrassment with his blocks. When we decided it would be good to talk about his stuttering with his third-grade class, he drew a poster-sized version of the rock in his throat and showed it to his class and he and I talked about how they could help him. For Alison, a 9-year girl who was quite reserved and didn't like to talk about her stuttering, the graduate student who was her clinician made a video with her to share with her family and friends—and maybe someday, her class. In the video, Alison is shown making her clinician hold onto a stutter and dance around in a circle as she did it. Then the roles were reversed and the clinician had Alison stutter and dance while timing how long she could do it. On the video, Alison engaged in a variety of other activities playing with her stuttering, all accompanied by music. The overall impact of the video was to help Alison feel that she was in control of her stutter and free to stutter or not, as she chose. At the end of the video, Alison shows off her prowess with a ping-pong ball gun shooting empty containers representing stutters, with uncanny accuracy.

For me, these activities that release feelings about stuttering help release the tension and holding back that affect speech as well. They give the child the experience of "letting go"—both of feelings and of speech. But they also give the child a chance to play. Stuttering therapy becomes fun for a while, a diversion from the hard work of becoming more fluent.

Procedures to Reduce the Frequency of Stuttering

Operant conditioning procedures are often part of treatment approaches for achieving this goal and typically involve reinforcement for fluency and, occasionally, tactfully calling attention to stuttering and allowing a "do-over." Rewards may be verbal, such as the clinician's praise or approval, or tangible, such as tokens that can be redeemed for snacks, prizes, or an opportunity to take a turn in a game. Rewards for fluency and gently highlighting stuttering can be the primary tools used for treating beginning stuttering and are sometimes coupled with a hierarchy based on the complexity and length of utterances. In this case, clients move from producing one or two words fluently, moving on to longer phrases and then to spontaneous speech. Reward and highlighting stuttering may also be used as "shaping" tools for intermediate- or advanced-level stuttering, in which clients begin by speaking in a way that produces instant fluency, such as speaking very slowly, and then progressing to more and more normal-sounding speech in more and more difficult situations. This approach—sometimes called "prolonged speech"—was foreshadowed in remarks by Francis Bacon in the late 1700s (Siegel, 2007). Here are Bacon's words quoted by James Boswell (1819):

> *In all kinds of speech, either pleasant, grave, severe, or ordinary, it is convenient to speak leisurely, and rather drawlingly than hastily: because hasty speech confounds the memory, and oftentimes, besides the unseemliness, drives a man either to stammering, a non-plus, or harping on that which should follow; whereas a slow speech confirmeth the memory, addeth a conceit of wisdom to the hearers, besides a seemliness of speech and confidence.*

The general term for treatments such as prolonged speech that focus on increasing fluency rather than decreasing the abnormality of stuttering is "fluency shaping."

Procedures to Reduce the Abnormality of Stuttering

These procedures are appropriate for clients who have developed struggle, tension, escape, and avoidance behaviors that make their stuttering obvious and sometimes alarming to the listener and the client himself. Therapies that target the abnormality of stuttering often use reward and mild punishment to change long, tense stutters into increasingly briefer and more relaxed ones and to diminish clients' use of escape and avoidance behaviors. To meet this goal, reward and punishment are often accompanied by a systematic program for reducing negative emotions. Such programs are founded on the belief that negative emotions elicit increased tension, escape, and avoidance behaviors and that these behaviors are maintained by the fact that they are rewarded when the stutterer finally gets the word out by squeezing and pushing on it. These approaches are often referred to as "stuttering modification."

A classic stuttering modification approach is that of Van Riper (1958, 1973, 1975b), which begins first by reducing negative emotions through (1) objective study of the stuttering, then focuses on (2) desensitization to the frustration and embarrassment of it. Next, the clinician teaches the client to self-correct his stuttering after a stutter, where the self-correction is an easier form of stuttering, not a fluent utterance. Then the clinician helps the client change to an easier form of stuttering while it is happening, ending the stutter in an easier way that is rewarded by its release. Gradually the client starts to begin his stutters in this easier fashion, in a way that makes the stutter much more like normal speech. Stuttering modification often results in a modified style of speaking that contains brief disfluencies produced in a slightly slower than normal way of talking. In an early description of this therapy, Van Riper (1957) sketches out how his therapy combines psychotherapy with behavior modification to help the client accept his stuttering as well as accept himself as he learns to stutter easily in more and more challenging situations.

Some therapy approaches—both fluency-shaping approaches for older children and adults as well as therapy approaches for preschoolers—don't aim to reduce the abnormality of the stuttering behavior directly, but instead focus on increasing fluency with the assumption that as fluency increases, stuttering diminishes to negligible levels.

Procedures to Reduce Negative Thoughts and Attitudes about Stuttering and Speaking

A number of therapy procedures can help clients become more realistic about how listeners perceive them and what this may mean to them. Cognitive therapy, for example, can be an excellent technique for helping clients think and feel more positively about their speech, listeners, and the situations that have elicited negative emotions in the past. Clients can learn to examine their thought processes and understand how what they *think* influences what they *feel* and how they *act*, particularly in regard to such maladaptive behavior as muscular tensing that leads to more stuttering. Some clinicians use **cognitive behavior therapy (CBT)** as their sole treatment and others as a supplement to techniques for learning to speak fluently or to stutter in an easier way. The book, *Cognitive Therapy: Basics and Beyond* (Beck, 1995), is a good source for learning this approach, and I discuss cognitive therapy in the chapter on advanced stuttering. An excellent introduction to this approach with stuttering are two Stuttering Foundation DVDs: (1) *Tools for Success: A Cognitive Behavior Therapy Taster* and (2) *Implementing Cognitive Behavior Therapy with School-Age Children* (www.stutteringhelp.org).

Procedures to Reduce Avoidance

Some clients have very little avoidance, and once they learn to speak fluently they enter speaking situations freely without expectation of difficulty. Others, however, because of temperament, learning, or both, have a strong tendency for avoidance that may be almost "hard-wired" because it is learned so well. Avoidance behaviors are usually serious issues that must be addressed in individuals who are school age (intermediate stuttering) or older (advanced stuttering). Treatment to reduce avoidance should begin by reducing negative emotions, particularly fears of stuttering and of listeners' reactions. Fear of stuttering can be tackled by a systematic program of rewarding clients with praise, support, or tangible reinforcement for "catching" a stutter, holding onto it and accepting it, and releasing it slowly and loosely. Fear of listeners' reactions can be lessened by clients' voluntarily stuttering to acquaintances and strangers. When a person who stutters can deliberately imitate his typical stuttering pattern and pretend to stutter, he finally feels in control during a stutter; this and the feeling of "stuttering" while also feeling in control is highly rewarding. Perhaps even more important than voluntary stuttering is the success and reward an individual feels if he is able to drop avoidance behaviors and go right into a feared word, stay in the stutter (showing it "who is boss"), then release it in a slow, controlled fashion.

Reducing fear is not enough, however. Studies of animal behavior have shown that, even when avoidance symptoms disappear after fear is reduced, fear eventually returns and so do its symptoms—conditioned avoidance behaviors (Ayres, 1998; Bouton, 2016). Thus, new responses to the old stimuli must be taught. In stuttering therapy, an example of learning a new response to an old stimulus is for a stutterer to slow his speech rate as he says a word he expects to stutter on. This is an aspect of the "preparatory set" used in many stuttering modification approaches, as well as what I call "downshifting" to a slower speaking rate before attempting a difficult word, taught in fluency-shaping programs.

Avoidances are not confined to the moment just before a difficult word. Individuals who stutter may also avoid opportunities to speak by pretending to be busy when the telephone rings or by waiting for someone else to make introductions of new acquaintances. These avoidances can be treated by helping a client construct a hierarchy of easy-to-difficult speaking situations, in which he can use newly learned stuttering modification or fluency-shaping techniques. Clinicians can also motivate clients to continue seeking out new situations in which they can be open about their stuttering and can use their new strategies to manage stuttering. At meetings of the SpeakEasy Associations of Australia and the United States and conventions of the National Stuttering Association (https://westutter.org/), there are always impressive testimonials by clients who have sought out public speaking opportunities, joined Toastmasters (an international organization of people who want to practice public speaking), or found other ways of increasing their approach behaviors and decreasing their tendency to avoid stuttering and speaking.

Procedures to Increase Overall Communication Abilities

For many children, adolescents, and adults, communication blossoms when fears of stuttering and listeners' reactions are reduced, and ease of speaking is increased. For others, long-standing habits of avoiding speaking situations and the accompanying lack of social experience have stunted the growth of their communication skills. For still others, concomitant problems, such as attention deficit or extreme shyness, may have prevented them from learning how to communicate well. Communication skills should be addressed in treatment whenever it appears that they are not appropriately developed. Observations of a client's communication and reports from a school-age child's teachers will indicate the areas that may need to be addressed. Specific skills that can be worked on include eye contact, turn taking, maintaining a topic, making relevant contributions to conversation, speaking intelligibly, clarifying and repairing what was said, and developing a willingness to initiate and maintain communicative interactions with others (Kent, 1993; Smith, McCauley, & Guitar, 2000). Although these skills can be worked on individually, group therapy provides excellent opportunities for clients to practice them. Direct instruction, modeling, role-playing, and video-recorded feedback with discussion can be used to teach and refine communication skills.

Procedures to Create an Environment that Facilitates Fluency

Preschool-age children, especially those on the borderline between normal disfluency and stuttering, may need only a little change in their environments for their stuttering to disappear permanently (Starkweather, Gottwald, & Halfond, 1990). Treatment focuses on parents: counseling them to reduce their anxieties, modeling for them, and continuing to support the changes they make. Parent-child interactions are usually the key element of the environment that can be changed to facilitate fluency. Video recordings and playback of these interactions in the clinic or observations at home, coupled with parent counseling, can help parents improve how they communicate with their child (Guitar, 1978; Guitar, Kopff-Schaefer, Donahue-Kilburg, & Bond, 1992; Kelman & Nicols, 2008; Rustin, 1991). Parents usually work on creating a facilitating environment (slower speaking rate, frequent pausing, and increased attention to the child) during brief, one-on-one daily sessions with the child. In some families, other aspects of the environment may need to be changed, such as a home's hurried pace of life, stressful life events, and the communication styles of other family members. Older preschoolers may also benefit from a direct approach, involving contingencies for fluent speech and stuttering.

For school-age children, the creation of facilitating environments may include working with the child's family, but the school setting may be equally important, if not more so. Clinicians often work in partnership with a child or adolescent to make school a "fluency-friendly" environment. The clinician may arrange meetings with the child and his teachers to improve the teachers' understanding of his stuttering and to open lines of communication between the child and teachers. A child's peers can be invited to treatment so that they may improve their understanding of the child's stuttering, while the process of the child's openness about his stuttering with other children is begun. Freely discussing his stuttering with other students is one of the most powerful ways for a school-age child to make his environment more fluency-friendly. For some children, a powerful boost can be given to therapy's progress if they are able, with the clinician's help and support, to make a presentation to their class about the nature of stuttering in general and their stuttering in particular. A good example of a child and her clinician presenting to the child's class is shown in a video on *thePoint* for Chapter 11: "Child Presenting to Her Class."

For adults, openness about stuttering is also a major way in which they can create a supportive environment. By commenting on their stuttering, by showing a sense of humor about it, and by sharing what techniques they're working on, adults who stutter can create environments in which their listeners are quite comfortable with the adults' stuttering. This helps them feel free to use various fluency-enhancing techniques.

My own treatment for each age and the treatments of several other clinicians are presented in the next four chapters. Descriptions of the other clinicians' approaches include their beliefs about the nature and development of stuttering as well as rationales for their choice of goals and procedures to treat each level. Both my own approaches and those of other clinicians have been developed and refined, usually over several years' of trial and error. When possible, supporting data are provided for each treatment, but in many cases, where such data are not available, I suggest what data would be appropriate to gather.

Motor Learning Principles for Treatment

Most of our treatments involve working with the client in a relatively structured environment for a short period of time and then hoping for generalization to an unstructured environment between treatment sessions. The motor learning literature—cogently summarized by Verdolini and Lee (2004)—suggests that certain principles must be followed for generalization to take place. Table 10.1 summarizes some of their ideas and suggests how they might apply to the treatment of stuttering.

TABLE 10.1 Principles of Motor Learning and Their Applications to the Treatment of Stuttering

Principles of Motor Learning (Verdolini & Lee, 2004)	Application to Stuttering Treatment
In the first stages of motor learning, feedback is important, but then the client must evaluate his own performance in order to achieve for long-term change.	When teaching a technique such as easy onsets or pullouts, the clinician should let the client know when he has done well, but gradually diminish feedback and replace it with asking the client to evaluate how he felt his easy onsets and pullouts were. A 1–10 scale could be used for rating them.
Rather than instructing the client, the clinician should facilitate the client's own discovery of new behaviors that work. In doing so, the clinician should utilize the client's sensory processes to discover helpful changes.	As the client is trying to change old habits of tension and struggle, he should be urged to feel, hear, or see what he is doing as he searches for ways to change. An example is Dean Williams's (2004) question to clients: "What are you doing to interfere with talking?" and his admonition to "feel what you're doing."
As new habits are acquired, old habits must be suppressed by conscious inhibition.	Before speaking, a client should pause and tell himself not to use an old habit (such as tensing larynx, lips, and/or jaw) and be aware of how that change feels.
In order for responses to become automatized (and therefore stable in the face of distracters), the client needs to consistently use the new behaviors in relevant stimulus situations.	Clients need to consistently use new behaviors, such as easy onsets in place of habitual tense stuttering behaviors in order to build up automaticity in their use so that they will be available under stress.
Clients should use variable practice with different stimuli and in different environments.	Clients should practice new behaviors (e.g., light contacts or slow rate) with a wide variety of words and sentences, in different types of speech tasks, and outside the clinic room as well as on the telephone in the clinic.

SUMMARY

- The clinician's attributes are a vital ingredient in treatment success.
- Empathy, genuineness, and warmth are three clinician attributes that have been considered important by Van Riper (1975a) and are discussed in Lieberman (2018).
- An important component of best clinical practice is choosing evaluation procedures and tools that have been shown to be valid and reliable.
- Best clinical practice dictates becoming aware of evidence of effectiveness for treatment procedures that you use and adapting treatment procedures to fit clients' needs, as well as continuous assessment of improvement in attributes that have been chosen as goals for treatment.
- Continuing education is vital to keep abreast of new approaches and new evidence of effectiveness of current approaches.
- Clinicians should develop an informed set of beliefs about the nature of stuttering and fit assessment and treatment procedures to those beliefs.
- Goals for treatment and for continuing assessment should come not only from the clinician's beliefs but also from the client's (or family's) informed choices.
- Treatment procedures for meeting these goals can include methods of reducing frequency and severity of stuttering and secondary behaviors, reducing negative emotions and thoughts that interfere with fluency, increasing communication abilities, and developing environments that facilitate fluency.

STUDY QUESTIONS

1. What are the three important characteristics of a clinician described by Van Riper?
2. How might each of these characteristics facilitate progress in treatment?
3. What are the characteristics of evidence-based practice?

4. How might two clinicians' beliefs about the nature of stuttering result in two very different treatment approaches? How might these beliefs result in two similar treatment approaches?
5. Which of the treatment goals described in this chapter are appropriate for borderline stuttering?
6. Which are appropriate for beginning stuttering?
7. Which are appropriate for intermediate stuttering?
8. Which are appropriate for advanced stuttering?
9. Describe the differences between "fluency-shaping" and "stuttering-modification" approaches to treatment.
10. How might reducing negative emotions reduce stuttering frequency?
11. How might reducing stuttering frequency reduce negative emotion?
12. Which goal would you start with and why?

SUGGESTED PROJECTS

1. Video record yourself and a client during an evaluation or a treatment session. The first time you watch it, note only the things you think you do well. The second time you watch it, note two things you would like to improve. Meet with a colleague or supervisor and discuss how to improve the things you would like to and then work on those in another session and videotape yourself again. Watch this new tape for improvements in the behavior(s) you have chosen to work on.
2. Choose a test you use in your evaluation procedures and then try to find evidence of its validity and reliability.
3. Choose a treatment procedure you use and then search the literature to see if you can locate any information about its effectiveness.
4. Find a stuttering treatment approach that is described in detail and determine what the goals of treatment are, what the procedures are to reach these goals, and whether there is a description of how to measure progress on these goals. Examples are (1) Acceptance and Commitment Therapy for Adults who Stutter (Beilby, Byrnes, & Yaruss, 2012; Beilby & Yaruss, 2018), (2) Avoidance Reduction Therapy for Adults who Stutter (Sisskin, 2018), (3) The Lidcombe Program (Onslow et al., 2017), and (4) Stuttering Prevention and Early Intervention (Gottwald, 2010).
5. Describe in detail your own beliefs about the nature of stuttering applied to children with intermediate stuttering. Given these beliefs, what therapy goals do you have for a child with intermediate stuttering?

SUGGESTED READINGS

Bothe, A., (Ed.). (2004). *Evidence-based treatment of stuttering: Empirical bases and clinical applications.* Mahwah, NJ: Lawrence Erlbaum.

This text, available in hard copy or electronic format, contains chapters dealing with data on stuttering treatments and the scientific basis of treatment approaches.

Gendlin, E. (1981). *Focusing.* New York, NY: Bantam Books.

This is an unusual book. The author, who was on the faculty at the University of Chicago, was a protégé of Carl Rogers, the well-known psychotherapist. Focusing is a technique developed by Gendlin and his colleagues to help clients "listen" to their bodies to discover new feelings and insights. The technique is supposed to lead to a feeling of relief from worries and anxieties that have been plaguing them. When I was in graduate school I was bothered by uncomfortable feelings in my stomach and abdomen related to a difficult statistics course I was taking. Having read an essay by Gendlin about focusing, I tried it and found quick relief from my discomfort and subsequently "aced" the course.

Levine, P. (2010). *In an unspoken voice: How the body releases trauma and restores goodness.* Berkeley, CA: North Atlantic Books.

A colleague who is also interested in the psychosomatic aspects of stuttering recommended this book to me. I am finding it quite relevant to one of my theoretical perspectives that some individuals with persistent stuttering may have stored in their bodies (in a mind-body sense) the effects of childhood distress when their stuttering began and felt out of their control. Some of the therapeutic suggestions may be relevant to the treatment of some stuttering.

Manning, W., & DiLollo, A. (2018). *Clinical decision making in fluency disorders* (3rd ed.). San Diego, CA: Singular.

The first chapter describes many aspects of the clinician as well as of the clinical interaction in stuttering therapy. Also relevant to the topics in the current chapter is Chapter 7: Counseling and People Who Stutter and Their Families which contains an excellent description of the therapeutic alliance and other aspects of helping the person who stutters change his behaviors, thoughts, and feelings. In Chapter 8, Therapeutic Process: Facilitating a Journey of Change, Manning and DiLollo describe goals for treatment and subtleties of how and when to work toward them.

Shapiro, D. (2011). The clinician: A paragon of change. In *Stuttering intervention: A collaborative journey to fluency freedom.* Austin, TX: Pro-Ed.

This textbook contains two excellent chapters on clinician characteristics. One deals with the "magic" of the client-clinician relationship and touches on many of the attributes needed by effective clinicians. Another discusses the processes of students becoming qualified clinicians. The author talks about many aspects of supervision and analysis of clinical interactions.

Van Riper, C. (1957). Symptomatic therapy for stuttering. In L. E. Travis (Ed.), *Handbook of speech* (pp. 878–896). New York, NY: Appleton-Century-Crofts, Inc.

Although this is an old chapter, it is an excellent description of how Van Riper combined psychotherapy with behavior therapy to create what we now call "stuttering modification" therapy. It is unparalleled in its explication of how his therapy motivates the client to confront his stutter and his "self" at the same time. Because of the emotional support and acceptance Van Riper provided, his clients were often able to reduce the abnormality of their symptoms and develop a "fluent stuttering" that passed for fluent speech.

Van Riper, C. (1958). Experiments in stuttering therapy. In J. Eisenson (Ed.), *Stuttering: A symposium* (pp. 273–290). New York, NY: Harper & Row.

This chapter describes the stuttering treatments that Van Riper experimented with in his first 20 years after leaving University of Iowa and setting up a speech clinic at what became Western Michigan University. Of particular interest is the systematic changes he made in treatment protocols year by year to develop the most effective methods and the five-year follow-ups he made to measure long-term progress.

Van Riper, C. (1975a). The stutterer's clinician. In J. Eisenson (Ed.), *Stuttering: A second symposium* (pp. 453–492). New York, NY: Harper & Row.

This chapter is still a useful description of the attributes that may be important in clinicians who treat people who stutter. It also contains excellent sections on clinicians' roles in motivating clients and discusses the subject of whether clinicians who themselves stutter should treat clients who stutter.

Zebrowski, P. (2007). Treatment factors that influence therapy outcomes of children who stutter. In E. Conture, & R. Curlee (Eds.), *Stuttering and related disorders of fluency* (pp. 23–38). New York, NY: Thieme.

This chapter has some excellent summaries of research relating to variables that can affect therapy outcome, including information about the relationship between the client and clinician.

11

Treatment of Younger Preschool Children: Borderline Stuttering

Chapter Objectives

After studying this chapter, readers should be able to:

- Understand the difference between indirect and direct treatment
- Be able to plan and carry out indirect and—if needed—direct treatment of a younger preschool child
- Learn about data collection in the clinic by the clinician and at home by the parents, both of which can be used to guide treatment
- Learn the basics of treatment approaches to preschool children advocated by three other groups of authors

Key Terms

Direct treatment: Therapy that works directly on the child's speech by having him or her speak more fluently, stutter more easily, or both

Easy stuttering: A very mild type of stuttering characterized by slow and relaxed repetitions or prolongations of sounds that are brief and smooth. This can be a target of direct treatment, with the goal being to change stuttering into normal disfluency.

Indirect treatment: Therapy that involves alleviating stresses that the child might be experiencing in communication at home and in other situations

Maintenance: The process of fading treatment while continuing to support the child and family so that fluency achieved in treatment does not diminish

One-on-one time: A period of about 15 minutes each day during which one parent is alone with the child and follows the child's lead in play and conversation. In this time, parents can practice new behaviors such as using a slower speech rate with pauses, and children can experience their parent's full attention.

Percentage syllables stuttered (%SS): This is one measure of stuttering frequency that is often used as data to determine how much a child is stuttering at a particular time. We suggest using %SS along with SRs as an indication of whether treatment is working.

Playing with stuttering: Pretending to stutter in a way that deliberately changes some aspect of the stutter, such as how many repetitions are produced. This activity is thought to decrease the child's frustration and fear of stuttering and thus reduce tension and struggle.

Severity ratings (SRs): Numbers on a 0 to 9 scale given daily by parents to describe their child's fluency. The SR scale is shown in Figure 8.5 and described in detail in Chapter 8.

Spontaneous fluency: A child's natural fluency that occurs without work or thought on his part

Younger preschool children: Children between 2 and 3.5 years

In this chapter, I will describe a number of different approaches to treatment of younger preschool children. I will begin by describing the approach I have been taking with this age group for more than 30 years.

AN INTEGRATED APPROACH

I would describe the stuttering in **younger preschool children** (2–3.5 years) to be at the "borderline" level with loose and relaxed repetitions. Treatment for them should be **indirect**, aimed at changing the environment. The presumption is that an indirect approach will decrease environmental stress on the child and, at the same time, will not call too much attention to her stuttering and will thereby not interfere with natural recovery. However, a small number of children this young are a little more severe. They are starting to add tension to their stuttering and may be aware of and frustrated by it. Nonetheless, I would refrain from formal **direct treatment**, such as the Lidcombe Program described in Chapter 12. Instead, I use play-based "slightly more direct treatment" for more severe younger preschool children. I aim at having them learn to stutter more easily and then gradually become fluent. Paramount in my approach is to make sure they feel good about talking and increasingly confident that they are in control of their speech.

In this chapter, I use the terms "family" and "parent" or "parents" interchangeably to indicate the important adults with whom the child commonly interacts. Cultures and families differ in who should be involved in the child's treatment. When I imply that one parent is the major player in the interaction patterns I describe, the reader should freely adapt the treatment to suit each situation—one parent or two, older children or cousins, nannies, grandparents, or other caregivers.

Most treatment of stuttering at this age is indirect because it involves working with the family environment to decrease stress and to increase fluency, rather than working directly on the child's speech. The initial focus is decreasing the family's concern, trying to understand their feelings, and helping them change selected aspects of the family-child interactions. If a child's family can discover ways to facilitate the child's fluency, they become confident in their ability to effect change and are able to assume long-term responsibility for the child's fluency. If this is not effective, then slightly more direct work on the child's speech by the clinician, with some help from the family, is appropriate. Figure 11.1 depicts the flow of treatment for most children using my approach.

I illustrate our approach to treatment with the case example of Ashley, the 2.5-year-old preschool child whom I introduced in Chapter 1.

An Integrated Approach

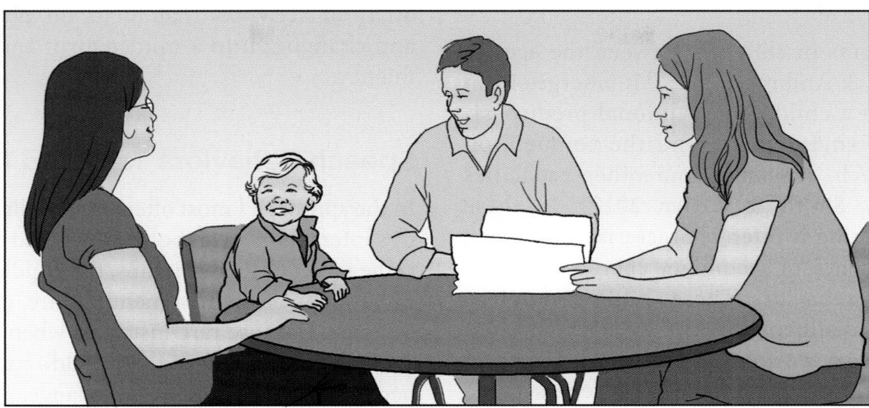

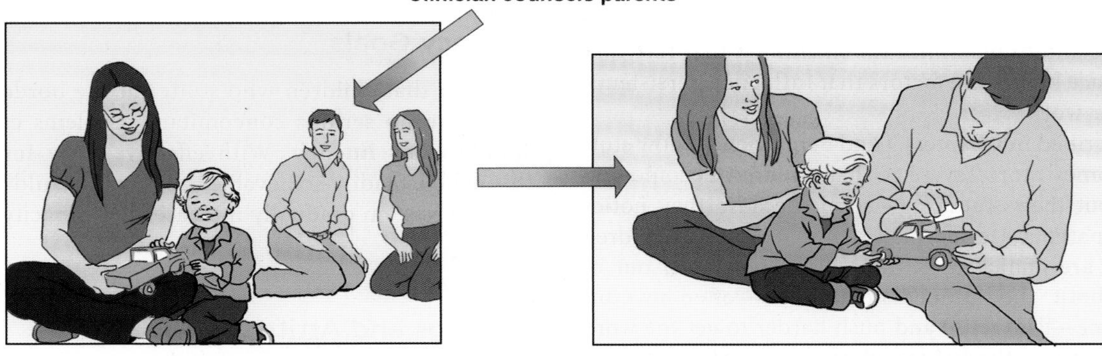

Figure 11.1 Treatments for younger preschool children who stutter.

Case Example

Ashley

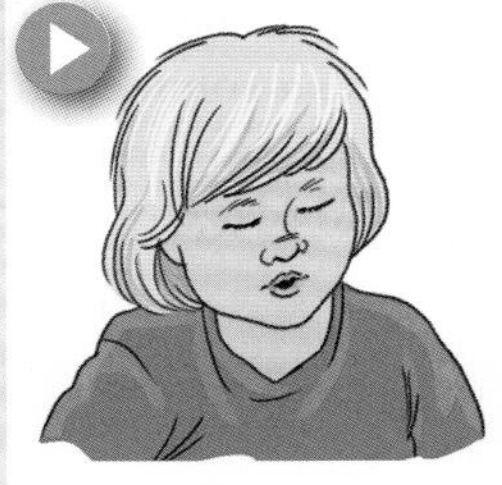

Ashley's stuttering, as you will remember from the video clip in Chapter 1, was characterized by multiple part-word and single-syllable whole-word repetitions. Two-and-a-half-year-old Ashley gave little indication that she was aware of her stuttering. Because her stuttering was quite frequent and gradually worsening, Ashley underwent treatment despite her young age. Indirect treatment was carried out via once-weekly home visits by a clinician with experience in stuttering. The clinician began by playing with Ashley on the floor with a variety of toys including dolls and a dollhouse. The clinician used a slow rate of speech with many pauses, as we describe in this chapter. She did not ask Ashley to change her own rate but only modeled the rate for Ashley and her mother, who observed. Gradually, the mother took a greater and greater part, but the clinician continued to be part of play so she could observe the mother's own use of slower speech rate with more pauses. After each session, the clinician and mother talked about how the mother was doing. The clinician was careful to praise the mother for what she was doing well before suggesting ways she could improve. In addition to slowing her speech rate and pausing more frequently, Ashley's mother also learned to turn most of her questions into comments. The clinician took data on the child's stuttering in each session.

This play therapy continued for about 8 weeks. Ashley's stuttering in the sessions disappeared, and her mother reported that she was more and more fluent in situations outside of the sessions. Recently, we video recorded an interview with Ashley at age 8, completely fluent and with no recollection of ever having stuttered.

Author's Beliefs

Nature of Stuttering

Stuttering usually begins in children between the ages of 2 and 3½ years (Yairi & Ambrose, 2005). It emerges from the interplay between a child's constitutional predispositions, stresses in the environment, and the competition for resources as speech, language, and other capacities develop rapidly (e.g., Smith & Weber, 2017). In these young children, stuttering is often characterized by a lack of tension and an absence of secondary characteristics—escape and avoidance behaviors. These children are often barely aware of their disfluencies. And even in children who show some signs of tension early in their stuttering development, their stuttering and their awareness come and go. Because many children recover spontaneously, our aim in treatment is to prevent stuttering from becoming more severe and to maximize the likelihood that recovery will take place before the factors that influence persistence can do their work.

As I described in Chapters 5 and 6, my view of how stuttering becomes more severe is that children become distressed about their stuttering—either because they notice that their parents are alarmed about it, or the children themselves are panicked as their disfluencies feel out of control, or both. Their immediate response—often not consciously done—is to tense and push harder to get the word out. I liken this to the harder effort we use when we have a key in a lock that refuses to open. Soon after, escape and avoidance behaviors may develop. If this escalation can be prevented, the plasticity of normal neural maturation will allow most of these children to develop neural networks like those of fluent children or to compensate for constitutional anomalies that create stuttering. To promote such flexibility in development to blossom into normal fluency, however, the clinician and family must provide an environment that fosters fluency and diminishes negative experiences with speaking.

In view of the presumed causes of borderline stuttering, our treatment focuses on four goals:

- Facilitate fluency by having family members speak slowly with pauses, change questions into comments, and listen attentively to the child.
- Reduce the parents' anxiety about their child's stuttering, thereby reducing the likelihood that they will convey distress about their child's stuttering to her.
- Reduce the child's alarm at his stuttering, in part by asking parents to comment acceptingly if the child seems at all frustrated when stuttering occurs.
- Reduce general stresses felt by the child.

If indirect therapy is not effective in reducing stuttering after 6 weeks, or if the child's stuttering proves to be more advanced than initially thought, I add more slightly more direct procedures. My slightly more direct approach for stuttering in younger preschoolers consists of a hierarchy of activities that focus on playing with stuttering and changing it to a milder form and then gradually into fluency.

Speech Behaviors Targeted for Therapy

In the approach I most often use—indirect therapy—the family's interaction style (both speech and nonspeech behaviors) is the target of therapy. Thus, the child's speech behaviors are not a focus of the treatment but are, of course, periodically assessed. In those rare instances when this approach doesn't soon decrease stuttering, the child's stuttering behaviors and her emotions are targeted for change.

Fluency Goals

I believe that children who stutter at the borderline level who have no serious concomitant problems can achieve **spontaneous fluency**. With effective early intervention, this goal is readily achievable because the child's maturing nervous system gradually increases her capacity for fluent speech.

Feelings and Attitudes

Although the main focus of treatment is on the behaviors of family members and others who interact frequently with the child, a parent can do a great deal to reduce the child's negative feelings about stuttering when she shows signs of frustration or dismay with her speech. This will be described in detail in the Procedures section, but I will make a few brief comments here. Usually, family members can tell if a child is showing signs of frustration or other distress about her disfluencies. They need to observe facial expressions, pitch increases, or whether the child stops in the middle of a stutter and changes what she is trying to say. When these or other signs of distress occur, a parent can make a comment, in a relaxed and accepting manner to reassure the child. It could be something like "I know it's hard when words get stuck, but it's ok. You're doing fine."

Maintenance Procedures

Many younger preschool children achieve fluent speech soon after their families have made some environmental modifications, and most maintain fluency without further treatment. However, it is important for the clinician to keep in contact with the family, even after formal treatment has stopped, to check on whether the child is reverting to older, more stressful interaction patterns. This support for **maintenance**, through telephone calls or e-mail, is gradually faded.

Clinical Methods

Working with stuttering at this level involves a variety of therapy procedures. I educate families by providing them with DVDs and reading material (such as that available from the Stuttering Foundation) to help them understand the nature of stuttering and the ways in which they can help the child become more fluent. The clinician should be familiar with the material before giving it to the family so that the clinician and the family can discuss it after the family has read or viewed it. I counsel families by listening to their concerns and by trying to understand their hopes, desires, fears, and frustrations. I brainstorm and problem-solve with families when I help them choose aspects of their interaction patterns to modify. I collect data on the child's speech and on the family's perceptions of his stuttering and fluency. And finally, I provide support as the child's stuttering decreases and the family strives to maintain their new styles of interaction.

Clinical Procedures: Indirect Treatment

This section describes the stages of indirect treatment, including continuing assessment of the child's speech at home and in the clinic, introduction of a slower speech rate with pauses, and introduction of other changes that the clinician and the family choose.

Severity Ratings

As I explained in Chapter 9 on assessment, during the closing interview the family is given a copy of the **Severity Rating (SR) Scale** (Fig. 8.5), and its use is explained to them. Although the scale was originally designed for use with the Lidcombe Program (see Chapter 12 for details), it is excellent for use with families of younger children who will be receiving indirect treatment. As you will remember, it is a 10-point scale that the family completes at the end of every day. Ratings range from 0 = no stuttering and 2 = extremely mild stuttering all the way to 9 = extremely severe stuttering (which may never be seen in a particular child). At each clinic session, after a baseline of the child's speech is collected in the first 10 minutes, the clinician and parent compare their SRs for the child's speech during the baseline measure. Agreement is defined as the parent and clinician's SR for that sample not differing by more than one point. If the difference between the ratings is greater than a single point, the clinician's rating is assumed to be accurate, and she discusses her rating with the parent to help the parent better understand the rating system and become "calibrated." The parent uses the scale to make a daily rating of the child's speech at the end of every day and brings or e-mails the week's SR chart to the clinician for discussion in each clinic meeting.

Baseline Speech Measures

At the beginning of each clinic visit, the clinician video records and observes the first 10 to 15 minutes of parent-child play. Attending to both the child's speech and the parent's interaction style, the clinician's first task is to decide on an SR for the child's speech in this parent-child play period. As noted, this will be compared with the parent's SR for the same sample. The clinician also notes aspects of the parent-child interaction, especially those on which the parent and clinician have agreed the parent will work on.

Family Interaction Patterns

As described in the section on assessment of the younger preschool child in Chapter 9, my approach to treatment involves study of and experimental change of parent-child interaction patterns. The change is described as experimental because not every change will have positive effects on the child's fluency; therefore, a change may be tried and discarded if the result of the "experiment" isn't positive. Here is a list of some conversational interaction patterns observed in some families that may need to be changed to facilitate the child's fluency.

1. High rates of speech
2. Rapid-fire conversational pace (lack of pauses or too-short pauses between speakers)
3. Interruptions
4. Frequent open-ended questions or questions that demand an answer
5. Many critical or corrective comments
6. Inadequate or inconsistent listening to what the child says
7. Vocabulary far above the child's level
8. Advanced levels of syntax

Table 11.1 gives some detailed suggestions for evaluating these parent-child conversational variables. Table 11.2 provides ideas for changes that families can make to facilitate their child's fluency. The clinician should study the family's interaction patterns and suggest one or two most relevant changes rather than give a long list to the family. Clinicians may also want to watch (and share with the family) the Stuttering Foundation video "7 Tips for Talking with the Child who Stutters" (https://www.stutteringhelp.org/content/7-tips-talking-child-who-stutters). This will provide ideas that the clinician can selectively suggest to the family.

Although other clinicians may begin treatment focusing on other family-child interaction variables, my own preference in most cases is to begin by helping families reduce their speech rate and increase their pausing. Supporting data on the effectiveness of parents slowing their speech rates and pausing more often are provided at the end of this section. In the next few paragraphs, I will describe how to help parents slow speech rate and increase pause time.

Slower Speech Rate with Pauses

For most families, the clinician starts by helping the parents reduce their speech rate and increase their pause time when talking with their child. The evidence reviewed in Chapters 2 and 3 suggests that individuals who stutter have constitutional

TABLE 11.1 Suggestions for Quantifying Family-Child Interaction Patterns

High rates of speech	Count the number of syllables spoken by each family member interacting with the child. Next, using a stopwatch, measure the amount of time each individual speaks. Be sure to stop timing whenever they stop speaking or pause for more than 2 s. Resume timing as soon as the speaking continues. Then, calculate the time in minutes to hundredths of a minute (e.g., 1 min and 13 s would be 1.22 min). Divide the total number of syllables spoken by the time in minutes to obtain the number of syllables per minute (SPM). For example, if a family member speaks 366 syllables in 1.22 min, their rate of speech is 300 SPM. Normal adult speaking rates are 165–230 SPM (Andrews & Ingham, 1971). Thus, this is a fast rate of speech.
Rapid-fire conversational pace (lack of pauses between speakers)	Using a stopwatch, measure intervals from when the child stops speaking to when another family member begins. If these intervals average less than 1 s, the pace of conversation is rapid.
Interruptions	Count the number of sentences or sentence-like utterances the child speaks during the sample and the number of times a family member interrupts the child. Divide the number of interruptions by the total number of sentences. If more than 10 percent of the sentences contain interruptions, the child may feel pressure to speak quickly.
Frequent questions	Count the number of sentences spoken by family members to the child and the number of sentences that are questions. Divide the number of questions by the total number of sentences. If more than 25 percent of the utterances are questions, the child may feel pressure from having to answer questions.
Many critical or directive comments	Each sentence of the family members should be characterized as being either "critical/directive" or "accepting/nondirective." Sentences characterized as critical/directive would be (1) those that convey a slight or stronger criticism of what the child is saying or doing, (2) those that pressure the child to speak or direct the child's activity, and (3) those spoken with a tone of voice that is stern or negatively incredulous. The number of sentences that is critical should be divided by the total number of sentences. If the percentage of critical/directive comments is higher than 50 percent, the child may feel stress from high standards in the family.
Inadequate or inconsistent listening to what the child says	Assess the content of family members' sentences during each speaking turn. Note whether family members are responding to the content of the child's utterances. If more than 50 percent of family members' utterances ignore the topic the child has been speaking about, the child may feel he is not being heard.
Vocabulary far above the child's level	Compare the vocabulary level of family members' speech with that of the child. If more than only a small amount of the family members' vocabulary exceeds the child's receptive level, the child may feel pressure when trying to understand family members' vocabulary.
Advanced levels of syntax	Assess the syntax used by family members when speaking to the child. If more than only a small amount is considerably above the child's current receptive level, the child may feel not only pressure by difficulty understanding family members but also pressure to use syntax that he has yet to master.

deficits that make it challenging for them to produce speech at rapid rates. If parents provide a model of slower speech with plentiful pauses, this model alone will probably influence children to speak more slowly (Guitar & Marchinkowski, 2001). More importantly, a model of slower speech with adequate pauses has been shown to reduce children's stuttering (e.g., Guitar, Kopff-Schaefer, Donahue-Kilburg, & Bond, 1992; Stephanson-Opsal & Bernstein Ratner, 1988; Zebrowski, Weiss, Savelkoul, & Hammer, 1996). The clinician emphasizes that parents should not instruct the child to slow his speech rate; such direct instruction tends to be ineffective and annoying to the child. Simply speaking in the style of television's Mr. Rogers will have the desired effect. Parents and clinicians can refresh their memory of this speaking style by watching YouTube videos of Mister Rogers, including his 2002 Commencement speech at Dartmouth College (see link in Table 11.2).

Teaching Slower Speaking Rate with Pauses

After rehearsing a slower speech rate with pauses, you can meet with the parents, model this style of speaking, and ask them to try it. Sometimes, beginning with a reading passage is easier than having a conversation. Most parents find it slightly embarrassing to speak this way at first, but your modeling this style will make it easier for them. Strongly reinforce them

TABLE 11.2 Things Families Can Do to Help the Younger Preschool Child Who Stutters

Listening time	All children benefit from feeling that what they have to say is important. This is especially true for the child who is beginning to stutter. Set aside some time each day as "listening time" with your child. Make it at least 5–10 min (or longer if you can) at about the same time each day, so your child can depend on it. Try to have it be a time when you can be alone with your child, free from distractions. During that time, refrain from making suggestions or giving instructions. Merely "be there" for the child, listening attentively to what he or she says or quietly playing alongside the child if he or she chooses not to talk. The book on listening by Shafir (2000) is an excellent resource for improving listening skills.
Slow rate	It will benefit the child if family members reduce their conversational rate of speech to a slow, soothing style. Speech should sound relaxed and calm, with comfortable pauses throughout. Fred Rogers on "Mister Rogers's Neighborhood" is a good model. For a sample of his slow rate with pauses, watch the YouTube video "Fred Rogers' 2002 Dartmouth College Commencement Address." https://www.youtube.com/watch?v=907yEkALaAY
Pauses	The pace of conversation can be kept appropriately slow if the speaker pauses 1–2 s before starting to talk. This also helps to keep the speaker from interrupting another speaker.
Positive comments	Make many specific, positive, and accepting comments about what your child is saying and doing. Limit corrections or criticisms to important issues. Changes for the better usually happen more quickly when someone feels he is OK as he is. The child who feels good about himself will be better able to use "listening time," "slow rate," and "pauses" to gain more fluency.
Fewer questions	It is natural to ask a child many questions in order to encourage him to learn new things and to display that knowledge. However, this makes some children feel "under the gun." So it may be a good idea to decrease demanding questions and instructions. If you are worried that your child won't learn enough if you are too laid-back, keep in mind that learning comes naturally to children. They learn best from your interest in things, especially from your interest and positive comments about the things they do and say.
Taking turns in family conversations	All children find it easier to talk if family members take turns rather than interrupting and talking over each other. A student and I published an article about how effective this approach was for her son who stuttered (Winslow & Guitar, 1994). She found that having family members hold a "talking stick" (an object like a salt shaker) when they took their turn was a helpful reminder not to interrupt each other.

for the things they are doing well. Once they have a pretty good style, if you can video or audio record their speech and play it back to them, their experience of hearing and watching themselves speak this way will help them remember it. If you have a laptop with a camera, you can record a clip of them speaking this way and e-mail it to them so they will have it at home to refresh their memories from time to time.

Trying Slower Rate with Pauses in the Clinic

After the parents feel comfortable using the new speaking style, the clinician and a parent can carry out some play interaction with the child and use the slower rate with pauses (Fig. 11.2). If the child asks the parent why he or she is talking in a funny, slow way, the clinician or parent may explain to the child that the parent talks too fast and needs to learn to slow down. With some children, we enlist them to remind the parent to slow down if they think the parent is talking too quickly. Children delight in correcting adults, especially their parents.

Using the Slower Rate with Pauses at Home

If the clinician is not satisfied with the parents' ability to speak with the child using this new speaking style, home practice should be delayed until the parents have mastered it. However, most parents pick up the new style quickly, and they can begin using it at home immediately. One parent should try to spend 15 minutes a day playing alone with the child and using the new speaking style. *The best time is in*

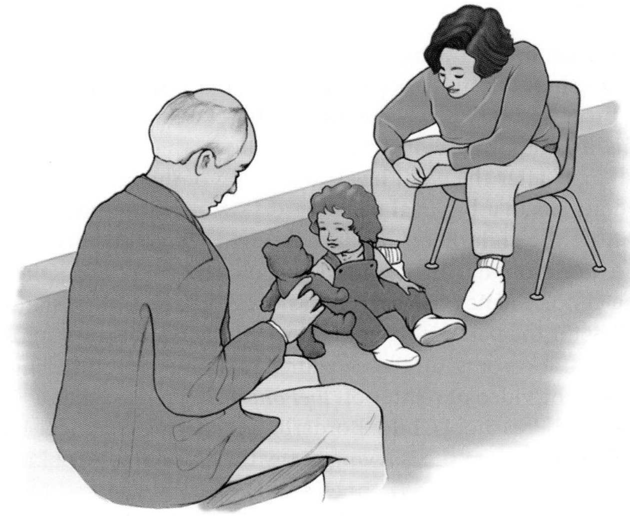

Figure 11.2 Clinician models interaction patterns while the mother observes.

the morning because it may influence the child for the rest of the day. Many families are too busy at this time, feeding and dressing their children and themselves; for them, one-on-one slow speech practice in the morning may be possible only on weekends. In this case, any 15 minutes per day of **one-on-one time** with the child is acceptable. Most important is that the parents do it every day. If one parent does most of the one-on-one play with slow speech, the other parent should also use the slower speech rate when talking with the child whenever he or she can.

Monitoring Parents' Practice of Slower Rate with Pauses

Most parents benefit from consistent support for any changes they are making in their interactions with their child. I often keep in touch with them between clinic visits via e-mail or telephone, but I always suggest that they keep a brief journal of their experience with the new speaking style by making notes on the SR chart they are completing every evening. When parents are willing and able to video record themselves at home using the new speaking style during their 15-minute daily interactions, the recording is a fine motivation for them to practice and a good way for me to monitor their progress. In any case, their interaction with their child at the beginning of each session allows me to be sure they are using an effective speaking style and allows me to collect data on the child's **percentage syllables stuttered** during this interaction. When I'm observing this, I can also read the SR chart with the parents' notes about their daily work between clinic visits. In the discussion that follows the parent-child interaction, I am careful to reinforce the parents for everything they are doing well. In all discussions, the clinician's role is first and foremost to be an empathetic listener, allowing the parents to take the lead in assessing their progress and formulating plans to work on change.

Commenting on the Child's Speech

If the child is showing signs of frustration or other distress during her stutters, I ask parents to begin commenting by first letting the child know when she is talking well. I demonstrate this for them by saying something like "That's really good talking!" after the child has had a string of fluent sentences. I don't make a big deal of it but do say it with enthusiasm so that the child hears it and is pleased. Don't do this very often to avoid having the child become self-conscious. Once the child's fluency has been occasionally praised, then she is ready for the parent to comment when the child shows signs of frustration or is nonplussed during a moment of stuttering. Watch the video of Ashley on *thePoint* (Chapter 1, Video 1-1: A Young Preschool Child: Borderline Stuttering, Segment 1). Notice that when she is trying to say the cat's name "Cookie," she repeats "Co-" many times and eventually you can hear her pitch increase and she is running out of breath. She is also looking around, slightly baffled at what is happening to her. After she gives up and has finished her utterance, a clinician or parent could then say "Oh, that word 'Cookie' was hard to say. Sometimes words just get stuck and that's ok." A parent or clinician shouldn't do this very often or else the child may resent it or be embarrassed. Observe how the child reacts. If she seems even more distressed than before, back off of the commenting for a while and try again with a briefer reassurance, like "mmm-hmmm" after the stutter and then a comment letting the child know she's been heard and understood even though there was a stutter. If all goes well, the child may have a look of slight relief after she hears that everything is all right, even though the word got stuck.

Working with Other Aspects of the Parent-Child Interaction

As the clinician works with the parents or other family members on their speech rate and pausing, and occasional comments, she continues to assess the child's progress toward normal fluency, as indicated by percent syllables stuttered (%SS) in the treatment setting, SRs at home, and discussions with the family. If these indicators of fluency do not portray a steady downward progression of stuttering in the first 3 or 4 weeks of treatment, the clinician and family should consider other aspects of the parent-child interaction that may be putting pressure on the child's fluency. Consider items 3 to 8 in Table 11.1.

Modifications of Family Communication Style

Remember that most of the interaction patterns in families of children who stutter are not abnormal or particularly negative. They usually are quite typical of the culture in which the child is being raised. However, a child sensitive to communicative pressure may benefit from some modification of family communication patterns in ways that facilitate her fluency. It is vital that the clinician help the family understand that they are not causing the child to stutter because of inappropriate communication patterns. Instead, their communication is normal, but they can help their child by changing a few aspects of their communication to facilitate fluency.

One of the first things I do if I sense some aspect of the family communicative style might need a little modification is to have the parents watch with me the video recording of their interaction with their child. As we watch together, I praise many things that the parents are doing well. Praise is vital in helping develop the parents' confidence and encouraging them to keep doing things they are doing well. As I praise the parents, I listen acceptingly to their comments even if they are self-critical. We watch together for things that the parents and I both feel might be putting pressure on the child. The best situation is when parents notice something to change—something that I also feel may be pressuring the child's fluency. Then together, we plan to change that aspect of the interaction and observe the results.

For example, in the 3rd week of treatment, a parent was doing a great job using a slower speech rate with pauses. However, the child's fluency—which had increased somewhat—had now plateaued. The parent and I watched the most recent video recording, and as we watched, I praised her slow speech with pauses. After a few minutes, the parent commented that she was surprised to see that she asked her child so many questions, rat-a-tat-tat, one right after the other. I agreed with her and we discussed alternatives, such as making comments instead of asking questions, and she tried this out during the week. The following week, the child's SRs showed further increases in fluency, and the parent's interaction at the beginning of the session revealed an impressive decrease in questions. This change, accompanied by the slower speech rate with pausing, was enough to increase the child's fluency to normal levels, which was maintained long term.

Changes in Family Routine

In addition to changing conversational interaction patterns, a family may identify other stresses on the child that need to be changed, such as the amount of individual attention the child receives and the "busyness" of the family's schedule. My main function in helping families work on such stresses is to give them information about changes that others have found helpful and to be a sounding board for their plans for changing. I encourage them to assess, informally, the effects of these changes on the child's fluency and his overall adjustment. Although my praise and appreciation may help, a significant change in the child's stuttering is the real motivator. Notes the parent makes on the chart of daily SRs will help you and the family identify factors that may facilitate fluency or cause upward spikes in a child's stuttering. A parent, for example, noted on her SR chart that her child's stuttering flared up if she left the room while he was playing. She alleviated this stress by being careful to let the child know ahead of time if she were about to leave the room and that she would be right back. This example is a reminder of the importance of parents' attention for a child's self-esteem. When a child senses that his mother or father understands her and genuinely cares about her (cares about what she likes to do, what she thinks about things, and how she feels), the child feels more comfortable with herself, is less anxious, and is better able to speak easily.

To emphasize what I've said earlier, for many younger preschool children who stutter, a little more one-on-one time spent with a parent every day, preferably in the morning, can boost fluency tremendously. Although the morning can be the most difficult time for parents who work outside the home, one-on-one "fluency time" in the morning can have a positive effect on the child's speech for the rest of the day. If mornings are too difficult, some one-on-one time in the afternoon can also be very helpful. The time does not need to be long, just 15 to 20 minutes, but the parent needs to be with the child in a place where, ideally, they won't be interrupted.

The child should choose what to play or talk about, and the parent should follow the child's lead, participating as the child directs. As a parent becomes more and more comfortable with this nondirective play, she may want to explore ways of helping the child feel really understood. One of the parents we worked with, for example, learned to "mirror" her child's momentary emotions as they built a tower of blocks together. When the child placed a block on the tower and it fell off, the parent would quietly murmur a sound of disappointment, echoing the child's facial expression. This child made impressive gains in fluency in only a few weeks, and I believe that this parent's deep attention to the child may have contributed significantly to this change. Although parents may vary in the level of empathetic response they can achieve, increased caring attention is probably a realistic goal for most families.

Attentive play can become child-directed conversations as a child grows older, and such conversations can continue the process of helping the child develop a sense of being loved, understood, and appreciated. In his article *Making Time for Your Child*, the child psychiatrist Stanley Greenspan suggested "In spontaneous, unstructured talk or play, try to follow your child's lead. The goal is to 'march to your child's drummer' and to tune in to the child at his level" (Greenspan, 1993, p. 111).

Course of Treatment

Sometimes families report that their attempts to make changes have been fairly successful. For example, they may have been able to slow their speaking rates and to simplify their language and may have seen improvement in their child. I let them know that their changes have been key factors in the child's improvement and stress the importance of continuing them. It is easy to resume old patterns after some improvement occurs, whether it's the challenge of losing weight or helping a child become more fluent.

Each child and each family is unique in how they respond to treatment, but it is possible to note some common trends. For example, some children become much more fluent soon after the family makes one or two changes in their environment. Occasionally, a child may become fluent immediately after an initial session, possibly because the family is less anxious about her disfluencies after sharing their concerns with a professional. Whatever the cause, early and immediate fluency gains should be viewed with cautious optimism. I share the family's pleasure at such dramatic change but suggest that their child's fluency may be fragile and will need to be nurtured by our continued efforts to create a facilitative environment.

Sometimes the path toward fluency is rough and irregular. The child may make little or no progress or may improve for a while and then return to his old pattern of disfluency. When this happens and the family or clinician feels frustrated by slow progress, further exploration of the family's feelings about the child's stuttering is called for. Many times family members worry about the child's future, afraid that stuttering will be a serious handicap for her. Sometimes there is lingering guilt about having caused her stuttering. Often it is hard for parents to accept the blemish they feel that stuttering creates on the family image.

Whatever the source of a family's anxieties, their concern about stuttering may easily radiate to the child in their reactions to her stutters. Unwittingly, family members may show their anxiety or disappointment through facial expressions or body language, which may make the child "hesitate to hesitate" and thus stutter more severely. Open and frank discussions with the family about their feelings and concerns are likely to be more helpful at this point than trying to change their reactions. In such discussions, the clinician's role is to make it easier for the family to talk about their concerns, so I listen carefully, try my best to understand them, and convey my understanding with acceptance and respect. When family members feel understood and accepted, it is easier for them to share their feelings and accept them. When this occurs, some feelings may change, and in turn, the child's stuttering may decrease, possibly because her stuttering no longer seems so terrible to the family.

Another barrier to changing a family's interaction patterns is the fact that some styles of interaction reflect important cultural values. For example, in the urban eastern United States, family members sometimes finish each other's sentences, conveying a closeness and solidarity within the family that is highly valued. If they are asked to speak more slowly and pause between speakers' turn takings, such changes would conflict with one of the family's implicit cultural values. Another example might be parents who frequently teach, correct, and criticize their children's behavior. This "instructional" mode of interaction may reflect the importance that the family's culture places on education.

I believe that it is important to explore how the family feels about changes they are considering. Often, they can find ways to change other variables that will be as effective, thereby leaving unchanged those interactions that are of value to the family. Some years ago, I worked with a parent who spoke very rapidly to her 4-year-old child who was beginning to stutter. She resisted changing her speech rate because "it isn't the way we talk." In addition, she was frequently critical of her child's behavior. Consequently, I encouraged her to use positive reinforcement for fluency, as described in the Lidcombe Program approach to treatment of beginning stuttering in Chapter 12. At that time, I had just read the article by Onslow, Andrews, and Lincoln (1994) and, borrowing just the positive reinforcement for fluency from that, asked this mother to let her child know with upbeat statements of praise that she liked his smooth fluency. The child's stuttering diminished almost immediately, and she was delighted with her ability to help her child.

Sometimes a family may resist change and doesn't fully participate in treatment. There may be psychological issues that need to be resolved through referral to a family counselor, or the family may have other, more serious problems with which to cope. In such cases, I talk with the family directly about my concerns. This usually leads to an open discussion of their situation, a referral to a family counselor, or, in rare cases, their decision to withdraw the child from stuttering therapy for the time being. If this happens, I let the family know that I remain available to them, and I try to stay in contact by occasional phone calls or e-mails to make it easier for them to resume the child's therapy if they wish to.

Maintenance

Indirect treatment of a younger preschool child is often effective within five or six sessions, over a period of 1 or 2 months. The child's speech becomes markedly less disfluent. Part-word repetitions become whole-word or phrase repetitions, which are more like typical children's disfluencies, and the family's concerns about the child's speech diminish. When this happens, I review with them the changes the family has made with them and the changes in their child's stuttering that reflect her improvement. Using this information, I help the family develop a plan to deal with periods of increased stress that may prompt stuttering to reappear. Most families feel that they have a handle on how to reduce stress on their child at this stage of therapy and their experiences in observing and changing their behaviors have given them confidence. If their child's stuttering suddenly increases, they know how to examine their speech rates or attentiveness when talking to the child and how to examine other aspects of their interactions and implement needed changes.

Effective maintenance for stuttering in younger preschool children is the result of two things: (1) helping the family to view the child's stuttering more objectively with less anxiety, guilt, or panic and (2) building the family's confidence in their own ability to implement problem-solving skills they've learned to use when the child's disfluencies increase. Sometimes, however, despite a family's best efforts to respond constructively, stuttering returns. This may occur after an increase in stress from some trauma or from typical life events, such as moving to a new house, or it may accompany a growth spurt in the child's language. On the other hand, it may be inexplicable. Whatever the cause, the family should feel comfortable getting back in contact with the clinician. I let each family know at the end of therapy that relapse is possible, not abnormal, and that I would look forward to seeing the child again if help is needed.

Supporting Data

Many years ago, my colleagues and I published two papers that evaluated the effect of changing parent-child interactions with a 5-year-old child who stuttered (Guitar, 1978; Guitar et al., 1992). Although this child was an older preschooler, the principles of working with the family on their interaction style were similar to those described for the younger preschool child. Our approach to treatment was to video record parent-child interactions over five treatment sessions and then view the videos with each parent. When viewing the videos, we let the parent decide what to work on in the intervening week and then recorded a new parent-child interaction after a week of work on changing the behavior they had selected. After six sessions, the child's stuttering had diminished to the level of normal disfluency; we followed the child for 10 years, and the stuttering never reappeared. In an analysis of the parents' behavior and the child's stuttering, we discovered that the changes in parent behavior that were most related to the child's improvement in stuttering comprised two different changes. The first change in parent behavior was the mother's reduction in her speech rate. This change was most related to her daughter's decreases in "primary stuttering," in other words, easy repetitions. The second parent behavior change was the mother's increases in her accepting, supportive statements. This change was highly related to decreases in her daughter's tense blocks or "secondary stuttering."

A variety of other studies have shown that changes in parent's communicative interactions affect their children's stuttering. Stephenson-Opsal and Bernstein Ratner (1988) demonstrated that when the mothers of stuttering children slowed their speech rates, the children's stuttering decreased. Starkweather, Gottwald, and Halfond (1990) reported on 29 children they treated for an average of 12 sessions (some required as many as 40 sessions), all of whom completely recovered. Their approach involved primarily modification of the parents' behavior, including reduction of speech rate, having special speech time, matching parent language to child language, and reducing parents' negative reactions to stuttering. Zebrowski et al. (1996) showed that decreases in mother's speaking rate and pause time were associated with decreases in stuttering in some children.

Further supporting data on this approach are presented in the outcome measures of the Michael Palin Centre's treatment of preschool children, described later in this chapter. Moreover, yet more supporting data come from reports by Franken, Kielstra-van der Schalk, and Boelens (2005) and by de Sonneville-Koedoot, Stolk, Rietveld, and Franken (2015) that provide evidence of the effectiveness of parent-child interaction therapy (the RESTART Program). The study by de Sonneville-Koedoot et al. reported that 65 out of 91 children treated with this approach were no longer stuttering 18 months after treatment. In the next chapter on treatment of older preschoolers, the treatment approach described by Gottwald (2010) uses a great deal of indirect treatment but supplements it with direct treatment when needed. She reports that 26 of 27 children who were stuttering notably before treatment were speaking normally a year or more after treatment ended.

Clinical Procedures: Slightly More Direct Treatment

My approaches to therapy evolve as I learn more about children who stutter and treatment options. Earlier, my choice of an additional treatment approach for those borderline stutterers who didn't respond to indirect treatment had been the Lidcombe Program (LP), which I will describe in detail in Chapter 12. However, I would no longer use LP with children younger than 3.5 years, nor with children who have a very sensitive temperament. In regard to the age factor, research suggests that older preschool children who have been stuttering for a longer period of time need less treatment time in LP that those who are younger and have just begun to stutter (Jones, Onslow, Harrison, & Packman, 2000). This suggests that LP treatment may not be the most efficient approach for younger preschool children. Also, I am reluctant to use LP for very sensitive children because my own clinical experience suggests that these children may react negatively to contingencies for stuttering.[1]

The material in the following sections on slightly more direct treatment has been helpful for younger preschool children who need something more than indirect treatment. Because of my theoretical orientation, my slightly more direct treatment approach is guided by the principle that therapy must be fun for the child and should reduce negative emotions associated with her stuttering.

I don't use slightly more direct treatment with every child who is a borderline stutterer, but it is a good alternative to combine with indirect treatment when indirect treatment alone does not decrease the child's stuttering significantly after 6 weeks. The causes of failure with an indirect approach are often unknown. Sometimes, a family seems unable to modify the child's environment as planned, or they do, but the child's stuttering persists unchanged or increases. In these few cases, I try a slightly more direct approach, as described in the next section.

Slightly More Direct Treatment for Mild Borderline Stuttering

Most younger preschool children with borderline stuttering are often minimally aware of their disfluencies. Their repetitions appear relaxed, and they show no signs of defensive reactions to their stuttering or using extra effort to "fight" their stutters. They also are normally fluent a great deal of the time, and I think they have the capacity to develop entirely normal fluency. Consequently, when I use slightly more direct treatment for mild borderline stuttering, I focus on the child's fluency, assuming that she will easily be able to increase the amount of fluency she has and "outgrow" his stuttering with our help. As I described earlier when talking about a parent who didn't want to slow her rate, I followed some of the behavioral management strategies used by the Lidcombe Program, which is described in Chapter 12. In these cases, I train parents to respond to fluency with praise, and unlike the Lidcombe Program, I ask them to ignore

[1]It is possible that a very skilled clinician and a very creative parent can find contingencies for stuttering that don't bother even the most sensitive child.

stuttering unless the child is momentarily distressed by a stutter, in which case, I suggest the parents comment acceptingly on it as I have described earlier. Thus, it is not, strictly speaking, a Lidcombe approach.

I usually begin by training one of the child's parents to use praise for fluency during the daily one-on-one time with the child. The parent might say, "Gee, that was really smooth talking" or "I like the way you said that." The clinician and parent should decide how frequently to use positive reinforcement, but most children are annoyed by praise if the parent gives it too often. These fluent utterances do not need to be consecutive. A few children are annoyed by any praise at all given by the parent. In this case, the parent and the clinician can talk with the child about using something besides typical praise. Some children prefer their own phrase. One child wanted his parent to say "That was good monkey talk!" Another child asked for a gesture (thumbs up) instead of words.

As in parent-child interaction therapy, parents keep daily logs of the child's overall fluency for each day, using the 0 to 9 SRs described earlier. When the child has made substantial progress in decreasing severity, the clinician guides the parent in gradually replacing praise for fluency in the daily one-on-one sessions with praise used occasionally during other activities during the day. While the parent is carrying out this slightly more direct therapy, it is important for her or him to attend weekly meetings with the clinician to demonstrate using the procedure, to share SRs, and to discuss progress and problems. It is also important for the family to continue one-on-one sessions with the child and *to continue the changes made in their interactions and family lifestyle.*

Slightly More Direct Treatment for More Severe Borderline Stuttering

Some younger preschool children who stutter are beginning to have negative feelings about their disfluencies but are not showing the full-blown signs of struggle or escape behaviors that characterize beginning stuttering. Still, they may occasionally express real frustration with their stuttering.

Typically, I work with children having more severe borderline stuttering for about 45 minutes each week. I also continue to provide encouragement and support to the family in helping them make the child's environment as facilitating to fluency as possible. Our slightly more direct treatment activities are presented in a hierarchy that the clinician and child ascend as far as is necessary to bring the child's disfluencies into the "typical disfluency" range. Progressive steps are taken when the clinician senses that a child is feeling competent at the current step. Thus, progress may be rapid or slow and sudden or gradual, depending on the child's feeling of comfort and mastery with the tasks at hand. There is no need to hurry this process. It should take place within the context of games and activities that make the focus on stuttering casual and, above all, fun. The clinician needs to remain alert to the child's immediate sense of confidence and self-esteem in selecting the moment to move the child to the next step in the treatment hierarchy.

Modeling Easy Stutters

I begin slightly more direct treatment rather indirectly by providing models of **easy stuttering** in my speech. If the child's repetitions are fast and abrupt, my models are slow with gradual endings. If the child has many repetitions or long prolongations, I repeat or prolong sounds briefly. These models are done casually during play with the child. I don't produce them immediately after the child stutters but insert them randomly, about once every two or three sentences, as if I were stuttering as I talked.

Once the child has become acclimated to the models of easy stuttering after 10 or 15 minutes of play, I begin to make, occasionally, accepting comments about them. I might say, for example, "Hmmmm, I used slidey speech on that word, didn't I?" or "That word stuck a little, but that's OK, I slid right out of it." Most children appear to be shyly interested in what I am talking about, and slightly more direct therapy can continue to develop. A few, however, may react negatively and say such things as "Don't do that!" or "I don't like it when you do that." For them, even slightly more direct therapy needs to proceed slowly to allow my acceptance of them as they are and my support during play activities to gradually counteract the child's anxiety.

If the child has begun to experience the first pangs of frustration from stuttering, which can be inferred from her questions or complaints about getting stuck on words, I will try to help her express this. Even though I am making comments that show acceptance of my own stuttering, I occasionally may produce a longer than usual stutter and say, "Sometimes they go on for a long time. That makes me mad." I continue to try to sense what the child is feeling and to empathize as naturally as possible. I use this empathic focus not only when I am modeling easy stutters but throughout slightly more direct treatment.

For children who evidence periods of acute frustration with their stuttering, parents should be coached on how to make empathetic statements in a calm, soothing, slow style when the child is going through a difficult time. As I do direct therapy, I try to involve the parents in appropriate activities both at home and in the clinic. If their indirect treatment has not been effective, I need to be sure the parents do not feel pushed aside by my direct therapy with the child. They need to remain active participants.

The Child Begins Active Participation: "Catch Me"

When I sense that a child is comfortable with my easy stuttering models, I see if the child will take part. I may say, for example, "Can you help me? Sometimes when I get stuck on a word, it goes on and on. Then I try to make my stuck words real slow and loose, and it helps me get unstuck. But sometimes I forget. If you hear me go on and on like thi-thi-thi-thi-thi-this, just say, 'There's one,' and I'll try to make it slow and loose with slidey speech." When the child catches me, I will change a fast, tight repetition to a slow, loose one. As I model stuck words, I choose a style of stuttering similar to the child's.

Praise should flow liberally when the child catches one of my modeled stutters. This provides the child with a sense of accomplishment that is associated with something she previously felt to be out of control, even though now it is in my speech. For many children, tangible rewards, such as small snacks or turns at a game, are important motivators and should be used along with praise to establish the child's ability to catch the clinician's stutters.

The Child Begins Active Participation: Play

This stage can either follow or precede "Catch Me." It depends on the clinician's judgment about which activity would be more comfortable for the child. Sometimes you may start one of these stages but find the child is not ready and you switch to the other. The **playing with stuttering** stage engages a child in following the clinician's lead in playfully imitating disfluencies that are similar to her own, such as repeated or prolonged sounds. The purpose is to desensitize the child to the frustration that sometimes arises in more severe borderline stuttering. It is a process that may take place because play can give a child a sense of mastery without the risk of failure. The concept of play is quite interesting. Scientists speculate that children's play is an opportunity for them to practice and master skills that are needed in adulthood. Playing with stuttering may take advantage of children's natural tendency to play and provide them with the pleasure of mastery and control over something that has been frustrating and sometimes even frightening.

Take, for example, the child who stutters primarily in a repetitive fashion. The clinician might say, "Let's play a game of saying some sounds over and over and see how many times we can say them. I bet I can say a whole bunch of times! Watch this. Ba-ba-ba-ba-ba! Can you do it that many times?" Or it can begin by making sounds for animals, puppets, or other toys: "Hey, this is a zebragella! It goes 'lllllla! llllla!' (using prolongations). Then it jumps around like this (clinician jumps around) and chews the carpet (clinician pretends to chew the carpet)."

The clinician and child can keep incorporating such play into their routine as long as the child finds it fun and the clinician can free herself to enjoy uninhibited play. From playing with repeated or prolonged sounds, the clinician can build a bridge to playing with repeated or prolonged sounds in conversation and, in time, to the child's actual stutters.

The Child Produces Intentional Stutters

After the child is able to catch the clinician's stutters and appears comfortable doing it, the clinician should begin looking for opportunities to ask the child to produce a stutter intentionally. This can be done most easily by pretending to have trouble producing slow, loose stutters. For instance, the clinician might say, "I can't seem to make this one slow and loose. Can you show me how to do it?" Again, this should be done intermittently and casually mixed in with other activities that are fun for the child.

Praise and, if needed, tangible rewards are used to help the child build confidence. When the child is able to produce slow and loose stutters, the clinician can let the parents know, in the child's presence, about this accomplishment, focusing on the child's ability to teach the clinician. If the child seems proud of this accomplishment, the clinician can take advantage of this opportunity and have the child show intentional stutters to the parents. This not only desensitizes the child to stuttering with the parent, but it also desensitizes parents to the child's stuttering and models acceptance of the child's stuttering for them.

The Child Changes His Own Real Stutters

For many young children (younger than 3½ years) whose stuttering fluctuates between mild and severe levels, these slightly more direct therapy activities, combined with a facilitating environment provided by parents, may be enough to advance their fluency into the typical range within a few months. For those whose stuttering persists, still another stage of direct therapy may be necessary. In such cases, I look for opportunities when the child seems ready to modify her own stutters.

I begin by responding to a few of the child's real stutters with accepting comments to help the child feel comfortable with his stutters. I might say, with an accepting voice, "Oh, that one was a little bumpy on 'my-my-my car…,'" and then return to the business of playing. After further play, when the child stutters again, the clinician can model an easier and slower style of stuttering on the same word and comment positively about it. I then ask the child to imitate my easier stutter and praise her for doing so, using reinforcements and guidance to shape her stuttering to a slow, relaxed style.

I look for slightly slower and easier stutters in the child's speech and reward them. Even if the child intentionally stutters, but in an easier way than he stuttered previously, I reward her. From this point on, the clinician uses a combination of modeling and reinforcement to shape the child's stuttering. It is the deliberate slowness and "easiness" with which the child produces repetitions or prolongations, along with the sense of playing with stuttering, that make it possible for the child to begin feeling a sense of control. This in turn should reduce her frustration and fear, further diminish tension, and enable her to move through stutters with minimal effort.

After the child is able to make her stutters slower and easier in the clinic, generalization may occur away from the clinic without the need for formal transfer activities. Such "spontaneous" generalization may be a result of the child's increased self-esteem from gaining mastery over behavior she previously felt uncomfortable about and felt was out of her control. Consequently, emphasis should be placed on the stutters that a child handles successfully, rather than when she loses control.

If generalization is not occurring automatically, I work with family members to make the child's ability to play with and modify stutters a point of pride at home. Initially, the child can teach parents and siblings to stutter in the clinic under the clinician's guidance. Then the clinician can work with the child at home and involve family members if possible and if needed, so that the parents learn to use positive reinforcement selectively to increase the child's slow and easy stutters and let her know that she is appreciated. Even though the emphasis here is on slow and easy stutters, the effects of speech and language maturation and the increasing confidence that the child feels in her speech as a result of reduced frustration should result in normal fluency.

One final note about slightly more direct therapy with young children who stutter: Van Riper once told me that one of his daughters began to stutter quite severely at a young age and he found a way to help her, using (slightly more) direct therapy. Van Riper and his wife used what now might be called "rhythm therapy." They had their daughter speak short sentences in a rhythmic manner, accompanied by clapping her hands. In fact, all the family talked this way for several weeks, after which his daughter became completely fluent, despite a minor relapse or two.[2]

OTHER CLINICIANS

The approaches of several other clinicians are described here. Many of these approaches are used not only for borderline stuttering in younger preschool children but for beginning stuttering in older preschool children as well. I have selected them because they all involve the child's family, which I consider of major importance when working with preschool children. The nature of intervention ranges from monitoring the child's stuttering to helping parents change their interaction patterns to direct work on the child's way of speaking, if needed.

Even though some of these approaches present data on their effectiveness, clinicians using any approach should collect their own data on progress and outcome. As suggested in Chapter 8, baseline measures of the child's stuttering at the beginning of treatment should be made in a valid and reliable way. Because the fluency of preschool children is highly variable, recordings of the child's speech should be made at home as well as in a clinical setting. The Stuttering Severity Instrument-4 (Riley, 2009) should be used to assess frequency and severity. When treatment begins, weekly measures of progress should be made; percentage of syllables stuttered in the clinic and daily SRs of speech at home made by a parent are effective and efficient. When the child has achieved fluent speech (SRs at home of 0 [normal fluency] and less than 1%SS in the clinic), a maintenance program should be started, involving continued measurement at home and during gradually faded clinic visits. Children with borderline stuttering can be expected to achieve stable, normally fluent speech within 6 months. Clinicians should assess how long a child is in treatment before fluency is achieved and how well the child maintained that fluency a year after treatment ends.

Edward Conture and Colleagues

Conture's indirect therapy for preschool-age children (Conture, 2001; Conture & Melnick, 1999; Richels & Conture, 2007) is carried out in parent and child groups that meet separately each session and then as a combined group. The parent group observes portions of the children's therapy and is provided information, suggestions, and opportunities to help them facilitate their child's fluency outside the clinic setting. The parents and clinician also discuss child-rearing issues that directly affect the child's ability to receive maximal benefit from treatment. The children's group helps the child learn the skills of effective communication.

During the initial phase of treatment, the groups meet once per week to establish the child's fluency. When the child's stuttering in the clinic is below 5%SS for 4 consecutive weeks (which usually takes about 12 weeks of treatment but for some longer), the family then meets less frequently—but still regularly—with the clinician so that the parents can continue new behaviors more independently and the child's increased fluency can be transferred to home and beyond. This is followed by a maintenance phase, to be described.

Conture and his colleagues stress the importance of data to guide treatment. Richels and Conture (2010) describe their evaluation procedures and the important relationships between pretreatment information and the outcomes of treatment, for example, understanding that a slow-to-warm-up child may require a longer period of treatment before becoming successful. They typically collect measures of the child's stuttering frequency at the beginning of every clinic visit and are beginning to use a rating scale on a monthly basis to examine parents' perceptions of their children's disfluencies and children's responses to stuttering beyond the clinic to determine how well treatment effects are generalizing and to guide dismissal.

Specifics of Treatment

Children's Group

The children's group begins with conversation led by the clinician. Samples of 100 words of conversation are obtained from each child to provide disfluency data for each session. Activities in the children's group then begin with rules that foster good communication, which include listening when someone else is talking, taking turns in conversations, and not interrupting. These rules are described to the child

[2]Compare this with the syllable-timed speech approach for preschool children who stutter, reported by Trajkovski et al. (2009).

verbally and augmented by brightly colored pictures depicting each of the three rules. Children are reinforced for using the rules appropriately. After rules are reviewed, the clinician engages the children in "story time," during which reading of an age-appropriate story is intermingled with questions asked of the children that match each child's language and fluency abilities (e.g., "forced-choice" questions—such as is this a rabbit or a skunk?—are asked of a child who is fluent only at this level of linguistic demand, while open-ended questions are asked of a child who is ready for that level of demand). Story time is followed by a craft or game activity that blends turn taking and verbal responses consistent with each child's abilities. The clinician models the interaction strategies with which the parents are being familiarized in their group (see below).

Parents' Group

Many of the parents' group activities are focused on improved communicative interactions that dovetail with the turn-taking rules and adaptation of linguistic demand based on a child's demonstrated fluency, so that parent-child conversations at home increasingly facilitate the child's development of fluency, related speech and language behaviors, and ease of communication. The parents learn the following strategies over the course of treatment:

- Speaking more slowly (but still normally) to the child
- Adjusting the length and complexity of utterances to meet the requirements of the communicative situation—generally talking to the child using shorter, simpler sentences when appropriate
- Pausing for a second after the child speaks to give the child plenty of time to finish speaking and to slow the overall pace of conversation
- Decreasing the number of interruptions and questions when conversing with the child
- Decreasing the number of corrections of the child's speech, language, and related communicative behaviors

Parents in the group are asked first to observe their speaking behaviors with their child, as well as the child's speaking behaviors, and then encouraged to discuss their observations with the group. Subsequently, parents learn how to make changes in these behaviors and practice them in a single setting, once a day for about 5 to 15 minutes (depending on the situation and the parents' comfort level with new strategies). This helps them experience and learn these changes in a relatively controlled setting, such as nightly bedtime rituals, before trying them in more spontaneous situations, such as during conversations at the dinner table. The first new behavior parents are asked to practice is to speak more slowly but normally to the child and to pause for 1 second after the child finishes speaking before they start speaking. This change is thought to create a speaking environment that facilitates the child's fluency and overall conversational turn taking. This approach also attempts to produce a communicative environment in which the child is more likely to feel that he doesn't have to hurry to speak and helps to reduce how often parents are interrupting their child. The parents' pause after their child talks will also reduce the extent to which parental communicative behavior may encroach on the time during which the child may be planning and producing spoken language. Another important change for parents is to learn to use shorter and simpler sentences, not continually but when appropriate. Parents' modeling of this behavior encourages children to decrease the speed of initiating and maintaining speech as well as more easily adjust the length and complexity of their utterances to communicative requirements, enhancing their fluency. Similarly, parents learn to adjust the level of demand of their inquiries of their child according to their observations of the child's fluency in particular situations (e.g., keeping it simple, forced-choice questions when children are more disfluent, and using more open-ended inquiries when children are more fluent).

Parents discuss and practice other new behaviors on the list and are encouraged to use the group to support each other in planning situations in which they can try out these changes and then share the results of their efforts. Parents are most successful when they don't try to change all of their behaviors in all situations but work on only one or two at a time in such specific situations as talking with their child while playing a simple board game or playing alongside the child (e.g., building with blocks, playing with Play-Doh, dressing a doll, etc.) or reading a bedtime story. It is stressed to the parents that smaller periods of practice, almost every day, are more effective than longer periods of practice once or twice a week.

Throughout treatment, parents are provided with graphic descriptions of how their child is doing (Figs. 11.3 to 11.5). These "therapy graphs" depict three pieces of information: (1) total disfluencies per 100 words, (2) total stuttered disfluencies per 100 words, and (3) total nonstuttered disfluencies per 100 words. These graphs are used during therapy sessions as well as during parent-clinician counseling sessions to help parents understand expected variations in disfluencies and their child's progress over time, as well as to help the clinician plan short-term and long-term goals for each child. Parents are taught to differentiate nonstuttered disfluencies from stuttered disfluencies with many examples from their child's speech. This is important so that as the child improves, parents can accept the nonstuttered disfluencies as part of the child's "normal" speech—that is, speech that a typical child of that age would have.

Dismissal

Conture stresses that once a child is ready for dismissal, treatment is not abruptly terminated but gradually faded. First, the child's treatment changes from once a week to once every other week, then to once a month, once every 3 months, and, finally, once every 6 months for a year. If stuttering reappears at any time during this period, the child can be brought

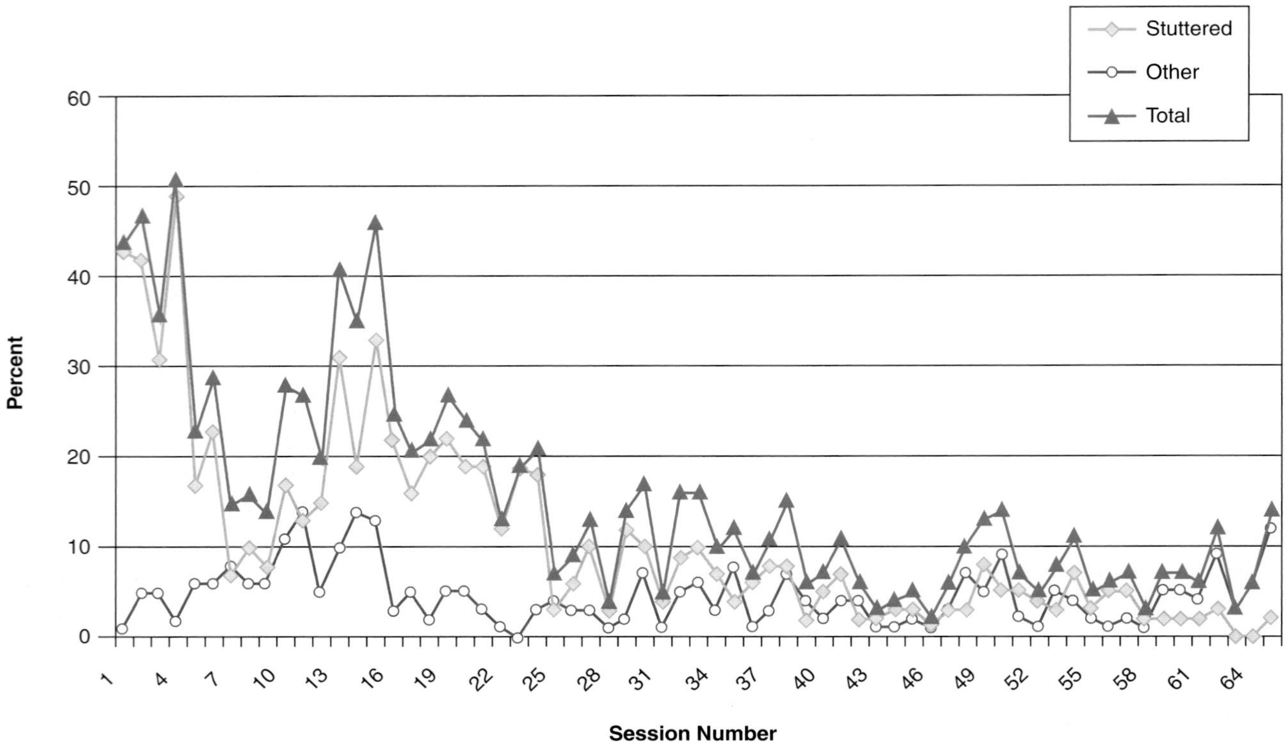

Figure 11.3 Example of a child whose treatment was successful. (Reprinted from Conture, E. G., & Curlee, R. F. (2007). *Stuttering and related disorders of fluency*. New York: Thieme, with permission.)

back into treatment until he regains fluency. Although this schedule of fading is the best approach, the time of a child's dismissal is sometimes negotiated with the parents. Some parents want to continue with regular treatment longer than may be necessary, which is only allowed if it is believed to be in the child's best long-term interest (typically as a means of helping the parent(s) prepare for independence). Other parents want to discontinue treatment after the child has become fluent but before gradual fading of treatment has been completed. In these cases, parents' wishes are granted, and the door is left open for them to return if necessary. Based on his experience, Conture rejects a one-size-fits-all approach to determining the length of treatment and criterion for termination. Instead, he considers the individual needs of each child, the nature of his problem, the child's learning history, the parents' concerns, perceptions of their child's progress, and the extent of their involvement in therapy, in determining each child's pace in moving from skill acquisition to maintenance to dismissal (i.e., establishment of normal disfluency).

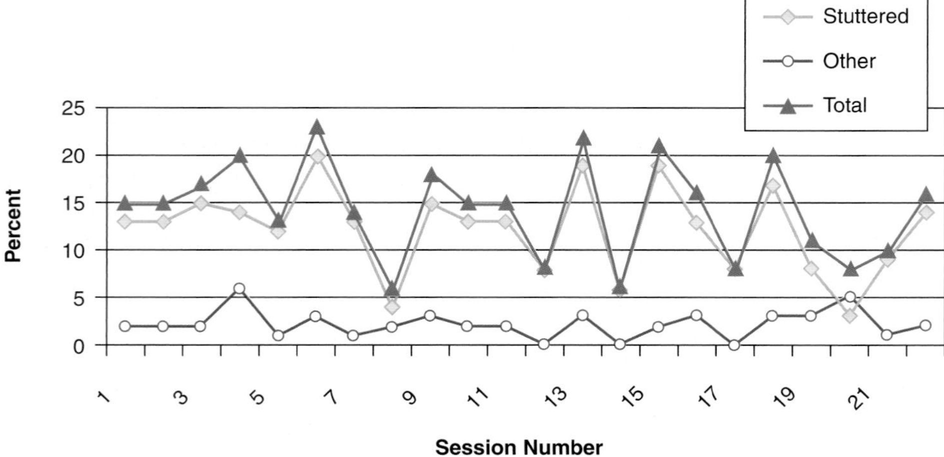

Figure 11.4 Example of a child with highly variable performance during treatment. (Reprinted from Conture, E. G., & Curlee, R. F. (2007). *Stuttering and related disorders of fluency*. New York: Thieme, with permission.).

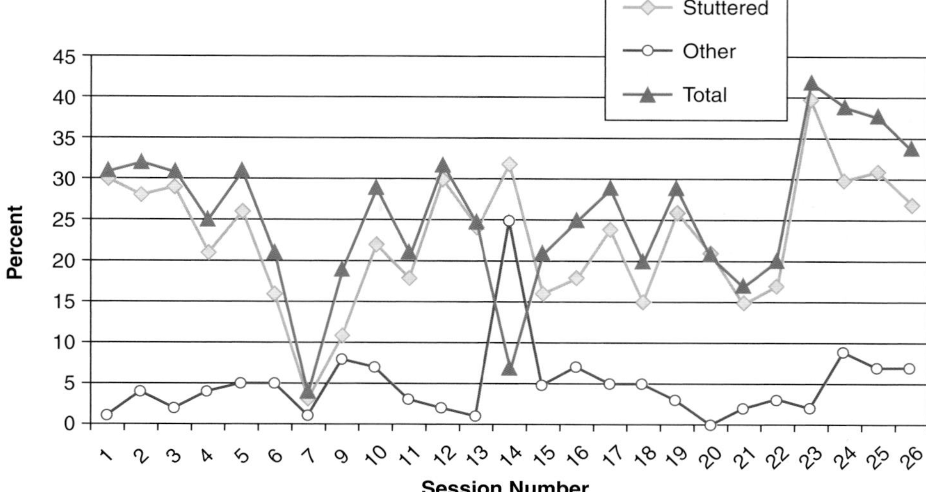

Figure 11.5 Example of a child not responding to group treatment. (Reprinted from Conture, E. G., & Curlee, R. F. (2007). *Stuttering and related disorders of fluency*. New York: Thieme, with permission.)

Supporting Data

Richels and Conture (2007) reported on 32 children (ages 2–9 to 6–0) who stuttered on an average of 10 words per 100 (stuttering-like disfluencies), averaged 21.3 on the SSI-3 (moderate severity), and whose time since onset of stuttering averaged 15.5 months. All of the children had received at least 12 treatment sessions—enough time to have shown some response to therapy, according to their experience. Results indicated that on average, these children decreased their stuttering-like disfluencies by 31 percent in 12 sessions.

Palin Centre Parent-Child Interaction Treatment

The team at the Michael Palin Centre for Stammering Children has developed a treatment for preschoolers who stutter based on the therapy of Lena Rustin (1991). This approach rests on the premise that the vulnerabilities that underlie the breakdown in children's fluency also make it harder for them to cope with typical adult-child interactions (Miles & Ratner, 2001). Therapy uses video feedback to help parents identify interaction styles that support their children's fluency and then develop these styles in structured practice sessions at home. While the research indicates that changes in interaction style can be associated with increased fluency (Guitar, 1978; Guitar et al., 1992; Kasprisin-Burrelli, Egolf, & Shames, 1972; Millard, Nicholas, & Cook, 2008; Stephenson-Opsal & Bernstein Ratner, 1988), parent-child interaction styles are not considered to be causing the breakdown in fluency. Indeed, some studies have found that interaction styles change after rather than before the child started to stutter (Kloth, Janssen, Kraaimaat, & Brutten, 1998; Meyers & Freeman, 1985a, 1985b).

A detailed description of the Palin Parent-Child Interaction therapy program has been published in Kelman and Nicholas (2008; 2017), and illustrative video clips can be found in Botterill and Kelman (2010). The approach begins with a thorough evaluation of a child's strengths and needs. The child's receptive and expressive language, articulation, speech rate, social communication skills, and sensitivity are evaluated. This gives an indication of any vulnerabilities that may be contributing to the stuttering. A video recording is made of the parents and child in a play situation, and this is analyzed later to establish which interaction styles are likely to be facilitating fluency and which styles need to be developed further. A detailed parent interview elicits information about the child and his fluency in the context of the family, and the parents' ideas are sought about what facilitates the child's fluency. The parents may have observed, for example, that the child is more fluent when she has had plenty of rest but less fluent when she is competing for speaking time, such as at the dinner table. The parents' ideas are valued and incorporated into treatment.

The assessment findings are presented to the parents in terms of the child's strengths and needs in a formulation in which the clinician first summarizes which factors may be contributing to the stuttering as well as those that are helpful for fluency development then suggests therapy options. The clinician stresses to the parents that nothing they have done has *caused* their child's stuttering but that their participation in treatment is vital in helping the child.

Parent-child interaction therapy involves both parents with the child attending once weekly for 6 weeks. Therapy begins by identifying interaction strategies that parents are already using and finding ways to increase them. In the session, the clinician views a video of the interaction with the parents, inviting them to comment on the helpful things they are already doing, such as speaking more slowly or pausing for a few seconds when the child finishes a speaking turn rather than talking immediately. If the parents observe that they are talking too fast, the clinician finds examples on the video of when they are talking slower, at a more facilitating rate. The overarching principle behind changing parents' interaction behaviors is to find ways of giving the child more time to plan and execute speech. Together, the parents and the clinician decide on a target, such as increasing the parents' pause time after the child speaks. The parents work on the new target daily in 5-minute practice sessions at home with the child.

In subsequent sessions during the initial 6 weeks of treatment, the clinician reviews the parents' homework and then records each parent interacting separately with the child. The clinician then reviews the two videos with both parents together. While watching his or her own videotape, each parent picks out several interactions with which he or she is pleased and one behavior that they might develop. The rationale for this is discussed, exploring how an interaction style can affect the child's fluency. Although much of the emphasis is on their communication interactions, the parents also learn to use "family strategies" that include praise of other skills to build up the child's confidence. The book *How to Talk So Kids Will Listen and Listen So Kids Will Talk* by Faber and Mazlish (2016) is used for teaching parents to praise their child once each day for something specific the child did. Other "family strategies" are also introduced, such as family members all taking turns speaking and managing the child's sensitivity or perfectionism. Also, families are encouraged to talk openly with the child about stuttering so that it becomes an acceptable behavior even as the family helps the child become more fluent.

After 6 weeks of meeting with the clinician, the parents work on their own at home for a second 6-week period of "consolidation" of their new behaviors. Parents send homework record sheets to the clinician each week and continue the daily 5-minute interaction times that each parent has with the child. The clinician responds via e-mail, phone, or regular mail. At the end of this 6-week consolidation period, the family meets with the clinician for a review of progress. If the child's fluency is significantly better and continuing to improve, the parents are asked to continue working on the changes they are making, and another review is scheduled 6 weeks later. If the child's fluency is not improving, more direct treatment (using *child strategies*) is introduced. These include teaching the child to use a slower rate of speech, including pausing, and increasing eye contact. If at all possible, the child's fluency is monitored for a minimum of 1 year.

Supporting Data

Data have been published for 13 children, showing short-term (5 weeks) (Matthews, Williams, & Pring, 2010), medium-term (6 months) (Millard, Edwards, & Cook, 2009), and long-term (12 months) (Millard et al., 2008) efficacy. Using experimental single-subject methodologies, the clinician-researchers at the Michael Palin Centre have demonstrated that the indirect components of this approach (interaction and family strategies) can be effective in reducing the frequency of stuttering in children (Matthews et al., 1997; Millard et al., 2008, 2009). In addition, there is evidence that the approach can reduce the impact of stuttering for both the children and the parents and increase parents' ratings of knowledge and confidence in managing the stuttering (Millard et al., 2009). By including only children who had been stuttering for more than 12 months, collecting data over a baseline phase prior to therapy, and using statistical analysis that compared change against variability in the baseline phase, the researchers concluded that improvements were attributable to the therapy.

In a study involving 55 children who were treated and followed for a year, Millard, Zebrowski, and Kelman (in press) showed that the children showed significant reductions in frequency of stuttering and in the impact of stuttering on their lives. The authors also found that the children's perceptions of themselves as communicators improved and their parents were relieved of much of their worry about their child's stuttering and became more confident in how to support their child.

Stuttering Foundation Approach

The Stuttering Foundation (SF) has advocated a general approach to children who are beginning to stutter—a treatment that can be carried out by parents, ideally with guidance from a trained clinician. The SF's online store on their Web site (www.stutteringhelp.org) currently has available a number of items designed for parents of preschool-age children who are beginning to stutter. Two excellent SF videos for parents are listed in the "Suggested Viewing" section at the end of this chapter. In addition, Ainsworth and Fraser's booklet, *If Your Child Stutters: A Guide for Parents*, eighth edition (2010), helps families differentiate between normal disfluency and stuttering and provides guidelines to help them create fluency-facilitating environments.

Conture's *Stuttering and Your Child: Questions and Answers*, fourth edition (2010) published by SF, provides families, teachers, and others with information about stuttering and how children who stutter can be helped. It covers a wide range of issues, including stuttering versus normal disfluency, the possible causes of stuttering, changing the home environment, dealing with others' responses to the child's stuttering, and treatment. Although formal aspects of treatment are left to professionals, specific advice is given in highlighted pages about how parents, babysitters, day care centers, and teachers can help children who stutter. Parents are instructed how to be good listeners, how to increase the times when the child feels he is being heard, and how to reduce both conversational and lifestyle pressures on the child. Babysitters and day care centers are advised to react as normally as possible to the child and to treat him like other children, while ensuring that he has plenty of time to say what he wants to say without feeling rushed. Teachers are encouraged to give the child support for oral recitations, allow him the same speaking opportunities as other children, and help the entire class develop good speaking and listening practices.

One of the SF's most popular publications on the treatment of stuttering in young children is the video *Stuttering and Your Child: Help for Parents* (Guitar, Guitar, & Fraser, 2010). It is available free as streaming video on the SF Web site and as a DVD that can be purchased inexpensively. This video, in both English and Spanish, was designed to be used by families working alone, as a preliminary tool, as well as by those who are in treatment with a speech-language pathologist. The video teaches families to make changes in the child's environment, primarily in two areas: communicative interaction and family lifestyle. It also describes when to get help from a speech-language pathologist and what to expect in an evaluation and from treatment. The SF Web site quotes an American Speech-Language-Hearing Association book review that refers to this video as "perhaps the best buy in the nation for information on children and stuttering."

All of the SF's publications emphasize that families are not the cause of stuttering but that families can create an environment that facilitates the growth of fluency. The following suggestions for changes in families' conversational interactions are described in detail in both publications, and parents demonstrate them in the video:

- Talk more slowly.
- Use plenty of pauses in your speech after the child finishes talking.
- Ask the child fewer questions.
- Spend time physically close to the child, such as having him in your lap when you read to him.
- Allow silent time in conversations so that the child doesn't feel compelled to talk and isn't interrupted.
- Help the child learn to take turns talking.

The following suggestions are for families wishing to change some aspects of their lifestyle to facilitate their child's fluency:

- Try to find an opportunity each day, preferably in the morning, when special attention can be given to the child so that he is getting one-on-one time with a parent or another caregiver. During this time, the focus should be on listening to the child and letting him direct the play. The best interactions at these times are those when the parent is talking little and is primarily there for the child as he talks and plays.
- Slow the pace of life, when possible. Give the family more time to do fewer things.
- Develop regular, consistent times for meals, naps, and bedtimes.
- Use reasonable and consistent discipline.
- Make sure the child gets plenty of rest.
- Provide plenty of time for the child to transition from one thing to another. For example, getting ready to go to a birthday party after playing quietly at home may require an extra 10 or 20 minutes because the two activities are so different. Parents might, for example, talk to the child about what the birthday party will be like, so the busy-ness of the party won't be so unexpected.

In addition to these ideas for changing a child's environment, the SF's publications suggest that parents should try to become aware of what events or situations are associated with the ups and downs of their child's fluency. Some children who stutter are more sensitive to common, everyday life stresses; things that may not bother most children may cause a child who stutters to become more disfluent. Some examples might be visits by strangers, holidays, a parent leaving for or coming home from work, or an argument between parents. If it can be predicted when more stressful events might occur, extra support can be provided to the child during such situations.

A family that is working with their child on their own is advised that if their child's stuttering does not show a gradual decrease after these changes have been in place for over a month, they should seek help from a speech-language pathologist who specializes in treating childhood stuttering.

In addition to an extensive online bookstore with many low-cost publications and video material, the SF Web site also has a page with guidelines from ASHA for seeking insurance coverage for stuttering evaluation and treatment (www.stutteringhelp.org/insurance.htm).

Restart

The RESTART program was developed in the Netherlands and is based on the Demands and Capacities Model (Gottwald, 2010; Starkweather et al., 1990). In Chapter 6 on Theories of this textbook, I describe the Demands and Capacities Model and explain relevant treatment procedures that derive from this theory. A good example of this treatment is given in Chapter 12 in the section describing Sheryl Gottwald's approach to working with older preschool children.

In essence, RESTART therapy involves training parents to decrease demands on the child, including those in linguistic, cognitive, emotional, and motor domains. Parents set aside 15 minutes a day, 5 days a week as a "special time" for the child, focusing on what the child wants to talk about or do. During this time, a parent focuses on reducing the demands—especially those related to communication—and providing support. If needed, more direct therapy is provided to improve the child's capacities for fluency, such as working on the child's speech-motor abilities and word-finding capacity. The manual for the RESTART treatment approach using the Demands and Capacities Model is available online at http://www.nedverstottertherapie.nl/wp-content/uploads/2016/07/RESTART-DCM.Method.-English.pdf/.

In 2015, several investigators associated with the RESTART program published a study that demonstrated the effectiveness of RESTART (de Sonneville-Koedoot et al., 2015) compared to the Lidcombe Program (LP) (see Chapter 12 for a description of LP). Results indicated that of the 199 children who participated (99 randomly assigned to LP, 100 to RESTART), approximately equal percentages had recovered completely when they were assessed 18 months after the beginning of treatment. Specifically, 70 percent of the children treated with RESTART and 76 percent of the children treated with LP were found to have less than 1.5 percent syllables stuttered at this follow-up measurement time. Although it may appear that the Lidcombe was slightly better than the RESTART program, given the variable of stuttering seen in each group, the 6 percent difference could have occurred by chance. Other measures of their recovery were also positive for both treatments at the final assessment. This study strongly suggests that both direct (LP) and indirect (RESTART) treatments are effective. Unfortunately, the effectiveness of these approaches could not be compared with natural recovery because ethical considerations prevented the use of an untreated control group.

SUMMARY

- Borderline stuttering in young preschoolers is characterized by an excess of normal disfluencies, particularly part-word repetitions and single-syllable whole-word repetitions. Although the child may have a high frequency of disfluencies and may repeat sounds many times, she typically is not frustrated or embarrassed by the disfluencies. If these emotional reactions do occur, they are usually transitory. Onset of stuttering is relatively recent (less than a year).
- The occurrence of borderline stuttering in young preschoolers is thought to be the result of an interaction between a child's neurodevelopmental predisposition and typical developmental and environmental stresses. The family is not to blame for the stuttering but can be vital in creating a facilitating environment that increases fluency.
- Treatment is usually focused on helping families make changes in their conversational interactions and in family routines.
- Changes in the family's interaction patterns include helping family members: (1) slow their speech rates; (2) pause for 2 or 3 seconds after the child finishes talking before they begin to speak and adding pauses in their own speech; (3) listen attentively to what the child is saying; (4) ensure appropriate turn taking by all members of the family, including the child; (5) ask fewer questions that require long answers; and (6) use vocabulary and sentence complexity that are close to the child's level when speaking to him.
- Changes in the family routine should include the following: Arrange a time, preferably in the morning, when one parent or caregiver can have 10 to 15 minutes of uninterrupted time with the child. During this time, the parent should be primarily there for the child, listening and paying attention to what the child is saying and doing, and appropriately reflecting the child's feelings. This can be a time in which a parent or caregiver practices the interaction patterns suggested earlier.
- The family should be encouraged to carry out the following changes in their lifestyle: (1) create structures and predictable routines to increase the child's sense of security; (2) slow the pace of family life, so that there are calm transitions from one activity to another; (3) ensure that the child's life is not too busy or rushed; and (4) use consistent, reasonable discipline with the child to ensure that she feels her family is in control.
- If a child's stuttering does not begin to decline within a month or 6 weeks, more slightly more direct treatment should be undertaken. In this approach, for mild borderline stuttering in young preschoolers, parents are taught to use occasional praise for fluency during one-on-one sessions with the child. For more severe stuttering in this age group, the child is taught to change harder stutters into easier ones, using modeling by the clinician, playing with stuttering, voluntary stuttering, and reinforcing slow, easy stutters in his spontaneous speech.
- Other clinicians' indirect approaches to stuttering in this age group include parent counseling coupled with changes in parent-child interaction patterns, group therapy, and work with families on changing family lifestyles.
- One other clinician's more direct approach teaches children to use slow and smooth speech and to take turns in conversation. Another approach assesses the linguistic level at which a child is fluent and then moves the child through a hierarchy of longer and more complex responses while keeping him fluent for longer periods of time.

STUDY QUESTIONS

1. What are some aspects of family conversational interactions that may put pressure on the young preschool child vulnerable to stuttering?
2. What changes can a family make in their home to relieve speech and language pressures?
3. Discuss how the clinician can facilitate changes in family routines that may help the child's fluency.

4. What are some of the barriers to change that are found in some families? How can the clinician help the family overcome these barriers?
5. Compare my slightly more direct approach to a young preschooler who stutters mildly with my approach to one who stutters more severely.
6. Compare one of the other clinician's more indirect therapies with one of the more direct therapies.

SUGGESTED PROJECTS

1. Conduct an informal ABAB study of the effect of slowing your speech rate on a conversational partner who is not aware of the purpose of your study. You will need to record your conversation so that you can analyze the data afterward.[3] In the first A condition, conduct several minutes of conversation at a normal rate; in the first B condition, conduct the same amount of conversation at a slower rate. Then repeat the two rates in two subsequent A and B conditions. Was your speaking partner affected by your speaking rate?
2. Pretend that you are the parent of a child who is beginning to stutter. Search the library and the Internet for advice about how to help your child, and determine whether there is consistency in the advice or whether conflicting information is given.
3. Examine the materials presented in this chapter from other clinicians and determine whether the approaches are designed just for stuttering in young preschoolers or whether the authors intend them for older children as well.

SUGGESTED VIEWING

7 Tips for Talking with the Child Who Stutters (Stuttering Foundation; www.stutteringhelp.org). Also available on YouTube. This free video provides excellent suggestions for both clinicians and parents, appropriate for helping preschool children who stutter when an indirect approach is used or is combined with a direct approach.

Stuttering and Your Child: Help for Parents (Stuttering Foundation; www.stutteringhelp.org). Available on YouTube by putting in title. Chmela, K. (2004). *Working with preschoolers who stutter: Successful intervention strategies*. **(Video) Memphis, TN: Stuttering Foundation.** This is a video of a convention presentation designed to teach clinicians how to work with preschool children who stutter, using modeling of easy, relaxed speech when talking to children and counseling parents to develop a fluency-friendly environment.

[3]You should ask your conversational partner's permission to record her or him, but without explaining the purpose of your "experiment." Perhaps you could tell them—before you start—that you are studying your own speech characteristics. Then, after you have analyzed the data, you could share it with them, explaining your true purpose.

SUGGESTED READINGS

Ainsworth, S., & Fraser, J. (2010). *If your child stutters: A guide for parents* (8th ed.). Memphis, TN: Stuttering Foundation of America.

This inexpensive booklet gives advice to parents who think their child is beginning to stutter.

Conture, E. (Ed.). (2010). *Stuttering and your child: Questions and answers*. Memphis, TN: Stuttering Foundation of America.

This booklet provides answers for parents to commonly asked questions about stuttering in young children.

Gottwald, S. (2010). Stuttering prevention and early intervention: A multidimensional approach. In B. Guitar, & R. McCauley (Eds.), *Treatment of stuttering: Established and emerging interventions*. Baltimore, MD: Lippincott Williams & Wilkins.

This is a very useful detailed description illustrated by video clips of the direct and indirect treatment for preschoolers who stutter developed by Gottwald and Starkweather over the past 25 years.

Guitar, B., & Conture, E. (2015). *The child who stutters: To the pediatrician* (5th ed.). Memphis, TN: Stuttering Foundation.

This free booklet provides information about the nature of stuttering and signs to look for in deciding which children should be referred for treatment. Handouts with suggestions for parents are also provided.

Guitar, B., Kopff-Schaefer, H. K., Donahue-Kilburg, G., & Bond, L. (1992). Parent verbal interaction and speech rate. Journal of Speech and Hearing Research, 35, 742–754.

This article describes therapy with parents of a young child who stutters and the analysis of parent-child interactions. The analysis of parent variables affecting the child's stuttering demonstrates that her stuttering can be categorized as either easy repetitions (tension-free) or blocks (tense). These two different types of stutters are affected by different parent behaviors (speaking rate or nonaccepting comments).

Kelman, E. & Whyte, A. (2012). *Understanding stammering or stuttering: A guide for parents, teachers and other professionals*. London, UK: Jessica Kingsley Publishers.

This book's title comes from the fact that both "stammering" and "stuttering" are used in the United Kingdom for what is called "stuttering" in the United States. It provides an explanation of the nature of stuttering as well as guidelines to help the child and to find professional treatment.

Richels, C., & Conture, E. (2010). Indirect treatment of childhood stuttering: Diagnostic predictors of treatment outcome. In B. Guitar, & R. McCauley (Eds.), *Treatment of stuttering: Established and emerging interventions* (pp. 18–55). Baltimore, MD: Lippincott Williams & Wilkins.

A very thoughtful description of the use of diagnostic data to predict short- and long-term outcomes. Interestingly, successful short-term outcomes appear to be related to less severe stuttering at the beginning of treatment, but successful long-term outcomes are more related to diagnostic indicators of expressive (rather than inhibited) temperament and to lower language scores at the beginning of treatment.

Starkweather, C. W., Gottwald, S. R., & Halfond, M. H. (1990). *Stuttering prevention: A clinical method.* Englewood Cliffs, NJ: Prentice-Hall.

This book details a program of assessment and treatment for children who stutter and for their parents. It is the basis for treatments based on the Demands and Capacities model.

Walton, P., & Wallace, M. (1998). *Fun with fluency.* Bisbee, AZ: Imaginart International, Inc.

Although published several years ago, this manual provides accurate information about working with both borderline and beginning stuttering. The manual covers both indirect and direct treatment, information, and materials for working with parents and teachers and includes many activities for children aged 2 to 7.

12

Treatment of Older Preschool Children: Beginning Stuttering

Chapter Objectives

After studying this chapter, readers should be able to:

- Describe the characteristics of a child who has beginning stuttering
- Describe the author's beliefs about stuttering, targets in treatment, goals for treatment, how much to involve feelings and attitudes in treatment, and maintenance procedures
- Delineate the procedures involved in the Lidcombe Program, the stages of therapy, and the criteria to complete each stage
- Explain how formal training may be obtained for using the Lidcombe Program
- Outline the components of Sheryl Gottwald's "multidimensional approach"
- Describe a number of different approaches to working on stuttering and concomitant speech or language problems

Key Terms

Concomitant speech and language problems: Difficulties with articulation/phonology and/or difficulties with language that sometimes accompany stuttering. When this occurs in some children who stutter, it poses a problem of which disorder to work on first.

Demands and capacities: The perspective that the factors associated with the onset and persistence of stuttering are the demands placed on the child by her environments balanced by the child's innate capacity for fluent speech

Lidcombe Program (LP): An operant conditioning-based approach to stuttering treatment, delivered in the home by a parent or other caregiver and guided via weekly meetings with the clinician

Older preschool children: Children between 3.5 and 6 years of age

Operant conditioning: A type of behavior modification that uses rewards and punishments to increase or decrease the frequency of a behavior

Severity Rating (SR) Scale: A scale from 0 to 9 used daily by parents to assess a child's stuttering. May be used by clinician as well during weekly clinic sessions.

Stage 1 (of LP): The initial step of LP in which the child becomes normally fluent. Criteria for completing Stage 1 are 3 consecutive weeks in which (1) the parent's weekly SRs are 0-1 during the week before the clinic visit and 4 of the 7 SRs are 0 and (2) the clinician's SR for the entire session is 0-1.

Stage 2 (of LP): When the child meets the fluency criteria to complete Stage 1, this maintenance stage is begun. Weekly clinic meetings are faded systematically so that the parent and child meet with the clinician in this sequence: 2, 2, 4, 4, 8, 8, and finally 16 weeks apart. The child must continue to meet fluency criteria.

Unambiguous stutter: A moment of stuttering that is so clear and evident that the parent or the clinician has no doubt that it should be categorized as a stutter

Verbal contingencies: Comments to the child made immediately after an event (e.g., fluent utterance; stutter) that are intended to change the frequency of that event

AN INTEGRATED APPROACH

Children with beginning stuttering are usually between 3.5 and 6 years of age. To distinguish them from children with milder, borderline stuttering, I refer to them as **older preschool children**. They have probably been stuttering for at least several months, and their parents may well be concerned that it is not a transient problem that will disappear on its own. What follows are some details on the core and secondary behaviors of their stuttering, as well as feelings and attitudes that often characterize stuttering in this age group. These children's most common core stuttering behaviors are part-word repetitions that are produced rapidly, usually with irregular rhythm. Some prolongations may also be present. Both the repetitions and prolongations may contain excessive tension, which can be heard as abrupt endings to the repetitions and/or as increases in vocal pitch in repetitions and prolongations. Blocks may also be present, with evidence of tension and struggle. Secondary behaviors are typically escape devices, such as eye blinks, head nods, and increases in pitch as the child tenses her vocal cords trying to get the word out. A few avoidance maneuvers may be observed, such as starting sentences with extra sounds like "uh" or changing words when a stutter is anticipated may be observed. In many cases, when the frequency of stuttering becomes high, these children may put their hands to their mouths to push words out or may momentarily avoid talking. Children with beginning stuttering usually feel frustrated and sometimes panicked with their difficulty in talking but have not yet developed a strong anticipation of stuttering or learned to be ashamed of their speech.

I will illustrate our approach with a description of Katherine's treatment. She is the 3-year-old child I introduced in Chapter 1. The course of her treatment is depicted in Figure 12.1.

Case Example

Katherine

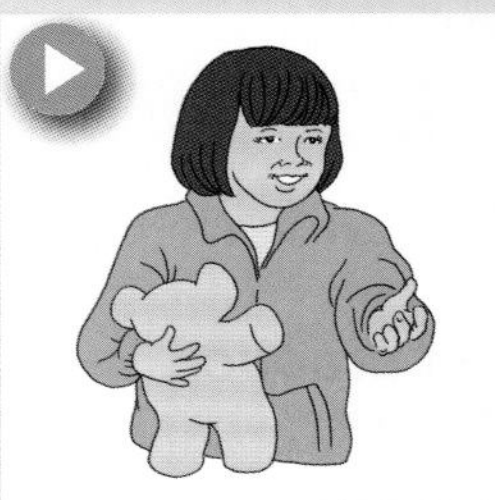

Katherine's therapy began when she was 3 years old and stuttering severely—on 21 percent of her spoken syllables. As you may remember from our description of her stuttering in Chapter 1, Katherine's pattern was characterized by repetitions, prolongations, and blocks, with a predominance of blocks with much struggle behavior. She had changed from bubbly and talkative to withdrawn and reluctant to engage in conversation.

At the time she came in for an evaluation, two other clinicians and I had just been trained in the Lidcombe approach—the treatment described in this chapter. Several weeks after the evaluation, we began Katherine's therapy by training her mother in using **verbal contingencies** (praise) for Katherine's fluent speech during daily, 15-minute practice sessions at home. We also trained her in making daily ratings of the severity of Katherine's stuttering. During our weekly clinic meetings with Katherine and her mother, we measured the frequency of Katherine's stuttering in conversation at the beginning of each session. The rest of each session was spent on problem-solving any issues that came up during practice sessions and training Katherine's mother in the next steps of treatment. These next steps included using verbal contingencies for stuttering and then using verbal contingencies during natural conversations throughout the day.

After several weeks went by, we saw notable improvement in Katherine's stuttering, shown by both our weekly measures of her stuttering frequency in the clinic and her mother's daily ratings of the severity (SRs) of Katherine's stuttering at home. The steady decline in Katherine's stuttering continued, interrupted by an occasional spike upward when a stressful event occurred, such as a visit by relatives or a family trip. At one point, Katherine's stuttering shot up for several days, and we worked with Katherine's mother to figure out the source of the problem. We discovered that Katherine's father, in his eagerness to help, began to use verbal contingencies without training when he was alone with Katherine and overdosed her with several hours of contingencies each day, instead of the recommended 12 or 15 contingencies per day. Once that was resolved and Katherine's father was trained to use contingencies judiciously, her stuttering continued to decline steadily. Katherine became fluent after about 6 months of treatment. Over the following year, the clinicians continued to stay in touch, but Katherine and her mother came in to the clinic less and less frequently.

Seven years after therapy had been completed, we contacted Katherine and her parents to assess her status. She had been completely fluent ever since treatment ended and today is highly verbal with only dim memories of ever having stuttered. Her parents have become a valuable resource for other parents of children who are beginning to stutter as they contemplate treatment.

Author's Beliefs

Nature of Stuttering

As I've described in chapters in the "Nature of Stuttering" part of this book, I believe that beginning stuttering arises when children's neurodevelopmental sensorimotor difficulties related to speech production interact with their temperament and other developmental and environmental influences to produce or exacerbate repetitions, prolongations, and blocks. This is essentially the position taken by C. S. Bluemel in his book *The Riddle of Stuttering* (1957). It was further articulated by Wendell Johnson and colleagues (1959), who suggested that the problem of stuttering arises as a result of interactions among (1) the amount of the child's disfluency, (2) the reaction of his listeners to the disfluency, and (3) the child's sensitivity to his own disfluency and to listeners' reactions. I would add to Johnson's list of interacting factors any pressures that a child may feel internally (e.g., to speak quickly and in long, relatively complex sentences) and any anxieties the child may experience as the result of moving, the birth of a sibling, or other life events.

In some children, beginning stuttering emerges gradually after they have gone through a period of borderline stuttering as younger preschool children. As these children get older and if stuttering continues, they begin to respond to negative experiences of repetitive disfluencies with increased tension. However, in some children, beginning stuttering appears suddenly, close to the onset of stuttering. They may be easily frustrated or highly distressed when many of their speech attempts result in repetitions or prolongations that feel out of their control. As these children respond, at first nonconsciously, to these core behaviors, they increase tension and develop a variety of escape behaviors that are reinforced. Their eye blinks, head nods, and pitch increases are rewarded because they often result in the release of stutters. Gradually, classical conditioning influences when and where

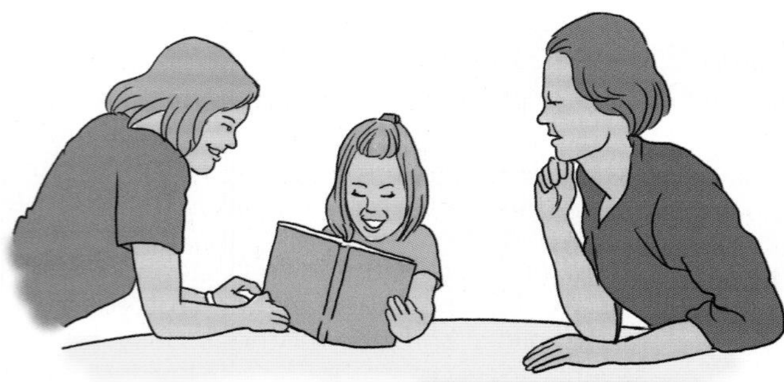

Mother and child in clinic session

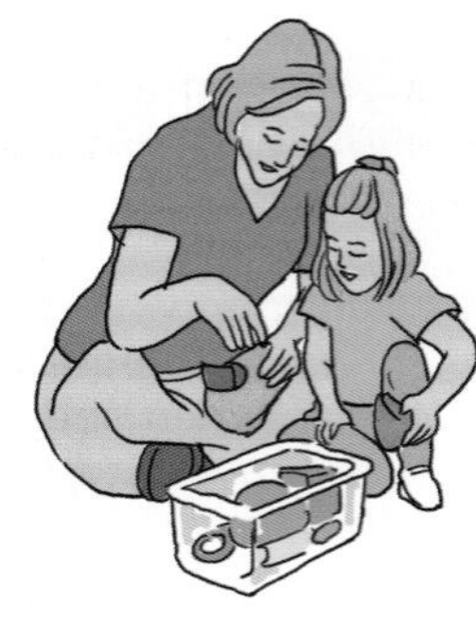

Mother and child in practice session at home

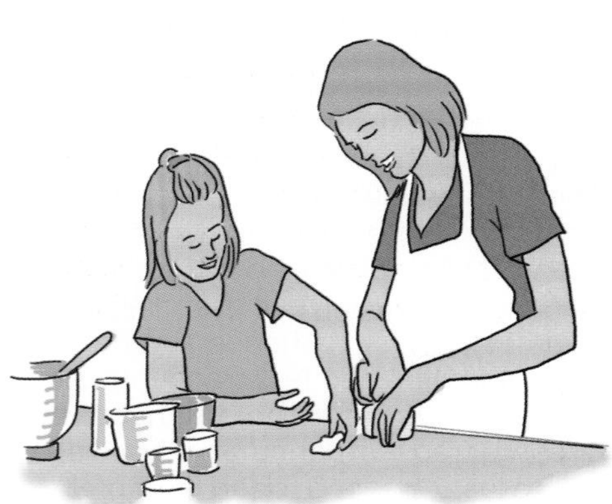

Mother and child in natural conversation at home

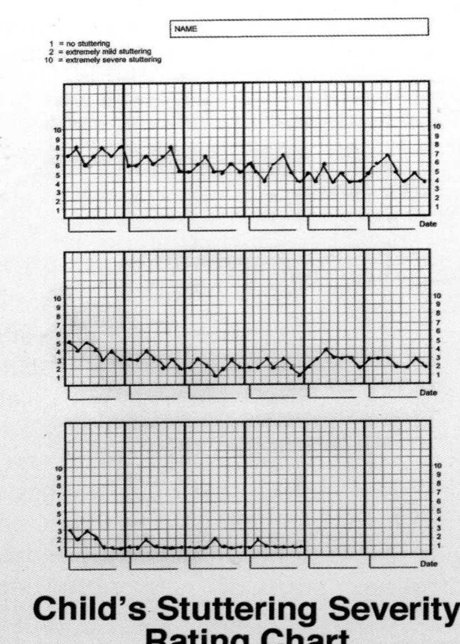

Figure 12.1 An overview of treatment through the Lidcombe Program.

the child's stuttering occurs. Specifically, negative emotional experiences that are associated with stuttering become etched into memory and associated with various contexts, such as the telephone, impatient listeners, or particular sounds and words. As stuttering spreads and becomes more pervasive and more consistently present, these children become aware of their stuttering, although at first they may have little shame of it and do not dread speaking situations. Because of the plasticity of the brain at this age, some children with beginning stuttering develop better sensorimotor control of speech production, and their stuttering goes out the door it entered. Their stutters diminish in frequency and severity and disappear or become a minor nuisance. Other children, perhaps those with more widespread sensorimotor deficits, a more sensitive temperament, or larger doses of other developmental and environmental stresses, continue to stutter and often develop more advanced symptoms.

Like Oliver Bloodstein (1975), I believe that if we can provide a child with beginning stuttering a sufficient number of positive, fluent speaking experiences during treatment, fluency will replace stuttering. Bloodstein, whose 50-year career was focused on the nature and management of childhood stuttering, strongly advised treatment that would ensure that "the child experiences daily successful, pleasant, and rewarding speech with a minimum of stuttering" and that these daily experiences be created by the parent at home (Bloodstein, 1975, pp. 61–62).

Neurodevelopmentally, the daily, structured practice of fluency, in the approach I often use, reinforces the neural pathways for fluent speech so that they become more robust, more automatic, and more resistant to stress. Echoing Bloodstein, I believe that this may happen best when treatment is administered by the parent at home, where it can be done 7 days a week. It also appears effective if natural fluency is elicited at first in highly structured situations, systematically reinforced, and then carefully transferred to more and more real-life situations in which stuttering has been occurring.

The increased fluency gained through this treatment reduces the opportunities that a child might have to experience stuttering as distressing because most of her speech is fluent and becoming more so every day. Preventing this distress prevents the tension and struggle that would follow, heading off a cycle of increasing tension and struggle begetting more fear speaking leading to even more tension and struggle accompanied by escape and avoidance behaviors. Also important is the aspect of treatment that makes the child aware that she is fluent—explicit reinforcement for fluency. I have more than once heard children undergoing this treatment say, proudly, "I'm a good talker!"

Keeping the child and her family in treatment for an extended period, with carefully phased out maintenance sessions, allows time for the child's neurological system to mature and for typical fluency patterns to become stabilized.

Speech Behaviors Targeted for Therapy

Which speech behaviors are targeted for the child with beginning stuttering? In the approach I advocate in this section, the **Lidcombe Program (LP)**, the clinician teaches the parent to first reinforce the child's fluent speech and then respond, less frequently, to stutters. The parent uses appropriate and varied verbal contingencies immediately after fluent utterances but comments gently on stutters much less frequently or occasionally asks the child to try the word again immediately after she stutters. It is critical that the parent's responses to the child's stutters do not elicit negative emotions (emotions that would trigger defensive tension responses) from the child. Thus, parents must be taught, under the clinician's mindful guidance, to apply contingencies to stutters carefully and to observe the child's response. If the child does appear to resent these contingencies, they should be immediately changed or treatment must use a different approach.

Fluency Goals

Almost all children who are treated with effective therapy for beginning stuttering will gain or regain spontaneous, typical fluency. In most cases, a year or two after treatment ends, the children will have little or no recollection of having stuttered and will not have to monitor their speech or work at being fluent.

Feelings and Attitudes

As noted earlier, a child with beginning stuttering has only occasional frustration and intermittent concern about talking. She has only mildly conditioned fears or avoidances of stuttering. Thus, it is unnecessary to focus directly on feelings and attitudes in therapy—in most cases—for a child with beginning stuttering.

The feelings and attitudes of these children are, however, influenced by the family. The clinician teaches the family member providing the at-home treatment to be matter-of-fact about the child's "smooth" and "bumpy" speech. The clinician and family member openly discuss the child's stuttering during their weekly meetings when the child is also present. These aspects of treatment are intended to reduce any embarrassment or shame that was associated with stuttering and foster the child's acceptance of stuttering as just a little mistake, like bumping into a table or tipping over her tricycle. This is a far cry from the "conspiracy of silence" that formerly characterized the treatment of children who stutter.

Maintenance Procedures

Systematically fading contact with the child and her family is vital for maintaining fluency. In my experience, if families leave treatment after fluency is achieved without having participated in a maintenance program, stuttering may return. Thus, it is important for clinicians to stress the importance of maintenance procedures at the outset of treatment. Moreover, the clinician and family should continue with careful data collection as contact is faded, so that the family can return to regular weekly meetings and discuss appropriate contingencies for fluency and stuttering if any relapse occurs.

Clinical Methods

Clinical Procedures: Lidcombe Program

For the past 25 years, I have been using the Lidcombe Program (LP) (Onslow, Costa, & Rue, 1990; Onslow, Packman, & Harrison, 2003) to treat preschool children with beginning stuttering. I was initially trained in using this program in a workshop led by Rosalee Shenker of the Montreal Fluency Centre. Subsequently, I developed more expertise through consultation and mentoring from Rosalee and my colleagues, Julie Reville, Melissa Bruce, and Danra Kazenski. Follow-up training with Elisabeth Harrison further sharpened my skills. For readers interested in using this approach, I urge you to obtain formal training at one of the many workshops offered around the world by the Lidcombe Consortium. More information on LP is available at http://www.lidcombeprogram.org. On this Web site, there are links to pages that provide information in the following categories: Families and Caregivers, Speech Language Pathologist, and Teachers and Health Professionals. The information for Speech Language Pathologists includes copies of materials needed for using the Lidcombe Program including the treatment guide that can be found by clicking on the Research and Publications link. An excellent chapter in Guitar and McCauley (2010), written by Harrison and Onslow, gives a detailed description of LP. Fourteen short video clips on *thePoint* (Chapter 12 videos) show Harrison (a master LP clinician) treating a preschool child using LP.

Overview

The Lidcombe Program uses **operant conditioning** procedures, which are administered by a parent in the home during conversations each day and guided by weekly meetings with the clinician. Treatment begins in structured conversations designed to elicit a maximum of fluent speech by the child so that the child receives mostly positive reinforcement. Approximately every fifth fluent utterance is followed by *praise* (e.g., "That was really good, smooth talking!"), *acknowledgment of fluency* (e.g., a very low-key "That was smooth"), or *request for self-evaluation* (e.g., "Was that smooth?"), which is used only after a fluent utterance. When the child stutters, the parent provides an occasional *acknowledgment of the stutter* ("That was a little bumpy") or *a gentle request for self-correction* (e.g., "Can you say 'truck' again?"). Table 12.1 lists verbal contingencies for fluency and stuttering.

The ratio of **verbal contingencies** for fluency to verbal contingencies for stuttering is kept very high (about 5:1) to make the program a positive experience for the child. As the child's stuttering decreases, practice sessions are faded and gradually replaced by contingencies during natural conversations each day. Verbal contingencies for fluency and stuttering continue, but in more casual, natural situations, such as when the parent is talking with the child in the car, in the kitchen, or at a store. Once the child is fluent in all situations, treatment is gradually faded in a systematic fashion. Throughout the program, the clinician and parent regularly assess the child's stuttering and use those measures to make treatment decisions.

Stage 1: The First Clinic Visit

Stage 1 of the Lidcombe Program begins with the first clinic visit when the clinician meets with the parent (or other caregiver) and child to accomplish three goals: (1) to explain severity ratings (SRs) to the parent, (2) to assess the child's stuttering, and (3) to teach the parent to conduct daily practice sessions. Stage 1 clinic visits are typically 1 hour in duration.

Assessment of Stuttering Using the SR

Assessment of the child's stuttering is carried out primarily by using the **Severity Rating (SR) Scale** (see Chapter 8). This is a 10-point scale that the clinician and parent use in each clinic meeting. In addition, the parent records SRs at the end of every day, reflecting his or her judgment of the child's stuttering severity that day. The daily SRs are crucial data used to assess the child's progress and make decisions about contingencies. On the SR Scale, a 0 represents no stuttering, a 2 represents extremely mild stuttering, and a 9 represents extremely severe stuttering.

TABLE 12.1 Verbal Contingencies for Fluent Speech and Unambiguous Stuttering

	Examples of Verbal Contingencies

Fluent speech	■ Comments should be specific to speech (i.e., "nice" or "very good" is too general).
	■ Always give at least five praises before a contingency for stuttering.
	■ Adjust the types of praise to those that the child seems to enjoy. Here are some examples:
	  ■ "That was smooth."
	  ■ "Great, your words are smooth!"
	  ■ "Nice smooth talking!"
	  ■ "No bumps there, excellent."
	  ■ "I didn't hear any bumps."
	  ■ "Wow, that whole story was totally smooth."
	  ■ "Was that smooth?" (The answer should always be "yes" and followed up with another instance of praise.)
	■ Also praise for spontaneous self-evaluation (i.e., if the child says "I was really smooth today" or remarks on his own smooth or bumpy talking).

Unambiguous stuttering	■ Use low-key delivery and move quickly to a praise.
	■ Use one request for correction after every five praises (approximately six contingencies for stuttering a day).
	■ Some children become so smooth during a session they do not need any contingencies for stuttering. This is okay because the goal is practicing stutter-free speech.
	  ■ "Oops, I heard a little bump."
	  ■ "That was a little bumpy."
	  ■ "There was a bump."
	  ■ "You got a little stuck there."
	  ■ "You only need to say ______ once."
	  ■ "Say ______ again." (Use if child is comfortable with repeating stuttered word.)
	■ Remember only to praise smooth speech; it's important not to praise bumps!

In the first clinic meeting, after discussing the scale in detail with the parent, the parent and I play and talk with the child to obtain an adequate, representative sample of the child's stuttering. I then ask the parent to tell me what SR she would give the child's speech in that sample, which I compare with my own judgment of the child's SR. It is usually possible with only a little discussion to ensure that the parent is using the scale appropriately. On the rare occasion that the parent's rating differs from mine by more than 1 point, I explain how I came up with my rating and then try to determine if the parent seems to understand my rationale and is likely to be accurate in her future ratings. If I have doubts, I use video clips of the child's speech to help teach the parent how to use the scale. I typically ask the parents to make videos of the child's speech at home during the first few weeks of treatment so that I can continue to "calibrate" the parent's ratings. Once I'm sure the parent understands the scale, I ask him or her to rate the child's speech at the end of every day and to bring the ratings to our weekly meetings. The standard Lidcombe procedure has the parent bring in a chart that displays each day's SRs of the child. I encourage the parents to add comments to the chart if the child has gone through a period of increased stuttering, sickness, or other event that the parent feels may have an impact on severity or the child's response to treatment.

Assessing the Child's Percentage of Syllables Stuttered

The use of %SS to assess the child's stuttering is optional. When I am conducting LP treatment, I usually assess the child's %SS at the beginning of treatment and at other important points in the program such as when the child moves from Stage 1 to **Stage 2**. For a formal assessment using %SS, I typically video record the first clinic session and later score the child's stuttering from her speech in that sample, which should be at least 300 syllables.

Teaching the Parent to Conduct Daily Practice Sessions

A critical part of the first clinic visit is to show the parent how to conduct the daily practice sessions. It is most important to create situations that not only are fun but also stimulate a lot of fluent speech in the child. This enables the parent to begin treatment using a great deal of positive verbal contingencies for fluency. To demonstrate for the parent, I begin by using a picture book or picture cards with the child to elicit short, fluent words. To keep the child's interest, I talk with a lot of enthusiasm and move through the pictures quickly. I usually name a picture or two myself as a model for the child and then ask her to name some pictures. After the fifth fluent utterance, I praise her fluency immediately by saying something specifically about her speech, such as "That was really smooth talking!" or "You said that really smoothly!" It is important to make the praise directly relevant to the child's fluency, rather than general praise. After modeling for the parent, I ask him or her to work with the child, and I coach the parent if necessary.

With children who have more severe stuttering, I may need to begin with single-syllable words or have the child repeat the word after me. Children who have milder stuttering can

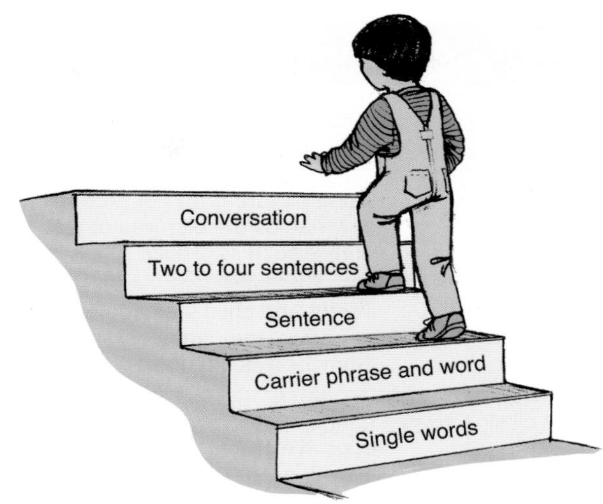

Figure 12.2 Linguistic hierarchy used for practice sessions at the beginning of Stage 1 in the Lidcombe Program.

progress quickly from single words to carrier phrases (such as "I like ______") and words to short sentences of three or four words. Figure 12.2 shows a linguistic hierarchy that most children can quickly climb on the way to natural conversations in the beginning of Stage 1.

One of the mistakes parents often make when they first begin is to use positive verbal contingencies for fluent speech that are too general. They might say, for example, "That's good" or "You're doing well." In this case, I simply restate the need for specific praise and observe the parents doing it.

Another common error is for parents to let the child make longer responses than are appropriate, thereby allowing more stuttered than fluent utterances to occur. Fortunately, a little discussion and lots of modeling will usually clear this up. For those children who need to start at the one- or two-word utterance stage, specifically praising their use of one or two words will help keep them at this level until it is appropriate for them to move to longer utterances.

As I mentioned earlier, it is crucial that the parent make the practice sessions fun for the child. It may be helpful to suggest games and activities for the sessions. Table 12.2 lists some of the activities that parents can use with the child in these practice sessions.

At the end of the first clinic visit, I review the activities and tasks the parent will be doing over the coming week and respond to any questions she has. Some parents benefit from taking notes or being given a written description of things they will be doing; others like to have a follow-up e-mail. In all cases, I encourage them to call or e-mail me if they have any questions or concerns during the week.

Stage 1: Subsequent Clinic Visits

Most subsequent clinic visits have three goals: (1) to assess the child's stuttering, (2) to discuss the current progress, and (3) to introduce new procedures when appropriate. Each session begins with the clinician and parent assessing the child's

TABLE 12.2 Suggested Games and Activities for Structured Treatment Conversations

Grab bag	The parent puts interesting items into a large cloth bag or pillowcase, and the child guesses what each is by reaching into the bag and feeling the item.
Picture naming	Using picture books or picture cards, the child names each picture. At the one-word level, the child only names the pictured object. As longer utterances are permitted, the child can use a carrier phrase such as "That's a ______," or she can name the item and its color, such as "red rabbit."
Reading a story	Parent and child look at a familiar book while the parent reads or tells the story. To elicit a word or phrase, the parent asks the child to complete a sentence, such as "Then Goldilocks said, 'Somebody's been sleeping in my ______.'"
Rhyme closing	Parent makes up a rhyme and leaves the last word blank, like "Once there was a man—he cooked his eggs in a frying ______."

stuttering using the SRs. This assessment is made from the child's conversational speech when talking with the parent and the clinician until a representative sample of the child's speech has been obtained (about 300 syllables or 10 minutes). The clinician gives the child's speech a rating on the SR Scale and asks the parent for her rating of that sample. If the parent and clinician ratings differ by more than 1 point, a discussion ensues that helps the parent align her ratings with those of the clinician. Accurate parent SRs are essential to the integrity of the treatment program. These ratings, along with the clinician's ratings, determine whether treatment is progressing successfully and signal when to fade practice treatment conversations and transition to treatment in natural conversations. They also indicate when to move from Stage 1 to Stage 2 of the Lidcombe Program.

After the clinician and parent complete their ratings of the child's speech, they discuss the week's SRs and the progress of the home treatment. As they talk, the child usually plays by herself in the same room, with some interaction and encouragement from the parent and the clinician. The openness with which discussions of the week's progress take place is a hallmark of the Lidcombe Program. There is no attempt to keep the child from overhearing the parent and clinician discussion of the child's stuttering. The matter-of-fact manner in which the clinician and parent discuss the child's speech seems to me to make it more likely that both the parent and child will feel less anxious about the child's stuttering and may reduce any shame the child might feel about her difficulty. During the parent and clinician's discussion, some children often make noise to call attention to themselves. In my experience, this is not because the child objects to the discussion of her stuttering but is only an attempt to get the focus back on herself. At such times, it may be helpful if the clinician simply asks the child, "Right now, I want to talk to your mommy for just a minute; then we'll play again!" or she may take a minute to play with the child.

As the clinician looks over the parent's weekly SRs, the clinician may ask about the days in which ratings are higher or lower than average, or the clinician and parent may brainstorm solutions to problems that may be indicated by lack of change in the ratings. This is often a time when videos of the practice sessions from home are useful, so that the clinician can assess how they are being conducted. It is also helpful to have the parent demonstrate during each clinic visit how he or she is conducting the treatment at home by doing a few minutes of a practice session with the child using the verbal contingencies (Fig. 12.3). When adequate progress is being made and home SRs and clinic assessments indicate that the child is becoming more fluent, new treatment procedures can be introduced.

Once a parent is appropriately reinforcing fluency, he or she may be taught to use verbal contingencies for stuttering in practice sessions. The mildest is verbally acknowledging the occurrence of an **unambiguous stutter**. Only unambiguous stutters should be acknowledged because normal disfluencies should not be treated as stutters. The descriptions of normal disfluencies and stuttered disfluencies in Chapter 7 clarify this difference. I typically model an acknowledgment of stuttering for the parent, which is given after about five or more instances of contingencies for fluent utterances. It

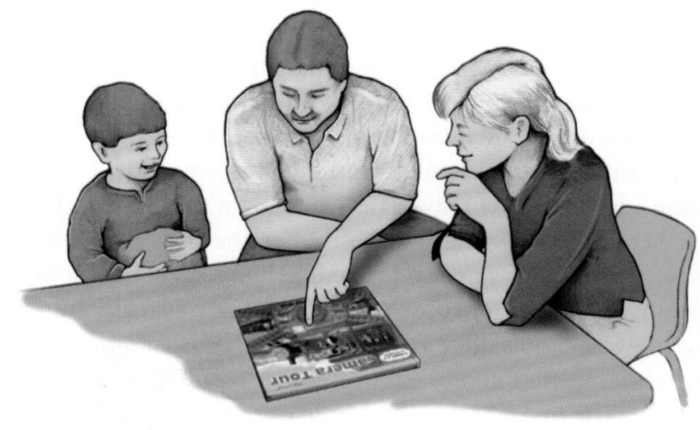

Figure 12.3 Clinician observing a father demonstrating a practice session with his child.

is important that the parent learn to use contingencies for fluency several times before using a verbal contingency on stuttered speech. When I demonstrate acknowledgment of stuttering, I use comments like "a little bumpy one there" or "that one was a little bumpy." I make the statement quietly, immediately after the stutter and without any negative inflection in my voice. After I have modeled how to acknowledge stutters, I ask the parent to try it, but only after he or she has praised several of the child's fluent utterances. Most children hardly seem to notice the acknowledgment, although some may stop momentarily and look at the parent when it is given. Typically, I ask parents to continue using contingencies for fluency and begin using acknowledgment of stuttering for a week before introducing further verbal contingencies for stuttering.

In the following weekly meeting, I introduce requests for self-correction of unambiguous stuttering. This verbal contingency asks the child to say the stuttered word again with a phrase such as (if the child has stuttered on "I") "Can you say 'I' again?" *Such requests are made in a positive, supportive manner*, and it is important that the parent practice this contingency after the clinician demonstrates it. Some parents may be hesitant to request a self-correction and may convey their concern to the child. Others may inadvertently use a slightly negative or impatient tone when asking for a correction. However, a clinician's patient modeling and subsequent coaching can do wonders to shape parents' responses into helpful, supportive requests.

After the child has repeated the word fluently, the parent should praise the self-correction with comments like "Nice job of making that word smooth." If a child ignores a parent's request for self-correction or refuses to self-correct, the parent just moves on. If the child says the word again but stutters again, the parent may say something supportive like "That's OK; sometimes those words are hard."

In the subsequent weeks, the clinician monitors the child's progress and ensures that the parent is delivering verbal contingencies effectively. The clinician also checks to see that the child is enjoying the practice sessions and is responding well to the contingencies for both fluency and stuttering. Every child and every family are different, so the program must be individualized in each case. For example, some children may indicate they are uncomfortable with such praise as "That was really smooth talking." In this case, the parent can ask the child what she would like the parent to say when she is talking smoothly. Alternatively, the parent can use one of the other verbal contingencies for fluency. Some children who don't react well to praise will happily respond to requests to self-evaluate their fluency. One child I worked with preferred that the parent put a penny in a jar, which made a nice "plink" sound, rather than verbally praise her fluency. Another child who loved the Boston Red Sox asked his mother to say "That's Red Sox talking!" after fluent speech. You can guess what the child asked the parent to say after the child stuttered. It had to do with a New York team.

Stage 1: Introducing Verbal Contingencies in Natural Conversations

When treatment has progressed well for 2 or 3 weeks, and SRs indicate improvement, a gradual transition can be made from practice sessions to natural conversations. Thus, verbal contingencies of praise, acknowledgment of stutters, and requests for correction can now be given in typical daily conversations, such as during meals, riding in the car, shopping, and playing. When treatment is first introduced in natural conversations, practice sessions usually continue for a time to make the transition easy. When contingencies in natural conversations have been going well for a week or two and stuttering continues to decrease, practice sessions can be faded gradually. For example, each week, one or two practice sessions may be dropped until they have all been discontinued and replaced with contingencies in natural conversations.

There are several reasons why practice sessions may subsequently be reinstated. The first reason is if stuttering increases for a day or more, in this situation, practice sessions may be conducted until the child's fluency has returned to earlier levels. Another reason for continuing or reinstating practice sessions is if the child asks to continue practice sessions for a period of time as the transition to natural conversations is made. Sometimes parents feel that things are going so well in practice sessions that they believe the transition to natural conversations should be made slowly.

Several issues may warrant consideration when using contingencies in natural conversations is just getting underway. Parents may wish to begin with just praise for fluent utterances and then add acknowledgment for fluency and for stuttering, requests for self-evaluation, and, finally, requests for self-correction of stuttering. If problems appear in response to any of these verbal contingencies, they can be solved immediately. It is also important that verbal contingencies not be given relentlessly throughout each day but are used selectively at first, so that the parent can judge how the child is responding. If the child reacts well, which is usually the case, the parent can begin using verbal contingencies in more and more conversations, but at the same time, the parent should make sure that the child is not overwhelmed by too-frequent attention to her speech. The child needs to experience the normal flow of conversation for its own sake, rather than feel that everything she says is being evaluated. This is essential for sensitive children.

Another issue that may arise relative to contingencies in natural conversations is who is giving the verbal contingencies. Although only one parent may have been conducting the practice sessions, both parents, and even other family members, may be involved in the natural conversations. When this is done, it must be done very carefully and be individualized for each family. Other adults in the home or older siblings may be appropriate in some cases, whereas a sibling close to the child's age may not be. If a child is responsive to the contingencies given by one parent in natural conversations, I usually try adding another family member and evaluate the child's response. I recommend that the clinician meet with any family members who are giving verbal contingencies to ensure that they understand how crucial it is that much more praise for fluency be given than requests for self-correction of stuttering and that requests for self-correction be done in a supportive manner. Also, the focus on the content of the conversation rather than its fluency needs to remain a top priority.

Contingencies in natural conversations at home and weekly meetings in the clinic continue until the child is essentially fluent and can move to Stage 2. This point is reached when two criteria are met: (1) the parent's SRs for 3 weeks in a row are all 0s and 1s, with at least four of the ratings being 0, and (2) the clinician's SRs *for the entire clinic visit* are 0s or 1s for these same 3 weeks. Meeting these criteria is vital if the child is to remain fluent after treatment. If the clinician has any doubts about the reliability and validity of the parent's SRs, she should request that the parent bring an audio or video recording of the child's speech at home to confirm that the criteria are met.

Stage 2: Maintenance

One of the most important components of the Lidcombe Program is its maintenance procedure. Because relapse is common in stuttering treatment, parents are cautioned when they begin Stage 1 of the Lidcombe Program that it is essential that they continue to work with the clinician through the end of **Stage 2**. They are reminded of this throughout Stage 1 so that the procedures of the second stage are expected. Stage 2 consists of 30-minute clinic visits that are scheduled at gradually greater intervals. Typically, there are two visits at 2-week intervals, then two visits at 4-week intervals, then two visits at 8-week intervals, and, finally, one visit 16 weeks later. During this period, parents continue to provide verbal contingencies for fluency and stuttering just as they did during Stage 1 and continue to record SRs, but the clinician guides the parents in gradually decreasing their verbal contingencies until they are completely discontinued.

To progress through this schedule of visits, the child must maintain the same level of fluency achieved to begin Stage 2 (clinician SRs of 0 or 1 for the entire clinic visit and parent SRs beyond the clinic visit of 0s and 1s, with at least four ratings of 0 during any given week). When the parent and child come in for a scheduled clinic visit, they have a discussion of how the child's speech has been since the previous visit. This discussion, as always, is focused on the parent's SRs and reports of how the child is responding to verbal contingencies. At each visit, the clinician and parent decide whether to continue decreasing the frequency of clinic visits or to make some changes, such as keeping to the current frequency of visits, resuming or increasing contingencies in natural conversations, or reinstating both practice sessions and contingencies in natural conversations. It is also possible that some aspect of the verbal contingencies may need to be adjusted. For example, sometimes a child becomes so fluent that when stutters do occur, parents or other family members apply contingencies to stuttering without concurrently giving the appropriate number of contingencies for fluency. Sometimes, making this adjustment will solve a problem of stuttering re-emerging or increasing in frequency. In other cases, stuttering reappears because of momentary stress. In such cases, reinstating weekly visits may help the parent and clinician get the child back on track.

Stage 2 takes about a year to complete for most children. Although minor relapses may occur, parents are usually able to accurately assess what changes need to be made to bring the child back to essentially fluent speech.

Problem-Solving

In general, the Lidcombe Program runs smoothly without much difficulty if clinicians follow the program carefully. However, it is common for minor problems to arise during Stages 1 and 2. This section describes some common problems that may occur and their possible solutions. For more detailed descriptions of troubleshooting and special cases, see *The Lidcombe Program of Early Stuttering Intervention—A Clinician's Guide* (Onslow et al., 2003) or the Lidcombe Program Treatment Guide, available on the Lidcombe Web site.

Sometimes, progress toward fluent speech is stalled for several weeks, or previous gains are momentarily lost. If so, I usually begin by talking to the parent about what he or she thinks might be occurring. Parents are often able to pinpoint something they have changed about the way they are doing treatment. Or it may be that a parent misunderstands some aspect of treatment. Thus, it helps to have parents demonstrate how they conduct treatment, and it may be even more helpful to have them bring in a video of treatment at home. Examples of things that may go wrong include the following: (1) parents are less attentive to praising fluent speech regularly so that fewer positive reinforcements are made than requests for corrections; (2) parents become lax about the consistency of practice sessions so that many days are missed; (3) other family members, while trying to be helpful, make mistakes in providing verbal contingencies because they have not been trained; (4) the child is overly sensitive to verbal contingencies and asks parents to stop using them; and (5) some children who stutter severely at the beginning of treatment have trouble generating adequate fluency in structured sessions.

The problems that arise from misunderstanding the parameters of treatment can usually be resolved by supportive feedback and guidance of the parent and modeling of appropriate behavior. Other issues, such as conducting treatment inconsistently, may require brainstorming with the parent about how treatment can be conducted more regularly. If a child isn't enjoying conversations, progress will be stalled. But it is not difficult to coach parents in delivering treatment in ways that are enjoyable, effective, and fun for both parent and child. Clinicians who have worked with preschool-age children have usually learned how to keep a child interested and achieve therapy goals at the same time. It may be appropriate for other family members to become involved in practice sessions, but they must be trained by the clinician to deliver contingencies effectively. Practice sessions may be shared by both parents and other caregivers, but the clinician should ensure that whoever is delivering treatment is doing so accurately, and direct training is the best way to achieve this.

If a child objects to the parent's verbal contingencies after treatment has gone on for some months, it is usually helpful to ask the child how he or she would like the parent to respond to fluent speech and to stuttering. Some sensitive children prefer nonverbal contingencies such as a wink or a "thumbs up" after several fluent utterances and just a quick eye contact after a stutter.

With children who have moderate or severe stuttering, it is critical to structure their treatment conversations so that the child is largely fluent and only stutters occasionally. One way to do this is to ensure that in practice sessions, the child is, at first, using only short utterances (which are more likely to be fluent). Short fluent utterances should be reinforced, but not longer ones. This "differential" reinforcement of shorter utterances will teach the child to make short, fluent utterances for the first part of the training. Then, after the child is reliably experiencing mostly fluent speech in the practice sessions, longer utterances can be stimulated. With the help of the clinician's instruction and modeling, the parent can learn how to move the child up a linguistic hierarchy of increasingly longer and more complex sentences while preserving fluency.

The Lidcombe Program is an effective treatment approach but should be used only after attending a training workshop conducted by the Lidcombe Program Trainers Consortium. Information about workshops, research articles on treatment outcome, and a treatment manual are available on the Lidcombe Web site. After training, the clinician can join an online Lidcombe discussion group, which provides a wealth of information about various challenges that may arise in treatment.

Outcome Data

A number of studies have reported that the Lidcombe Program is effective in eliminating stuttering in most preschoolers. A long-term outcome study of 42 children treated with the program showed that their stuttering was at near-zero levels 4 to 7 years after treatment (Lincoln & Onslow, 1997). Other research reported that the mean number of clinic visits needed to complete Stage 1 treatment in a sample of 29 children was 18 clinic visits (median = 16) (Rousseau, Packman, Onslow, Harrison, & Jones, 2007). In response to concerns expressed by critics that the Lidcombe Program might produce negative psychological effects, Woods, Shearsby, Onslow, and Burnham (2002) compared pre- and posttreatment measures of the *Child Behavior Checklist* (Achenbach, 1988) and the *Attachment Q-Set* (Waters, 1995) and found no ill effects of treatment on the children's psychological health. In fact, the *Child Behavior Checklist* showed improvement in the children's behavior after treatment.

An important research tool for assessing treatment effectiveness is a randomized controlled trial. To use this procedure to test stuttering treatment, a group of children who stutter would be divided in half. One-half would be given a treatment, and the other half would be given no treatment (the untreated group would eventually be treated once the study data have been collected). Just such a study was carried out in New Zealand (Jones, Onslow, Packman, Williams, & Ormond, 2005). When the Lidcombe-treated group (n = 29) was compared with the untreated group (n = 25), a significantly (p = .003) greater improvement was seen with the Lidcombe-treated group. The "effect size" was 2.3 %SS. This means that the difference between the treated group and the control group final levels of stuttering relative to their variability in stuttering was very large; in fact, the authors indicate that it was more than twice the minimally clinically significant difference stated in their treatment protocol before the study was done.

While the majority of research on the Lidcombe Program has been done in Australia, publications from researchers in the United Kingdom, Canada, and other countries have appeared. For example, Miller and Guitar (2009) showed that Lidcombe can be very successful when implemented by supervised graduate students with excellent outcomes for 15 preschool children. Duration of treatment (number of sessions required to reach the end of Stage 1) was predicted by scores on the Stuttering Severity Instrument (Riley, 2009); children who stuttered more severely before treatment took longer to become fluent. This is important information for clinicians so they can let parents of children with more severe stuttering know that treatment may take 20 sessions or more. In a later study, Guitar et al. (2015) combined the data from these original 15 children and added 14 more children, all of whom were assessed pretreatment and 2 years after treatment. Long-term outcome indicated that most children showed near-zero stuttering, and for the few others, stuttering was substantially reduced. Stuttering severity before treatment was a strong predictor of outcome, such children who were more severe before treatment had slightly more residual stuttering at long-term assessment. Girls did slightly better long term than boys. Latterman, Euler, and Neumann (2008) assessed the outcome of Lidcombe treatment in Germany, showing it to be quite effective, and Femrell, Avfall, and Lindström (2012) reported on its success in Sweden.

The Lidcombe group in Australia has also published data on conducting the Lidcombe treatment in a group setting (Arnott et al., 2014) as well as webcam delivery of Lidcombe to parents over the Internet (O'Brian, Smith, & Onslow, 2014). In both of those treatment environments, the Lidcombe approach was found to be effective compared to traditional delivery procedures.

ANOTHER CLINICIAN'S APPROACH: SHERYL GOTTWALD

I present Sheryl Gottwald's approach to working with stuttering in preschool children because it has good outcome data indicating that it is effective. In addition, it is different from the Lidcombe Program because both the child and his environment are treated, whereas on the face of it, the Lidcombe Program focuses treatment only on the child.

Gottwald (2010) has refined an approach first developed at Temple University by Starkweather, Gottwald, and Halfond (1990) and extended by Gottwald and Starkweather (1999). They designed it for children ages 2 to 6 who stutter. This treatment popularized their concept of "**demands and capacities**," described in Chapter 6, that ascribed stuttering to a combination of the demands placed on a child by her environments (internal and external) interacting with her innate capacity for fluent speech. Because there are many factors maintaining the child's stuttering, Gottwald terms her approach "multidimensional." Among the dimensions are treatment focused on the parents to reduce stresses in the child's environment and treatment focused on the child to strengthen the child's fluency. Gottwald carries out her assessment and treatment by working to understand the family's and child's needs, working with their strengths, and supporting them deeply as they deal with their challenges.

Modifying the Environment

Gottwald is very sensitive to each family's needs as she works with them to help them modify the child's environment. She describes her orientation this way: "Families bring their own individual needs for emotional support; until their feelings of sadness, guilt, frustration and other emotions are addressed and acknowledged, it will be so much more difficult for them to make the changes necessary to support their child's fluency. We discover what families need by talking with them about their hopes, observations, feelings and needs" (Gottwald, personal communication, July 2018).

The initial component of treatment—parent counseling—provides parents with what we currently know about the nature of stuttering. Figure 12.4 was drawn from a video clip of Gottwald counseling a mother and father whose child is stuttering. A series of video clips illustrating Gottwald's approach is available on thePoint, in the video links for Chapter 12.

Some of the information that Gottwald shares is that stuttering is highly variable and that many factors may influence its ups and downs, including factors that they may be able to change. The family is also introduced to an etiological model of stuttering, which explains stuttering as emerging from interactions between the child's capacities and the demands placed on the child. The clinician also helps the family find ways of talking about stuttering with their child. They learn to support the child by commenting sensitively when she has difficulty getting a word out. Open acknowledgment of stuttering is intended to reduce the child's and the family's negative feelings about stuttering. For example, a parent might say to a child who has just stuttered and appears frustrated or ashamed, "Sometimes those words really get stuck. It's OK. I'm here to listen." This conveys to the child that the parent has the time and is focused on listening patiently.

During individual counseling, families are also taught to change other aspects of their behavior that may be affecting their child's fluency. For example, family members may learn to respond to the child's stuttering without interrupting, looking away, or otherwise conveying impatience. To decrease pressure from the family's speech and language environment on the child, family members may be taught to

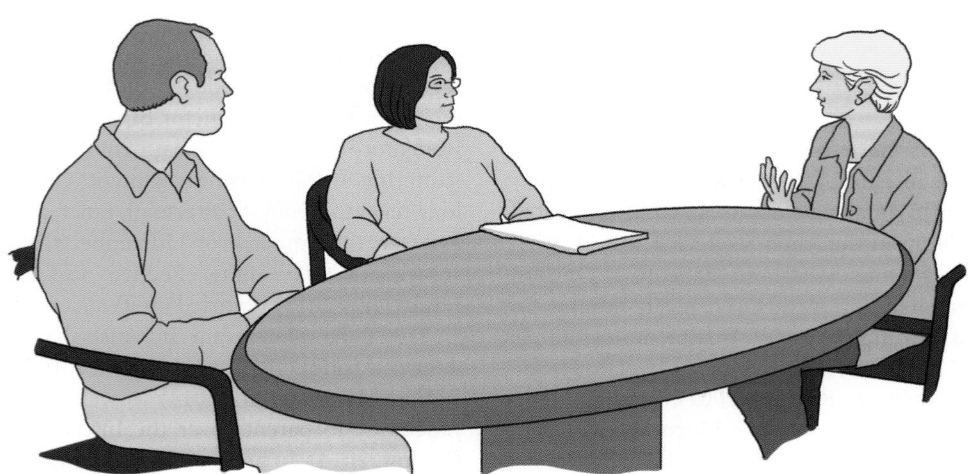

Figure 12.4 A clinician counseling a family about treatment for their child.

TABLE 12.3 Modifying the Speech and Language of Family Members

1. Use a speech rate that more closely matches the child's.
2. Pause between conversation turns.
3. Eliminate questions requiring long, complex answers.
4. Respond to the content of the child's message regardless of fluency.
5. Acknowledge struggled stutters by using meaningful words, such as "That's okay."

slow their speech rates, pause more frequently, and simplify their language when talking with the child. To increase the child's self-esteem, families may be urged to create times each day when the child has a parent's full attention. Sometimes, family members may be bombarding the child with questions or otherwise pressing him to speak. As a remedy, they are shown how to talk about what they are thinking and doing as they play with the child, thereby modeling the behavior they want to encourage. Table 12.3 lists some of the things that family members can do to facilitate fluency.

In addition to changing behavior directly related to speech, families are also counseled about other stresses in the home. For example, Starkweather et al. (1990) have noted that a hectic family lifestyle can exacerbate a child's stuttering. Once parents understand that a too-busy family schedule may be a factor in their child's stuttering, they are often able to reduce the hustle and bustle in the home and are gratified when their child's stuttering subsequently diminishes. In addition, a slower pace and more relaxed lifestyle can often provide increased satisfaction for all family members.

Gottwald sometimes supplements individual family counseling with group therapy in which two to four other couples whose child stutters are incorporated, when that can be arranged. This gives families an opportunity to share experiences and ideas and to support one another. As members of a group, parents receive support from one another and can share ideas for helping their children. The clinician's role is to help the group members develop a sense of mutual trust by modeling concern, acceptance, and respect for all group members and their ideas and feelings. Generally, the group talks about topics they select, although the clinician may also suggest topics that are often concerns of most members, such as regression during treatment and termination of treatment.

Modifying the Child's Speech

The other major component of Gottwald's therapy—besides working with the parents or caregivers to change the child's environment—is modification of the child's speech. This involves parent and clinician modeling and reinforcement, as well as the clinician's instruction when needed. Instruction in changing stuttering with older preschool-age children is a natural outgrowth of the parents and clinician talking openly about stuttering with the child. The procedures that the authors use to modify a child's speech are as follows.

Children Who Stutter with Minimal Struggle

First, the clinician talks and plays games with the child in a very fluency-enhancing setting. This situation includes the clinician talking slowly in a relaxed way with plenty of pauses and silences. Then the clinician teaches the child to talk in a slow, relaxed way. This is done with very little linguistic demand on the child; for example, a game they play may require only simple short sentences. Gradually, as the child becomes more and more fluent in this situation, demands are gradually increased. This may entail games and conversation involving longer and more complex utterances, or the clinician may speed up her speech rate. For those children who continue to stutter in this low-pressure situation, Gottwald teaches them to stutter using "easy bounces" at the beginning of an utterance, li-like this.

Children Who Stutter with Moderate to Severe Struggle

For those children who stutter with noticeable tension and struggle, Gottwald begins therapy by talking with them about stuttering, so that they will recognize what they are doing when they stutter and thereby increase their acceptance of it. By playing games that reward stuttering, the child changes her feelings about her stuttering and may even begin to stutter on purpose. This then leads to changing the stutters so they become gradually looser and looser. Gottwald encourages these children to use bouncy speech (re-repeating sounds easily and loosely) or stretchy speech (lllllllllike this) in which easy, loose prolongations take the place of struggled stutters. As she works on helping the children change their stutters, Gottwald also works to help them express their feelings as a way of leading to improved attitudes about their stuttering and a better understanding of it.

Termination

Individual and group parent counseling and modification of the child's speech continue until the family environment and the child's speech have met the following two criteria. First, the environment has changed enough so that major stresses have diminished and the family seems to understand the dynamics that may exist between environmental stresses and the child's stuttering. Second, the child's stuttering has decreased to the point at which she is normally disfluent, with an occasional mild instance of stuttering.

Supporting Data

Starkweather et al. (1990) reported that most of the children they have treated have regained normal fluency. Of 39 children whom they treated using this approach, 7 dropped out, and of the remaining 32 children, 29 recovered completely, and 3 were still in treatment at the time of the report. The average child requires about 12 sessions of therapy using this approach, although some children require much more before therapy can be terminated.

Gottwald and Starkweather (1999) treated an additional 15 families with their approach. Although 1 family dropped out, the children of the remaining 14 families achieved normal fluency and reported maintaining it a year after the children were dismissed from treatment. Further data on her approach were provided by Gottwald (2010) involving the children of 27 families. Again, 1 family dropped out, but 26 families reported their children had normal fluency 1 year or more following dismissal from treatment.

TREATMENT OF CONCOMITANT SPEECH AND LANGUAGE PROBLEMS

One of the clinical issues that should be considered, especially with beginning stuttering in older preschoolers, is the management of **concomitant speech and language problems**. Research has indicated that some children who stutter are delayed in their speech and language development, especially in their articulation or phonological development (Bloodstein & Ratner, 2008). Moreover, meta-analysis of 22 studies of language abilities in children who stutter suggested that children who stutter, compared to children who don't, are likely to have language difficulties, either subtle or notable (Ntourou, Conture, & Lipsey, 2011). These findings make it clear that children who stutter should be assessed for phonological and other language problems before treatment. When concomitant problems are found, the challenge is to plan how best to work with these other problems as treatment of stuttering is planned.

Let me begin this section by describing how clinicians using Lidcombe deal with concomitant problems. When using the Lidcombe Program, it is imperative that only stuttering be treated during Stage 1, when the parent and child are highly involved in working on fluency. Typically, the Lidcombe Program up to the end of Stage 1 is conducted first, and then any other speech or language problem would be treated. In some cases, however, when another problem is particularly severe, treatment can be focused on that problem first until appropriate improvement is made. Then, Stage 1 of Lidcombe can be implemented, and treatment of the other problem(s) can be resumed when Stage 1 is finished. During treatment of the Lidcombe Program, it is crucial that parents understand that the focus is on fluency only, so that their SRs are not affected by the other disorder(s). Placing the priority on the treatment of stuttering is recommended because of its greater likelihood of chronicity and exacerbation as children grow older. This contrasts with most other developmental problems that tend to improve a little or at least not worsen appreciably if treatment for them is delayed.

A number of clinicians not using the Lidcombe Program have recommended a variety of ways of responding to other concomitant speech and language problems in beginning stutterers. One approach is to work on phonological problems at the same time as they work on fluency, if they are severe enough to warrant intervention. When doing this, Conture, Louko, and Edwards (1993) use an indirect articulation treatment. Avoiding the traditional "corrective" type of therapy, they provide the child with plenty of models of target phonemes through extensive auditory stimulation and opportunities for improved production. This is done in an accepting environment rather than correcting the child when she is wrong and asking her to try again with more attention and effort. Diane Hill (2003) begins with receptive training and then follows with a sequence of working on phonological change, sound play, sound approximation, and rehearsal of correct sound production in a few target sounds. If language is an issue, the clinician again begins with receptive training, followed by integrating practice with proper syntactic forms into the fluency hierarchy of more and more complex language. For example, the clinician provides appropriate instructions and materials and has the child practice a specific syntactic structure while using easy, relaxed speech.

Wall and Myers (1995) recommend that concomitant problems be treated after fluency has been stabilized if the child's other disability is mild and not interfering with speech intelligibility. However, if the disability is interfering with intelligibility, the problem should be dealt with immediately because it may be adding considerable stress to the child's communicative attempts. If treatment of a phonological or articulation disorder is begun, Wall and Myers recommend that the phoneme or class of phonemes selected for treatment be one that is the easiest for the child to produce—usually those that are acquired relatively early in development by most children. Words and syntactic structures selected for practice material should be ones with which the child can easily cope. Work on speech sound production can be integrated with work on fluency. For example, practice of a new sound in a word can be integrated with practice of easy speech.

Finally, the "cycles" model alternates fluency treatment with language or phonology therapy over the course of the year (Hodson & Paden, 1991; described in Bernstein Ratner, 1995). Bernstein Ratner points out that this provides children with initial periods of concentrated learning of new skills (for a specified amount of time irrespective of whether or not the client meets criteria for finishing the treatment), followed by opportunities for spontaneous generalization of these skills to other settings while the other treatment is cycled in. This alternation continues until one of the problems is resolved so that all attention can then be given to the remaining issue.

SUMMARY

- I believe that beginning stuttering arises from an interaction between children's constitutional predispositions and developmental and environmental influences to produce primarily repetitive disfluencies with increased tension. Escape behaviors are also an important component of the disorder as children experience increasing frustration with their inability to complete a word.
- I believe that a key element of treatment for children this age is to prevent them from having negative emotions associated with their stuttering. When children have negative experiences, the danger is that they will react to stuttering (and anticipated stuttering) with tension and struggle that will begin a cycle of increasingly negative feelings and increasingly tense stuttering, coupled with escape and avoidance behaviors. Focusing treatment on increasing fluency and building the child's confidence in her fluency will prevent this cycle.
- Fortunately, children with beginning stuttering usually have a large amount of fluency that can be reinforced and generalized to situations that previously elicited stuttering.
- The Lidcombe Program is a parent-delivered, operant conditioning program for preschoolers in which the parent is guided to conduct daily treatment conversations and apply verbal contingencies to fluency and stuttering. Treatment begins in practice sessions and quickly moves to natural conversations throughout the day, so that treatment is conducted in the child's natural speaking environment, promoting generalization to all aspects of the child's world. Once the child is fluent in all situations, the clinician manages a phased withdrawal of clinic contact with careful monitoring of progress so that the family can respond to any relapses by reinstating needed features of treatment and then return to the fading process.
- Another clinician, Sheryl Gottwald, uses an approach based on the "demands and capacities" concept and treats both the family and the child. Gottwald uses an individualized treatment in which the clinician gets to know each family and each child so that their needs can be met in a way that plays to their strengths and supports their challenges.
- In the Lidcombe Program, work on other communication disorders precedes or more typically follows Stage 1 of treatment. In other treatment approaches, clinicians often integrate work on fluency with other concomitant speech or language problems. Several approaches to the challenges of treating stuttering and concomitant disorders exist.

STUDY QUESTIONS

1. Describe Stage 1 and Stage 2 of the Lidcombe Program for the beginning stutterer. What is the goal of each phase?
2. Describe practice sessions and natural conversations in the Lidcombe Program.
3. Describe the two major ways of collecting data on the child's progress in the Lidcombe Program.
4. Describe how data are used to guide the child's progress in the Lidcombe Program.
5. Compare the Lidcombe Program with Gottwald's approach. In what ways are they similar, and in what ways are they different?
6. Describe how the treatment of beginning stuttering and other speech and language disorders can be managed.

SUGGESTED PROJECTS

1. Develop a hierarchy based on length and complexity of utterances that could be used by a clinician who is working with beginning stuttering and wants to move from single words to conversational speech.
2. Develop a hierarchy, based on increasing social complexity, for a child with beginning stuttering. Design it for use by a typical, two-parent family with older and younger siblings and grandparents who visit frequently. In other words, design a series of interactions that a parent could take a child through that would have her practice fluency in more and more challenging social situations with the family members listed.
3. Interview the family of a child with beginning stuttering who was treated successfully. Find out what they perceived to be the most helpful aspects of treatment and what advice they would give to other families just beginning treatment.

SUGGESTED READINGS

Bernstein Ratner, N. (1995). Treating the child who stutters with concomitant language and phonological impairment. *Language, Speech, and Hearing Services in Schools*, *26*, 180–186.

In this insightful overview of the treatment of children with concomitant disorders, Bernstein Ratner identifies several models that have evolved.

Conture, E., & Curlee, R. F. (2007). *Stuttering and related disorders of fluency*. New York, NY: Thieme.

Chapter 4 gives a description of the Lidcombe Program including case studies. Chapter 5 presents a group approach to treating stuttering in preschool children and parents.

Guitar, B., & McCauley, R. (2010). *Treatment of stuttering: Established and emerging interventions.* Baltimore, MD: Lippincott Williams & Wilkins.

Several interventions described in this book are applicable to older preschool children, and each is accompanied by video clips illustrating treatment. Of particular importance to the current chapter is the chapter by Harrison and Onslow.

Packman, A., Onslow, M., Webber, M., Harrison, E., Arnott, S., Bridgman, K., …, Lloyd, W. (2016). The Lidcombe Program Treatment Guide. Available under Research and Publications using the link for Speech Language Pathologists at http://www.lidcombeprogram.org

This manual gives detailed information about the procedures that clinicians use in administering the Lidcombe Program. The manual is frequently updated as new information is obtained about how to make the program effective.

Shapiro, D. (2011). *Stuttering intervention: A collaborative journey to fluency freedom* (2nd ed.). Austin, TX: Pro-Ed.

The section on direct intervention in the chapter on intervention with preschool children has many excellent suggestions for treatment, including ideas for building up resistance to fluency disruptors and encouraging expression of emotion. In addition, there is an excellent section on working with children who stutter and have concomitant disorders.

Zebrowski, P. M., & Kelly, E. (2002). *Manual of stuttering intervention.* Clifton Park, NY: Singular.

The chapter on treatment of the preschool child, particularly treatment of those children who are likely to persist in stuttering, contains many excellent ideas for direct work on stuttering. Many case examples are given. The authors are both world-renowned stuttering therapists.

13

Treatment of School-Age Children: Intermediate Stuttering

Chapter Objectives

After studying this chapter, readers should be able to:

- Describe the characteristics of a child who has intermediate stuttering
- Describe the author's beliefs about stuttering, targets in treatment, goals for treatment, how much to involve feelings and attitudes in treatment, and maintenance procedures
- Outline the goals and activities of these components of treatment: exploring goals, beliefs, and feelings, as well as changing stuttering behaviors, being open about stuttering and accepting it, performing voluntary stuttering, reducing fear and avoidance, coping with teasing, maintaining improvement, and learning and generalizing fluency skills
- Describe important aspects of working with parents and working with teachers to help the school-age child who stutters
- Describe the treatment procedures of (1) Yaruss, Pelczarski, and Quesal; (2) Harrison, Bruce, Shenker, Koushik, and Kazenski; and (3) Walton

Key Terms

Acceptable stuttering: Stuttering that is mild enough that it doesn't bother either the speaker or the listener and doesn't interfere with communication

Cognitive behavioral therapy: Working with thoughts and beliefs that may give rise to the negative emotions associated with stuttering

Desensitization: Helping the individual become less sensitive to negative experiences such as stuttering or negative listener reactions

Exploring: Approaching and getting to know something you may have been afraid of

Fluency disrupters: Stimuli that put pressure on someone's speech so that he or she stutters. Examples are interruptions and fast-talking conversational partners.

Fluency skills: The elements of superfluency, such as slow rate and easy onset of phonation

High-quality stutter: These are stutters that are held without any avoidance until fear and tension are reduced. The stutters are then released slowly and loosely. They are the results of learning to "stay in the stutter."

Proprioception: This is one of the "fluency skills," referred to above. It involves closely attending to sensory feedback associated with speech movement (such as the feeling of the jaw and tongue moving) to guide speech. This attention to proprioceptive feedback may reduce the impact of faulty auditory feedback that may hinder fluency.

School-age children: Children between 6 and 14 years old

Staying in the stutter: Going right into the stutter, without any avoidance behavior, and prolonging the articulatory posture and sound associated with the moment of "stuckness," with the purpose of extinguishing the threat and fear associated with the experience of being stuck

Superfluency: A style of speaking that incorporates fluency-shaping components such as slow speech rate and gentle onset of phonation

Voluntary stuttering: Deliberately stuttering or pretending to stutter so that one loses some of the fear of stuttering

AN INTEGRATED APPROACH

The typical **school-age child** who stutters (intermediate stuttering) is usually an elementary or junior high school student between 6 and 14 years of age who has been stuttering for several years. I use the word "child" or "student" to refer to the client, but I am aware that when a youngster is 10 years or older, in many ways he is more like an adolescent than a child. This student will probably exhibit tense part-word and monosyllabic whole-word repetitions, as well as tense prolongations. However, blocks with tension and struggle are also common in these students. They are the most disruptive aspect of his stuttering, both to him and to listeners. The student may also use escape devices, such as body movements or brief verbalizations (e.g., "uh"), to break free of stutters once he is stuck in them. If his stuttering has advanced further, he may use avoidance strategies such as starters, word substitutions, circumlocutions, and evasion of difficult speaking situations. The very same "uh" that began as an escape device *during* the moment of stuttering may suddenly appear *before* a moment of stuttering, as learning does its sinister work of teaching the child maladaptive behaviors. What has happened is that the torment of being jammed in a stutter creates negative emotions that spread when the student anticipates a word or sound that he has had trouble on before. If he's like me, he will end up using a multitude of "uhs" until his feared word or sound finally feels like it can be said fluently.

Another notable feature of the student's disability is the shame and embarrassment he feels because he stutters. Humiliations have piled up like concrete blocks, squashing his self-esteem. He is afraid of getting stuck in a stutter and afraid of real or imagined rejection because of it. Shame becomes a constant companion, dogging him when he must speak. Because he is in school and must talk in class as well as on the playground, he is constantly experiencing humiliation because he can't talk like other kids. He even may be teased and mistreated by his peers because of his stuttering.

There are exceptions. A few school-age children who stutter are not humiliated by their occasional difficulty. They may have grown up in unusually accepting and supportive homes. They may have compensating talents—like superb athleticism. Or they may just have resilient temperaments that keep them from feeling bad for very long when bad things happen. These students will benefit from a therapy strategy different from that used for children with more common intermediate stuttering. This approach—teaching fluency skills—will be described in a separate section after I give details about treating the majority of the students you will be working with: those whose stuttering is accompanied by fear, shame, and avoidance.

The treatment approach I will describe in the next section is for most of the school-age children who stutter. This approach aims to first reduce their negative emotions and then teach them easier and easier ways to stutter that are close to typical fluency. Some steps in this approach are depicted in Figure 13.1.

I illustrate our approach to treatment with the case example of David, the 6-year-old elementary school student whom we introduced in Chapter 1.

Author's Beliefs

Nature of Stuttering

In intermediate stuttering, anomalies in the neural pathways supporting speech production, combined with a child's vulnerable temperament, interact with developmental and environmental factors to prevent natural recovery and produce or exacerbate the core behaviors of repetitions, prolongations, and blocks. School-age children respond to these disfluencies with increased tension that then makes stuttering worse. As students experience more and more of these increasingly severe core behaviors, they become distressed because their speech feels out of control and they can't fix it. In desperation, they blink their eyes or nod their heads to break out of a stutter. They feel embarrassed as their stuttering becomes more severe and noticeable, and they often realize they are the only kids doing it—they are unlike their peers or anyone else they know. And if they do happen to know others who stutter, for example, a father or cousin, they may have learned that these individuals are not open about it.

The more they stutter when talking to family and friends, the more these students dread it happening again. These moments of anticipatory fear spread via classical conditioning—that is, through the repeated pairing of negative stuttering experiences (emotions) with various sounds, words, and speaking situations. As more of their talking is infected with stuttering, they try to cope by avoiding—dodging feared words and difficult situations, saying "I don't know" when asked a question, or throwing in extra sounds to get a stuck word moving. Avoidance behaviors are reinforced when these tricks are intermittently successful in preventing stuttering. Because longer and more abnormal stutters lead to more negative listener reactions, children with intermediate stuttering develop the belief that stuttering is bad and, therefore, they are bad when they stutter. Shame about their speech becomes a feature of their daily life.

Because the tension response, escape and avoidance behaviors, and negative feelings and attitudes are all learned, they can be modified by new learning. The context for this change must be an accepting, supportive environment that focuses on the child as a person, rather than just on his or her stuttering. Many students with intermediate stuttering feel that they have failed in previous therapy and thus have disappointed their parents and teachers by not becoming fluent. Thus, I try to help these children feel accepted with their current level of stuttering as well as help them experience mastery and success with their speech *and* with their communication.

If treatment can provide a student with a sufficient number of emotionally positive speaking experiences in therapy, such as experiences in which he feels "in control" of his speech, the increased fluency and positive feelings associated with speaking will generalize to other environments. The clinician can use operant and classical conditioning principles to achieve this increased fluency and generalization, rewarding beneficial changes in stuttering and associating speaking with pleasure. Furthermore, because predisposing neurophysiological factors may contribute to the core behaviors in the speech of many students who stutter, it is also important to help them cope effectively with any remaining disruptions in their speech. These twin goals of coping with the remaining stuttering and gaining positive speaking experiences can be achieved using a combination of reducing negative feelings,

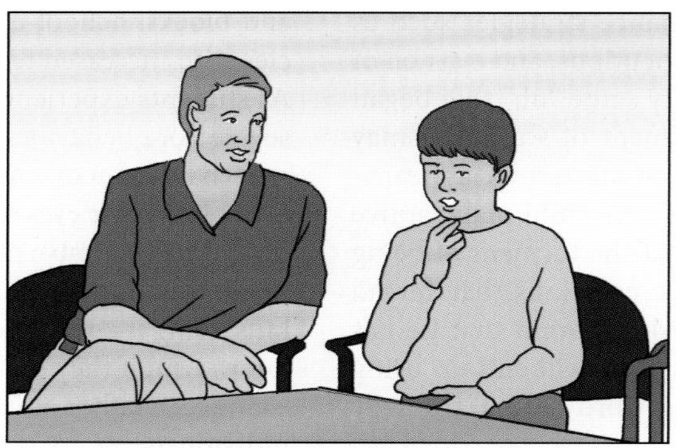

Student Explores His Stuttering

uh-uh-mmm-uh-uh-my
Not quite

Try it with me...mmmmmyyy
mmmmy
Nice job!

Mmmmmmyy stutters are easier now that I'm no longer afraid of them.

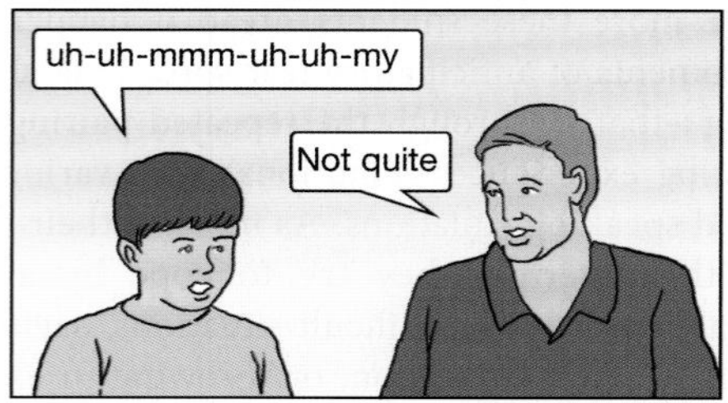

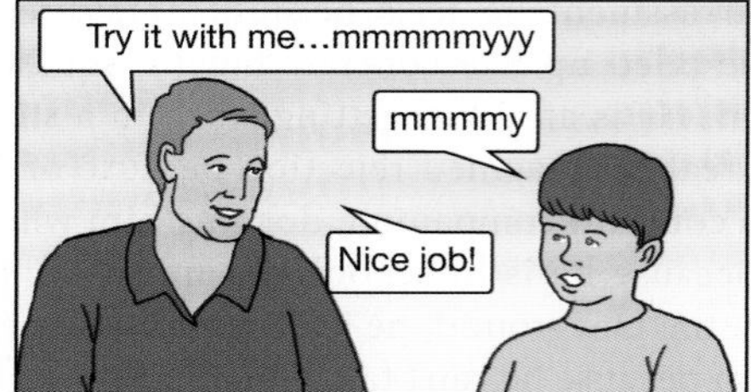

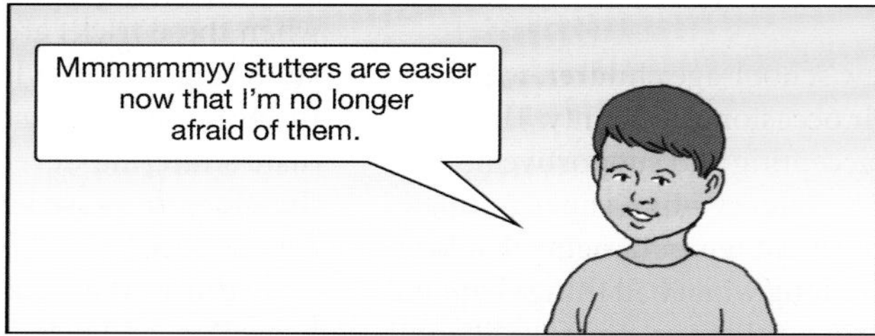

Student Learns to Make His Stutters Easier

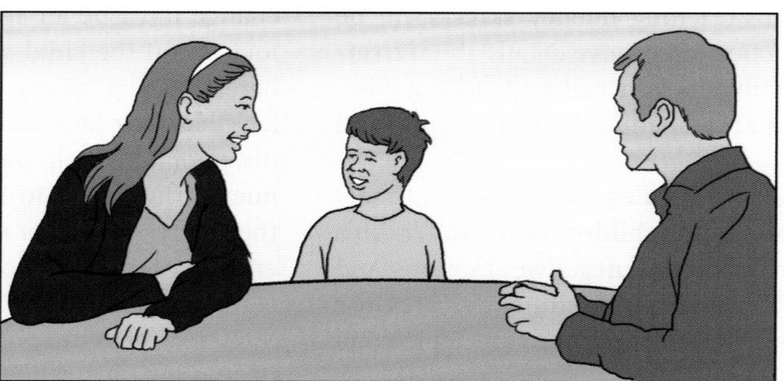

Student Generalizes His Fluency Skills to New Listener

Figure 13.1 Overview of the chapter.

increasing self-confidence, and teaching students to stutter more and more easily. In implementing these goals with a school-age child, I find that the child's age and maturity influence the selection of clinical procedures.

Finally, it is important to reduce developmental and environmental influences that may be contributing to the child's stuttering. I can do this by working with the child's parents, his classroom teachers, and his class, helping them create an environment that accepts the child regardless of his progress with speech, thus helping him feel free to work on his speech with the further outcome of facilitating change. In addition, I help the child communicate directly with his parents and teachers about how they can best help him deal with his stuttering.

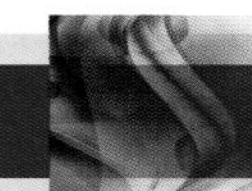

Case Example

David

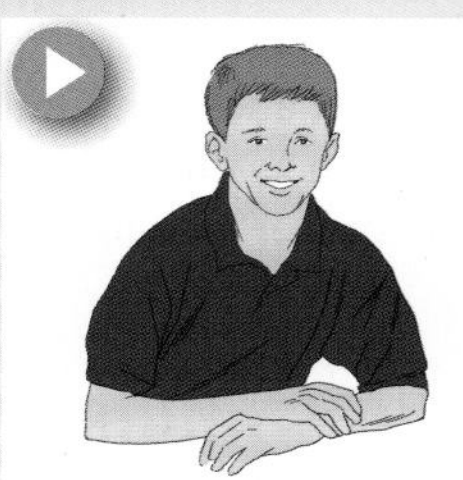

When David was 6, he began weekly treatment with me (and a graduate student), when I was using an early version of the treatment described in this chapter. In those days, I used primarily stuttering modification, but the modified stuttering became a fluency skill for David. In other words, he used his modified stutters on both stuttered words and some fluent words as well.

In the first months of treatment, David was extremely sensitive about his stuttering and unwilling to work directly on it during the exploration stage of treatment. In fact, he wouldn't even discuss his stuttering and would often walk out of the therapy room when I brought it up. My response to his reluctance was to pepper my speech with easy stutters (slightly drawn-out onsets of words lllliiike this). I'd occasionally probe whether he was willing to talk about his stuttering (he wasn't). Our activities were confined to shooting hoops with a basketball net attached to the back of the door and bowling with plastic pins and balls as I kept up a steady flow of easy stutters. I would sometimes comment that I needed to use easy stutters to control my stuttering (David later said he never believed I really stuttered but was just pretending). One day, David spotted a jar of candies on my desk and asked if he could have one. I traded him one in exchange for him trying an easy stutter. Thus began a steadily effective therapy strategy. Over the next year, he increasingly warmed to the idea of changing his stuttering from hard blocks to easy "slide-outs" (as he called them) while earning candies. The candies always went home in a bag that his mother put away in a drawer and then surreptitiously returned to me for recycling as rewards for easy stutters.

David learned other **fluency skills** such as slowing and proprioception but always favored slide-outs. We practiced them with many listeners in many different situations. At some point, David decided on his own to keep a score sheet of the number of slide-outs he used in the therapy room and outside. Perhaps because he received a reward for each slide-out, at first, David began to put in slide-outs even on words he wasn't stuttering on. Slide-outs became a fluency skill for him. Soon, David would give himself a check mark for each slide-out without my having to tell him; I intermittently praised him after he used a slide-out and reinforced himself. I think this self-reinforcement was an important part of his therapy that he invented himself.

In addition to working on the ease and fluency of his speech, David improved his attitudes about speaking, largely through talking with his class about his stuttering. Always a bit of a ham, David was happy to make presentations to his classes in third, fourth, and fifth grades. He showed posters and video clips he had made, answered questions, and had other students come up and "learn how to stutter." During his elementary school years, the course of therapy was full of bumps and detours, as well as great gains in fluency. Once when his family sold their house and built a new one in a different neighborhood, he was thrown for a loss and started to stutter more severely again. During this time, he was also teased by another student who was having his own problems at home and school. A few months' work with David, his parents, his teachers, and his friends, as well as the child who teased him, brought him through this relapse stronger than ever, and he continued to gain confidence in his speech throughout junior high and high school without further therapy. When he graduated, he was essentially fluent with a few minor repetitions and prolongations.

I should add to this account that David's parents were a major help to his therapy. They were always willing to come to our clinic and talk over his progress (even in the early days when he wasn't making any), as well as promoting therapy activities at home (such as buying him a punching bag to release his frustrations during a relapse). At my suggestion, they tried to reinforce his fluency at home, particularly at the dinner table. This lasted all of 2 weeks and came to a screeching halt when David declared he just wanted to talk and not do therapy at home as well as at the clinic. What he wanted was just his parents' general support of him, which they gave unstintingly.

David's sister and brother were very sympathetic to him when he was going through a bad patch, and David was surprisingly open to talking with them about his stuttering. David was also open with many others about his stuttering, including my class and a local television show. I think another key aspect of his recovery was his participation when he was in high school as a mentor in group therapy for younger school-age children. He was a much-loved "older brother" to the group and helped them immensely by modeling his slide-outs as well as leading them into situations outside the clinic. He even threw in some voluntary stutters to give them courage to try it too.

Recently, David read the above description of his therapy and thought it was accurate, but he said this: "One thing you might want to add was once I kind of 'owned it' as my thing that made me different, that changed my attitude a lot and helped me become more open about it."

Speech Behaviors Targeted for Therapy

The speech behaviors targeted for intermediate stuttering therapy are primarily stuttered speech. Unlike treatment of beginning stuttering, which focuses on increasing fluent speech, this therapy begins with a focus on stuttering behaviors that are first approached, explored, accepted, and then changed. But for those children who are hardly bothered by their stuttering, fluent speech is the target. Fluency is shaped using various tools, such as easy onsets and light contacts.

Fluency Goals

Which fluency goals are realistic for school-age children? Some intermediate school-age children who stutter may become typical or spontaneously fluent speakers. This is more likely for younger than for older school-age children. Those who don't become completely fluent need to develop tolerance and acceptance of their remaining stuttering and thus be able to stutter in a looser, milder way because fear less often triggers tension and all its attendant escape and avoidance behaviors. Essentially, we are asking the child to stutter in an honest, straightforward way without the ducking and dodging that so often interfere with communication. In short, a realistic fluency goal for many intermediate school-age stutterers is **acceptable stuttering**, that is, fluency mixed with mild or very mild stuttering.

Feelings and Attitudes

How much attention should be given to the student's feelings and attitudes about his speech? A lot. When a child is frustrated, embarrassed, and afraid of stuttering and of speaking, the clinician must help him feel okay about himself and his speech. Furthermore, because these children are starting to avoid certain words and speaking situations, it is important to reduce these avoidances and fire up the "approach" neural systems in the brain. For all this to happen, the child must feel the clinician's acceptance of him *as he is now*. This acceptance is conveyed, especially at the beginning of therapy, by the clinician's evident curiosity about what the child is doing when he stutters, why he does it, and whether that helps him. It is also conveyed by the clinician's genuine interest in the child, even apart from his stuttering and fluency.

The client-clinician relationship is one of the most important things in therapy (e.g., Wampold, 2015). Thus, if the child wants to talk about something other than his stuttering, this can be very healthy and the clinician should listen attentively. Many school-age children have told me, years after therapy, that one of the most helpful things I did was to let them talk about whatever they wanted, and I listened without stopping them to have them work on their stuttering. Your therapy room should be a place where a student can have some time to talk about personal issues and not worry about whether he stutters or not.

I have an additional thought about the importance of the clinical relationship. In Chapter 5—on Learning and Unlearning—I suggested that the reaction that becomes the fear of stuttering starts out as a nonconscious perception of threat: the threat of being out of control and helpless to stop it. An accepting clinician may be the antidote to the perceived threat. As the school-age child repeatedly experiences the clinician as an interested and nonpunitive listener—an adult who is on the same team as the child—the child may then let go of some of his or her nonconscious defensive responses.

Maintenance Procedures and Relapse

As I described in Chapter 5 on Learning and Unlearning, our primary treatment approach to changing stuttering behavior in schoolchildren is to decouple the link between the conditioned stimulus (stuttering or anticipated stuttering) and the conditioned response (increased tension and struggle and accompanying escape and avoidance behaviors). We do this by helping the child tolerate and accept his stuttering as it is happening and then let him experience the release of tension and the new ability to finish the word easily. In learning terms, we are "extinguishing" the threat/fear that was triggered by the stuttering. However, research reveals that behaviors that were eliminated by extinction can reappear (1) when some time has passed since the extinction treatment was delivered and (2) when the individual is in a context different from that in which he received the extinction treatment (Bouton, 2016). The effect of the passage of *time* can be seen when individuals are treated in an intensive therapy format and then discharged. Commonly, their stuttering returns, slowly or suddenly, several weeks after treatment ends. The effect of *context* is evident when a child is treated in a therapy room by an accepting clinician and becomes quite fluent but stutters when he goes back to his classroom. Change of context had sudden effect on my own speech. When I received stuttering therapy from Van Riper, I left his treatment group prematurely (and against his advice) and started to hitchhike around the country to test my newly fluent speech. I stood on the edge of the highway going out of town with my thumb in the air. The driver of the first car that stopped to pick me up asked me "Where are you going?" I answered, "Chi-chi-chi……Chi-chi-chi……" My stuttering was back, for Round 2. It hadn't given up. But neither had I.

To prevent relapse, treatment must include strategies designed to keep the extinction of the old fear active for the long term. Treatment should be tapered off gradually rather than end suddenly, and the clinician should maintain intermittent contact with the child for a time afterwards. Some students who end therapy with improved fluency can be enlisted as mentors to younger children who stutter. This can help them remember what they did to achieve greater fluency as well as increase their self-esteem.

Clinical Methods

In the first stages of therapy, to help the student reduce negative emotion, I use a combination of (1) listening acceptingly as we talk together about the student's stuttering, including his feelings about being seen as someone who stutters, and (2) joining the student in playing with stuttering—to make therapy fun, to reduce anxiety, to reward hard work, to approach the fear associated with stuttering, and to learn to reduce tension and struggle. When the student is less afraid and not so ashamed of his stuttering, I use modeling and coaching to teach him a different response to the anticipation and experience of stuttering.

I also work with his parents and the teachers to create "stuttering-friendly" environments that increase the student's comfort using the techniques we learn together in treatment. The measures I use to assess progress are described in the section titled "Progress and Outcome Measures."

Clinical Procedures: Working with a Child

Okay, now let's get down to the nitty-gritty of doing therapy. My clinical methods for intermediate stuttering have been influenced by many people, but Charles Van Riper has been my prime inspiration. Many of the techniques and much of the philosophy in my approach come both from therapy with Van Riper for my own stuttering and from the chapter in his treatment book entitled *Treatment of the Young Confirmed Stutterer* (1973). I am also indebted to Julie Reville, who shared her intuitive clinical approaches with this age group. Many activities that she and I developed for treating children with intermediate stuttering are presented in our workbook, *Easy Talker* (Guitar & Reville, 1997). More recently, I have been influenced by Danra Kazenski, my former Ph.D. student and now a colleague in our department at the University of Vermont. She has an exceptional understanding of stuttering and of school-age children. She works with children individually, in small groups, and in large ones.[1] We share so many ideas and strategies that I never know which ones she came up with and which ones I did.

Beginning Therapy: Exploring and Changing Stuttering

I start treatment by getting to know the child—who he is, and what he likes to do after school and on weekends, and all about his family and his pets and his favorite snacks and drinks, and games he likes to play, and anything else that comes up naturally in our conversation. I let my real interest in him reveal itself. Most of the time I'm paying attention just to what the student says and conveying that I'm appreciating him as we talk. His daily life, his favorite activities, and his experiences all provide the metaphors and analogies that we will use as we work together. Some of the time I'm also quietly observing his stuttering, to the extent that it shows up in our conversation. As we talk, I convey my comfort with his stuttering by my relaxed attention during his moments of stuttering. At first, I just watch and listen carefully to learn what he does when he stutters; eventually, when he seems to be ready, I help him explore his stutters, as described in the following sections.

Exploring

Exploring is the opposite of avoiding; it is an "approach" behavior that can reduce negative emotions. When I proposed a theoretical background for persistent stuttering in Chapter 6, I speculated that the temperament of many children who have developed intermediate-level stuttering might be biased toward avoidance and withdrawal from threatening stimuli. To help them ignite their "approach" neural circuitry (Gray, 1987; Kinsbourne & Bemporad, 1984), I use play to make stuttering approachable. This idea is put into practice by engaging such youngsters in appealing, enjoyable activities that counteract their natural tendency to avoid.

For some students, you may want to use the first "explorations" (goals of therapy, beliefs about stuttering) to help them understand the nature of what you and he will be working together on. For others—those who seem tentative or impatient—you may want to dive right into exploring the core behaviors of their stuttering (see the section with that title further along in this chapter) and then show them how they can change these behaviors. Students who are unsure about being in therapy need an immediate taste of success if they are to buy into the process.

Exploring the Goals of Therapy

A student needs to know where he's going in therapy and to know that the clinician has a map to guide him on his trip through sometimes difficult territory. Depending on his age, I will ask him about past therapy, what he learned, and what he'd like to get out of therapy. Most school-age children will probably answer that they would like their stuttering to be totally gone. I might respond that we can work toward that goal, but then I would ask him if it would be okay if he had a little stuttering sometimes when he's excited or in a hurry. I let him know that at first, he and I will be working to get to know his stuttering and what makes it happen. Then we'll work on helping him change his talking so that it will be easier. I might tell him this at the very beginning of therapy or after several sessions. It's often helpful to draw some pictures or diagrams to make the activities and sequence of therapy easier to grasp. Figure 13.2 illustrates the sequence of therapy for our approach. It may help the student you are working with if you and the student redraw the sequence as you explain what the student will be doing in each stage.

[1]Danra was recently selected by the National Stuttering Association (NSA) as Chapter Leader of the Year. Check out the Web site she created, with help from NSA: www.burlingtonstutters.org.

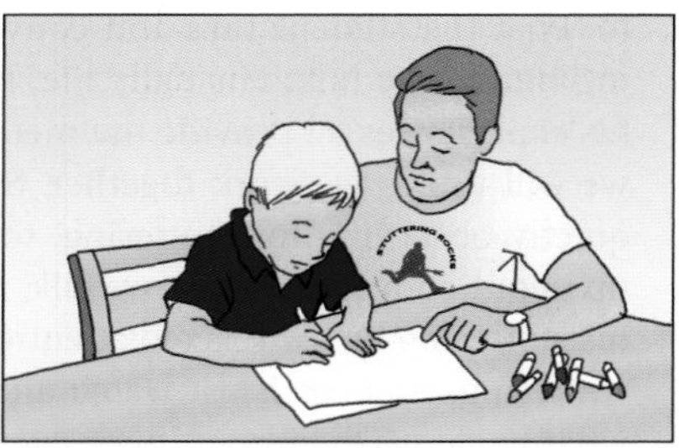

Exploring goals, beliefs, and feelings

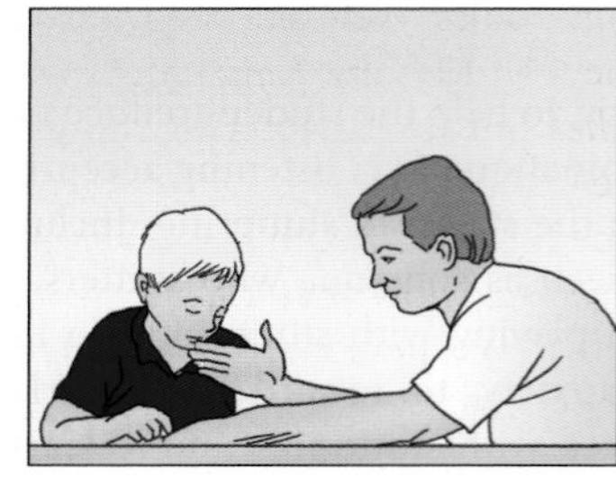

Exploring and changing core behavior

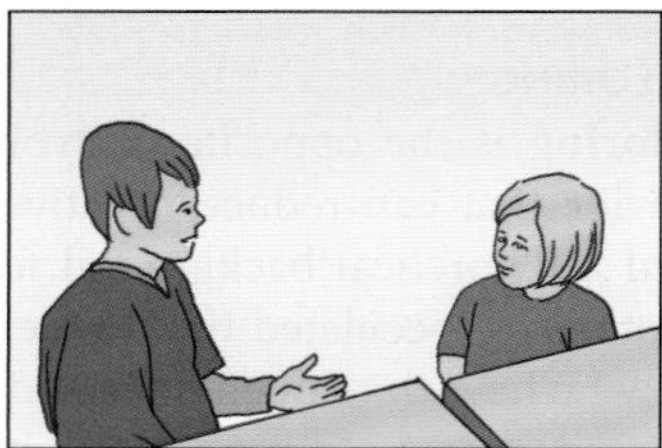

Openness

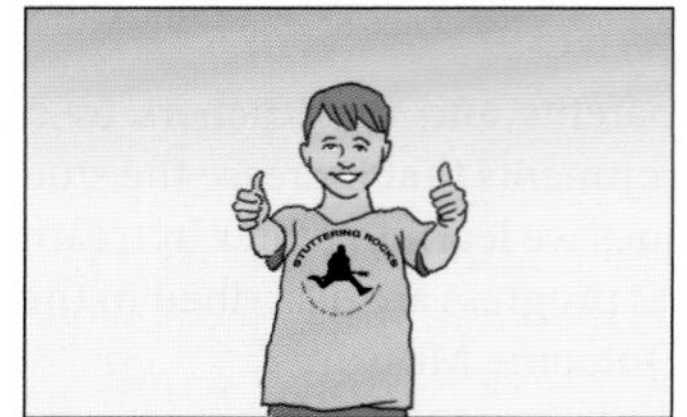

Acceptance

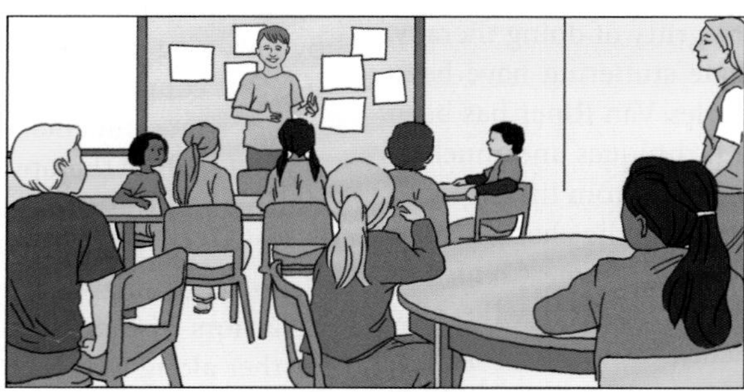

Transfer

Figure 13.2 The sequence of therapy.

Exploring Beliefs about Stuttering

A student with intermediate stuttering must be given some explanation for his stuttering. He knows he stutters and has been stuttering probably for a number of years, and he needs to have an explanation for why he talks differently from his friends. So, what do I say to this youngster?

Choosing words that are appropriate for the child's age and comprehension level, I let him know that stuttering is not his fault and that much of it is learned and can be unlearned. I let him know that he must already be a good learner to have learned all the things he does when he stutters. This means he will be good at learning some new, easier ways of handling his stutters. To help him realize that stuttering is not his fault, I may say that just like some kids have trouble drawing pictures of things or other kids find it hard to play a musical instrument, he has a little more trouble getting words out smoothly if he is talking fast and has lots of ideas to get out. I let him know about famous people who also have the same problem, like Ed Sheeran, Bruce Willis, James Earl Jones (the voice of Darth Vader in the original *Star Wars* trilogy), Samuel L. Jackson, and Nicholas Brendon (star of the TV show "Buffy the Vampire Slayer"). Many sports stars also stutter (or used to), such as Shaquille O'Neill and Tiger Woods. Lots of famous people stutter, but they have learned to change their stuttering so it is hardly noticeable, and so can he. The Stuttering Foundation home page (www.stuttering-help.org) has a long list of famous people who have stuttered and have lived fulfilling lives despite it.

I go on to explain that any inborn tendency to stutter accounts only for the fact that sometimes when he talks fast or is excited or tired, he finds that he stumbles over words. This is the part I call natural stuttering. Other parts, the most bothersome parts, like getting really tight when he stutters or putting in extra sounds or eye blinks, are learned. If they are learned, he can change them. One tool I sometimes use to help teach intermediate stutterers about stuttering is the video, *Stuttering: For Kids by Kids*, which is available from the Stuttering Foundation (Scott & Guitar, 2004). This DVD has great examples of kids who stutter talking about the difficulties they face and how they have worked on their speech.

One of the videos on this book's Web site shows a child describing how useful the *For Kids by Kids* video was to him (see video clips on *thePoint* for Chapter 9: Diagnostic Evaluation of a School Age Child).

In helping a child to better understand his stuttering, I think it is beneficial for him to know that a lot of children stutter and that he is not the only person in the world who stutters. Often, a child may not know any other children who stutter and may believe that he is one of only a very few who have this problem. So, I tell him that about 1 in every 100 kids stutters and that there are over 2 million people in the United States who stutter and millions more around the world who stutter. I believe this sort of information helps a child to feel less alone because of his or her stuttering. Both Friends (https://www.friendswhostutter.org) and the National Stuttering Association (www.westutter.org) have Web sites that provide information about stuttering for kids and parents and also have annual meetings in which kids who stutter meet other kids who stutter. These meetings are often life-transforming experiences.

Exploring Feelings about Stuttering

Most students who stutter find it hard to talk about the hurt and shame they feel from not being able to talk like their peers until the student and I have worked together for a while and a trusting relationship has built up. Nonetheless, I try, early in therapy, to see if they will share a little of what they have experienced as they try to navigate a very verbal world with broken words. Van Riper (1973) suggested that school-age children who stutter are able to talk about difficult situations even if they can't identify difficult sounds and words. He believes that talking about situations in which they have had bad experiences provides comfort and even inspires hope. When I think back to my own childhood, I can imagine feeling relief in being able to share, with an accepting clinician, how hard it was for me to talk with the class about my favorite TV shows and radio programs and what I liked to do after school and on weekends. The class sharing time was mostly a time of dead air for me and probably for most children who stutter.

I ask kids about the times that are hard for them because they stutter. If they are willing to share, I listen attentively and praise them for talking about hard times. I often comment on the experiences and feelings that other children have when they stutter, such as the angry and sad feelings that result from being teased, being told by adults to slow down, having words finished for them, and being interrupted. Together, we go onto the Internet and find places where other kids have shared their stuttering experiences, like the "Just for Kids" link on the Stuttering Home Page (http://www.mnsu.edu/comdis/kuster/stutter.html).

I find that some children express their feelings more freely through drawings. Thus, I may ask them to draw pictures of what stuttering is like. I begin by telling the child that some stutters are like a stuck door (or whatever is most relevant to his type of stutters), and I draw something that represents the feeling. I usually make jagged lines to represent frustration and talk to the child about how stutters like that might feel. Then, I ask the child to draw a picture showing how it feels when he gets stuck on a word. In explaining his drawing, the child is often able to express how he feels. Therefore, I use drawing throughout therapy to help the child deal with old feelings of hurt and new feelings that are encountered during various stages of therapy. My experience has been that children's feelings often affect their fluency. The more practice they get in expressing their feelings, the less those feelings interfere with talking.

Another way in which drawings can be used to explore feelings is by using a metaphor proposed by Joseph Sheehan (1970) called the "Iceberg of Stuttering." Clinicians from the Michael Palin Centre make great use of the iceberg analogy by having children draw their own icebergs showing their stuttering behaviors as the small top part of the iceberg above water and their feelings in the large underwater portion. A good depiction of this can be seen in the video mentioned earlier, *Stuttering: Basic Clinical Skills* (Guitar & Fraser, 2007), available from the Stuttering Foundation.

Most students who stutter feel at least a smattering of shame, and some students feel a lot of it. Being ashamed of stuttering means you feel you are bad or stupid or incompetent because you stutter. You feel your parents are disappointed in you and your peers think you are not very cool. You want to hide your stuttering and hide yourself in a closet until it goes away. As you can imagine, the burning urge to hide your stuttering does not help you work on it to change it and make it go away (or at least to decrease it). Because shame wants you to keep your stuttering under wraps, it is hard for students to share their feelings of shame with anyone. But there is a place to start. If the student is able to talk about difficult situations, he or she may be able to talk about teasing. And how he or she feels about being teased for stuttering is one of the faces of shame. If you can tell the child about what other kids have said about being teased, this may get the flow started. Sometimes, I have been able to get a child to draw a picture of being teased. Drawing the teaser as particularly ugly can provide a little comic relief. Humor is always a balm to hurt. There are some links to a section on teasing in the Just For Kids section of the Stuttering Home Page. By looking at them, a child who stutters may realize how most kids who stutter get teased, and he can see what other kids have said to teasers.

Another key to relieving hurt feelings and shame is for a student to let the world (or at least a few friends) know about his stuttering. Being able to tell his class about his stuttering, with the clinician's help, is immensely helpful. It can relieve shame and reduce teasing. If you go to this book's Web site, you can watch a video showing a class presentation that a child did with her therapist (see Chapter 13 videos on *thePoint*). Also, especially for children in a support group, wearing a shirt that proclaims "Stuttering Is OK!" can be fun. In fact, as

I write these words, I'm wearing my T-shirt that shows a leaping guitar player and says in big words "Stuttering Rocks!"[2]

By now, the child has shared with me his moments of stuttering and his feelings about them. Moreover, he has found me to be an understanding and accepting listener. Some deconditioning of speech fears has already occurred. Thus, some basic groundwork has been laid in preparation for the following stages of treatment.

Exploring and Changing the Core Behaviors of Stuttering

I guide a child to approach and explore the core behaviors of his stuttering using three principles taken from treatment research on anxieties and phobias in animals and humans (Mineka, 1985). I believe these are relevant to stuttering because Mineka and her colleagues (e.g., Mineka & Oehlberg, 2008) suggest that the uncontrollability of aversive events is an important aspect of the threat they pose to the subjects. You can see the parallel with stuttering. These principles of treatment, adapted for stuttering, are (1) the clinician must be unafraid of stuttering, (2) the child must explore and study his or her stuttering, and (3) the longer the child is able to remain in contact with moments of stuttering, the more his or her fear will be reduced.

First Principle: The Clinician Must Be Unafraid of Stuttering

Taking the first principle and applying it to stuttering, the clinician can demonstrate her lack of fear of stuttering by showing her curiosity about the student's stuttering. She can listen carefully to what he is saying but at the same time be noticeably attentive to what he is doing when he stutters. After getting to know the child and with introductory remarks about wanting to learn about the child's stuttering, the clinician can comment on the child's stuttering. She might tell the child she needs to learn as much as she can about his stuttering in order to help him. Then she would ask him if it's okay if she makes comments on his stutters as she tries to study them. Most kids will give at least a reluctant assent. If one particular stutter is more tense or longer than others, she can say "Oh, there was a good stutter. Seems like you really squeezed your tongue when you said that word." This comment has the effect of letting the student know the clinician is more than okay with his stutters and even curious about them. Later on in therapy, the clinician can ask the child to teach her how to pretend stutter like he does, having him coach her to improve her stutters so they are more like his. She can also show the child she is unafraid of stuttering by taking the lead in practicing in all situations (unless the child wants to take the lead). When I worked in a school system in Washington, D.C., I often asked a student to stutter on purpose or make changes to his stuttering when going into the administrative assistant's office. I always went first, modeling for the child some pretend stutters in my own speech. The clinician should cultivate and renew her own lack of fear of stuttering. She should be able to pseudo-stutter comfortably when talking with the child alone as well as in public to acquaintances and strangers.

Second Principle: The Child Must Explore His or Her Stuttering

Exploring is the beginning of changing. In this stage of treatment, the clinician helps the child get in touch with what he's doing when he stutters, and that is the doorway to being able to modify it. Depending on the sensitivity and reluctance of the child, I might begin to discuss the child's stuttering with him when we are drawing pictures, playing a game, or doing something else the child enjoys. Thus, I can alternate between helping the child explore his stuttering and moving back to an activity that is fun. To start, I simply comment on the child's stuttering in an accepting manner. I take note of how he responds and whether he appears uncomfortable or whether he acknowledges his stuttering even subtly and nonverbally when I comment on it. This first approach to stuttering may go quite easily if I have won the child's trust and he is not excessively embarrassed by his stuttering. Those who are very sensitive can be helped to face their stuttering by proceeding slowly.

For an especially sensitive child, I begin by providing him with a feeling of mastery over something else, such as a board game, drawing, or "shooting hoops" in the therapy room. I then alternate between exploring his stuttering and giving him relief through other activities of his choice.

As I explore a child's stuttering with him, I not only comment on it but also ask him to describe what he's doing when he stutters. For example, I might say, "Okay, there was an interesting one. What did you do when you stuttered on that word? Where did you feel that stutter?" Then, I help him feel and identify what he actually does when he stutters. For many children, this focus on stuttering behavior—especially if they are rewarded for it—creates an openness about stuttering that can begin to change their emotions from shame and helpless confusion to a more hopeful and objective outlook. For many children, this might be the first time anyone has openly talked with them about their stuttering.

Let me pause for a moment here to say more about rewards. Most students under the age of 10 or so are delighted to have frequent rewards for their work. Therapy must be fun, and rewards help make that so. Therefore, when I first begin to work with a child, I ask him about his favorite candies or sodas or other things he'd like as little rewards for his hard work. I also check with the child's parents, when possible, to make sure they are okay with soda or candy as rewards. As they get older, some children are not so hot to get candy or soda rewards. Some students can work out with their parents

[2]T-shirts that say "Stuttering Is OK Because What I Say Is Worth Repeating" are available from the Stuttering Foundation (www.stutteringhelp.org) for $10.

a credit system in which a student gets points in treatment as reinforcements for accomplishments. Points are later cashed in for something the parents agree to buy for the child. One example of a point system was developed by a student named Cameron (who agreed to have his name used). When therapy began, when he was 7 or 8, he was happy to get candy rewards; then, when he was older, he said let's drop the candy. He and his parents agreed to a point system that eventually netted him (after many, many points) an electric guitar. Both reward systems (and the electric guitar) can be seen in the videos of his evaluation (see Chapter 9 video clips of a diagnostic evaluation of a school-age child on *thePoint*) and videos of his treatment (see Chapter 13 video clips on *thePoint*).

Going back to the early exploration of a child's stuttering, I teach him about "speech helpers," which are the lungs, larynx, and articulators, and their involvement in speech production. A cardboard or plywood cutout of a head, neck, and chest with speech helpers drawn on it may help. For examples, see Exercise 1-1 in *Easy Talker*, our workbook that is listed in Suggested Readings at the end of the chapter; also watch the "Exploring Talking and Stuttering" part of *Stuttering: Basic Clinical Skills*, a DVD available from Stuttering Foundation (Guitar & Fraser, 2007). This part of the video includes having the child get to know his stuttering (and therefore being less afraid) as well as learn to change it.

For a more sensitive child, I start with instructions about how speech helpers work during fluent speech and later explore what the child does with his speech helpers when he stutters. For children who are a bit less emotional about their stuttering, I might incorporate instruction about speech helpers into our exploration of what they are doing when they stutter. In this part of treatment, the child learns the parts of his speech mechanism, what he does when he talks, and what he does when he stutters. The child is also learning that stuttering is not a scary monster that attacks him but simply things he does that hold back his speech as he tries *not* to stutter.

As the student and I talk about his speech helpers, I ask him to *feel* what he is doing when he stutters. I ask him to pretend to stutter and make the pretend stutter as tight as a real stutter would be. This is an important moment in therapy. If he can stutter voluntarily (pretend stutters) and be rewarded for it, his fear of stuttering will diminish a little.

If the student is able to do some pretend stutters, we then try to make stuttering fun, crazy, and weird. We have contests to see who can have the longest stutter, the loudest stutter, or the craziest stutter. My colleague Danra Kazenski takes kids through exercises in "silly stuttering" where they play with stuttering and reduce the fear and shame associated with it by having fun with stuttering.

Figure 13.3 shows an example: Danra is having a child show how a monkey might stutter. They are both enjoying this play, and it is loosening up the child so that he can experiment with changes in his stuttering, going from tense and struggled stutters to looser and easier ones that feel in control.

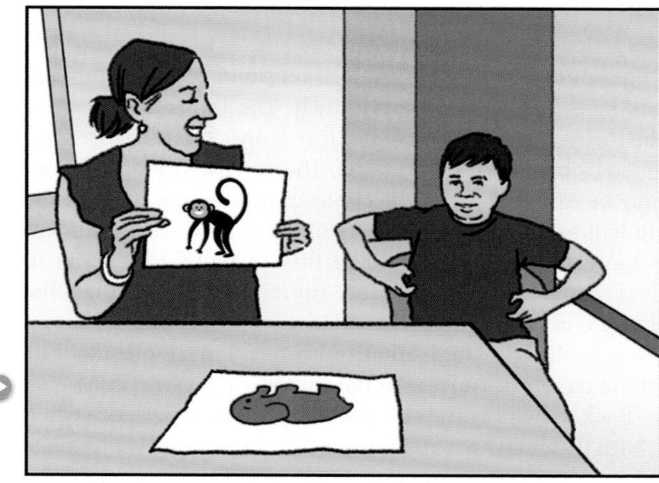

Figure 13.3 Danra and her client Aden Gagne doing "silly stuttering."

Once a child is comfortable with discussing his stuttering and even playing with stuttering, I move to having him reduce his fear of being stuck in a stutter—this is the heart of changing the behavior. I begin by having the child try to "catch me" stuttering. This can be done earlier in the flow of therapy, but whenever it is done, it should be adapted to how sensitive the student is. Some children don't immediately like the idea of catching my pretend stutters right at the beginning of therapy, so I may delay this work until after we've explored his stuttering. To start, I throw in a few pretend easy stutters and ask him to let me know, by signaling (pointing at me or saying "there's one"), whenever he notices a stutter in my speech. Easy stutters can be repetitions, prolongations, or blocks, but they are produced slowly and without much tension. In these pretend (or, for me, sometimes real) stutters, I try to stay in (prolong) the actual moment of stuttering (holding onto the posture of the articulators when the stutter is "stuck"), even if it means slightly distorting a stuttered plosive or two. I reward the student when he successfully catches my easy stutters, and I sometimes talk about what I did when I pretended to get stuck. This lets him know that I am not afraid of stuttering and in turn provides a model of talking objectively about stuttering. Clinicians can do this "legitimately" even if they don't stutter. For an older child, it might be useful for the clinician to explain that she doesn't stutter and ask the student if he minds if she puts some pretend stutters in her speech. Most children know that the clinician's stutters are voluntary and are okay with it. This is especially true if the child has previously coached the clinician to pretend stutter in a way similar to his real stutters.

After several minutes of putting easy stutters in my speech (where I stay in the moment of stuttering) and having him catch me, I ask the child if it's okay if I try to catch his stutters.

As I prepare to describe catching the child's stutters and having him stay in them, let me spell out what "**staying in the stutter**" means and why I use it. The phrase "staying in the stutter" refers to holding onto the stuckness of the stutter—the articulatory posture when the stutter is tense—and letting sound or airflow continue as tension decreases and then ending the word loosely and slowly. The aim is to extinguish the threat (nonconscious) and fear (conscious) that are triggered by being stuck in a stutter. These negative emotions can only be extinguished if the clinician praises and rewards the student as he continues to stay in the stutter. As the student is more and more successful at this, he will find it easier to do. I also use the phrase "easier stuttering" to mean the same thing. With apologies to the reader for excessive terminology, when I refer to a "**high-quality stutter**," I mean one that hits all the targets of "staying in the stutter."

Back to helping the child have a positive experience when I, with the child's permission, catch his stutters: I try to make this as positive an experience as possible for the child, by being pleased with his stutters and sometimes rewarding his stutters when I catch them, helping the child feel good about himself and his work. As I suggested in Chapter 10: Preliminaries to Treatment, I think the relationship that the clinician has with the child can be a powerful force in helping the child reduce negative emotions (both nonconscious and conscious). The overall goal here is to change how the student feels about the stutters *as he is having them*. Thus, when I catch one of his stutters, I use coaching and modeling to help him *stay in the actual moment of stuttering*—the core behavior. Stutters go by very quickly and the student won't particularly enjoy staying in the heart of the stuckness, so it may take a considerable amount of modeling, persuading, and reinforcing to have him stay in the stutter and tolerate it. Also, some sounds don't make it easy to stay in the stutter. For example, on a stuttered plosive, it is hard to stay in it and keep some sound or airflow going. On a stuttered /b/ in "Barry," you need to keep your lips together, vibrating, while the /b/ sound is steadily coming out. Yes, this distorts the typically exploded /b/, but it achieves the goal of learning to tolerate and transcend the fear that initially permeates the heart of the stuckness. The sound /p/ can be even more challenging because only the sound of airflow is heard as the posture is held and the lungs continue to expel air. Particularly difficult are laryngeal blocks that shut off all sound and airflow. You must help the child stay in the posture and gradually get sound or airflow going. For voiced sounds, the laryngeal block can be released and eased out of by using vocal fry. Once the child learns to tolerate the discomfort of staying in the stutter, *in an environment that accepts and even rewards his staying in the stutter*, the fear begins to diminish. And because it's the fear that triggers the tension, the stutters themselves become easier and looser.[3] This experience—of being able to tolerate being in the stuckness of the stutter—done over and over and rewarded by the clinician, leads to easier stutters. Then, the child anticipates easier stutters—*stutters that feel in control*. So begins the happy spiral of easier stutters begetting anticipation of easier stutters, leading to more and more and more easy stutters and increased freedom to talk. Once "staying in the stutter" (and having the tension melt away) has been learned fairly well in the therapy room, generalization can begin. Or it may begin to happen spontaneously as the child feels success.

Before I talk in detail about generalization, I thought it would be good to share an example of a school-age child learning to stay in the stutter, keep good eye contact, and release the word slowly once the tension has melted. Recently, when I was looking through old folders for examples of children's work on staying in the stutter, I came across my notes from a session made on May 23, 1993, when working with a child I'll call "Charlie." Here they are:

> *A good session on Thursday. We began with a chat. He didn't mention stuttering. He asked to have candy. Yes, two pieces. I said I needed help on my book; he described what was going on when he stuttered and moved through it easily. After a little of this, he reiterated how it made him worse to focus on stuttering too much. He asked to play bowling and I said okay if we can make it a reward for holding a stutter and looking at me and then moving through it slowly. We bowled and I rewarded him verbally and with candy when he stuttered. This really took off. He really got a kick out of getting candy so easily and piling it up; he got 10 pieces of candy, had great "managed" stutters with good eye contact, and good easy releases. He even rewarded me when I had some easy ones. At the same time, he was teaching me about bowling and I did really well and he accepted being beaten by me. At the end of the session, as we said goodbye, his mom tried to ask a lot of questions about what he had worked on. When he said bowling and candy, she said she hoped he'd worked on his speech as well; he kind of ignored this, and went on about something else. I must find a tactful way of talking to her about this—I think she'll bring it up.*

In addition to making notes after each session, I sometimes video record parts of therapy, with the child's permission. After he does some particularly good work, I ask him if he'd like to see the video clip of it. Video playback works particularly well if the child can be put in charge of recording and playback. Some students will get a kick out of learning to edit their videos so they look and sound pretty good. This book's Web site contains a video called "Cam's Popcorn Video" in videos for Chapter 13 that shows what a school-age client and his graduate clinician can put together to show his family and his friends what he's doing in therapy.

[3]In the video clips for evaluation of school-age children, in Chapter 9, one clip called "Trial Therapy" demonstrates how a clinician can coach a child (Cameron) into staying in the stutter and letting it go easily.

Third Principle: The Longer the Child Is Able to Remain in Contact with Moments of Stuttering, the More His Fear Will Be Reduced

The third principle taken from the phobia treatment literature suggests that extended amounts of time in contact with feared object (stuttering) will help reduce fear of it. The idea of being "in contact" with stuttering behavior may have an important meaning in the context of speech motor control. A child who has been stuttering persistently for several years may have lost easy access to proprioceptive awareness (nonconscious physical feeling) of his speech or may never have had it to an appropriate degree. This may make it difficult for him to use proprioceptive information to coordinate speech movements. Therefore, as a child explores his stuttering, I help him increase his conscious awareness of what he's doing when he stutters, particularly for more severe moments of stuttering. If I can guide him to stay in the moment of stuttering until it's likely that he *can* release the block, he can feel what he's doing and then will realize that he can control the tension and movement of his speech structures. *The shift that he will feel as he holds on to stutters for an extended period of time will seem like a change from being out of control to being in control.* It is, as we say to our kids, "Showing the Stutter Who's Boss." The feeling of being in control may indeed result from a change in the activity of brain areas that control speech movements. It may be a shift from a motor area of the brain that is not well supplied with sensory feedback to a motor area with better sensory information that controls movement. This shift in brain areas has been shown to be a correlate of motor movement that is under the subject's control (Guitar, Guitar, Neilson, O'Dwyer, & Andrews, 1988; Humphrey & Reed, 1983).

Openness, Acceptance, and the Beginning of Mastery

At this point in therapy, the student is starting to feel less embarrassed and ashamed about stuttering. He is not so terrified when his articulators seize up and his listener looks down. Now, he is on his way toward mastering what was once, to him, a fatal flaw. For a child with intermediate-level stuttering, working for this mastery is a lifelong process. At first, it takes immense effort and attention—his stuttering has been Darth Vader, Voldemort, and Goliath, all rolled into one. But when teaming up with a strong clinician, supportive parents, empathetic peers, and caring teachers, stuttering can be sent packing or at least cut down to size. Gradually, success is no longer measured in fluency but in little moments of manageable stuttering.

Being Open about Stuttering

A major milestone for the child traveling along the road toward mastery is becoming more open about stuttering. The clinician, by her own models of **voluntary stuttering** in public places, can inspire the school-age child to talk about stuttering casually with friends, to refer to it in humorous ways when it happens, and to educate people about it. Children differ widely in their readiness to be open about their stuttering. However, once most of them feel some sense of mastery over what has made them feel helpless in the past, they are much more able to let people know about it. If a child stutters in class, I rehearse casual comments that he can make about his stuttering when he is giving an oral report or answering a question in class. He might say, for example, "My report is about how maple syrup is produced. Before I begin, I just want to say that I'll probably stutter sometimes while I'm talking, but don't let it bother you. I'm dealing with it." Or he might say, "I'll probably stutter, but it's no big deal." Basically, it is not so much the content that is important as the fact that the child acknowledges his stuttering and that he's working on it. He feels good that he has acknowledged it, and his audience is more comfortable than if he stutters and tries to hide it. One vehicle a child can use to be open about his stuttering with family and friends is a zany video about stuttering that he makes with his clinician. Take a look at the music video clip of Alison and her clinician dancing with stuttering. It's in the Chapter 13 videos on *thePoint*, titled "Alison's Video."

A child may also benefit from developing a repertoire of casual comments to make about his stuttering if he gets particularly hung up on a word while talking to friends, relatives, or strangers. He might learn to say, "Wow! I really got hung up there," or "I'm really running into a lot of blocks; I'd better slow down a bit." In my experience, the most effective comments are those that the child comes up with spontaneously when he feels comfortable with his stuttering. These are unforced, often funny remarks that put the child and his listeners at ease, like saying "Who burped?" after you have an unexpected burp.

Teaching other children and his teachers about stuttering can be a powerful tool in combating the shame and embarrassment that often accompany a school-age child's stuttering. Although this can be done with small groups of students brought into the therapy room or in meetings with the child and his teachers, our experience has been that eventually sharing information about stuttering in front of the entire class is extremely effective for many children. When and if a child is ready to do this, we work together to prepare, rehearse, and then give a presentation that informs the class about stuttering in general and the child's own stuttering in particular. A question-and-answer period is a crucial part of the presentation because it gives the child's classmates a chance to express their curiosity about stuttering. It also gives the child an opportunity to become an expert in the very behavior that previously made him feel so helpless. We usually bring along some item of interest to share with the class, such as slides of famous people who stutter or a video we've made or a cell phone with a delayed auditory feedback app so the child can let his peers experience the kind of stuttering that results from trying to talk with the delay.

Here is an example of how this can work. A second grader who was very sensitive about his stuttering was also rather proud of a brief segment on a local television station that showed him working on his stuttering. He was willing to show a video of this segment in class and answer questions about his stuttering. The following year, I accompanied him to class for a full-scale presentation about stuttering. This presentation included posters he had made, demonstrations of therapy techniques, and a question-and-answer segment. A year after this program, the child had a particularly rocky beginning to the school year because his stuttering had returned full force after his family moved to a new house in a new neighborhood. However, he was still willing to do another presentation with me. This time, he used more video clips of himself talking, because he was more reluctant to talk at length; however, he talked to the class about some of the "ups and downs" in his progress with stuttering.

Another example is a second grade student, Nejla, who came to therapy in our clinic, accompanied by her public school clinician. Together, they produced a brief video with jazzy music to show to her class as the centerpiece of a live presentation she made with both the school clinician and the graduate student she worked with in our clinic. The presentation to her teachers and peers can be seen in the video clips on *thePoint* for Chapter 13 titled "A child talks to her class about stuttering."

Accepting Stuttering

The therapy, up to this point, has usually made the student a tiny bit more accepting of his stuttering, but the road to acceptance is long. In fact, true mastery of managing stuttering includes being able to accept failure some of the time. As you have gotten to know the student, you and he will probably be able to come up with some helpful analogies for acceptance of failure in the world of performance. What does the student admire? Ballet? Soccer? Baseball? Music? Farming? Car racing? Cooking? In any performance—in any endeavor that humans try to master—there is some failure. Mastery comes not from intolerant perfectionism but from being able to miss the target at times and keep on trying. As LeBron James (four-time most valuable player in the National Basketball Association) has said, "You have to be able to accept failure to get better." (https://www.quotezine.com/lebron-james-quotes/).

When the California State Fullerton baseball team started out with a losing season in 2004, a professor of kinesiology at the university got the team together and gave them advice to forget any bad plays or poor at-bats they'd had in the past, "flush them down the toilet," and concentrate on now. To keep them from forgetting his advice, he gave the team a miniature toilet that they put at the top of the dugout during each game. When they won the College World Series at the end of that season, their championship rings were engraved with the words "Next Pitch" (Witz, 2018). A child who stutters can be taught to forget past bad experiences and just concentrate on what he is doing now. Even if he fails, he can focus on the things he did right.

The clinician can be vital in helping the student accept his failures and find the little successes. This will come up frequently as the student is trying to master staying in the stutter, letting the tension release, and ending the word slowly. When the clinician provides a model that the student isn't able to match, she can find some things about the student's try that she can praise. For most people, feeling good about a try helps them use feedback about what they need to adjust their aim. So when a student stays in a stutter for only a brief moment and then ends the word quickly, let him know enthusiastically that he made a good try. Then give him another model and have him produce the stutter *along with you*. That will usually provide enough guidance that he will deserve more praise for coming much closer to the high-quality model you provided.

I'll return later in this chapter to the idea of accepting stuttering and missed targets, especially when we talk about transferring new skills to the world beyond the therapy room. For now, I'll recommend some very informative reading relevant to this topic. In the book *More Than Fluency* (Amster & Klein, 2018), there are two chapters that will give you many ideas about helping students deal with stuttering that happens even when they are trying not to. "Avoidance Reduction Therapy for Stuttering" is one chapter and "Acceptance and Commitment Therapy for Stuttering" is another.

Another idea about accepting stuttering came from a poem about stuttering that started us helping children develop positive responses to their stuttering. Several years ago, a graduate student and I were helping a 10-year-old girl learn to stop fighting her stutters and learn to handle them with grace and ease. One of the steps in her exploring her stutters was to get to know her stutters and "make friends with them." The graduate student, Charles Barasch, wrote a poem for the girl to help her accomplish this:

Getting Unstuck

for a young girl who stutters

When breath hides in your stomach
like a fish under stone,
and when it's hooked thrashes
and teases, dive down and follow,
let it think it's pulled you in
while you swim past swaying weeds,
through the shadow and light
inside yourself. And when it thinks
it owns you, sing to it like a mermaid,
it will fall in love with you
and do whatever you want.
It will follow you home
and be your liveliest companion,
it will dance for you
and do tricks for your friends,
you will think you've never met anyone

so intelligent or funny.
The house you set up together
will be happy until the end of your days.

We have found that if students can have a creative response to their stuttering, by making their own poems about stuttering, drawing pictures of their stuttering, or making models of what stuttering is like using Play-Doh, the hurt is somewhat healed. One of the school-age children we have worked with recently sent a letter and drawing to the Stuttering Foundation web site to have it displayed for other children to see. If you have a student who would like to have his or her creative endeavor displayed on the web site, go to this page: https://www.stutteringhelp.org/drawings-and-letters-kids/.

Transferring New Skills to the Real World

If you have taught your student who stutters to go right into the stutter and hold onto it (with intermittent praise and rewards from you) until the tension is reduced, ending it slowly, and if he can do it reliably in the treatment room, it's time for transfer. Your student may be already transferring his skills to his speech with his family, especially if his parents have been supporting and reinforcing his practice. Now is the time to prepare for transfer by planning hierarchies and engaging in voluntary stuttering and **desensitization**.

Voluntary Stuttering

Voluntary stuttering has been around for a long time, at least since Van Riper's therapist (Bryng Bryngleson) taught him to use it in the 1930s. Bloodstein and Ratner (2008) have a good description of the origins and evolution of voluntary stuttering. One of the uses I make of it when working with school-age children is to have the child voluntarily put in his speech the target we started shooting for during the exploration phase of treatment: staying in the stutter. Once the student has been able to emulate my model of holding onto the stuttered sound, letting the tension release, and ending it slowly, I ask him to put in pretend stutters using that technique of stuttering. In fact, many of the students I work with will spontaneously use voluntary high-quality stutters to earn rewards. When I dole out rewards, I don't discriminate between real and voluntary stutters, in part because I often can't tell the difference. And the child may not be able to discriminate either. Getting rewarded for these voluntary high-quality stutters makes them feel like little victories. As we transfer these skills, the positive feelings associated with these stutters help to counteract the discomfort of being perceived as a kid who stutters in real-world situations, like when talking with friends.

Desensitizing Student to Difficult Situations and Challenging Words

Most students who stutter have some bugaboo situations in their daily lives that trigger stuttering. For me, it was reading Bible verses aloud in Senior Boys' Sunday School as we went around a room, in an old barn that was heated only by a woodstove. Sometimes we read the New Testament and so the sound /ʤ/ was often a challenge because it came at the beginning of many verses. For kids I've worked with, difficult situations often included being called on in class, being asked to say your name, and telling a joke or a story about something that happened to them. We begin desensitization by developing a hierarchy of situations in which we will practice high-quality stutters.

Planning a Transfer Hierarchy

I think it would be too daunting for most children to plan a hierarchy filled with all the situations that are hard for them, so we just begin with a few not-too-hard ones. Desensitization means simply working on high-quality stutters in situations that are challenging. Thus, you and the child think of a situation that is slightly hard, plan what the child might say in this situation, and then start by role-playing the situation in the therapy room. For example, the transfer hierarchy might begin with a situation called "Someone asks you your name" (if that's a challenging situation for the child). At first, the clinician asks the child his name in the therapy room and the child has a high-quality stutter, either real or voluntary (pretend). Then they might go into the hallway outside the room and repeat the situation. At some point, the child might feel comfortable enough to do this with another adult, such as a parent or a school staff member. Once the work is being done outside the therapy room, rewards and praise might be saved until the child and clinician are alone together, unless the child is happy getting praise or a tangible reward "in public."

An example of a hierarchy involving some of the steps in therapy that we have described in this chapter is shown in Figure 13.4.

Transfer Activities

Reducing Fears Related to the Classroom

Let's consider the situation of a student being afraid to speak aloud in the classroom. In this case, I would invite, with the child's consent, one or two of his classmates into therapy. I would play the role of the classroom teacher and have this small group of two or three children ask and answer questions. When the child began to feel comfortable doing this, I would expand the group to three or four classmates. Next, it might be helpful for the child and the rest of us to go to his classroom during the noon hour or at recess. After explaining our goal and therapy procedures to the classroom teacher, I would have the child sit at his desk and have the teacher ask questions about his lessons. These activities are about as far as I can go in simulating a child's fear of this situation. The child needs to take the last step of these therapy procedures by himself. He has been successful in a series of situations that successively approximate his feared situation, and his classroom teacher is now sensitized to his problem and understands his therapy. The chances are that after some initial ambivalence, he will overcome his reluctance to talk in class.

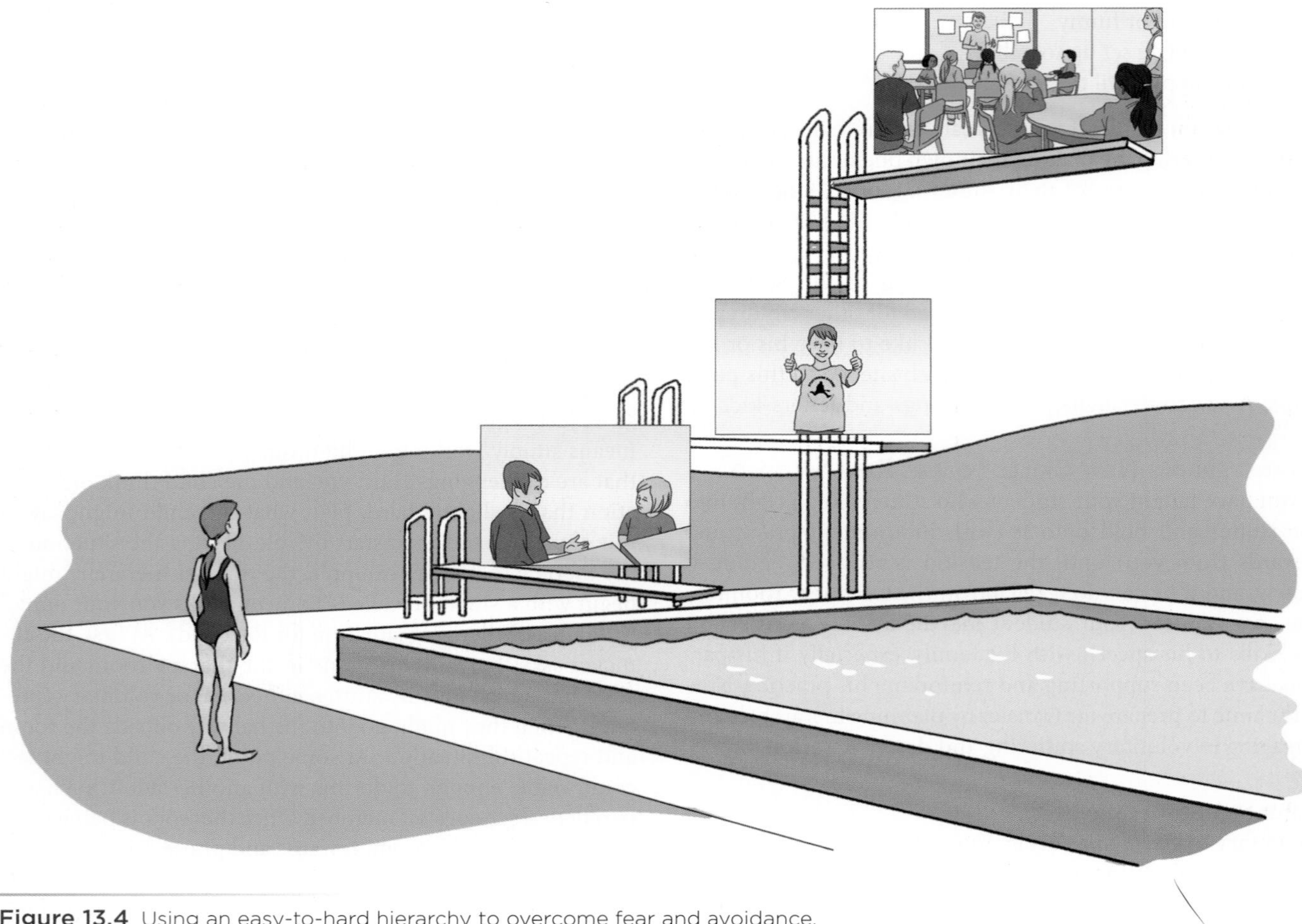

Figure 13.4 Using an easy-to-hard hierarchy to overcome fear and avoidance.

Scaffolding

I have found it useful with some children to "scaffold" their staying in the stutter during transfer activities by creating a stuttering-friendly environment, letting the listener(s) know that *we* are working on *our* speech. I use some voluntary (pretend) stuttering, staying in the stutter and ending loosely, as a model and encouraging the student to do the same. I am always careful to plan this beforehand with the student and ensure that he is comfortable with it. For example, I may tell a stranger in a mall that the child and I are working on our speech and we'd like to ask him some questions. Depending on the child's readiness, I may ask the first question or the child may. If the situation has been difficult in the past, I may coach the child in his use of staying in the stutter, as he speaks, by giving him subtle signals that we have worked out beforehand.

Transfer on the telephone lends itself to a great deal of scaffolding, which can be faded as the child is more and more successful. For example, the clinician and child may plan a variety of gestures or signs that can provide support as the child makes telephone calls to practice stuttering more easily. If we are practicing voluntary stuttering, which is always a good thing, I'll make the first phone call and have the child signal me to stay in the stutter whenever he wants. Then we will reverse roles. Sometimes, physical contact helps focus a child on his speech even in the face of some fear. If you and the child are comfortable with it, you could place your hand on the child's arm and squeeze it to let him know you notice that he is staying in the stutter or to remind him to do so.

More on Reducing Fear and Avoidance

Some children take a little longer than others to transfer their ability to stay in the stutter and let the tension melt before finishing the word slowly. They may have learned fears and avoidances that will require a concerted effort to overcome. It helps many children in this situation to deal with their fears if the right analogies or comparisons can be found. I get them to think about other fears they have overcome or about people they know, such as family members, who are afraid of such things as the dark, bugs, snakes, spiders, or swimming in deep water, and I enlist the child's help in listing ways they might overcome their fears. I also look for examples in pop culture, like Harry Potter, Spiderman, or Ninjago. By analyzing how people get over their fears and describing the rewards of facing fears and conquering them, I am often able to motivate children to tackle their fears of difficult words and situations.

Sometimes, we forget that fears are very natural, and perhaps some fears—like a fear of crocodiles—are important to help us survive. Let the child know that it's natural to be worried about words or situations that have given him trouble in the past. But he should also know that the fear of these things itself causes him to tense up and stutter. Here are some steps to help him to reduce his fears: (1) be okay with having some fear; (2) study the words or situations so he can learn about them; (3) practice his ability to stay in the stutter over and over before going into real-life challenging situations; and (4) get rewarded for going ahead and trying something despite his fear, even if he's not completely in control of his stuttering. In fact, if the child can just shoot for making his stuttering gradually less and less tense, it will be an easier target to hit, and he will succeed more and more.

Reducing Word Fears

It is usually easier to help a child overcome his fear and avoidance of particular words than of particular situations. This is because I can provide the child with more support in confronting word fears in the therapy room than I can provide when he confronts his situational fears in daily life. I can also use feared words over and over again within the therapy situation. For example, I worked with a young school-age child who stuttered who consistently substituted "me" for "I." This was not because of a language disorder but because he consistently stuttered on the word "I," and his parents reported that he had used "I" appropriately for a number of years before he began using this substitution. With this child, I began to practice saying "I" in unison with him, while we both pretended to stutter on it and stayed in the stutter. Next, we used "I" with high-quality stutters many, many times in carrier phrases while playing games. Gradually, the child regained his confidence in saying "I." Within a week or two, his avoidance of "I" was eliminated in therapy, and his parents reported that he was again using this pronoun appropriately at home.

Developing an Approach Attitude

In working on his fears and avoidances, the child must understand (as we've suggested before) that he doesn't have to be completely successful in using high-quality stutters in all situations all of the time. In fact, as he first tackles feared words and situations, he may stutter in his old way many times. Even so, he should be rewarded for trying. The "approach attitude," which we sometimes refer to as "seeking out" (Guitar & Reville, 1997), may reduce fear and tension so that high-quality stutters are more obtainable. Repeated exposure to the feared words or situations, when supported by the clinician, will make a big difference in applying new skills to feared words and situations.

Coping with Teasing

It is important to minimize any teasing that a child is receiving because of his stuttering. The clinician can deal with this at any time, but it may be helpful to address teasing after the child has mastered some fluency skills and is transferring them. (I address this issue in more detail when I discuss counseling parents and classroom teachers.) Regardless of how hard parents, teachers, clinicians, and friends may try to eliminate teasing, I doubt that it is possible to eliminate all of it. Thus, I try to give a child some defenses against the teasing that he is likely to receive.

I agree with Van Riper (1973) that the best defense against teasing is acceptance if a child is emotionally mature enough to feel and express acceptance. For example, if a child can say, "I know I stutter, but I'm working on it," or some similar statement, this will disarm most teasers. Nobody likes to tease someone who does not appear to be bothered. Running away, on the other hand, just reinforces teasing. Nevertheless, I have found that it is difficult for a school-age child to calmly accept and admit his stuttering when he talks to his tormentors. When I have been successful, I have done the following things.

First, I discuss the importance of calmly and openly admitting stuttering to teasers, rather than saying nothing. I explain how this type of response usually discourages teasers. I then explore with the child the sorts of statements he can imagine himself making. The words he uses must be words with which he feels comfortable. Next, I initiate role-playing with the child. As I play the role of the teaser, the child's task is to respond calmly to my heckling. He practices saying the types of statements he has chosen to use to counteract the teasing. I role-play this many times until the child feels comfortable with his response and can see himself doing this in a real-life situation. Finally, the day comes when he tries out this new behavior. I hope it works, but if it does not, I will be available to give the child support and encouragement in our next meeting.

I have also found that if I have two or more children who stutter or if I can form a group of several children who have speech or language problems, we can write and perform a play together about a child who stutters who triumphs over teasing.

Some children are especially sensitive to teasing and need patience and understanding as they work to develop effective responses. These children may have more inhibited temperaments, and their first reaction to a threatening situation is to withdraw or avoid. Hence, these children need practice in asserting themselves. In our role-playing, I experiment with a variety of ways in which the child can feel that he confronted the teaser. For some children, it might be teasing back; for others, it might be reporting the teaser to a teacher or the principal. A tactic taught by Bill Murphy, an experienced speech pathologist who also stutters, is to have children say "So?" back to the teaser after every taunt. Because it's a short utterance, children who stutter can often say it fluently and with gusto. Other excellent advice is contained in publications by Murphy, Quesal, Reardon-Reeves, and Yaruss (2013) and Yaruss, Reeves, and Herring (2018). A good list of resources related to teasing of children who stutter can be found at http://www.mnsu.edu/comdis/kuster/infoabout-stuttering.html#teasing/.

Maintaining Improvement

By this point in therapy, a child is usually speaking well in most situations. He is having a great deal of natural fluency in many situations and high-quality stuttering in others. His speech fears and avoidances have been eliminated or significantly reduced. I do not dismiss the child from therapy at this point but gradually phase him out of therapy. I see him for therapy on a weekly basis for a month or so and then on a twice-monthly basis for another month or so. If all continues to go well, I see him for a series of "checkups" over the next 2 years, first monthly, then bimonthly, and finally once a semester.

During these checkups, I obtain samples of the child's speech and oral reading and discuss with him how he has been talking in everyday speaking situations. I also interview his parents and classroom teacher about his speech at home and school. If I find that the child's fluency has regressed or that he has begun to use avoidance behaviors again, I re-enroll him in therapy. My experience is that a number of children may have one or two mild regressions before their fluency stabilizes. Such regressions are often associated with the beginning of a school year or with transfers from one school to another or with other disrupting factors.

When I return a child to therapy, it is usually for only a month or two. During these "booster" sessions, he may need to have his stuttering management skills "tuned up." He may need a brief refresher course on the importance of not avoiding, or he may just need an opportunity to talk to an understanding listener about his stuttering. In time, these regressions and our reevaluations become further apart until finally the day arrives when the child, his family, and I decide to dismiss him from treatment. My hope is that even though "dismissal" sounds rather final, the child realizes that he has an ally in me and in other SLPs who know about stuttering. That attitude could help him return to treatment if he thinks he needs some additional help—in a month, a year, or a decade.

Clinical Procedures: Teaching Fluency Skills

Some rare school-age children are more like beginning stutterers in their relative lack of fear toward stuttering. They don't need the procedures described at the beginning of this chapter: exploring stuttering, staying in the stutter, and other strategies aimed at extinguishing fear. Instead, these "low-fear" youngsters targeted in this section may need only a small amount of desensitization, and they can begin therapy by learning fluency skills to replace stuttering. Other children may indeed fear stuttering but be unable to make progress in desensitization until they have increased their fluency and thus may benefit from *starting therapy* with fluency skills training and then work on desensitization.

This focus on fluency in school-age children has a long tradition. In *Treatment of the Young Confirmed Stutterer*, Van Riper (1973) advocates building up a school-age child's fluency: "We always try to increase the amount of fluency in these children, and we want them to feel it and recognize it when it does occur rather than to focus their attention only on the stuttering" (p. 434). Following Van Riper's lead, I teach children without notable fear of stuttering to increase their fluent speech by using a variety of skills. Once a child has learned these skills, he can use them to replace stuttering with what I call "**superfluency**."

Specific Fluency Skills

The skills described in this section are also described in the workbook, *Easy Talker* (Guitar & Reville, 1997), which includes reproducible worksheets for each skill. There is no magic to the order in which these skills should be taught. In this section, I will begin by describing what skills I think are the easiest before going on to those that are a little harder or more abstract. They may be taught in any order or all at once; with the latter option, the clinician models fluency with flexible rate, easy onsets, light contacts, and proprioception and then shapes the child's responses. Video clips of a school-age child using superfluency are available on *thePoint* under Chapter 13.

Flexible Rate

Flexible rate is simply slowing down the production of a word, especially the first syllable (Boehmler, personal communication, 2003). Slowing is thought to be effective in reducing stuttering by allowing more time for language planning and motor execution (see "Fluency-Inducing Conditions" in Chapter 1). This skill is called "flexible rate" rather than "slow rate" to emphasize that only those syllables on which stuttering is expected are slowed, not the surrounding speech. I also think that "flexible rate" is more acceptable to school-age children who may be tired of hearing people tell them to "slow down."

Flexible rate is taught first by having the clinician model production of words in which the first syllable and the transition to the second syllable are said in a way that slows all of the sounds equally. Vowels, fricatives, nasals, sibilants, and glides are lengthened, and plosives and affricates are produced to sound more like fricatives without stopping the sound or airflow. After the clinician's model, the child produces the word with flexible rate, and successive approximations of the target (i.e., improvements) are reinforced. Practice should include all the sounds of the language; you can use a search engine to find interesting word or phrase lists, such as animals and the sounds they make (http://www.abcteach.com/free/l/list_animal_sounds.pdf). Younger children may be helped to learn flexible rate by running an obstacle course of chairs and tables in which they have to slow down as they move around obstacles but can speed up in parts of the course without obstacles. As you and the child run the obstacle course, you can tell a joke or a story and slow down both your speech and your movements as you negotiate the obstacles. Older children can get the idea by using analogies from their areas of interest. For example, some video games have race cars that can be slowed down on curves and sped up on straightaways.

Pausing

Winston Churchill, who stuttered, gave many fine speeches and most are notable for their pauses. Listen to his "Their Finest Hour" speech, especially the end. You will hear that although Churchill used pauses to reduce his stuttering, he also achieved great dramatic effect with them. The school-age child who stutters—as well as the adult—can use pausing to reduce muscle tension and allow the brain to stay at a processing speed that is comfortable.

I use pausing when I use flexible rate to downshift in preparing to say a feared word a little more slowly. You can teach it to children by having them act out a pause in running an obstacle course as mentioned in the preceding section. Then, they can transfer pausing to appropriate places in their conversational speech. One of the youngsters I worked with recently told me he pauses after being called on in class before he begins his answer to a teacher's question, to take charge of the pace of speaking.

Easy Onsets

These are labeled as "Ee-Oo's" in our *Easy Talker* workbook (Guitar & Reville, 1997); they refer to an easy or gentle onset of voicing. My perception of my own stuttering is that if I begin a "feared" sound with a rapid onset of voicing (i.e., a hard glottal attack), I get myself into a "stuck" posture that feels like I can't move it. But if I start my vocal folds vibrating gently at first, I can usually get voicing going without stuttering. For me and probably for many others who stutter (but not all), vowels in word-initial positions are easier to use with an easy onset than are consonants. Vowels following a word-initial voiceless consonant, however, are fairly difficult for me. For example, I might prolong the "s" in "sun" and may block on the "u" unless I consciously employ a gentle onset on the /u/.

Again, teaching easy onsets is like teaching flexible rate. You model the target behavior on lots of different sounds and then have the child imitate your models and reinforce his successive approximations. Some children, particularly younger ones, may be helped to get the concept by performing an action, such as bringing their hands together slowly, as they produce an easy onset.

Light Contacts

Light contacts mean producing a stop consonant by just brushing the articulators together, keeping airflow going as the stop is produced.

Just as a hard glottal attack can trigger stuttering, hard articulatory contacts can also bring it on. When someone who stutters anticipates difficulty with a sound, he'll often "preset" his articulators into a stuck position before starting a word, or he may even rehearse the stuttering behavior (Van Riper, 1936). Producing consonants with light contacts prevents the stoppage of airflow and/or voicing that can trigger stuttering. Light contacts are taught by modeling a style of producing consonants with relaxed articulators and continuous flow of air or voice, depending on the consonant. Plosives and affricates should be slightly distorted so that they sound like fricatives but are still intelligible. For example, when I produce the /b/ in "Barry" using a light contact, I slow down the movement into and out of the lip "closure." Instead of stopping the airflow and voicing by closing my lips, I let my lips loosely vibrate and allow the /b/ sound semiclosure continue for a little longer than normal. For a /p/, my lips barely touch and air flows out of my not-quite-closed lips, creating a slight turbulence so that it sounds a little like an /f/. For those readers who are phonetically minded, I'm actually producing fricative cognates for the /p/ and /b/ sounds. Because these sounds aren't used contrastively in English, my listeners don't notice, but my stuttering does!

Teaching a child to use light contacts is accomplished by modeling a variety of words with initial consonants and reinforcing the child's successive approximations of the target. To make the concept more interesting and perhaps clearer, you can use a variety of games to demonstrate light contact. For example, you might try catching soap bubbles or throwing and catching water balloons or raw eggs. You can also use games that build towers or require you to gently pick up an object (like jackstraws, also called pickup sticks) without disturbing other objects. These activities enable the child to use a light, gentle touch in a vivid way. Once a child gets the basic idea of using light contacts in speech, you can combine flexible rate, easy onsets, and light contacts together in practice on multisyllable words while using these skills on the first syllable and the transition to the second syllable and then finishing the word at a normal rate.

Proprioception

In the present context, **proprioception** refers to sensory feedback from mechanoreceptors in muscles of the lips, jaw, and tongue (Abbs, 1996). This feedback may be crucial in controlling speech movements, and its use as a concept in stuttering therapy may have originated from Van Riper (1973, p. 211), who suggested that "... some of the stutterer's difficulties seem to originate in the auditory processing system. [Therefore,] if we can get him to concentrate upon proprioceptive feedback rather than auditory feedback, we can bypass these difficulties." Recent brain imaging studies reviewed in Chapter 2 support Van Riper's contention that the auditory systems of people who stutter may be dysfunctional (e.g., Budde, Barron, & Fox, 2014; Ingham, 2003; Stager, Jeffries, & Braun, 2003), but there is also evidence that other sensory systems may not be functioning normally either (e.g., De Nil & Abbs, 1991). The work of Cykowski, Fox,

Ingham, Ingham, and Robin (2010) and Chang, Zhu, Choo, and Angstadt (2015) suggesting that people who stutter may have inadequate density in left-hemisphere fiber tracts that connect sensory integration areas and motor planning areas is another sliver of evidence suggesting problems in sensory processing. The effectiveness of teaching proprioception may be that it promotes conscious attention to sensory information from the articulators, perhaps bypassing inefficient automatic sensory monitoring systems and thereby normalizing sensorimotor control.

Children can be taught to use proprioception in a number of ways. One of my former students, David Stuller, has taught proprioception by having a child first hold a raisin in his mouth and report on its taste, shape, size, and other attributes. This activity tunes the child into sensations from his mouth before introducing speech, which may have negative associations for more severe or more sensitive intermediate stutterers. Children can also learn proprioception by picking a word from a list and then closing their eyes and silently moving their articulators for this word and being rewarded when the clinician guesses the word. During this game, children can be coached to feel the movements of their lips, tongue, and jaw as they say a word. Proprioceptive awareness can also be enhanced by using masking noise or delayed auditory feedback to interfere with self-hearing. Although it is not always easy to judge accurately whether or not a child is using proprioception, I look for slightly exaggerated, slow movements to verify that a child is trying to feel the movements of his articulators.

Once a child seems to have acquired proprioception skills, they can be combined with flexible rate, easy onsets, and light contacts as described in the next section. I call using the combination of all these skills "superfluency."

Replacing Stuttering with Superfluency

The use of superfluency to replace stuttering begins with practice on fluent speech. I start with three-word sentences like "I am great!" and have the child practice putting superfluency on the first syllable and the transition to the second. Using multiple letters to represent superfluency, I would depict its production like this: "IIIIaam great." By first modeling the production and then listening and watching the child imitate it, the clinician shapes the child's superfluency skills. Clear and enthusiastic feedback to the child will help him learn; a reward system will make learning fun.

At first, it is important to ensure that all the elements (flexible rate, easy onset, light contacts, and proprioception) are present. Later on, when a child has learned to use superfluency successfully, he may develop his own version that may use only those elements necessary for him to be fluent. Some children become quite fluent and may need to use superfluency only rarely because, for them, having a tool that replaces stuttering with fluency gives them confidence and replaces anticipation of stuttering with anticipation of fluency. Thus, they appear to no longer need to put their articulators in anticipatory postures or have anticipatory tension that triggers stuttering.

After starting with a simple three-word sentence, the clinician continues having the student practice superfluency using both long and short sentences with a variety of initial sounds and with superfluency used in a variety of positions. At first, she has the child imitate her model but then fades the strength of that cue. The more successful the child is in learning good quality superfluency, the less the clinician needs to model the sentences. For those sentences not imitated after the clinician's model, the child can read the sentence from a list, using superfluency on words that are circled. Here are a few sentences to use: "Just do it!" "Show me the money," "Yes, we have no bananas," and "Step away from the car." Develop your own practice sentences by finding phrases from a child's favorite video games or movies. Video or audio playback of the child's successful utterances can be helpful in creating an auditory target in the child's mind to guide him.

After a youngster has mastered the use of superfluency on fluent utterances at the phrase or sentence levels, the focus should be on conversation. At first, the clinician should model superfluency on many of her utterances, both on sentence-initial words and on initial sounds of other words in sentences. The child should be rewarded for superfluency during the time he is working to master it in conversation, but systematic fading of his rewards should be used to make the skill independent of the clinician's feedback. In any case, the activity must be fun for the child, especially if he is taken out of class for therapy. I often use rewards that release frustration toward past stuttering, such as shooting a ping-pong ball gun or throwing a stuffed rat at cans and bottles that have pictures of "stutters" taped to them. A burp gun that shoots ping-pong balls is available from www.HammacherSchlemmer.com.

Some children respond well to concrete representations of new skills they are trying to learn. To help them get the idea of shifting into superfluency from normal speech as they attempt a difficult word, I use the idea of "downshifting" a car or truck. In Vermont, it's easy to have kids imagine they (or an adult) are driving a four-wheel drive truck and need to downshift when they see deep snow ahead. In other geographic areas, south of Vermont, downshifting may be needed before driving through deep mud or up a steep hill. Downshifting can be acted out by the clinician and child by talking and changing into superfluency as they talk when encountering pretend snow, mud, or a hill while walking around the therapy room. Some children may have trouble perceiving when they might stutter on an upcoming word. These children can often be helped in two ways. First, they may be given a little training on the side, using reinforcement for stopping after a stutter, then during a stutter, and finally before a potential stutter, shifting into superfluency on the feared word in each case. Second, they may benefit from massed practice of superfluency on fluent words—just using superfluency on every word, whether or not they expect to stutter on it. This may help them automatize the shift into superfluency before an anticipated stutter.

During the conversation, because superfluency on fluent utterances is being rewarded, the child will probably get into a mindset that will make it easy for him to use superfluency with words on which he expects difficulty. Sometimes you can tell when a child uses superfluency on an expected stutter rather than an expected fluent word, and sometimes you can't. However, the child can often tell you when he is actually using it on an expected stutter, and you should give him an extra reward for these times. There is no harm done when the child uses superfluency on an "expected" stutter that was really just a fluent word. The more practice the better. When the child has replaced stutters with superfluency in the therapy room and superfluency is comfortable for him to use, he can begin using it in structured situations.

Transferring Superfluency to Structured Situations

This section describes not only the specifics of transferring fluency skills but also additional elements, such as being open about stuttering, which will help make transfer successful and aid in maintenance.

Transfer of superfluency to replace stuttering with other listeners and in other situations begins by setting up a hierarchy with the child of easy to difficult situations, in which the child and I can use voluntary downshifts to superfluency together. I use the word "voluntary" here to mean that superfluency is used on nonfeared words—that is, words on which the child doesn't expect to stutter. In the context of using voluntary superfluency, anticipated stutters will eventually occur, and the child will be primed to replace them with superfluency. We begin each session by working together to plan a hierarchy and determine the number of reward points for each accomplishment. At this time, I am getting information from the parents about the child's progress at home.

At an appropriate level of difficulty in the hierarchy, I bring the parents into therapy and have the child teach them about downshifting into superfluency and then develop a plan to have the child use both voluntary and real (when stuttering is expected) downshifts at home. One or both parents, depending on the child's preference, should help him keep a log of the number of downshifts he makes each day. However, involving parents as therapy helpers is not effective for some children. They prefer not to have their parents function in this way but merely want their parents to be supportive listeners. In such cases, I sometimes telephone the child at home and have him record himself talking to me with superfluency from his home. If he's motivated, he can listen to the recording on his own.

By now, the child may be speaking with little difficulty in many situations, but some situations are probably still giving him problems. As I continue the transfer process, I turn more attention to those situations in which the child is having trouble using superfluency successfully to replace his stuttering.

Clinical Procedures: Working with Parents

I have five goals in mind when working with parents of an intermediate stutterer: (1) explaining the treatment program and the parents' role in it, (2) discussing the possible causes of stuttering, (3) identifying and reducing fluency disrupters, (4) identifying and increasing fluency-enhancing situations, and (5) eliminating teasing. I will discuss each of these goals in turn.

Explaining the Treatment Program and the Parents' Role in It

First, I discuss the stages of our therapy program with the child's parents, letting them know how I hope to take the mystery out of stuttering for the child by exploring with him what he does when he stutters. I also tell them about our goal of teaching the child to hold onto stutters and learn to tolerate the previously feared stuckness of stuttering in order to release the tension. To the parents, it may even sound like their child is stuttering more when he uses staying in the stutter and reducing the tension. It's important that I not only demonstrate this strategy for the parent but also have them try it and get good at it so they will know what to be pleased with in their child's speech. Second, I tell them that therapy may take time, perhaps 1 to 3 years and in some cases even longer. Third, I inform them that communicating with their child about his stuttering is important and that they should express their acceptance of his stuttering and acknowledge their understanding that it is often difficult for him to work on it.

Explaining the Possible Causes of Stuttering

I believe it is important for the parents of a school-age child who stutters to be given an explanation of the possible causes of stuttering. I explain current thinking about the nature of stuttering. In some cases, parents have no information about the causes of stuttering. Since I want them to participate in their child's treatment, they need to understand the rationale for our treatment program. Many parents feel guilty about their child's stuttering because of some outdated or inaccurate information they may have. They may have been exposed to an explanation that is no longer considered valid, or they may have been given some erroneous information by a well-meaning but misinformed friend or relative. Such parents then blame themselves for some supposed misdeed on their part. They need good, current information about the nature of stuttering. Often, just supplying this information relieves them of their guilt. The following materials have been helpful supplements to parent counseling:

1. On the "Stuttering Home Page" Web site (http://www.mnsu.edu/comdis/kuster/stutter.html), there is a link titled "Information about Stuttering," which leads to another link for parents of children who stutter. Articles, essays, books, and other materials for parents are provided directly there or are described so that parents can find them elsewhere.
2. On the National Stuttering Association Web site (http://www.westutter.org/whoWeHelp/NSA-Family-Programs/parents/School-Age.htm), there is a wealth of information for parents of school-age children who stutter.
3. On the Stuttering Foundation Web site (http://www.stutteringhelp.org/), a link titled "For Parents of School Age Children" leads to many useful items including "If You Think Your Child is Stuttering: 7 Ways to Help"—a video that provides useful information to parents. The Foundation also has other videos, *Stuttering: Straight Talk for Teens* and *Stuttering: Straight Talk for Teachers*, that can be helpful for parents.

Using language that is appropriate to the parents' level of understanding, I provide the type of information that I presented in the early chapters of this book. I describe how developmental and environmental influences may interact with predisposing physiological and constitutional factors to produce or exacerbate a child's initial repetitions and prolongations. The child responds to these disfluencies with increased tension in his effort to inhibit them. In time, the child also learns a variety of escape and possibly starting behaviors to cope with his repetitions and prolongations. I go on to suggest that predisposing physiological factors are most likely neurological in nature and are related to a child's deficits in speech production. I suggest that the child may have problems in timing the fine motor movements required for fluent speech. I add that children who stutter may also have a more sensitive temperament, and that could compound the stuttering by making the child more likely to have learned emotional reactions to his speech difficulties. I also note that in many cases, the predisposing physiological factors may be genetic in origin. Thus, there are many possible sources for his speech difficulty. I also suggest that because of the way the brain may be organized—with perhaps a very active right hemisphere—the child may have special talents in the areas of drawing, music, engineering, and other visual and creative endeavors.

I explore, with the parents' assistance, the developmental and environmental influences that may be interacting with the child's predisposing factors to affect his stuttering. These are reviewed in Chapter 4. In some cases, I may not identify any developmental or environmental factors that seem to be contributing to the problem; however, when I do identify one or more possible factors, I attempt to lessen their influence. My experience suggests that in most cases, the solution to reducing the impact of developmental and environmental influences is fairly straightforward. In a few cases, when it may be more difficult, I have suggested that counseling by a family therapist may be helpful.

I also talk with parents of a school-age child who stutters about avoidance behaviors. I describe these behaviors to them and explain how the child's word and situation avoidances are behaviors he has learned to use in coping with the embarrassment and fear of talking. I also explain how, in therapy, I will be helping the child eliminate his use of these avoidance behaviors. I will also point out that avoidance learning is unfortunately a rather tenacious form of learning so that they will need to model patience as the child "unlearns" avoidances.

Some parents feel responsible for their child's stuttering and may feel they need to find a cure for it. While I'm discussing the possible causes of stuttering and after I've mentioned the possible neurological differences in children who stutter, I often bring up the possibility that their child will always stutter but that it needn't interfere with his life. Because this can be such an important issue for parents, I try to judge whether this moment is the right time to discuss it. For example, if this is an initial phone conversation, I might not bring it up at that time. But if this is a face-to-face meeting and we have some time to talk about their concerns, I find it helpful to let parents know that a child who is still stuttering after age 9 or 10 years will probably continue to have at least a little stuttering throughout his life. In saying this, I am sure to indicate that most individuals who stutter into adulthood don't let their stuttering get in the way of their goals, and I will cite some examples of famous people who have achieved success even though they stuttered. At this point, I am careful to let them respond to this information. Parents sometimes envision difficulties in academic, social, and career areas for their child who stutters, and it is important for them to express these concerns and for me to listen deeply to them.

Identifying and Reducing Fluency Disrupters

As I explained in other chapters, environmental influences are often critical factors for managing beginning and borderline levels of stuttering in preschool children. Intermediate-level stuttering in school-age children is more complex and requires direct treatment of a child's behaviors and attitudes, but environmental factors are important for this level of stuttering as well. The home environment of a school-age child who stutters may involve stresses and **fluency disrupters** that can be substantially alleviated if the clinician can join forces with an interested, motivated family. I begin by asking family members to observe when the child stutters most and when he stutters least. With this information, I brainstorm with them various ways to reduce potential stresses and to observe the effects on the child's stuttering. For example, some children stutter a lot when there is competition for attention at the dinner table or when several children arrive home from school at the same time, all wanting to talk to their parents. In other cases, changes in a family routine may spark an increase in a child's stuttering. Whatever the sources of stress, I encourage the parents and other family members to take the lead in identifying them and in planning ways of reducing such stress. Even in cases in which stress may result from relatively abstract sources, such as a family's attitude that stuttering is shameful, the family is unlikely to change unless they feel that they and their points of view are respected and understood by the clinician. In an accepting environment, a trusting relationship can be developed, and a family may be open to seeing the child and his stuttering in new ways.

Increasing Fluency-Enhancing Situations

During the process of identifying the times when a child stutters more frequently, families also discover there are times when a child is extremely fluent. These may be specific situations or just days or weeks when the child is particularly fluent. Whatever the case, families can find ways of increasing factors that promote fluency and giving a child plenty of opportunities to talk when he is fluent. For example, a child may be especially fluent when he is talking to a parent at bedtime, when he is sleepy and relaxed. This provides a parent an opportunity to comment on the child's "smooth speech" and to let the child know that they can imagine how good it must feel to talk easily. The clinician can help parents find ways of increasing fluency-enhancing situations and of reinforcing their child's fluency without implying that the times when he stutters are bad. Encourage the family to empathize with the child about fluency being great but that stuttering just can't be helped sometimes.

For those children who are willing to work on their fluency with members of their family, a program of home therapy can be developed cooperatively by the child, parent(s), and clinician. Regular contact between the clinician and family members is important to facilitate and guide this component of treatment. Face-to-face meetings are ideal, but phone calls, journals, or e-mail will also suffice. A typical home program would include severity ratings made by both parents of the child's speech at home and by the child of his speech at home and at school. The specific behaviors to be rated and an effective reward system are negotiated by the child, parents, and clinician.

Eliminating Teasing

If any of an intermediate stutterer's siblings are teasing him about his stuttering, his parents need to stop it. I have found the best way to do this is to have parents have a serious talk with the teaser. They need to explain that teasing makes stuttering worse and must be discontinued. Usually, this is sufficient. If it is not, I have found it effective for me as the child's clinician to talk to the sibling about the importance of not teasing his or her brother or sister. In fact, the teaser can be taught what behaviors on his or her part can be really helpful to the child who stutters. Having an adult other than a parent talk seriously about this matter sometimes carries more weight with teasers.

Another important issue for parents is their reactions to teasing by other children at school. Although this is a serious matter, parents may do more harm than good if they are overly upset by teasing. The child who is teased will take his cue from his parents. If parents are anxious or distraught about their child's being teased, the child will be more deeply affected by it. If parents let the school take care of the incident and convey to the child that they have faith in his ability to handle it but are also empathetic to his concerns, they will help the child maintain a good perspective on it. However, if the teasing continues without further reaction from the school or the school is not sympathetic to begin with, the clinician can offer to talk with the principal or classroom teacher, depending on where the stuttering is occurring and being dealt with.

Clinical Procedures: Working with Teachers

I believe it is very important to have an intermediate stutterer's classroom teacher(s) involved in the student's treatment program (Fig. 13.5). After all, the child spends as much, if not more, time with the teacher than any other adult. In the remainder of this section I'll use "teacher" to mean both one of the child's teachers and many. I have four goals in mind when I am working with a classroom teacher: (1) to explain the treatment program and the teacher's role in it, (2) to facilitate the teacher talking with the student about his stuttering, (3) to help the student and teacher work out the child's class participation, and (4) to help the teacher eliminate teasing.

The students in the University of Vermont 2017 summer camp program for school-age children who stutter created a "survival guide" for both students and teachers. It would be useful to share this both with the child's teacher and his parents as well as the child himself. It's available via this link: http://westutter.org/wp-content/uploads/2017/08/BTS-Survival-Guide.pdf/.

Explaining the Treatment Program and the Teacher's Role in It

Involving the student's classroom teacher(s) in treatment works best if the student gives his permission for this to take place. Even the most reluctant students usually agree to let me make a contact with the teacher. If the student has several teachers, I always ask which teacher(s) the student would like me to talk to. Sometimes, a meeting with several teachers at once is efficient. When I worked as a speech-language pathologist in junior high and elementary schools, I gave in-services about stuttering to teachers at the beginning of the

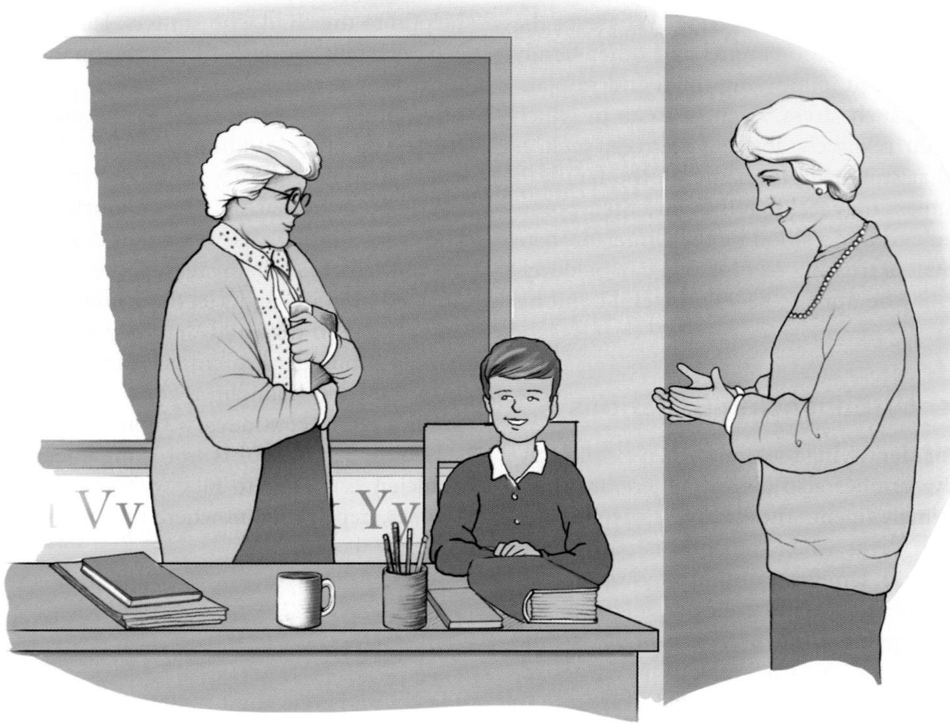

Figure 13.5 It is important to have the classroom teacher involved in the child's treatment.

school year. If such in-services can be arranged, the Stuttering Foundation DVD *Stuttering: Straight Talk for Teachers* (Scott & Guitar, 2012) makes a powerful addition to a presentation on the problems faced by school children who stutter and how teachers can help them. Or consider showing another of the Foundation's DVDs: *Stuttering: For Kids, by Kids* (Scott & Guitar, 2004).

It is beneficial for classroom teachers to have an overview of the student's treatment program, so I discuss how I am helping the student increase his fluency, eliminate his avoidance behaviors, and improve his overall communication ability. I want the teacher to understand the rationale behind these procedures. Therefore, I am careful to answer any questions the teacher may have, believing that helping the teacher understand our goals will have at least two benefits: (1) the teacher will have a better understanding of how to interact with the student and (2) the teacher will be better able to give me feedback regarding the student's fluency in the classroom. I use the Teacher's Assessment of Students' Communicative Competence (TASCC) (Smith, McCauley, & Guitar, 2000) described in Chapter 8 to measure the student's baseline levels and progress. I also explain the teacher's role in the student's therapy and discuss why and how I would like the teacher to implement the three goals of how to talk with the student about his stuttering, how to help him cope with oral participation, and how to eliminate any teasing he may be receiving. I discuss each of these in the following paragraphs.

Teachers' Talking with the Child about His Stuttering

A friend of mine recalled going all the way through school from kindergarten through high school without any teacher ever mentioning his stuttering. He stuttered severely year after year, and everyone knew he stuttered, but nobody ever acknowledged it. This silence, he said, was very painful. I believe that it is better for a classroom teacher to sit down with a student who stutters and talk calmly with him about his stuttering, letting him know that she is aware of his stuttering and would like to help him in any way possible. The teacher should tell the student that she will not interrupt or hurry him when he is talking. Just this sort of acknowledgment and acceptance of the student's stuttering by a teacher will make the child feel more comfortable in the classroom.

Coping with Oral Participation

The teacher should also talk with the student about his oral participation in class. I believe it is important for a school-age child who stutters to participate orally in class. It is also important for him to feel comfortable participating, and the teacher should seek the student's input on this matter. Possibly, some classroom procedure, such as calling on students in alphabetical order, is creating apprehension for the student who stutters and could be modified. For example, the student may prefer to be called on early, before his apprehension builds up. With an understanding of the student's feelings and flexibility in procedures, most teachers can help a student who stutters become much more comfortable in his oral classroom participation.

Reducing Teasing

It is not unusual for children who stutter in elementary or junior high school to be teased about stuttering at school. If a classroom teacher becomes aware of teasing, she should attempt to stop it. As I indicated during my previous discussion of teasing in the home, I believe the best way to do this is to have a serious talk with the teaser. The teacher needs to explain that the child's teasing is making the stutterer's speech worse and that he needs to discontinue it immediately. The teacher should make it clear that this behavior will not be tolerated. Some teasers are themselves troubled children and will need help from the school counselor to change their behaviors.

Progress and Outcome Measures

Measures of progress and outcome, as described in Chapter 8, need to be taken to assess the effectiveness of treatment. Data on stuttering and fluency (%SS, Stuttering Severity Instrument [SSI-4], measures of attitudes [CAT and A-19], and assessment of communicative competence [TASCC]) can be used to measure progress during treatment and outcome after maintenance.

This concludes the description of my approach to treatment of a school-age child with intermediate stuttering. I now describe the clinical procedures of some other clinicians. As you have seen, the major focus of my approach is to reduce the negative emotions associated with stuttering and then teach a strategy to manage stuttering. Relatively little emphasis is put on teaching fluency skills. The approaches described in the next section are more focused on teaching fluency skills from the beginning of treatment, and they have other additional dimensions not covered in my approach.

APPROACHES OF OTHER CLINICIANS

J. Scott Yaruss, Kristin Pelczarski, Bob Quesal, and Nina Reeves: Treating the Entire Disorder

These clinicians differ from me in their focus on fluency skills from the very beginning of treatment. They also incorporate **cognitive behavioral therapy** as well as acceptance and commitment therapy. In addition, much of their work on generalization is aimed at increasing the child's participation in social and academic situations.

This intervention is described in detail and illustrated with a 20-minute DVD in Yaruss, Pelczarski, and Quesal (2010). The goal is to help the child become the most effective

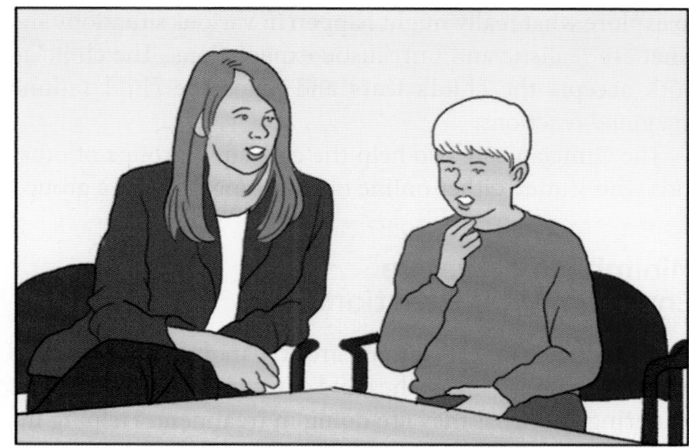

Figure 13.6 A clinician like Kristin Pelczarski helping a student feel what he is doing when he stutters.

communicator he can be. Subgoals include (1) increasing the child's fluency and reducing his stuttering, (2) reducing the child's and the environment's reactions to the child's stuttering, and (3) helping the child increase participation in social and academic activities (Fig. 13.6).

Minimizing the Impairment (Increasing Fluency and Decreasing Stuttering)

The clinician begins by working directly on the child's fluency—for example, by helping him learn to reduce speaking rate and increase pause time. This is done in such a way that the changes in the child's speech are enough to promote fluency but not so much that the style of speaking sounds abnormal. As the clinician helps the child make changes in his speaking rate and pausing, she also teaches the child to reduce physical tension in his speech mechanism. For this purpose, light contacts and easy starts are incorporated into the child's speech, especially at the beginnings of utterances.

This more fluent style of speaking is taught in easy-to-more-difficult hierarchies. For example, the child uses this style of speaking while reading and then progresses to more and more natural conversations in the treatment room. Then, the child practices this speaking style in gradually more challenging real-life situations, using a progression that the child and clinician design together.

Minimizing Negative Personal Reactions

To help the child decrease his negative reactions to his stuttering, the clinician helps the child use voluntary stuttering in easy-to-more-difficult situations. The clinician also uses strategies drawn from cognitive therapies such as cognitive-behavioral therapy and acceptance and commitment therapy (Beilby & Yaruss, 2018; Scott, undated) to help the child change his thoughts about his stuttering and his imagined listener reactions to it. This is assisted by role-playing situations to explore what really might happen in various situations and what are realistic and unrealistic expectations. The clinician both accepts the child's fears and helps the child rethink imagined reactions.

The clinician can also help the child find groups of other kids who stutter, either online or by arranging such a group.

Minimizing Negative Environmental Reactions

To reduce negative reactions from parents, teachers, and peers, the clinician helps the child educate these groups about stuttering and what they are doing in treatment. Helping the child reduce his negative emotional reactions to his stuttering will also help the child respond to bullying, teasing, or other hurtful responses from peers by making matter-of-fact responses to provocations. Class presentations by the child and the clinician can also be used to educate peers and create a more stuttering-friendly environment.

Helping the Child Participate More Fully in Social and Academic Situations

To achieve this goal, the hierarchies that the child and clinician constructed while working on speaking strategies are adapted to help the child participate in more and more social and academic situations. The authors advocate a "generalization scavenger hunt" to organize and motivate this part of treatment. In a nutshell, the child and clinician develop a list of important speaking situations that the child may face during a typical day. These usually include conversations with family, classmates, and friends outside of school. The hierarchy is arranged in an easy-to-harder matrix with a list of strategies to choose from for each situation to enhance fluency and reduce stuttering to choose from for each situation. As the child goes through a typical day and enters a planned situation, he picks which strategy he'll use in that situation. This whole procedure, practiced as frequently as possible, enables the child and clinician to track progress and decrease the amount of limitation and restriction that stuttering puts on the child's life.

Assessment of Progress and Outcome

Because this treatment is aimed at the overall effect that stuttering may have on a child's life, a major assessment tool is the *Overall Assessment of the Speaker's Experience of Stuttering* (Yaruss & Quesal, 2016). Yaruss et al. (2010) encourage collection of data on the effectiveness and efficacy of this approach using these measures.

Harrison, Bruce, Shenker, Koushik, and Kazenski: Lidcombe Program for School-Age Children

This approach is very programmatic, meaning that the steps are laid out ahead of time, like a recipe. However, they are adjusted to the individual child's progress and his individual preferences. I have taken most of this description of the Lidcombe Program (LP) for school-age children from a chapter by Harrison, Bruce, Shenker, and Koushik (2010). The LP for preschool children described in detail in Chapter 12 forms the basis of LP for school-age children. The principles are, first, that the treatment has two stages: Stage 1, in which a stable level of fluency is established in the clinic and beyond, and Stage 2, in which fluency is maintained, but clinic visits are systemically faded in duration and frequency. The second principle is that the treatment is parent-delivered; in Stage 1, the parent and child meet with the clinician once a week for an hour, during which time the parent is trained, and progress is assessed (Fig. 13.7). The third principle is that the parent conducts daily structured treatment conversations

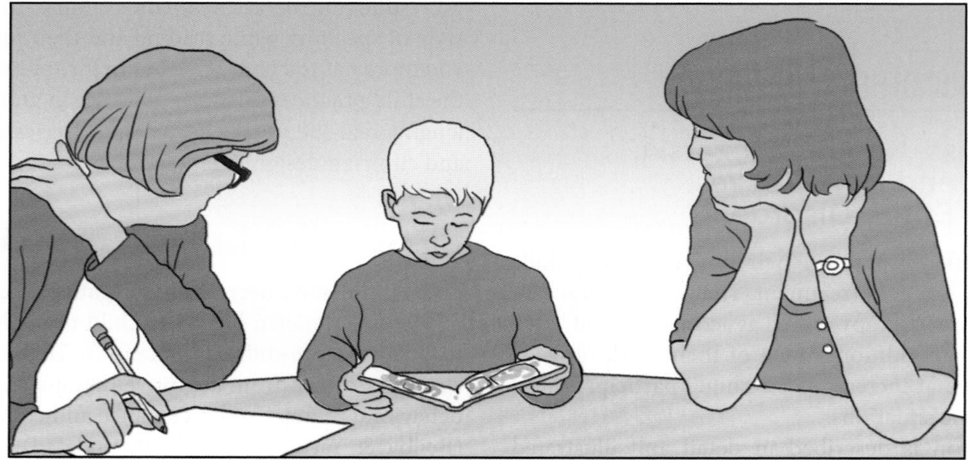

Figure 13.7 A clinician like Rosalee Shenker working with a student and his mother using the Lidcombe Program for school-age children who stutter.

with the child, and these gradually transition into unstructured treatment conversations.

During the treatment conversations with the child, the parent gives verbal contingencies (VCs) for stutter-free speech and for unambiguous stuttering. The VCs for both are the same as those in Table 12.1 in the previous chapter describing the LP for older preschool children. Another important principle is that Severity Ratings (SRs) are used by the parent and the clinician to track the child's progress. This is a 0 to 9 scale in which 0 = no stuttering, 2 = extremely mild stuttering, and 9 = extremely severe stuttering. The parent is taught to use the scale at home for daily ratings and is calibrated regularly by the clinician asking the parent to rate the child's speech during a clinic visit and comparing the parent's and the clinician's ratings. The parent's rating must not differ from the clinician's by more than 1 point. If it does, the parent must be trained further in the use of the scale. In addition to the parent's daily SRs, the clinician also assigns an SR to the child, rating the child's speech over the entire clinic visit.

Criteria for moving from Stage 1 to Stage 2 are three consecutive clinic visits in which the clinician's rating of the child for the entire visit is a 0 or a 1, and the parent's ratings of the child's speech over the past week are 0s and 1s with at least four 0s. Stage 2 is completed when the child maintains criteria-level fluency during the gradually faded clinic visits, spaced in this progression: 2, 2, 4, 4, 8, 8, and 16 weeks apart.

Some *adaptations for the school-age child* include the following, although these adaptations are optional. One adaptation is that the child may be taught to collect his own daily SRs. These may be useful because they may reflect the child's fluency in school. The child may enjoy charting his own progress, using a diary or a graph to keep track. However, the parent's SRs, along with the clinician's SRs, remain the primary measure of progress.

In another adaptation, the child should be encouraged to discuss with his parent the types of VCs he would prefer. Anything goes, as long as the VCs for stutter-free speech are reinforcing to the child and the VCs for unambiguous stutters call attention to the stuttering without rewarding it.

Some school-age children may prefer tangible rewards in addition to VCs. They may be used for progress in reducing SRs or just for participating in the program. Tangible rewards for fluent speech in many different situations will speed generalization.

My colleague Danra Kazenski, who has worked with school-age children using the LP for more than 5 years, has these additional suggestions:

- Develop VCs and tangible reward systems that take advantage of the child's interest (Fig. 13.8). For example, use a coin jar decorated with the child's favorite sports teams. Use code words that make the child feel really good about his fluency, such as "Now you're talking like LeBron James!"
- Encourage and reward self-corrections. Ask the child after he's been fluent "Was that smooth?" Give the child bonus points if he fixes a stutter without the parent having commented on it or if he identifies his fluent speech without prompting.
- The more independence you can give the child, the better, as long as the parameters of the LP are respected. For example, the child's SR's should be encouraged to keep his own SRs, and they should be taken seriously and discussed with him.

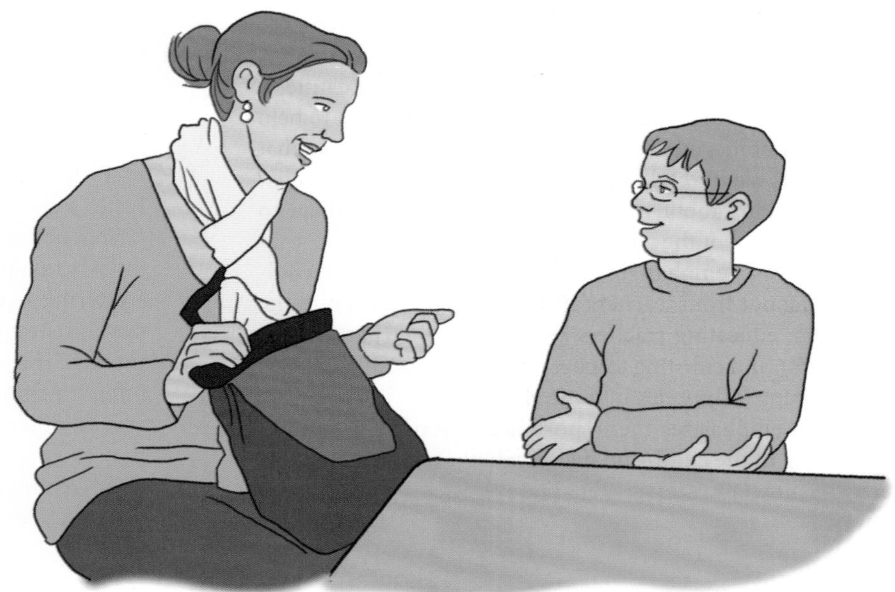

Figure 13.8 A clinician like Danra Kazenski using a mystery bag of toys as she reinforces a student in the Lidcombe Program for school-age children who stutter.

Patty Walton: Fun with Fluency for the School-Age Child

This approach differs from mine because it begins by teaching fluency skills. However, Walton is sensitive to the fact that some children need more work on their emotions and may need to manage stuttering that continues. In fact, she makes a statement near the beginning of her book that shows that she knows what treatment of school-age children who stutter is really like. She says "The greatest challenge clinicians face in treating school-age children who stutter is finding a balance between getting them to speak more easily and letting them stutter sometimes" (Walton, 2012). Walton is very realistic about the likelihood that most of these children will still have some residual stuttering even with the best treatment. She also realizes that the clinician must not be punitive toward any remaining stuttering, or she will lose the child's trust.

Walton's well-organized approach begins with a careful assessment that includes measures of stuttering severity, analysis of the child's stuttering pattern, assessment of the child's reaction to his stuttering, and his attitudes and emotions. She also assesses the parents' attitudes and behaviors toward their child's stuttering.

Her treatment plan varies for each child, but the following components are the core of her approach. She begins with "fluency-shaping" techniques, such as "stretching" out the first sound of phrases and including—only if necessary—easy onsets, light contacts, and other tools to increase fluency. Stuttering modification techniques are to be used if the child is reacting negatively to his stuttering: voluntary stuttering, pull-outs, and other ways of making the child feel more in control of his stuttering. She works with the child's attitudes and emotions, if the child perceives his stuttering to be negative or if he's being teased. In this area, Walton encourages the child to express his feelings about his speech, empowers him to take control of his stuttering, and helps him realize that success needn't be complete fluency but may be stuttering in a way that feels in control.

She believes strongly in parent counseling, which involves educating parents about stuttering and about treatment, teaching strategies that the parents can be involved in to help the child at home, openness about stuttering at home so that stuttering is okay to talk about, helping parents have realistic expectations about treatment, and encouraging them to reduce criticism of the child and his speech.

Walton also emphasizes working with teachers, including finding out from teachers about the child's speech in the classroom, educating teachers about stuttering (particularly this child's), and enlisting teachers' support to facilitate transfer of therapy techniques into the classroom.

Walton emphasizes the importance, throughout therapy, of listening to the child—no matter whether the child is stuttering or not—to validate what he says, what he thinks, and how he feels.

SUMMARY

- My approach to stuttering in school-age children includes two separate and distinct therapies: one for most children—who will have some negative feelings about their stuttering—and another for those few children who have little fear of stuttering.
- My treatment for the typical school-age child who stutters begins with an exploration of stuttering to decrease some of the negative emotions associated with it and then helps the student reduce the threat and fear of the moment of "stuckness" in stutters and thereby reduce the tension. After tension is reduced, the child then finishes the "stuck" word (which is now "unstuck") slowly and easily. As the child masters this strategy, he begins to have easier stutters that feel in control.
- For some students who stutter—those rare students with few negative emotions—"superfluency" can be taught. This type of speech incorporates flexible rate, pausing, gentle onsets, light contacts, and proprioception to enhance fluency and manage stuttering. Superfluency is then transferred to a variety of real-world situations.
- In the approach for most children, after learning to stay in the stutter (strongly reinforced by the clinician), reducing fear and tension, and learning to end the stutter slowly and loosely, the young client then works on continuing to reduce his fear and avoidance by (1) being open about stuttering, (2) accepting his stuttering, (3) learning to use voluntary stuttering, and (4) becoming desensitized to stuttering in a variety of situations. Following this, transfer activities take place.
- Other clinicians, whose therapies are described in this chapter, use many of these same techniques. Some reinforce fluency in a hierarchy from words to sentences to conversation in the clinic and then to everyday situations outside the clinic. Most of them foster a change in attitudes about speech and stuttering, not only to provide positive expectations for fluency but also to help clients accept any residual stuttering so that they will deal with it rather than avoid it. Many also prepare the child to deal with teasing. Thus, the core of these programs is similar, but each clinician adds innovations. I've included several different approaches to help readers see how they too may consider adding different elements to their treatment.

STUDY QUESTIONS

1. What is the "approach" attitude that I recommend for school-age children who stutter? What are some reasons why an "approach" attitude might help a child with intermediate stuttering?
2. What is the theoretical rational for "Staying in the Stutter?" In other words, why would staying in the stuckness of the stutter cause stuttering to become easier?
3. Many clinicians, including the Lidcombe group, believe that direct work on a child's attitude about speaking is not necessary because operant conditioning can change the child's speaking behaviors, which will automatically change his attitude. Do you agree? Give your rationale.
4. What is a "stuttering-friendly" environment, and how could you create one in a child's home and school?
5. Describe what the "exploration" phase of my treatment approach is designed to accomplish and how it meets that goal.
6. Suggest three ways in which you might assess to what extent the goals of the exploration phase of treatment have been met with a particular child.
7. Given what you learned about the nature of stuttering, explain why slowing speech rate (as in "flexible rate") might reduce stuttering.
8. When you are working on a transfer hierarchy and the child seems unable to transfer improved fluency to a particular situation, such as giving a book report, what can you do to achieve success on this step?

SUGGESTED PROJECTS

1. Avoidance reduction is an important component of the major treatment described in this chapter. Experiment with your own fears and avoidances to see if you can decrease them by using a "seeking out" attitude. For example, if you dislike making phone calls, devote a week to making extra phone calls and seeking out opportunities to make phone calls you usually wouldn't make. After the week is over, assess whether this experience decreased your dislike of making phone calls.
2. Watch the Stuttering Foundation video *For Kids by Kids*, and plan how you might use various clips from it to help a child explore his own and others' stuttering.
3. Draw a "road map" with pictures that you could use to help a school-age child at the beginning of therapy learn about what he will be doing over the course of therapy.
4. Develop new ways, new metaphors, and new activities to help a child learn to "Stay in the Stutter," let tension subside, and finish the word loosely and slowly.

SUGGESTED READINGS

Guitar, B., & Reville, J. (1997). *Easy talker: A fluency workbook for school-age children*. Austin, TX: Pro-Ed Publishers. Discontinued by publisher, but available used on Amazon.

This is a workbook for elementary school children that tells the story of several children at a camp working on their stuttering. Along with the story, sequenced concepts and techniques are presented, with workbook activities for children to complete. This book integrates stuttering modification and fluency shaping.

Harrison, E., Bruce, M., Shenker, R., & Koushik, S. (2010). The Lidcombe Program for school-age children who stutter. In B. Guitar, & R. McCauley (Eds.), *Treatment of stuttering: Established and emerging interventions* (pp. 150–166). Baltimore, MD: Lippincott Williams & Wilkins.

A detailed description (with video) of how the Lidcombe Program, originally designed for preschool children, can be adapted for school-age children.

Manning, W., & DiLollo, A. (2018). *Clinical decision making in fluency disorders* (4th ed.). New York: Delmar Publishers.

The chapter called "Treatment of Young Children" contains excellent information on approaches with children between 2 and 12 years old. The first author is an individual who stuttered throughout childhood and young adulthood but has essentially overcome it.

Ramig, P., & Dodge, D. (2005). *The child and adolescent stuttering treatment and activity resource guide*. Clifton Park, NY: Thomson Delmar Learning.

Goals of treatment, ideas for IEPs, steps in treatment, activities to teach elements of therapy, tips for involving parents and teachers, and a multitude of handouts (in Spanish and English) are some of the valuable contents of this book. Cluttering evaluation and treatment are also covered.

Van Riper, C. (1973). Treatment of the young confirmed stutterer. In *The treatment of stuttering* (pp. 426–451). Englewood Cliffs, NJ: Prentice-Hall.

In this chapter, Van Riper provides a comprehensive discussion of a classic stuttering modification approach to the treatment of the intermediate stutterer.

Walton, P. (2012). *Fun with fluency: For the school-age child*. Austin, TX: Pro-Ed.

This is a well-organized approach that combines stuttering modification and fluency shaping for the school-age child who stutters. This book provides a great deal of material that can be copied and used for each individual child.

Yaruss, J. S. (Ed.) (2003). Facing the challenge of treating stuttering in the schools. Part 2: Selecting goals and strategies for success. *Seminars in Speech and Language, 24*(1), February issue.

This journal issue is full of relevant and practical ideas for working with intermediate stuttering in a school setting.

Yaruss, J. S., Murphy, B., Quesal, R., Reardon-Reeves, N., & Flores, T. (2004). *Bullying and teasing: Helping children who stutter*. New York, NY: National Stuttering Association.

The philosophy behind this book is to empower children who stutter to take charge of teasing situations themselves. However, it also provides excellent suggestions for parents, teachers, SLPs, and school administrators.

Yaruss, J. S., Pelczarski, K., & Quesal, R. (2010). Comprehensive treatment for school-age children who stutter: Treating the entire disorder. In B. Guitar, & R. McCauley (Eds.), *Treatment of stuttering: Established and emerging interventions* (pp. 215–244). Baltimore, MD: Lippincott Williams & Wilkins.

This chapter and accompanying video provide an excellent illustration of a broad-spectrum approach to treatment that targets affective, behavioral, and cognitive aspects of stuttering.

14

Treatment of Adolescents and Adults: Advanced Stuttering

Chapter Objectives

After studying this chapter, readers should be able to:

- Describe some of the behavioral, cognitive, and emotional characteristics of stuttering in adolescents and adults
- Explain what components of advanced stuttering may be learned, thus making them candidates for unlearning
- Describe three fluency goals that are appropriate for adolescents and adults who stutter
- Explain how classical conditioning principles can be used to help individuals unlearn old responses that account for many stuttering behaviors and attitudes
- Explain why fears and other emotions must be dealt with in treatment, along with changing how the individual speaks
- Explain what is accomplished in the first stage of treatment, "exploring stuttering"
- Describe how the clinician can help the client deal with feelings associated with stuttering
- Describe and demonstrate the five components of controlled fluency
- Delineate some of the important principles that must be followed to transfer a

new behavior from the therapy room to outside situations

- Explain how voluntary stuttering may help a person who stutters
- Give several examples of how a person who stutters can be open about his or her stuttering
- Indicate some of the things the client must do to maintain fluency gains after treatment

Key Terms

Acceptable stuttering: A mild form of stuttering that neither interferes with communication nor bothers the speaker or listener

Approach behavior: Consciously going toward something that was previously feared (or still is feared). Part of the reason that stuttering persists is that the individual avoids stuttering and avoids saying feared words and entering feared situations, causing the fear to continue. By deliberately approaching feared words and situations again and again, fear diminishes and so does stuttering.

Becoming your own clinician: Near the termination of therapy, the client becomes more and more able to give himself assignments to maintain the fluency he achieved working with the clinician

Catch and release: A term some clients and clinicians use to label staying in the stutter and letting the fear and tension go

Controlled fluency: A highly conscious style of speaking that induces fluency by modifying certain elements of speech

Counterconditioning: A way of decreasing a response such as fear of stuttering by pairing the previously feared stimulus (e.g., stuttering) with a positive stimulus (e.g., praise). The Wikipedia description of counterconditioning has a link to one of the pioneers of counterconditioning, Mary Cover Jones. The description of Jones' use of counterconditioning to help a boy named Peter reduce his fear of rabbits is a gem and will help readers understand counterconditioning via a straightforward example.

Deconditioning: Similar to counterconditioning except that instead of a positive stimulus, the previously feared stimulus (stuttering) is paired with a neutral stimulus (no negative consequence)

Easy onsets: Beginning phonation by gently bringing the vocal folds together instead of bringing them together quickly and with force that is sometimes referred to as a hard glottal attack

Exploring stuttering: Activities that help the client get in contact with the experience of stuttering without the negative emotions usually associated with stuttering. It is a type of approach behavior that can achieve **deconditioning**, thereby decreasing fear.

Flexible rate: Slowing the beginning of a word, especially when stuttering is expected

Fluent stutters: Another term for the type of stutters described above as high-quality stutters. It is used to help clients realize that their high-quality stutters are very much like fluent speech and often are not noticed by listeners as abnormal.

High-quality stutter: These are stutters that are held without any avoidance until fear and tension are reduced. The stutters are then released slowly and loosely. They are the results of learning to "stay in the stutter," with an especially slow, loose release.

Light contacts: Touching the articulators together lightly while speaking so as to avoid "setting off" a stutter by pushing too strongly

Pausing: While speaking, inserting pauses at appropriate locations, with the aim of gaining control of one's speaking and processing speed

Proprioception: Attending to the movement of one's articulators, with the aim of using that sensory information to replace auditory input from one's own speech (which may be faulty)

Spontaneous fluency: Speech without stuttering that doesn't require thinking about it

Staying in the stutter: Going right into the stutter, without any avoidance, and then prolonging the articulatory posture and sound associated with the moment of "stuckness." The purpose is to extinguish the threat and fear associated with the experience of being stuck. The clinician's praise and acceptance of the client's staying in the stutter are very important in extinguishing these emotions.

Voluntary stuttering: Stuttering on purpose or at least producing speech in a way that mimics stuttering, with the aim of reducing fear of stuttering

AN INTEGRATED APPROACH

Individuals with advanced stuttering are usually older adolescents or adults who have been stuttering for many years. Their patterns, which are well entrenched, consist of blocks, repetitions, and prolongations that are usually accompanied by tension and struggle, as well as escape and avoidance behaviors. Typically, these individuals have developed negative anticipations about speaking situations and listener reactions. Sometimes, their stuttering has been such an important factor in their lives that they have chosen occupations beneath their abilities (Van Riper, e.g., worked as a farmhand, digging potatoes, after he earned his Master's degree in English literature). Adults with advanced stuttering sometimes turn down promotions if more speaking is required than in their present positions and will often not participate fully in group discussions, team meetings, and conversations. In rare instances, some adults who stutter hide their stuttering by avoiding words or situations so completely that they don't show the usual signs of stuttering. Their stuttering is sometimes referred to as "interiorized."

Because the complex patterns of advanced stuttering involve behaviors, emotions, and cognitions, treatment is most effective if it targets all of these areas. These patterns are so deeply etched into the brain that treatment is best if it is intense, is long-lasting, and provides training for long-term maintenance. My approach to treatment is a brew blended from many sources. I have tried to integrate these procedures so that clients reduce their negative emotions and avoidances and learn to respond differently, with more **fluent stuttering** to old cues that have always triggered tense and struggled stuttering (see Fig. 14.1).

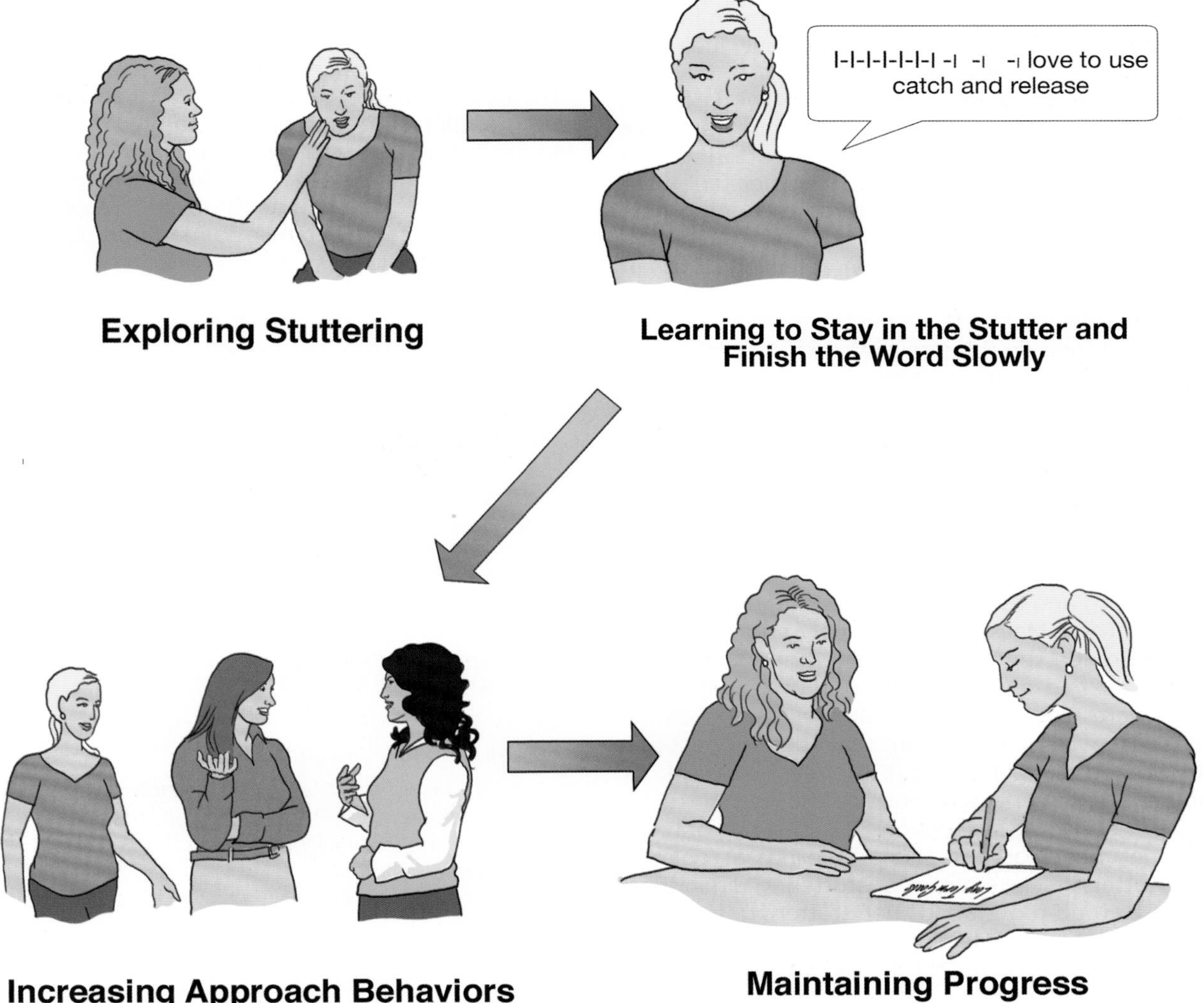

Figure 14.1 Elements of an integrated approach to treatment.

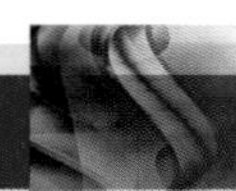

Case Example

Malisa

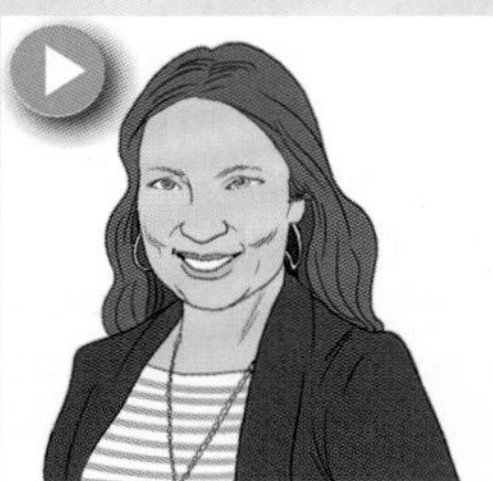

In the fall semester several years ago, a young woman named Malisa, an elementary school teacher in Vermont, came to us for treatment of her stuttering. She reported having difficulty talking to the parents of her students, introducing herself to new people, and making telephone calls. She also felt that her stuttering was keeping her from reading her poetry aloud at public gatherings. Malisa had a family history of stuttering and, in fact, had no memory of speaking without stuttering, even as a child. Our initial evaluation measures showed that her frequency of stuttering in conversation was 7.4 percent syllables stuttered, and her rating on the SSI-4 was severe. The Overall Assessment of Speakers' Experience of Stuttering (OASES, a measure of how much impact stuttering has on the individual's daily life) was moderate.

Two of my graduate students and I worked with Malisa during the fall and spring semesters. We began by helping her explore her stuttering and her feelings about it, through having her feel what she was doing when she stuttered, watching herself stuttering in the mirror, and discussing stuttering experiences and accompanying feelings, both in the past and present. After several weeks, we progressed to having Malisa stay in the moment of stuttering—learning to tolerate the frustration of being stuck—then gradually reduce the tension, and slowly finish the word on which she was stuttering. She practiced these high-quality stutters while watching herself in the mirror with us in the clinic, on video playback, and also in the nearby student center. When our work involved speaking to strangers in public, we would do the task first, using voluntary stuttering, as we stopped people on the sidewalk or in a building and asked questions using high-quality stutters. Then, Malisa would gamely choose someone, approach them, and try to employ staying in the stutter and ending slowly on her real stutters. There were plenty of failures as well as successes, but Malisa was quick to learn from our suggestions and worked diligently, in both her sessions with us and her assignments to practice at home.

The first five or six sessions focused not only on stuttering behaviors but also on feelings associated with stuttering. Malisa's fear of stuttering diminished as she learned more about her stuttering, explored past experiences and feelings, and repeatedly sought out opportunities to practice. Once Malisa was making changes in her overlearned stuttering patterns as well as in her feelings and attitudes, we introduced some elements of "controlled fluency"—easy onsets, proprioception, flexible rate, and pausing. After practice on using these in her fluent speech, we helped Malisa employ them to deal with anticipated stutters. Again, Malisa was a quick learner and was successful in turning some of her stutters into easier, briefer stutters so that she felt comfortably in control. Malisa also worked on voluntary stuttering and letting listeners know that she stuttered.

By the end of the spring semester, she was doing well, but still had some challenges when the stress was high or when she was caught by surprise. By the end of the spring semester, in May, after a total of 21 sessions, Malisa's percent syllables stuttered in conversation had decreased (from 7.4) to 1.4. Her SSI-4 score had decreased from severe to very mild, and her OASES score was "mild/moderate" (having been moderate). The percent syllables stuttered and SSI-4 scores may well have been influenced by the fact that we were now a familiar audience. In an eloquent letter of thanks to the clinic, Malisa wrote, "The last two semesters of work with you and (the two graduate students) have been pivotal in changing my outlook and stuttering behavior.... To be confident in 'voice' is a life skill with far-reaching effects." She added that she had just published a poem in a literary journal and was able to read it in public, not with complete fluency, but in a way that made her proud. Here is one of her poems about stuttering:

A stutterer introduces herself

or not, if the syllables come without sound
and the mouth pantomimes
the onset M in white gloves.

She begins with her lips open
so the penned up can slip out
to grass before morning's milking.
Let it always be a county fair in May.
Let moored breath beckon a wheedling wind
before the thunder of big-top speech.
Everyone will look up, necks exposed,
and wait
as the clouds roll in.

So the fluency's flexible,
may a maundering farm hand amble
the meandering mile, and consonants
become malleable when struck
or stuck by the jaw.

continued

But if blocked again again again,
the repetitions of Ma- Ma- Ma-
might call to mind the bleat
of judged goats in the grandstand and
you will feel ashamed
of your adolescent associations.
A trick trap door's underfoot
for moments like this.

Or, if you're kinder sort, maybe instead
you'll hear the infant summoning
Mother (the first sensible uttering)
and notice she's pretty
though her message is mazy.

And if the confusion continues
in this casual meeting of strangers,
I suggest you generously
let her build momentum or cancel
the conversation completely.
Some carousels are silent.
She's looking away.

Letting beginning be easy as ice cream—
licking maple creamees
melty at noon under the oak,
make light contact with your eyes
and her tongue will make light contact
in her mouth. And her larynx will release
the mechanical latch holding back
the tin tine that plays
the music of mute clowns.
The melody holds most of the meaning anyway
and red lipstick smears all the M's.

Reprinted from her book *Handing Out Apples in Eden* (2014, Wind Ridge Books) with permission of the author.

Our integrated approach to stuttering in adolescents and adults is illustrated above, using an example of a highly motivated young adult. If any of the terminology used in this description is not clear at first, it will become clear upon reading about the treatment process later in the chapter.

Author's Beliefs

The assertions that follow are not facts but rather my inferences about advanced stuttering and its treatment. The reader should keep in mind that it is filtered through my own experiences as a person who has stuttered since age 3, who received therapy at age 21 from Charles Van Riper, and who has had both successes and failures over the 50 years he has worked as a stuttering therapist.

Nature of Stuttering

As I described in Chapter 7, I believe that the origins of advanced stuttering arise from a physiological predisposition for inefficient neural activation patterns for speech and a vulnerable temperament interacting with environmental influences to produce and exacerbate core behaviors of, typically (but not always), repetitions. In the early stages, a child may react to these repetitions with a response of increased tension, pushing, and hurry. As a reactive child continues to experience and respond to the core behaviors, a negative spiral worsens the stuttering. Increased tension and struggle become more and more alarming to the child, and he then pushes harder to get words out. Soon, he tries to cope by adding a variety of escape behaviors, which are reinforced through operant conditioning, via the reward of finishing the word after deploying an escape behavior such as an eye blink or a head nod. During this same period, negative feelings—such as frustration, fear, and shame—become associated with stuttering. These feelings generalize through classical conditioning to more and more words and situations. Finally, the child begins to avoid feared words and situations, with fear then perpetuated through intermittent reinforcement. If these underlying processes continue until an individual reaches adolescence or young adulthood, the client will enter the stage of advanced stuttering.

Because increased tension, speeding up of speech rate, secondary behaviors, and feelings and attitudes are learned, they can be modified. Operant and classical conditioning principles are used to make these changes. However, because predisposing physiological factors contribute to these behaviors and also because many years of learning have reorganized the brain in people with advanced stuttering, *complete* unlearning may not be possible. Thus, it is crucial to help individuals with advanced stuttering learn how to cope with residual disruptions in speech if they are going to maintain improvements in fluency.

Speech Behaviors Targeted for Therapy

In this section, I include both *new* behaviors, which need to be learned, and *old* behaviors, which must be reduced or eliminated. In most individuals with advanced stuttering, well-learned tension and speeding-up responses are cued by anticipated and actual stuttering. They are typically accompanied by a considerable overlay of other learned secondary behaviors. To cope with these learned behaviors and to stutter more fluently, individuals with advanced stuttering must decrease their fear of stuttering and eliminate their escape and avoidance behaviors. Then, they must learn to respond to actual or anticipated stuttering by going right into the stutter without using starters or other delaying techniques. Once in the stuckness of the stutter, they need to learn to stay in the stuck posture while producing appropriate airflow and/or sound. When they are able to "be" in the stutter and—with much help from the clinician—tolerate the moment of "stuckness," the tension will release. Then they can move slowly through the rest of the word. The slow, loose finish of the word will be reinforced by the relief of finishing the word.

The above description is a *new* behavior that can be learned with guidance and support from the clinician. When learned and practiced, it gives the client a new feeling of being in control of his stuttering. Then, the client can relinquish more and more of his maladaptive *old* behaviors. These include escape and avoidance maneuvers that keep the stuttering "hot" and prevent recovery. But also as the client feels he has a tool that works and gives him some control, his emotions will change as well. Note that I advocate that only this one tool to respond to stuttering, making it easier for the client to decide what to do under stress. I will talk more about this in the sections to come on treatment procedures.

Fluency Goals

The ultimate goal that many people with advanced stuttering have in mind when they start therapy is spontaneous "fluency" in all situations or, in other words, normal speech. In my experience, most individuals with advanced stuttering do not reach this level of fluency. After treatment, clients may have periods of **spontaneous fluency**, lasting from a few hours to a month or more, but usually some stuttering returns, especially in stressful situations. At these times, I want clients to have options.

For those individuals who stutter who want to speak confidently, communicate easily, and feel comfortable in their speech, I want them to have the freedom to go directly into stutters, keep the sound or airflow going for a few seconds, and then end the word slowly. How they achieve **high-quality stuttering** will be explained when I describe the nuts and bolts of therapy.

Sometimes individuals who have been in therapy with me will have days and times when they can't get a handle on their stuttering. At those times, I would like them to just talk, without hiding their stuttering or avoiding. Ideally, at these times, they would just focus on communicating with their conversational partner, listening well, and saying what they want to say when they want to say it—stuttering be hanged!

Feelings and Attitudes

I believe that adolescents and adults with advanced stuttering typically have strong negative feelings and attitudes toward their stuttering and toward themselves when they begin therapy. I give these emotions and cognitions substantial attention throughout therapy. From the beginning, the client and I work together as a team to explore his fears of getting stuck on certain sounds and words, as well as fears of situations that have been humiliating to him in the past. We also work to uncover feelings of shame and inadequacy that years of stuttering have spawned. Even after many therapy sessions, these negative emotions and attitudes will rise up again as we transfer his newly learned tools of stuttering management to the outside world. Our direct work on feelings and attitudes, combined with his successes in feeling some control over his stuttering, reduces these negative emotions. This change is critical if our clients are to break free of morbid self-consciousness and be able to focus on the back-and-forth of good communication.

I believe that the clinician's major weapon for attacking negative emotions is *extinction*. As I described in Chapters 5 and 6, classical conditioning has linked many stuttering stimuli to negative emotions, and extinction will affect that link. For example, when an individual sees an upcoming "bugaboo" word (like his name, when he anticipates introducing himself), he dreads it. But when he is accompanied in this situation by a supportive clinician whom he trusts, and the clinician has taught him to use a tool that helps him stutter more fluently, he may feel substantially less dread. He knows the clinician is right there by his side and will accept him no matter what happens. He knows the clinician will praise him for even going into the situation and will applaud him for just trying to stutter more fluently. Thus, the link weakens. When this happens again and again—when he experiences a situation that has previously been humiliating but is now followed by a feeling of pride—he is more and more likely to not anticipate disaster when introducing himself.

You can see from this example that the client-clinician relationship is key. I think that when the client learns that the clinician is strong and knowledgeable, and that she has his best interest at heart, the client can move mountains, or at least he can learn to stutter more easily, both in the therapy room and outside, both for now and for the long term.

Maintenance Procedures

Despite its important role in therapy, it is clear from research that extinction of fear responses is vulnerable to "spontaneous recovery" (Bouton, 2016). Thus, maintenance procedures are vital to keep old tension, struggle, escape, and avoidance responses from returning under stress and with the passage of time. Effective maintenance depends, in part, on clients becoming their own clinicians, which should begin early in therapy. Clients learn to evaluate their own performance in mastering the skill of stuttering more easily and to monitor their fears and avoidances. I gradually shift more and more of the responsibility for therapy planning to clients as they improve, and it is important for them to have a realistic understanding of what they should expect in terms of their long-term fluency. Thus, clients need to understand the purpose of going right into the stutter and **staying in the stutter** until negative emotion and tension are reduced and then finishing the word slowly and easily. In this way, an easy stutter is reinforced by the relief of completing the utterance and the pride in controlling what had been uncontrollable before. It is also important that clients appreciate the relationship between conscientious practice of what they have learned in therapy and the attainment of their fluency goals.

Clinical Methods

Like the approach described for intermediate stuttering with school-age children, my management for advanced stuttering in adolescents and adults begins with exploring behaviors, cognitions, and emotions to decrease negative emotion associated with stuttering. My clinical relationship with the client is paramount in helping the client get in touch with his feelings and accept them. We work together on his emotional responses—particularly those that started in his childhood and are still strong. When the time is right, I teach the client to go right into the stuckness of the stutter and learn to tolerate the moment of stuttering to reduce the fear, and to finish easily. Then, I help the individual transfer and stabilize those skills with hierarchies of more and more challenging situations, voluntary stuttering, and seeking out feared words and feared situations. The measures I use to assess progress will be described shortly.

Clinical Procedures: Reducing Fear and Learning to Stutter More Easily

Procedures described here for working with advanced stuttering in adolescents and adults borrow liberally from many clinicians, especially my own therapist, Charles Van Riper (1973). I am also indebted to numerous colleagues in the field, as well as to my students and clients who have generously shared their ideas.

Key Concepts

1. *Treatment of adolescents and adults usually takes a long time, demands considerable motivation, and must maintain a focus on many fronts.* As you may remember from Chapters 11 and 12, treatment of preschool children can be as brief as a few months. But the older individual has been stuttering for many years, and much maladaptive learning has taken place. Therefore, as you will see, my approach has many stages, each subsequent stage building on the former and requiring continuing hard work on changing behaviors and emotions. There are exceptions; some clients are so ready to change and so emotionally robust that treatment feels like sailing with the wind at your back.
2. *Treatment should be tailored to each client's needs.* Although it would be easier if one sequence of treatment fit all clients, stuttering therapy is not so simple. Each person's biological makeup and life experiences differ; therefore, individuals require different therapy ingredients in the overall recipe for their success. Of the procedures presented in this section, *going directly into the stutter without avoidance, staying in the stutter, and releasing it slowly and loosely* are the heart of changing stuttering. But in order for it to work, the client must not be hampered by an overwhelming fear of stuttering and fear of listener reaction.

   To deal with these fears, most clients will need to confront, explore, and accept their stuttering with the clinician's support. However, individuals with mild stuttering who are not uncomfortable with their stuttering and who talk freely and easily with all types of listeners may not need to deal with reducing negative emotions as much. They may benefit from starting with fluency skills—which are described after the sections on exploring stuttering and achieving mastery of staying in the stutter, with their accompanying work on feelings.

   A clinician just learning how to carry out stuttering therapy may want to go through each step of treatment just as I have described them. An experienced clinician may want to reorder the steps to suit the client or may omit steps he believes the client doesn't need or add new steps of his own.
3. *Successful outcome of treatment depends, in part, on increasing approach behaviors and reducing avoidance.* Evidence from treatment outcome research suggests that successful long-term outcome is associated with positive communication attitudes and low levels of avoidance (e.g., Guitar, 1976; Guitar & Bass, 1978; Langevin et al., 2006). Work on attitudes, negative emotions, and avoidances takes two forms in an integrated approach to therapy.

   First, direct work on decreasing fear and avoidance can be effective in reducing stuttering (Van Riper, 1958). Neurophysiologically, the emphasis on approach activities may "kindle" emotional regulation by the left hemisphere, which, in turn, may "dampen" the avoidance and fear responses regulated by the right hemisphere (Davidson, 1984; Kinsbourne, 1989; Kinsbourne & Bemporad, 1984).

   Second, confronting stuttering by going right into the stutter, staying there with an attitude that reduces fear, and finishing the word slowly and loosely will positively affect attitudes and emotions through repeated experiences of feeling in control in situations where feelings of helplessness previously prevailed.
4. *Adults who stutter may continue to have speech-processing deficits after treatment and may need to continue to compensate for them.* Brain imaging research suggests that even after successful treatment, adults who stutter are likely to continue to show abnormally low activity in left-brain regions that are highly active for speech processing in nonstutterers (Ingham, Ingham, Euler, & Neumann, 2017; Neumann et al., 2003). Thus, the treatment program described in the following pages includes provisions for dealing with residual stuttering through long-term work on managing stuttering as well as work on new responses

to residual stuttering in a way that is comfortable for both the speaker and listener and thus doesn't interfere with communication.

5. *Measurements of progress and outcome are important.* I use two principal measures of behavioral change in treatment. As I noted in Chapter 8, "Preliminaries to Assessment," percentage of syllables stuttered (%SS) provides a useful measure of the frequency of stuttering for snapshots of progress during treatment. Frequency of stuttering is particularly handy for assessing audio-recorded samples of speech made outside of the therapy setting. At the termination of formal treatment and later, I use the SSI-4 (Riley, 2009) to assess overall severity of stuttering.

To assess a client's progress and outcome in terms of his feelings and attitudes about communication, I use the Modified Erickson Scale of Communication Attitudes (S-24), which was also described in Chapter 8. This measure has been adapted for repeated use and has been shown to be predictive of treatment outcomes (Andrews & Craig, 1988; Andrews & Cutler, 1974; Guitar & Bass, 1978). I use this measure before beginning the "Maintaining Improvement" stage of treatment so that I can assess the extent to which a client has generalized positive feelings and attitudes about communication situations. If a client shows more negative attitudes than the average normal speaker, it is a cue to continue working on approach behaviors and ensure that he has mastered the use of high-quality stuttering in all situations. Evidence for the validity and reliability of these measures can be found in Chapter 8. Recently, I have added to my assessment armamentarium the OASES-A (Yaruss & Quesal, 2016) to evaluate a client's perceptions of and his reactions to his stuttering, as well as how stuttering affects his quality of life.

Beginning Therapy

There are several issues I deal with in the first therapy sessions. The first is to understand what treatment goals the client has. The form "Personal Aims for Stuttering Treatment" (Fig. 8.1) gives me a glimpse of the client's initial hopes for what he can achieve in treatment. Frequently, we have discussed this in a preliminary way during the evaluation, but once treatment actually gets under way, it is important to revisit this topic and to clarify for both the client as well as the clinician what they are working toward. During this discussion, I bring up the options of spontaneous fluency versus a feeling of control of stuttering. I also discuss how important it is for him to communicate easily in various situations. In this discussion, we talk about various situations in his life that are likely to be affected by stuttering, and we explore what level of fluency is important in each of them. We look for situations in which the client is satisfied with his fluency and discuss what his speech is like at such times. We try to find levels of stuttering or fluency that would be good targets to shoot for.

A second issue the client and I deal with early on is to make a map of a possible course of treatment. Mindful of what the client's aims are, I provide brief descriptions of the stages of treatment we can go through, matching treatment to the client's present situation and his desires for improvement. The general plan I would describe is first for the client to get to know what he does when he stutters, including his behaviors, his thoughts, and feelings about his stuttering, and his listeners' possible reactions. I let him know that the next steps involve the confrontation of his stuttering with the aim of changing it to an easier form that would feel in control. Gradually, working more independently, he would seek out formerly feared words and situations and replace his old avoidance behaviors with a more assertive attitude and a more confident, more relaxed approach to those stutters that remain. Finally, in the later stages of treatment, I would help him work out a plan to use his new easier stuttering in more and more situations and to gradually become his own clinician so that he can diagnose and repair his speech if stuttering creeps back in.

Exploring and Changing Stuttering

The aim of this first phase of treatment is to help the client become more objective about his stuttering and to lift the clouds of dread and mystery that surround it. Objectivity is fostered through step-by-step procedures that help the client learn about his pattern of stuttering behaviors—what he does and why. As we do this together, it is my goal to begin to help him change how he feels about his stuttering as he sees it more objectively and feels more accepting of it via the clinician's acceptance, support, and encouragement. The clinician should keep in mind that as important as the steps are, the relationship with the client is even more important. As I've said before, the client must experience the clinician as accepting, but at the same time confident in the client's ability to change. Thus, the clinician shouldn't be afraid to challenge the client to try new ways of thinking and behaving. As this process goes on, the client becomes more optimistic. He realizes that stuttering consists of behaviors that he can control, and he feels supported by the clinician's belief in his ability to change.

Steps in the exploration process are outlined in Table 14.1.

Understanding Stuttering

The goals of this step are for clients to understand the rationale for exploring their stuttering and to become partners in planning therapy. I begin by giving clients a handout on Understanding Your Stuttering (see the box below).

As we discuss his stuttering, I find out from a client about other domains that he's worked on previously and improved, like skiing, painting, golf, photography, or anything else that required a positive attitude and practice. We discuss how

TABLE 14.1 Steps in Exploring and Changing Stuttering

Step	Activities	Goals
Understanding stuttering	Provide handout and discuss the elements of the client's stuttering with him. Clinician shows deep acceptance of client as he is now and shares the perspective that there is a logic behind what the client currently does in his core, escape, and avoidance behaviors.	To gain an understanding what has been mysterious and scary; beginning of desensitization
Approaching, exploring, and changing stuttering in the treatment room	Clinician and client examine client's stuttering behaviors. They then catch and hold stutters. Clinician showers client with positive feedback as he stays in a stutter and learns to feel what he's doing physically when he stutters. Clinician coaches client to feel tension reduce until the word can be completed. Via the clinician's modeling and coaching, client learns to end stutter slowly and loosely.	Continuing desensitization. Beginning of learning to modify stutters
Approaching and exploring stuttering outside of the treatment room	Client and clinician observe stuttering and client's reactions to it outside the clinic. As the stuttering is studied, client tries to catch, hold, and slowly release stutters outside of the treatment room. Continuing discussion of how client feels about his stuttering. Audio recording by client of his stuttering in various situations followed by discussions with clinicians.	Continuing desensitization. Client learns that he can tolerate his stuttering with more and more listeners. Client learns to stay in stutter until he can reduce tension and finish the word with a feeling of control

Understanding Your Stuttering

We want to better understand your stuttering ourselves, and we want you to do the same. You may not really know what you do or how you feel when you stutter. Because it's unpleasant, you have probably attempted to hide it from yourself as well as from others. Let's begin to explore your stuttering by discussing the following components of the problem. Once you explore and better understand your stuttering, it will lose its mystery, and you will be less uncomfortable with it.

CORE BEHAVIORS

These are the repetitions, prolongations, and blocks (getting completely stuck on a word) that you have; they are the core or heart of the problem. Core behaviors were the first stuttering behaviors you had as a child.

Why do you have these core behaviors? Research suggests that people who stutter may have "timing" problems related to their control of the speech mechanism. For fluent speech to occur, muscle movements involved in breathing, voice production (voice box), and articulation (tongue, lips, jaw) must all be well coordinated. Evidence suggests that people who stutter experience a lack of coordination among these muscle groups during speech. Furthermore, research implies that these physical timing problems are slight, but that they often show up as stuttering when feelings and emotions are strong enough to cause a breakdown in the coordination of the speech mechanism. In therapy, we will teach you techniques to assist you in coping more effectively with these core behaviors.

SECONDARY BEHAVIORS

Secondary behaviors are tricks you use to avoid stuttering or to help you get a word out. They are behaviors you have learned over the years to help you cope with the core behaviors, and they can be unlearned. These behaviors occur more quickly and less consciously than the development of superstitious behaviors, but they are not unrelated (e.g., wearing a lucky shirt). There are different types of secondary behaviors. Which of the following do you use?

Understanding Your Stuttering (continued)

Avoidance Behaviors

The category of avoidance behaviors covers all the things you might do to keep from stuttering. Word and situation avoidances include substituting words, rephrasing sentences, not entering feared speaking situations, and pretending not to know answers. You might also use "postponements," such as pausing before a difficult word or repeating another word or phrase over and over before trying to say a word on which you expect to stutter. Another avoidance trick some people who stutter use is called a "starter." This is when you might say a sound or word quickly just before a difficult word, as in saying "umwould you like to go to a movie?" Hand or body movements might be used in the same way.

Escape Behaviors

These behaviors are things a person who stutters does to get out of a word once he is stuttering, such as a head nod, jaw jerk, or eye blink. You may have developed escape behaviors that are so subtle that you don't notice them anymore. Some of them might be called "disguise behaviors" or "camouflaging" because they are attempts to hide your stuttering as it is happening. These include covering your mouth with your hand or turning your head when you stutter.

FEELINGS AND ATTITUDES

When you began to stutter as a child, you were probably unaware of your stuttering. Because you have been stuttering for many years, however, you may have experienced many frustrating and embarrassing speaking situations. Consequently, if you're like most people who stutter, you have probably acquired some negative feelings and attitudes about your speech. You may feel embarrassed, guilty, fearful, or even angry. Fear is the most common feeling. Individuals who stutter typically fear certain speaking situations and certain sounds or words. What feelings and attitudes do you have regarding your stuttering? As part of your therapy, we will help you reduce these unpleasant feelings and attitudes.

With my help, you will explore and describe the various components of your stuttering problem. Before you can change something, you need to understand what you are changing. And if you can break it down into manageable chunks, you can change it more easily.

emotions and attitudes can get in the way of new learning and may perpetuate old behaviors. I draw an analogy between the skills that the client has worked on and the task before us, which is to learn to modify stuttering and thereby increase fluency. We discuss the idea that if he can learn what he's doing when he stutters, then he may feel more objective and optimistic about his stuttering and be able to change what he's doing and become more fluent. I try to convey the idea, which will be repeated in many forms, that he has learned to speak in an inefficient way that is at least in part influenced by his desire not to stutter. However, despite years of tense and struggled stuttering, he can now learn to replace it with an easy, fluent form of stuttering. This process begins by his **exploring stuttering** and getting to know it and decreasing his understandable tendency to avoid or escape from it. I also discuss that, as with learning other skills, he will need to practice new techniques until they are second nature to him, and even after that.

Approaching, Exploring, and Changing Stuttering in the Treatment Room

The goal is for the client to make the first steps toward approaching his stuttering, rather than backing away from it. I also have the client, when I think he's ready, take the big step of changing how he stutters to make it easier and more fluent. As we begin studying his stuttering, I often use an illustration or model of the speech mechanism to show the client the structures associated with speaking and how they work in fluency and in stuttering. The client needs to learn about the core, escape, and avoidance components of his stuttering and, to some degree, why they occur. The client should also feel that the clinician is genuinely interested in him and in his speech. Because approach behaviors are thought to be regulated by the left hemisphere, they may dampen negative emotions that are right hemisphere based (Davidson, 1984; Kinsbourne, 1989; Kinsbourne & Bemporad, 1984). Hence, these approach activities are meant, in part, to decrease the client's fear of stuttering.

The activities associated with this step involve examining moments of stuttering as they occur in the treatment room. I explain to a client that to begin our work on his stuttering, we will work together to understand and explore what he is doing when he stutters. One of the aims of our work is to reduce the client's fear of stuttering. For years, he has been feeling "trapped" in the stuckness of stutters, helpless and struggling, with little or no reliable way to escape. I explain that he is like most people who stutter; the very act of struggling to escape from stutters increases his muscle tension and consequently the feeling of being stuck. But being able to stop struggling and tolerate his experience of being trapped reduces his

Holding onto the Stutter

The experience of being caught in a moment of stuttering (repetition, prolongation, or block) can be frustrating and scary. When your mouth doesn't do what you want it to, you feel out of control. If it goes on for several seconds or your listener is impatient or anxious, you may feel devastated. As unpleasant as these core behaviors are, you need to increase your tolerance for them to learn that you can experience them without panicking. If you can tolerate them and feel what you are doing in the moment of stuttering, your panic can diminish and the muscle tension can decrease. Instead of avoiding them or hurrying to get out of them, you need to learn to experience them and remain calm so you can change them.

So, how do you learn to remain calm while you're jammed (blocked) in a moment of stuttering? We'll use a technique called "holding onto the stutter" or "staying in the stutter." When you are stuttering and I signal you, I would like you to hold onto that moment of stuttering until I signal you to come out of it. If you are repeating a syllable, I would like you to continue repeating it; if you are prolonging a sound, I would like you to continue prolonging it; and if you are having a block, I would like you to maintain that articulatory posture and try to get or keep airflow or voicing going. While you do this, try to keep looking at me. Keeping eye contact with your listener will increase your "approach" brain activity and decrease fear. It's like the eye contact used by the leader of an animal pack to show that he or she is boss. Here, you are showing the stutter who is boss. You! You may also find that you can gain the sense that the listener (me) is on your side with your continued eye contact—another good thing! By experiencing these core behaviors of repetition, prolongation, and block over and over again while remaining relatively calm or becoming calmer as the stuckness continues, you will find your tolerance for them increasing. You will no longer become fearful at the thought of getting stuck on a word, and you will find the core behaviors becoming more relaxed. That is the key to change.

We will begin by reversing roles—in other words, you will signal me to hold onto a pretend stutter for several seconds when I voluntarily stutter. Then I will have you hold onto one of your real stutters for only a brief period of time, possibly 1 or 2 seconds. That is, when you get caught in a stutter, I will signal you to hold onto that stutter and keep it going, and I'll give a thumbs-up and then signal you to complete the word slowly. While holding onto a repetition, prolongation, or block, you are to try to stay as calm as possible. Just experience the stutter and be as calm and relaxed as you possibly can. As your tolerance increases, I will gradually increase the length of time you are to hold onto your stutters. Eventually, you will hold onto your stutters until the tension and struggle have dissipated and you can end them easily and slowly. This will involve you signaling yourself and me when you begin a stutter and when you will come out of the stutter. I will also have you watch yourself in a mirror as you are holding onto your stutters. Again, just experience your stuttering and try to remain as calm as possible. Remember that after you feel the tension ebb away, finish the word slowly and deliberately.

By experiencing these moments of stuttering over and over again in this manner, you will gradually lose much of your fear of them. You will find yourself feeling more comfortable when you are talking, and you will be talking more fluently. As this happens, you will develop an attitude of wanting to test yourself by taking on more and more situations that have been difficult in the past.

tension and perhaps provides more positive sensory feedback to the brain, allowing him to move forward in speech. I usually try to have the client feel tension at first and then notice that the tension gradually decreases while he's holding the posture and I am coaching him to stay in the sound and then finishing the word.[1] For some clients, this step in therapy is difficult and requires much practice and encouragement. The tension response is probably nonconscious, and reducing the tension is not so much an act of will and effort as it is an emotional "letting go." It may take much experimentation, as well as acceptance and support, when this letting go is hard to come by. If you can get some change in the tension as you encourage the client to temporarily accept the discomfort of the stutter, then spend some time exploring with the client what he did or what he felt or what he thought, as the tension went down.

Progress on this step can be assessed by the client's movement up the hierarchy for this activity. The hierarchy goes from him controlling my pseudostuttering with a hand signal (to give him a model of how to hold a stutter and feel in control while doing it), all the way to him holding onto a stutter for several seconds in a conversation with a friend or stranger while maintaining good eye contact and staying relaxed.

[1]Staying in a stutter but gradually reducing the tension before finishing the word is essentially what Van Riper called a "pullout." At first, emphasis is on staying in the stutter; then, once that is mastered, the client can learn to deliberately reduce tension and finish the word. Van Riper's pullout is a deliberate act of reducing tension, but, for me, staying in a stutter results in a (possibly) nonconscious letting go of tension, as negative emotion subsides.

I use the handout "Holding onto the Stutter" to provide the client the rationale for the activities associated with this step. Or I may just verbally convey the same information.

When I think the client understands the task, I talk about something of interest, such as our self-help group or the overall course of stuttering therapy. I put in some really obvious voluntary stutters that would be easy for me to hold onto, such as voiced continuant consonants like /l/ or /r/. The purpose of this is to model for the client a good example of holding onto a stutter the way I want him to do. If he doesn't immediately signal me to hold onto the stutter, I explain again how he should do that. Then I get back into stuttering, and when he signals, I prolong the sound and continue to maintain the tension I have while staying calm and relaxed. I emphatically praise his catching my stutters because even someone else's voluntary stutters may be hard for a sensitive client to bear. As we go along and discuss my stutters and what I'm doing physically when I stutter, I use a large array of different sounds and I try to stutter in the manner that he does. Then we reverse roles and I show him how to hold on to his stutters.

After I get the client's OK to interrupt him, I ask him to talk about his hobbies, his work, or his school—anything easy for him to talk about. As he talks, I watch for one of his more severe stutters and then signal him to hold onto it. I focus on severe stutters at first because mild stutters may go by so quickly that he cannot hold them as they occur. This process may take some coaching and practice because people who are not trained in our field (most clients) may not understand how to hold onto the exact sound that is being stuttered. Particularly hard are plosives, and the client may need extra coaching to stay right in a /b/ or /p/ that is stuttered (by producing it as the fricative counterpart to those stops), without going on to the next vowel sound. It is important, as you have the client hold onto a stutter, for him to have airflow and/or voicing appropriate for the sound he's stuck on. The clinician's model—when she shows the client how to hold onto a stutter—should demonstrate airflow and/or voicing. This is easier when the sound is a voiced continuant, as I indicated earlier. Plosives, such as /p/, can be held by keeping the lips only slightly in contact and allowing airflow to continue until tension is reduced and the transition into the next sound can be made slowly and loosely. A held-onto /p/ has the sound of air swishing through the lips. The sound /b/ can be held by also keeping the lips only slightly in contact and allowing voicing to happen while the lips vibrate. That sound will be sort of like the buzzing of a bee.

Some clients appear to have tight laryngeal closures as their major form of "stuckness" in a block. They may require a little extra work as you explore with them what they are doing to hold back sound and/or airflow. As they and you explore, they may find that your demonstrated acceptance and support of them during the stutter allows the block to release so that sound or airflow can begin. Remember, the tension in the block is happening because the client is fighting it, trying urgently not to stutter. Your acceptance of his being stuck will allow him to stop fighting it and accept momentarily the stuckness, and then the tension will subside. If necessary, you can help the client discover whether vocal fry (voicing that sounds like something frying in a pan on the stove and actually results from very slow vibrations of the vocal folds) can help get voicing going.

I show genuine interest in the client's stuttering and make observations about it such as "I noticed on that one it looked like you squeezed your vocal folds (or you may want to use the word 'throat' instead) trying to get the word out." I also ask questions like, "Is that how you usually stutter on words that start with 'B?'" As we explore stuttering together, I use my interest and acceptance to begin the process of *desensitization* or reducing the fear associated with stuttering. During this activity, I continue to teach the client about different components of stuttering, including core, escape, and avoidance behaviors, particularly as they apply to the client's stuttering. We have touched on components of his stuttering before, but our continued discussion of them, suffused with my acceptance and even humor about them, helps to drain some of the client's shame about his stuttering. This activity continues at a pace suited to a client's comfort talking about his stuttering. When the client is relatively comfortable examining his stuttering, I may use a mirror to help him explore and confront his stuttering, as depicted with a female client in Figure 14.2.

Another aspect of staying in the stutter is to maintain natural eye contact with the listener when holding onto the stutter. It creates a confident feeling in the speaker himself and enhances the social connection between speaker and listener. It enables the speaker and listener to assess the emotional state of each other. Thus, if the person who stutters maintains a calm demeanor and has natural eye contact with the listener, the listener is usually put at ease and is likely to telegraph that "everything is OK" back to the person stuttering.

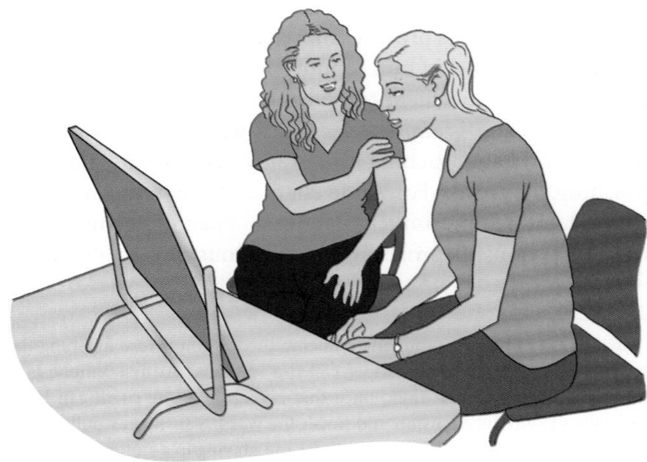

Figure 14.2 Exploring stuttering with the help of a mirror.

Note that while we work on approaching stuttering and exploring it, I am especially pleased when he can follow my instructions to "stay in the stutter."[2] When the client stays in the stutters, he learns that when he can tolerate the "stuckness," and stay in it, his physical tension drains away. This is a key experience. It is the discovery that he himself has the power to control what happens when he stutters.

As indicated earlier, an important sequel of learning to catch and hold onto stutters is to allow physical tension to be released to the point (and beyond) where the stutter becomes unstuck and the word finished. As I mentioned, some clients call this "**catch and release**," the phrase used to describe catching a fish and letting it go. It is not only releasing the block but it is letting go of the fear. Note that the release of the word must be done only after the tension is reduced to normal speech levels. This process involves powerful learning (operant conditioning). The relief felt by the client when he can release and finish the word using a high-quality stutter *reinforces* the reduction of tension to normal levels.

If the client is able to reliably produce high-quality stutters on feared words for a period of days or weeks, these become more automatic. Then, for many clients, because of the operant conditioning—the reinforcement of finishing the word with little tension—the reduction of tension occurs *just as they start* saying the word. Van Riper's term for this, when it is done deliberately, is "preparatory set."

Approaching and Changing Stuttering Outside the Treatment Room

After the client has many experiences in the therapy room "catching" his stutters, holding onto them, feeling what he's doing physically, and describing what he feels he's doing, we make plans to transfer this learning of high-quality stuttering to real-world situations. The client and I build a hierarchy of situations that begin with those that are least threatening. In the beginning, the clinician provides as much support as possible. It helps to emphasize to the client, as he transfers his catch and release strategy to the world outside the treatment room, that he only has this single tool to focus on.

In my experience with my own stuttering and with many clients, I have found that the transfer of high-quality stuttering to the outside world is made easier with the use of voluntary stutters. These are stutters done deliberately, using the familiar prolongation (holding) of the target sound and posture, followed by a slow release of the word. Voluntary stutters will be discussed at length in the next section. Not every client is willing to engage in voluntary stuttering before working on catching and releasing real stutters outside the therapy room. Thus, the clinician decides when and if to teach voluntary stuttering as a tool for transferring high-quality stuttering to a client's everyday life.

Using Voluntary Stuttering

One of the techniques I teach—at first in the treatment room—to prepare the client to transfer of high-quality stuttering to situations outside the therapy room is **voluntary stuttering**, touched upon in the previous section. This can be a very potent procedure for reducing tension and avoidance and thereby facilitating the transfer of catch and release. By using voluntary stuttering, the client is performing an **approach behavior**, which is intended to decrease fear and tension. This makes it more likely that the client will be able to use high-quality stutters successfully. Every clinician should be familiar with voluntary stuttering. The handout that I give to clients in this stage of therapy explains the whys and wherefores of voluntary stuttering.

When I first introduce voluntary stuttering to clients, many think I am crazy. After all, they came to therapy to rid themselves of stuttering, not to do more of it. At this point, I explain the rationale behind voluntary stuttering: stuttering is perpetuated by fear of stuttering, and reducing this fear will reduce the stuttering. An analogy often helps. For instance, suppose a person wanted to overcome a fear of dogs that causes him to freeze and be unable to move when in the presence of a dog. Overcoming the fear could not be done by running away from dogs. Instead, the person would have to begin seeking out contact with dogs with knowledge of how to approach them. The best way to do this would be to have the guidance of someone who was an expert on dogs and was not afraid of them and who would guide the person's contact with dogs in a series of small steps.

For example, the first step might involve only looking at puppies in a pet store; the next step might be talking to a clerk about the puppies. Then, the person might briefly pet a puppy and then perhaps pick up the puppy and hold it for a short period. This process would need to be repeated over and over again with gradually larger and larger dogs. Eventually, the person would learn how to approach a dog in a friendly way. As the person learned how to approach and make friends with dogs, his fear would gradually decrease.

This same process can be followed with stuttering. With your guidance, the client first learns to stutter on purpose with you in the safety of the therapy room and realize that he has nothing to fear. He'll learn that voluntary stuttering frees him from the need to be perfectly fluent and enables him to use easier stutters because he is less tense and no longer feels a need to avoid stuttering. The success of this process depends a great deal on the clinician being comfortable with stuttering. Thus, clinicians need to desensitize themselves to stuttering by practicing voluntary stuttering until the experience of voluntary stuttering and the experience of negative listener reactions do not bother them.

After explaining the rationale behind voluntary stuttering, I teach clients how to stutter voluntarily. First, I model

---

[2]When I ask a client to "stay in the stutter," I am borrowing a technique from the late Dean Williams, who was a master stuttering clinician at the University of Iowa. Dean was able to work temporary miracles by having a client stay in a moment of stuttering, feel what they were doing, and reduce the tension (or the tension just reduced itself). When a client did this, he often became suddenly very fluent.

Using Voluntary Stuttering

One of the most important goals for you to achieve in overcoming your stuttering is to reduce negative feelings associated with it, such as embarrassment, fear, and shame. The more embarrassed you are by your stuttering, the more fearful you are of getting jammed up in a stutter; the more ashamed you are of your stuttering, the more you will try to hide it. The more you try to hide your stuttering, the more tense you will become, and the less you will be able to use easier stuttering. This process needs to be reversed.

One way to reduce these feelings is to stutter voluntarily. If you are afraid of something and run away from it, you will always be afraid of it. The way to overcome fear is to confront it and discover that it's not as bad as you thought. By confronting your fear, you will learn that you are tougher than you think. By stuttering on purpose, first in easy situations and later in more difficult situations, you will learn that you can stutter without fear and shame. Using good eye contact with your listener(s) when you stutter will help you decrease fear and shame and give you a sense of being empowered.

You will begin using voluntary stuttering in the clinic, and I will help you start by putting easy repetitions and prolongations in your speech on nonfeared words. Don't be alarmed if you stutter on some of the words on which you use voluntarily stuttering. This is a common experience. Just keep on stuttering voluntarily until you can finish the word comfortably and without struggling. Ideally, you will voluntarily stutter with your usual amount of abnormal physical tension, but then you should consciously reduce the tension so that it is at a normal level when you finish the word slowly and loosely. We will continue to practice this until you are able to remain calm while voluntarily stuttering here in the clinic.

The next step will involve you going with me into the real world to do voluntary stuttering together. Again, you will use easy stutters released slowly and loosely while talking with strangers on nonfeared words. You may be surprised that most people are accepting of stuttering and will wait for you to say what you want to say. A few may frown or try to finish your sentence for you, but these will be trophies to collect, listeners we can discuss together later. While testing reality in this way, you will learn to tolerate your stuttering and any listener's reactions and to stay cool.

You will also need to use voluntary stuttering in your own environment to reduce your old fears. Old feelings die slowly! However, if you conscientiously do voluntary stuttering sufficiently often over a long period of time, with good eye contact with your listener, you will find your old fears decreasing. You will no longer be hiding your stuttering, you will be able to use high-quality stutters to replace your old, tense struggled stutters, and you will be talking more comfortably and fluently. When you are ready to do voluntary stuttering on your own in your everyday speaking situations, we will work together to help you prepare assignments.

the sort of "catch and release" that we have been working on, remaining calm and relaxed. Then, I encourage the client to attempt some voluntary stuttering on words that he would typically not stutter on, using the catch and release style of easy stuttering. If he comes close, I enthusiastically reinforce his efforts. If he finds this too difficult, however, I do it with him and have him shadow my voluntary stuttering using catch and release. With appropriate modeling and support, most people who stutter are able to do some voluntary stuttering within just one session. I continue giving the client lots of praise for his courage in doing something he may find difficult and am careful to point out that what had been so fearful at first no longer seems so scary.

After the client becomes comfortable using voluntary stuttering with catch and release in the clinic, it is time for him to move out into the world. First, the client and I establish a hierarchy of situations in which he can use voluntary stuttering. The clinician should always go into situations with the client and be the first to use voluntary stuttering during the beginning steps of the hierarchy. I ask him to rate my listeners on a scale that reflects a range of qualities. For example, a "10" might be someone who laughs or looks away, and a "1" might be someone who is attentive and listens patiently, or you could reverse it. The client may want to continue using this rating system when it is his turn to practice voluntarily stuttering as well because it can countercondition old emotions of feeling victimized and helpless. Clearly, when you are in the position of evaluating someone else (in this case, the listener), the power dynamic has changed in favor of the evaluator.

I voluntarily stutter in situations such as asking directions from strangers or getting information from store clerks, and I remain calm as I do it. If all of my listeners are patient and understanding, I ask the client to choose listeners for me whom he feels might be more difficult. After I've completed several of these, it is the client's turn to stutter voluntarily with strangers. We then continue to alternate turns, which provides additional **counterconditioning** as the client and

I compare our ratings of listeners and take turns choosing listeners for each other. In time, a client's feelings of assertiveness and exploration usually increase, which diminishes feelings of fear and avoidance.

I am careful not to allow a client to get in "over his head" with listeners who may be too difficult. I also lavish praise on each of the client's attempts, acknowledging how difficult it can be, and try to be sensitive to how much he wants to discuss each event. After a good workout with store clerks, for example, I may suggest that we take a break for coffee or a soda at a restaurant, where we can practice voluntary stuttering with the server and enjoy the counterconditioning effects of having a snack while doing something that was previously unpleasant.

The client and I continue working together on voluntary stuttering until he feels comfortable. Then he works his way through the rest of the situations in his hierarchy (such as voluntary stuttering with friends and relatives) on his own. He has to continue putting voluntary stuttering into his speech in each situation until his fear subsides before going on to the next situation. I check clients' progress during therapy sessions, commending them when they are successful while supporting, encouraging, and counseling them when they run into problems. Voluntary stuttering is a procedure that clients will continue to use throughout active treatment and maintenance.

Continuing to Transfer High-Quality Stutters to the Outside World

Once I'm satisfied that the client understands and can use voluntary stuttering, I begin transfer by making a phone call to a store to ask what their hours are. If the client is more afraid of making phone calls than face-to-face transfer activities, I might begin with something easier by bringing into the room someone whom the client doesn't know. If the client is OK with phone calls, I can begin with calls to randomly chosen stores. I put in a handful of voluntary stutters, similar to the client's real stutters, but with the catch and release strategy. We discuss my pseudostutters as well as the listener reactions. This works really well if I can do it on a speakerphone so the client can hear how the listener responds. When he's ready, the client makes a phone call and tries to catch his real stutters and release them slowly. Immediately afterward, we discuss his stutters and the listeners' reactions. Many listeners, of course, are patient and even encouraging. A few, who may be confused or anxious, may answer abruptly or even hang up. We celebrate these negative reactions, acting as though they were trophies given for high-quality stutters. This positive way of responding to what could be a negative experience puts a completely different spin on negative listener reactions. These experiences desensitize the client to his own stuttering and to listener reactions.

If a client is having a particularly hard time dealing with less than positive listener reactions, you may want to share with him an interesting video clip of a TED Talk about dealing with rejection.[3] The speaker describes how he desensitized himself to the pain of someone responding negatively to him. This video could lead to a fruitful discussion of listener reactions in which your client could express his feelings about them honestly.

The expressing of feelings is a vital part of therapy. As I work with an adolescent or an adult, I try to attend to the client's emotions so that therapy can keep moving forward. (Perhaps I should better say "lurching forward in fits and starts." *Therapy is rarely simple and predictable, and experienced clinicians know they must tolerate a messy process.*) I discussed dealing with emotions in Chapter 10, and some points are worth repeating. Wherever behavior change is going on, emotions bubble up. Stuttering therapy is no exception. The clinician should expect emotions and even try to elicit them so that she can listen and accept them, just as she accepts the person who stutters and his stuttering. Feelings of frustration, anger toward the self and toward the clinician, and hostility toward listeners are all common. When the client talks about his feelings, sometimes stuttering worsens, but the clinician should just accept whatever stuttering accompanies the expression of feelings, rather than "doing therapy" on the stuttering that comes out when feelings are vented. Not every clinician is a natural in dealing with feelings. It may take consistent reviewing of recordings of therapy sessions for most clinicians to recognize when a client is expressing feelings and to become alert enough to encourage the client to discuss them further. Sometimes emotions come in the disguise of resistance—refusing to work on stuttering outside the therapy room, doing assignments half-heartedly, and other signs of holding back. Such resistance is often a sign that, as Van Riper has pointed out, "the basic disorder is being affected" (Van Riper, 1958). You can often move a client forward, out of this emotional kind of "stuckness," by expressing acceptance of his holding back and letting him know that it's not uncommon for someone who stutters to have times when progress bogs down. It's almost as if his deeply learned habits underlying stuttering are fighting back, trying to preserve themselves. And he must make a determined effort to change them. As we'll see, as assignments move outside of the therapy room, resistance increases and the clinician's support becomes even more important than before.

I usually carry out assignments first, modeling the sort of conversational interaction I have in mind, modeling high-quality stutters. If we are walking outside on a sidewalk, I'll ask someone passing by what time it is or where a certain building or store is. I put in a few voluntary stutters and maintain a calm demeanor with good eye contact. Then the client and I discuss my stutters and the listener reactions. At this point if the client is game, we plan a speaking opportunity

---

[3]You can access the video online at https://ed.ted.com/featured/VdQTGGdx/

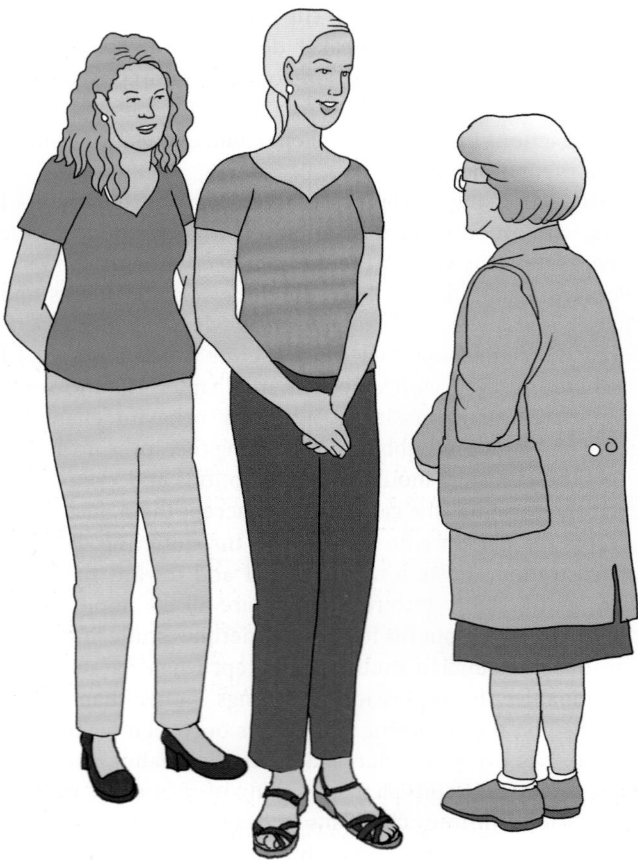

Figure 14.3 Transferring high-quality stutters in conversation with a stranger.

for him. Figure 14.3 illustrates the client using high-quality stutters with a stranger. If he's not game, then I ask him to pick a situation for me to do more stuttering in, and I carry out more voluntary stuttering while he listens and watches. Even if he's only observing, the client usually gains a lot by seeing my calm manner even while having severe (voluntary) stutters and by noticing that most listeners are very patient. If the client continues to resist approaching strangers and difficult situations, his feelings about this should be explored back in the therapy room. When the client is ready—either in this session or a later one—he goes into a planned situation and uses his typical speech, fluent or not. Most often, there will be some natural stutters that we can discuss immediately on the sidewalk or in a store.

When we go into situations outside the clinic together, I use my mobile phone to record our work for further discussion. Any small portable recorder will do. When the client is doing well, we record his stutters and listen to them again, back in the clinic. I always ask listeners if they mind if we record them, explaining what the client and I are working on. This not only makes the recording process very ethical but also promotes openness about stuttering. After we have recorded some of the client's high-quality (real) stuttering, we return to the clinic and listen to the recordings, discussing not only what the client was doing but also how he was feeling. If this goes well, I then ask the client to record some samples of his stuttering at home or at work and write down his observations about his stuttering when he later listens to it and finally shares it with me.

In the next session, when he brings a recording back, I respond enthusiastically. Remember that one goal of treatment is to activate "approach" behaviors and lessen avoidance behaviors. Recording stutters at home or at the office is, indeed, an approach behavior. If a client has been unable to carry out this task, he and I do the task together and record his stuttering in a situation outside the room or on the telephone.

During the sessions in which the client and I analyze his typical stuttering, I also look for stutters that are mild, brief, and forward-moving and call the client's attention to them. I ask the client to look for them in his samples collected outside and in his stuttering in the therapy room. As we attend to these, I let the client know that these are models of how he can learn to handle his stutters. In fact, he can make them more like fluent speech, so that neither he nor his listeners will particularly notice them or hear them as stutters. They will, in fact, become similar to the way persons who don't stutter would handle disruptions in their speech (Boehmler, personal communication, 2004). Another thing to watch for and praise is the client finishing his stutters with greatly reduced tension. In some clients, it happens naturally; in others, it must be practiced and reinforced.

The client and I develop transfer activities that continue to strengthen his approach attitudes and behaviors but that are not beyond his present capacity. He continues to record his stuttering in situations outside the clinic and take notes on listener reactions. It is important to ensure that the client is engaged in therapy activities on days when he is not attending treatment, and it helps if he and I keep in telephone or e-mail contact between treatment sessions. Not every client will stay in touch, but some will do it regularly and others will be in touch intermittently.

Teaching the Client to Evaluate and Reinforce His Behavior

An important component of treatment is helping the client learn to observe, evaluate, and reward (when appropriate) his own behavior. This is vital for generalizing the changes the client is making to his everyday environment, and it should start early in treatment. A chapter by Finn (2007) provides an introduction to this process. Finn describes the process as comprised of several steps:

1. Training the client to observe his behavior. In this stage of treatment, it is recording the stuttering and making notes on listener reactions. The clinician can work with the client in outside situations (with debriefing in the treatment room) to teach him how to carry out this assignment. They can decide together how many times the client should do this between sessions.

2. Training the client to self-evaluate his work. The client and clinician can together evaluate the frequency and quality of the client's recordings and observations of listener reactions.
3. Training the client to reinforce himself when he achieves a targeted goal. For example, he may want to reward himself each time he records his stuttering and take notes on listener responses. The client knows best what would truly be reinforcing, so deciding what to use for reinforcement should be a discussion led by the client. Finn suggests, as many have, that effective rewards are often things that the client is likely to do. Examples are drinking a favorite beverage, eating a favorite food, or taking the time to read a magazine or book. The client might want to give himself an instant reward such as a point or token that is counted toward a total that must be achieved before a tangible reward is collected. I keep myself motivated to run several miles every other day by eating a small pastry smeared with homemade red marmalade, after my run.

Positive reinforcers can be coupled with mild punishments to be most effective. The chapter by Finn (2007) and the references he provides are a rich source of ideas about how to incorporate self-management into treatment. Self-management can be used in each stage of treatment, and this will prepare the client to become his own clinician when treatment is finished.

Increasing Approach Behaviors

Reducing Fear of Listener Reactions

The goal of this step is for the client to continue to reduce avoidance, self-consciousness, and shame about his stuttering through further "approach" activities, such as being open about his stuttering. Until a few years ago, I had clients work on being open about their stuttering much earlier in therapy, but I have found that this is often a difficult step. It has been easier for clients to do this after they have made considerable progress increasing fluency and reducing the severity of their stuttering. The success of these activities can be assessed in terms of reductions in stuttering severity, increases in his speaking in situations that he previously avoided, and reports of greater comfort in talking despite stuttering. This step and the next can be the most difficult part of treatment for many clients, who often require encouragement and support from

Discussing Stuttering Openly

One way to become more comfortable with your stuttering is to discuss it openly with your family, friends, and acquaintances. When you get to the point of being open about your stuttering, you will lose much of your fear of it and be more relaxed. In most cases, your listeners already know you stutter, you know you stutter, but nobody ever says anything about it. It's like having a giraffe in the room and nobody mentioning it. You would feel much more comfortable about your stuttering if you could talk about it openly. Your listener would also be more comfortable if you were open and more accepting of your stuttering. Your listener often takes his cue from you regarding how to respond. If you look uncomfortable, he will probably feel uncomfortable, but if you are open and comfortable with your stuttering, your listener will probably feel at ease.

How can you be more open about your stuttering? Tell family and friends that you are in therapy and explain what you are doing and why you are doing it. After you have talked about it, encourage them to ask you questions about it. Create an opportunity to let them know how you would like them to respond to your stuttering. For example, some of your family and friends may finish words for you when you stutter. If you can, let them know at the appropriate moment that you would rather they wait until you're finished. Or some of your listeners may look away when you stutter. They may think this helps you. If this makes you uncomfortable, as it does most people who stutter, let your listeners know that it is helpful if they will maintain eye contact when you stutter. Some individuals who stutter find it easy to be open about their stuttering by wearing a T-shirt that says something like "Stuttering Rocks! What I have to say is worth repeating." The Stuttering Foundation Web site has a T-shirt that makes stuttering cool.

Another good practice is to make comments about your stuttering. If you feel like it, you can make a funny comment about your stuttering to put yourself and your listeners at ease. For example, if you have to introduce yourself and you think you will stutter on your name, you can say, "Make yourself comfortable, it may take me a few minutes to say my name." One of my friends who stutters says to a listener after he has stuttered when introducing himself, "If I stutter on my name, it's only because the witness protection program just changed it." Or just comment casually on a hard block you've had by saying, "Whew, that was a hard one." The more you do this, the less panicked you will feel when you stutter. Another opportunity for being open about your stuttering is when you are faced with making a speech or presentation to a group. Just before you begin speaking, let the audience know that you stutter. They'll find out anyway, but saying it upfront will put everyone, including yourself, much more at ease.

the clinician. It may help to remind them of where they are in the progression of treatment and to review the rationale for confronting fears associated with their stuttering. It may help even more if the client rewards himself generously after each time he is open about his stuttering.

The major activity of this step involves the client talking to others about his stuttering, which I initiate by giving him a handout on being open about his stuttering.

A few people with advanced stuttering will find these assignments easy, but most will not. I make sure that a client feels he and I are working as a team and that I am supportive and empathetic. I usually help him make lists of the situations in which he will begin to be open about his stuttering and then model an example for him. For example, if commenting on stuttering during a telephone call is on his list, I would call a store, produce a voluntary stutter, and immediately make a comment, such as "Wow, looks like I'm really stuttering more than usual today." Recently, when working with a young man who was quite sensitive and reluctant to talk openly about his stuttering, I had him video record me as I interviewed three different people on a busy shopping street. After getting permission to video record, I asked them a variety of questions about stuttering and found that each gave positive, supportive answers. The young man seemed impressed that the public was, after all, not uptight about stuttering. He then asked to do the next interview and carried it off with great success. Exercises such as this can help clients test reality and find out that much of their anxiety and disapproval about stuttering is in their minds rather than in those of the listeners. However, I prepare clients for the possibility that there will be a negative listener reaction (although this is rare) by expressing the hope that at least one listener will be impatient or rejecting so that we can see if we can retain our calm under stress.

Often, by using a hierarchy of situations, stress can be increased slowly. A client and I plan a hierarchy of tasks in which the client is open about his stuttering. We might go, for example, from a casual comment he might make to a store clerk about having a stuttery day all the way up to telling a group of people that he stutters and sometimes it's better and sometimes it's worse, but it's OK with him. In psychological terms, reductions in negative emotions that are associated with less stressful tasks will generalize to more stressful tasks. Consequently, when a client gets to the more stressful tasks, they will no longer be as difficult.

After the client completes the assignments on his hierarchy, he discusses the outcomes with me. I diligently give him a great deal of praise for confronting his fears and discussing his stuttering openly. At times, I may need to encourage or even push him to move on to the next step; however, I need to be sensitive to the intensity of his feelings so that I don't expect too much too soon. The client needs to feel he is in control of the amount of stress under which he puts himself.

The client will probably never completely finish with this activity because discussing his stuttering openly will always be an important, but perhaps intermittently difficult, strategy for him, not only during therapy but possibly throughout his lifetime. It can help him maintain his improved fluency long after therapy has ended. Thus, I get the client started on his hierarchy and then move on to the next step. Even as he works on other strategies, he will find it valuable to continue to be open about his stuttering. I encourage the client to keep a written record of his progress up this hierarchy so that he may refer to it if, after termination of therapy, he begins to hide his stuttering and old fears creep back in. Using his old records and seeing his old victories may motivate him to try anew to stutter openly, comment on his stutters, and re-establish his freedom to work (or strategically not work) on his stuttering in difficult situations.

Using Feared Words and Entering Feared Situations

Using feared words and entering feared situations are important approach behaviors that help clients continue their progress in managing their stuttering. Some clients will have accomplished a great deal in this area during the transfer of getting directly into the stutter and staying in it until tension is reduced. However, most will benefit from practice in seeking out remaining fears. I use a handout to begin teaching this step and supplement it with examples and discussion.

After the client has read the handout, I answer any questions he may have. I then encourage him to not use any postponements or word avoidances when in therapy from then on. If he does, I have him use a cancellation by redoing the sentence while using high-quality stutters on the word(s). When I think he deliberately uses a word that he appeared to want to avoid, I strongly reinforce this approach behavior. I also set up activities in which the client purposefully has to say feared words that we had previously identified and uses high-quality stutters when producing these words. These activities may involve him reading word lists and text that are loaded with his feared words or involve his composing sentences with these words. I warmly praise him each time he does not postpone or avoid a feared word, especially when he successfully uses high-quality stutters. Sometimes, he may be unable to stutter well and easily—his old habits may have shanghaied him. However, I am accepting of these occasions and let him know that I understand how hard it can be. This will help him become more comfortable saying these words and will reduce his tendency to want to avoid them.

To help the client eliminate his use of avoidances outside the clinic, I assist him in setting up a hierarchy of word and situation avoidances he commonly uses in daily life. Like most hierarchies, it should be sequenced from least to most difficult for the client. By using this strategy, his fears will be kept to a minimum. A typical step in the hierarchy is the client's deliberate use of certain feared words throughout the day. How often should he use these feared words? They have to be used over and over until he no longer wants or needs to avoid them.

Using Feared Words and Entering Feared Situations

An important goal for you to achieve in overcoming your stuttering is to reduce your avoidance of feared words and feared situations. In the past, you have probably changed words that you were sure you would stutter on and have also shied away from people and places that were very difficult for you. The problem in doing this is that avoidance perpetuates stuttering. It also perpetuates further avoidance, reducing your opportunities to communicate. To make real progress in therapy, you will need to change your avoidance mindset to one of approach and begin to seek out words you have stuttered on and situations you have found difficult in the past. These will be opportunities for you to make your controlled fluency stronger and more resistant to stress.

If you have not already developed this habit, you should now begin to approach words and situations that you previously avoided. It may help to use some voluntary or easy stutters on words you don't fear in difficult situations. Even though you may still stutter, the fact that you have an approach attitude will keep you from tensing and holding back as much as you usually do, and you will sometimes be surprised to find that you don't stutter as much as you expected.

This is hard work and very challenging for most people. It is certainly hard for most nonstuttering people who avoid some speaking situations, like talking on the telephone. But try to set yourself reachable goals and reward yourself when you accomplish each one. Buy something for yourself as a treat! Try to stop substituting easier words for harder ones, rephrasing sentences to get around feared words, and pretending you don't know the answer to questions when you really do. Instead of using these sorts of tricks, try to say exactly what you want to say, even if you stutter. If you are afraid you will stutter on a word you are about to say, commit yourself to saying that word, even if you stutter. Even better, of course, would be to use some high-quality stutters (holding onto the stutter and ending slowly). But you can't always do that. It's better to say what you want to say, even if you stutter. In time, you will find your old fears decreasing, and with this decrease in word fears, you will find your word and sound avoidances decreasing and your fluency increasing as well.

From today on, you should try not to avoid talking while in the clinic. In fact, talk as much as you possibly can. If you want to talk about a topic or ask a question, do it. If you think you are going to stutter on a word, go ahead and stutter. In the long run, this is much better than avoiding or postponing. You will learn that you can tolerate your stuttering, will be more comfortable with it, and will gradually become more fluent.

Eliminate your avoidance of feared situations by talking in all of those situations that you avoided in the past. For example, introduce yourself to strangers, start using the telephone more than you usually would, and look for opportunities to speak in groups. If you are aware of any fear of a speaking situation, take that as a sign to approach and enter that situation. Your willingness to speak in these situations will make things much easier for you in the long run. You will find your situation fears decreasing and your wanting to avoid these situations also decreasing; a by-product of this decreased fear will be increased fluency.

In addition to not avoiding speaking in the clinic, you should begin today to eliminate the use of word and situation avoidances in the real world. You will need to develop an approach attitude in your own speaking environment, and I will help you set up a series of outside speaking assignments from least to most fearful to help you overcome your use of avoidances. Now and then, old speech fears will be too strong, and you will use avoidances, but give it a try again the next day. In time, you will find the old fears decreasing and your tolerance for stuttering increasing. You will also be more comfortable with yourself as a speaker and speak more fluently. However, you will need to keep working on this approach attitude for a long time because it is very important that you conquer your avoidances and keep them vanquished.

Another step in the hierarchy has the individual entering situations that he usually avoids in daily life (Fig. 14.4). As before, he needs to enter these situations until he loses his motivation to avoid them. Many of the assignments can be completed as the client goes through his daily routine and will not take any extra time out of his day. For instance, he just needs to answer the telephone whenever it rings with the feared "hello" said using high-quality stutters or introduce himself to a different person each day. Other assignments may have to be created, and he may need to go out of his way to perform them. For example, the client may have to shop for an item whose name contains one of his feared sounds or fabricate reasons for making telephone calls to local businesses. When I was trying to get over my fear of words beginning with the /l/ sound, I went into many stores asking about *l*uggage, *l*ocks, and *l*ampshades.

To help the client get started on an outside hierarchy, it is helpful for me to join him for some of the assignments. Thereafter, he has to complete the assignments by himself and discuss his progress and any problems with me during

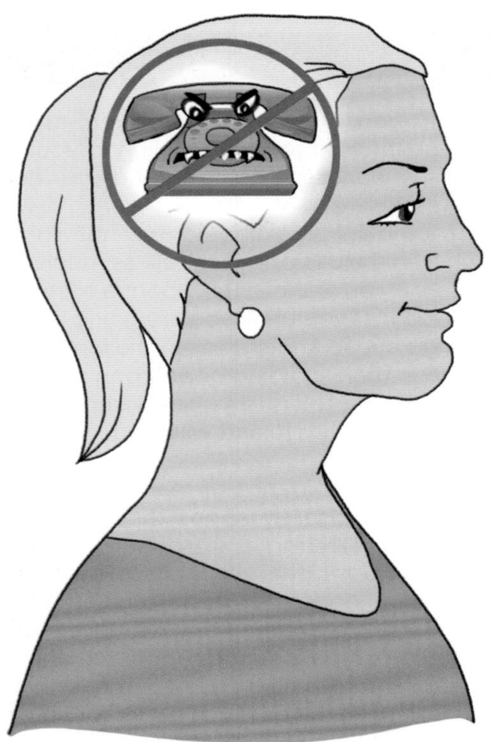

Figure 14.4 The client reduces fear and avoidance by approaching previously feared situations.

regular therapy sessions. I make sure that he keeps on track in completing his hierarchy and provide him with the necessary support and sometimes gentle nudging to help him do so. After the client has worked through as many situations as he and I think are sufficient, it is appropriate for him to complete the Modified Erickson Scale of Communication Attitudes (see Chapter 8). This will give me an indication of whether or not there are still situations that need to be approached and mastered.

Like discussing stuttering openly, eliminating the use of avoidances is a strategy that individuals will need to use throughout therapy and beyond. So, once a client has begun outside assignments successfully, it is time to move on to steps that will create the foundation for long-term change. Self-evaluation and self-reinforcement are crucial elements in a client's learning to decrease avoidance. As described in an earlier section, these behaviors need to be explicitly trained.

Maintaining Improvement

The goal of this last phase of therapy is to help clients generalize their improvement—that is, transferring their reduced negative feelings, attitudes, avoidances, and increased fluency to all remaining speaking situations and maintaining this improvement following termination of therapy. I introduce the following procedures during this phase: (1) **becoming your own clinician** and (2) establishing long-term fluency goals.

Becoming Your Own Clinician

If clients with advanced stuttering are going to generalize improvement to all speaking situations and maintain this improvement, I believe that they must assume responsibility for their own therapy. The literature on self-management provides helpful guidance for fostering this transition. The article "Self-Regulation and the Management of Stuttering" (Finn, 2003) is a good example. Finn points out that having clients set their own goals is a key element of success. I would also highlight the importance of teaching clients to formulate their own plans that target specific behaviors for specific changes. An article in *Time* (Ripley, 2005, 2008) on surviving disasters suggests that survivors of September 11 and other catastrophes often had developed a plan of action beforehand so that they were not affected by the common human response to unexpected stress—"freezing" or being unable to move. Plans made by clients before stressful situations arise will help them take action when they have opportunities to use catch and release and other strategies that will help them stutter more easily and feel in control of their speech.

I use the handout on "Becoming Your Own Clinician" shown in the box below to help clients learn how to combat avoidance and continue improving their fluency skills.

By this time, a client is probably getting close to completing his everyday speaking situation hierarchy. I point out to him, however, that completing this hierarchy is not enough and that he needs to pursue any other situations that are still giving him trouble. I ask him the following kinds of questions: Is he avoiding talking in any more situations? Is he still unduly afraid while talking in some situations? Is he unable to successfully use high-quality easy stuttering when anticipating stuttering in some situations? Is he hesitant to use voluntary stuttering in some situations?

If the client is still avoiding some situations, I remind him of the importance of using feared words and entering feared situations. It will also help him to prepare to be open about his stuttering in feared situations. I may have him reread the handout and then prepare assignments to overcome his current avoidances. I try not to assume any more responsibility than is necessary. I try to ask helpful questions but want him to figure out on his own what he needs to do. As time goes on, I will gradually have the client assuming more and more responsibility for planning his own assignments.

If he is having difficulties using high-quality stutters to replace his old tense stutters that he still pushes through too quickly in some situations, I explore the nature of his difficulties with him and help him determine what types of assignments he needs to work on to be successful. Maybe he needs more practice in some less difficult situations before he can reasonably expect to be successful in the more difficult situations. Perhaps he needs to further reduce his speech rate and

Becoming Your Own Clinician

Now that we have covered all the therapy techniques you will need to meet your therapy goals, it is time for you to become your own clinician. Although you have improved your fluency and reduced your emotional reactions to stuttering, you will probably still encounter some situations that will give you trouble. Thus, you will need to learn how to handle these situations as well as maintain the fluency you have gained.

Handling the difficult situations that remain will require you to be honest about where you think you may still stutter and what your fears are. Fear doesn't stand still; if you ignore it, it will grow, but if you pursue it, it will die. Therefore, you must be vigilant for words and situations that continue to spark fear in you and make you feel as if you won't be able to handle your speech the way you want. For these words and situations, you must be ready to use your techniques to work on these fears, techniques such as high-quality stuttering when you anticipate stuttering, openness about your stuttering, and voluntary stuttering. Up to this point, we have worked together to develop and carry out such plans, but now you will have to take more and more responsibility for them.

Working on feared words and situations is not limited to your initial course of therapy. It also involves maintaining the level of fluency you have now because adults who stutter often relapse or slip back somewhat after they leave therapy. Relapse is not inevitable, but neither is it surprising. After all, you have had years of practice in stuttering. In fact, you are an expert. You have avoided words and situations for a long time, and your negative feelings and attitudes about your speech are well learned. Because stuttering is deeply etched into your brain, you may always have some core behaviors and will need to cope successfully with them. Therefore, you need to become your own speech clinician. You will have to keep applying—on your own and long after you leave therapy—the techniques you have learned in therapy.

So, what is involved in being your own clinician? You will need to learn to give yourself assignments to overcome remaining difficult speaking situations and any new ones that crop up. If you still avoid speaking in a certain situation, you will need to design assignments that will eliminate this avoidance. If you are still fearful while talking in some situations, you will need to undertake assignments to reduce this fear. If you are still stuttering a lot in a given situation, you will need to plan assignments that will improve your fluency in this situation. At the beginning of therapy, I helped you create these assignments, but as you improved, more and more of the responsibility was turned over to you. We will continue to do this. With additional practice, you will be able to determine your therapy needs and to develop assignments to meet these needs. When you can do this, you will have become your own speech clinician.

I have found the following approach is effective in meeting this goal. Every day, you need to work on reducing any remaining speech fears and eliminating any remaining avoidances. For example, if you still feel fearful while talking in a certain situation, you could give yourself a daily quota of tasks to perform in that situation, including being open about your stuttering and using high-quality voluntary stutters in your fluent speech and when you find yourself stuttering. Every day, you will also need to work on improving your fluency. If you are still doing a lot of stuttering in a given situation, you could set a daily quota of talking time in that situation during which you will use controlled fluency. These are only examples; the important thing is for you to ask yourself every day which situations are still giving you problems and to give yourself assignments designed to overcome these problems. Now, let's get started in helping you become your own speech clinician.

muscle tension in these difficult situations so that his motor control does not break down as readily. I have found that some clients strive to be as fluent as possible in all situations; however, others are happy with some residual stuttering if it doesn't interfere with their communication. I am accepting of this because I realize that clients must set their own goals. During all of our discussions, I try to keep in mind that my goal is to help the client become independent. So, I gradually become less directive and gradually turn the responsibility for his assignments over to him. Throughout this phase of therapy, the client should be working daily on outside assignments and discussing his progress with me during therapy sessions. During this same period, I am more and more of a consultant, helping the client feel that he can go out and fly on his own.

Establishing Long-Term Fluency Goals

Before therapy ends, it is very important for a client to be aware of what he can expect in terms of fluency after termination from therapy. By having realistic goals, he can substantially decrease the possibility of becoming disappointed and frustrated with his speech and not developing feelings that may lead to relapse. To begin this topic, I share with him the handout on long-term therapy goals shown in the box below.

I make sure that the client understands the concepts of spontaneous fluency, high-quality easy stuttering, and

Establishing Long-Term Fluency Goals

You are at the point in your therapy when you need to consider your long-term fluency goals. Before you do this, I need to define three of the terms we will be using: "spontaneous fluency," "high-quality stuttering," and "acceptable stuttering."

Spontaneous fluency refers to speech that contains no more than occasional disfluencies, and there is no tension or struggle. This fluency is not maintained by paying attention to or controlling your speech. Therefore, you don't use controlled fluency to be fluent. You just talk and pay attention to your ideas. It is the fluency of normal speakers.

High-quality stuttering is done by going right into the word you might stutter on, holding onto the stutter while keeping good eye contact with your listener, and ending the word slowly and loosely.

Acceptable stuttering refers to speech that contains noticeable but mild stuttering that feels comfortable to you. You are not avoiding words or situations, and you feel OK about yourself as someone who stutters at times. You may have acceptable stuttering when you don't care about working on your speech. Or you may have it when you are trying to use high-quality stuttering but can't quite get a handle on it. It's healthy to feel OK about the occasional mild stuttering you have in either case.

Now, let's consider long-term fluency goals. A few adults who stutter become spontaneously fluent in all speaking situations on a consistent basis. They become normal speakers. In my experience, however, most adults who stutter do not reach this goal. Instead, they have situations, such as talking to close friends, in which they are spontaneously fluent. In other situations, such as speaking in groups, their stuttering tends to give them trouble. In these troublesome situations, I think it is important for these individuals—and possibly you—to have the following options.

First, *if* it is important to you to come over as confident in a specific situation, I want you to be able to use your high-quality stuttering. I know this is possible in most situations, especially if you have been "putting money in the bank" by practicing high-quality stuttering in your fluent speech. I also know that there will be some situations in which you will not be totally successful. In such situations, I want you to feel comfortable with acceptable stuttering.

Second, if it is *not* important to you to sound fluent in a situation, and you do not want to put the effort into using high-quality stuttering, I would like you to feel comfortable with acceptable stuttering.

These options or goals are both realistic and acceptable. In other words, you don't have to sound perfectly "in control" all the time or work on your speech constantly. Indeed, attempting to sound in control all the time can become burdensome. Where are you now with regard to these fluency goals? Are you satisfied with your present fluency? Where would you like to be in the future with regard to these goals? We should discuss these issues, and you should begin to make plans based on your answers.

acceptable stuttering. When I am convinced that he understands what is meant by these terms, I explore with him the types of fluency he currently has in various, everyday speaking situations. If he is unsure of whether he has achieved the levels of fluency he wants in various situations, he gives himself assignments to help him find out whether or not he is satisfied with the types of fluency he has in these situations. If he is satisfied, then he has met his goals, and the end of therapy is near. He can continue working along the lines discussed in the previous section on "Becoming Your Own Clinician."

I have observed a couple of problems that can occur with clients' fluency expectations or goals. First, many clients experience a great deal of spontaneous fluency at this point in therapy. They expect and want this spontaneous fluency to last forever without any effort on their part. It can last, but that will require continued work. A client will need to continue giving himself assignments—or push himself, as he encounters old fears—to keep his negative feelings and attitudes at a minimum and to extinguish his avoidance behaviors. He will also need to continue working on his easy stuttering so that he has confidence in his ability to use it when he chooses. Spontaneous fluency will be a by-product of these efforts, and I must help the client understand this. If he doesn't understand, he will be disappointed and possibly panicked when he begins to lose some of his spontaneous fluency, which could lead to relapse.

A second problem that can occur late in therapy involves clients with more severe advanced stuttering. These clients often fail to achieve a great deal of spontaneous fluency. If they are going to talk better, they need to use easy stuttering constantly and to have it kick in almost automatically. Even then, they often achieve only acceptable stuttering, which can be discouraging to them. It may be too much of a burden for them to constantly monitor and modify their speech. In time, they will become tired and give up doing anything at all, with relapse soon following. I need to help these clients accept and become comfortable with their stuttering as it is and be open about it. I also need to help them realize that they will need to expend effort to maintain this level of fluency. Clients with severe advanced stuttering may benefit especially from the support provided by a self-help group to help them maintain the motivation needed for continued self-therapy (Trichon & Raj, 2018; Yaruss, Quesal, & Reeves, 2007).

Once a client feels he is meeting his fluency goals and has become his own clinician, the frequency of his therapy contacts can be systematically reduced. I typically fade contacts to once a week for a month or two, then to once a month for several months, and finally to once a semester for 2 years. This gradual transition provides the client with some continued support. For example, if he is doing well, I reinforce his feelings, and if he is having a few problems, I can help him find solutions. Of course, if he has relapsed completely, he can re-enroll in therapy. Ultimately, as I say "goodbye," when we formally discontinue therapy, I commend him for all his hard work and let him know that if he ever needs me again, I am available to him.

Throughout the fading process, I assess his speech using the SSI-4 for samples gathered in the clinic on video and percent syllables stuttered for the samples he brings me from outside situations. I also use such measures as the OASES-A, the Erickson S-24, and the Stutterer's Self-Rating of Reactions to Speech Situations, which are presented in Chapter 8. The process of us mutually analyzing the client's fluency and working on areas that need further practice helps to keep him focused on using high-quality easy stuttering. It also increases the chances that he will become largely spontaneously fluent and his easy stuttering will become more and more automatic.

Clinical Procedures: Learning and Generalizing Controlled Fluency

This section is not meant for most clients, but for those rare clients who come to us with little fear of stuttering and good social-conversational skills. It describes the procedures to teach an adolescent or adult how to use a different speech pattern (prolonged speech) to generate fluency, which is then shaped to sound like normal speech and transferred to everyday life. If you are convinced that negative emotions and attitudes are not a problem for a client, you may want to try using "**controlled fluency**" with them. In my experience, an intensive period of therapy (e.g., 4–6 hours/day for several days in a row) can be a good way to teach controlled fluency skills and begin generalization.

An example of the effectiveness of teaching controlled fluency to selected clients comes to mind. I recently had a "reunion lunch" with a client I had not seen for more than 30 years. I'll refer to her as "Jean" although that's not her real name. Jean came to our university clinic for treatment for her severe stuttering, saying that she had recently undergone hypnotherapy that regressed her back to her childhood. In her hypnotherapy sessions, she learned about the circumstances surrounding the onset of her stuttering at age 5; however, that knowledge didn't change her speech. She continued to stutter as severely as ever and now wanted to manage her stuttering because it was interfering with her work and her social life. She seemed, to us, to be well adjusted, she had a good job with the state highway department as the only female draftsperson, and she drove a motorcycle for her transportation. My student clinicians and I used delayed auditory feedback (DAF) to teach Jean to speak very slowly and fluently during the course of 6 hours in 1 day. Jean came back the next day, speaking fluently but slowly. We then worked with her for another 6 hours to shape her fluency so that she sounded like a typical speaker, although her speech sounded a little precise and careful. That was at the end of the day on a Friday. We asked her to return to our clinic after the weekend, and we warned her that much of her stuttering would probably have come back by then, and we would work on that.

On Monday, Jean reappeared, saying that she was essentially fluent and many of her friends had commented on it. We just spent an hour or so reviewing her success and reinforcing her fluency. Subsequently, we saw her intermittently over the next 6 months and she continued to maintain her fluency. She moved out of state and married, but visited us 2 years later, demonstrating continued fluency. I lost touch with her after that, for 30 years, but saw her recently when she visited family in Vermont. She told me that those 2 days of therapy had changed her life and although she occasionally had a stutter or two, it was not an issue for her and she was able to speak well and easily in all situations. I think her success was at least in part due to her easygoing temperament and her lack of significant negative emotions associated with her stuttering even when she stuttered severely throughout her school years and on her job afterward, until she received our therapy.

Learning Controlled Fluency

The goal of these procedures is to have clients learn a controlled type of fluency to replace their stuttering. As a client works on controlled fluency, progress is assessed in the clinic by the clinician's judgment of whether the client can successfully produce speech with each of the components described in the following sections and whether he can use the components together in conversational speech that sounds natural. The fluency skills learned in this step are the same as those used with intermediate-level stuttering, but for the sake of review, I have outlined them in Table 14.2.

Once a client seems to have acquired the necessary **proprioception** skill, it can be combined with **flexible rate**, **pausing**, **easy onsets**, and **light contacts** into an overall style of speaking sometimes called "prolonged speech" or "smooth speech." I refer to this combination as "controlled fluency," which means the same as the term "superfluency," which I used in the chapter on treatment of intermediate stuttering. The clinician should feel free to use whichever term resonates with the individual client. When the client is first using this style of speaking, it requires concentration, which may activate left-hemisphere speech centers (De Nil et al., 2003).

TABLE 14.2 Fluency Skills

Fluency Skill*	Description
Flexible rate	Flexible rate is simply slowing down productions of a syllable, most commonly the first and second phonemes of a word (Boehmler, personal communication, 2003). Slowing is thought to be effective in reducing stuttering by allowing more time for the components of speech production to occur.
Pausing	Inserting brief pauses at grammatical junctures or before an important word or phrase. Pauses may reduce physical tension and allow more time for linguistic processing. Good examples can be heard in the audio recording of Winston Churchill's "Their Finest Hour" speech (http://www.youtube.com/watch?v=G4BVzYGeFOM).
Easy onsets	Easy or gentle onset of voicing. This seems to prevent stuttering by not allowing the speaker to close his vocal folds tightly before trying to start airflow through the glottis, as individuals who stutter often do.
Light contacts	Producing sounds by making articulatory contacts very gently or not fully making the contact. For example, a /k/ would be produced as a continuant rather than as a plosive by not completely constricting airflow. This may reduce the likelihood of a stutter because the speaker is not able to tightly squeeze one articulator against another.
Proprioception	Conscious attention to the movements of the articulators. May be taught by first having the client block out the auditory system using masking or talking at a normal speed while under delayed auditory feedback.† Then the client can learn to attend to proprioception without using any external stimulus.

*Skills that the client can use all together to produce more fluent speech. The client can also use only some of them depending on what suits him.
†You can turn your iPad or iPhone into a delayed auditory feedback (DAF) device by buying an app for under $20 from speech4good.com. Teach proprioception by having the client speak under DAF and try to "beat" the delay by attempting to talk at a normal rate, ignoring auditory feedback and just attending to the feeling of movement from his articulators (proprioception).

Transferring Controlled Fluency into Fluent Speech

The goal of this step is for clients to learn to use controlled fluency in their normally fluent speech to "put money in the bank," as Van Riper used to say. Thus, if a client can use the careful, deliberate style of speech that I call controlled fluency in his normally fluent utterances, he will benefit greatly from the practice. This will improve his chances that when he anticipates stuttering, he can call upon controlled fluency, and it will work for him. He may not always turn a stutter into a fluent utterance, but he may be able to produce the stutter with a feeling of being in control.

Once clients have mastered controlled fluency, they don't need to use it for the entire sentence. Using controlled fluency on the first word of a sentence or on a word within a sentence can be another way to keep this tool sharp. Some of my clients call these single-word uses of controlled fluency "slide-outs." Other clients and my graduate students refer to them as "slides," a term coined by Vivian Sheehan (personal communication, November 1999). Clients should be encouraged to develop their own names for the techniques they find helpful.

Assessing progress on this step is a matter of designing a hierarchy of speaking contexts in which controlled fluency can be used to replace normal speech and measuring a client's progress ascending the hierarchy. When I use the term "normally fluent" speech, I am not referring to perfect speech, which is not the goal of treatment, but to speech like that of people who don't stutter, which contains its share of normal disfluencies (e.g., whole-word and phrase repetitions) that the speaker handles easily.

To begin, the client and I design a hierarchy of speaking contexts that progresses from using controlled fluency on single syllables at the beginnings of sentences to using controlled fluency on various syllables in other sentence positions. It is important to remember that this is done only on words on which the client expects to be fluent. We start with conversations between ourselves in the treatment room and progress to outside speaking situations in which the client expects to be fluent. These may include simple telephone conversations in which the client asks what time a store closes, asking questions of store clerks, and stopping unfamiliar people on the street and asking them questions. The client and I then jointly design more transfer activities for a variety of natural situations in his life. At least some of these speaking opportunities should be audio recorded so that we can evaluate the quality of his controlled fluency outside the treatment situation.

One way to help the client practice controlled fluency on words in his normal speech is to help him set up a quota to meet by noon of every day. He should develop a tallying system, such as using a wrist counter like those used by golfers to tally strokes or carrying a box of 20 Tic Tacs® or other small candies and eating one for each word produced with controlled fluency on the first syllable. For my own self-therapy, I preferred to use a golf stroke counter because its noticeable presence on my wrist reminds me to practice controlled fluency on the initial syllables of many sentences throughout the day. Alternatively, I can set the alarm on my wristwatch (or smartphone) to chime once an hour to remind me.

Replacing Stuttering with Controlled Fluency in the Treatment Room

In this step, the goal is for clients to learn to use controlled fluency in response to old stimuli that were followed by stuttering. This means that the client needs to learn to use controlled fluency when he anticipates stuttering and before he finds himself stuck in a block. With lots of practice and success in many situations, he will develop confidence in his ability to speak with controlled fluency instead of stuttering. In time, he will learn to do it in such a way that his controlled fluency becomes more or less indistinguishable from normal fluency for both listeners and the speaker. Progress is assessed by measuring the frequency of stuttering in various situations.

I begin by having a client replace stuttering with controlled fluency during conversation in the treatment room. If he has practiced using controlled fluency in his natural speech, he knows what it feels and sounds like and has started to "groove" it. As a client begins to use controlled fluency to replace stuttering, he may benefit by looking in a mirror as he converses with me, watching for upcoming stutters, and focusing on what he is doing as he starts to respond. Then, as he works to use controlled fluency to replace anticipated stutters, the mirror helps him to monitor his speech in a more focused way. If a client has trouble "downshifting" to controlled fluency before stutters, I have him signal me when he anticipates a stutter and then plan his controlled fluency response. I sometimes use Van Riper's (1973) technique of having a client pantomime his target response before he begins it. Enthusiastic but gradually faded praise is helpful. I also use video recording and replay samples of his *successes* to help him learn. Early in this process, I ask the client to evaluate his response, sometimes providing feedback and sometimes not as I foster the goal of self-evaluation.

As a client is learning controlled fluency, I introduce "cancellations" (Van Riper, 1973) as a way of having him mildly punish himself when he fails to downshift into controlled fluency and stutters instead. Cancellations, which are taught by modeling, involve pausing for several seconds after a stutter (the pause functions as a "time-out"), having the speaker mentally prepare to use controlled fluency during the pause, and then using controlled fluency on the word just stuttered and continuing to talk. The opportunity to continue talking is a positive reinforcer for the controlled fluency. I am diligent in rewarding cancellations with verbal praise because they are one of the most powerful tools available for self-therapy. I gradually fade my praise and help the client to develop his own reward system. When used regularly throughout acquisition, transfer, and maintenance stages, cancellations can make controlled fluency a durable replacement for many episodes of stuttering.

I would like to highlight the point just made because it is important. Cancellations are an operant conditioning procedure. The pause after stutters is a "punishment" that decreases the frequency of stuttering, and the opportunity to continue speaking is a "reward" that will increase the use of controlled fluency. Cancellations are especially effective because they are self-administered operant procedures that a client eventually uses himself as he takes charge of his own treatment. A good description of cancellations by a fan of this technique can be found on pages 84–90 of the book *Forty Years after Therapy* by George Helliesen (2002), which is listed in the suggested readings for Chapter 1.

Transferring Controlled Fluency to Anticipated Stuttering

When a client seems confident in his responses during conversations with me in the treatment room, he and I design a hierarchy of increasingly difficult contexts in which to practice. Typical hierarchies involve (1) inside the clinic with me, (2) on the telephone while I'm with him in the clinic, (3) outside the clinic with me, and (4) everyday speaking situations.

The first hierarchy of inside the clinic with me varies the physical location and social complexity of therapy sessions in the clinic, which means conducting therapy in other locations in the clinic and bringing other people into therapy sessions. The size of the audience can be increased, and people from the client's world, such as family and friends, can also be brought into therapy. The client and I rank such situations from easiest to most difficult, and then he goes through these situations in sequence, using controlled fluency, both in his natural speech and when he expects to stutter, and cancellations if he does stutter. Usually, we work out a point system generating self-rewards to increase his motivation.

I have found that individuals with advanced stuttering need a separate hierarchy for the telephone. The same strategies or principles used in implementing the hierarchies discussed earlier are applied here as well. Thus, telephone calls, at first in the clinic with the clinician present, are arranged in a hierarchical order. The client practices using controlled fluency in fluent speech and on anticipated stutters or uses cancellations, if needed, during these calls until he meets the criterion for success, and the clinician continues to support and reinforce him during these activities. In time, the client will report successes in his daily use of the telephone outside of the therapy room.

Once a client has completed the in-clinic telephone hierarchy using controlled fluency, it is time to move on to nontelephone speaking outside the clinic during which I can accompany the client. We jointly select and sequence hierarchy situations and activities for this. Examples of these situations are asking directions from strangers or obtaining information from store clerks (Fig. 14.4). For some part of this hierarchy, a survey about stuttering given to strangers can be a powerful device to practice replacing anticipated stuttering with controlled fluency. Sample questions include the following: Do you know what stuttering is? Do you know anyone who stutters? How do you think you should respond to someone who is stuttering? Using this kind of survey has the side benefit of helping the person who stutters discover what prevailing attitudes about stuttering really are.

For any given situation, the criterion for success is that both the client and clinician agree that the client used these skills as well as he did in the clinic. This means that the controlled fluency he used to replace stutters and in fluent speech feels and sounds as good as it did when he used them in the clinic. Some instances of cancellation are acceptable in achieving success, but most stutters should be replaced by controlled fluency on the first try. This is a subjective evaluation, but realistically, it is the type of evaluation the client will use on his own in the future. It is also important that the client experience success in using controlled fluency in fluent speech. Then he must learn to replace anticipated stuttering in each situation a number of times so that he gains confidence in his ability to use controlled fluency. After gaining skill and confidence in using controlled fluency in outside situations with the clinician present, it is time for the client to move on to the next, more difficult hierarchy.

The everyday speaking situation hierarchy consists of situations from the client's environment and requires him to complete them on his own. Clients usually rank a dozen or more speaking situations that they encounter in a typical month, from least to most difficult. As a general rule, the client should feel that he has successfully used his transfer skills a number of times in the immediately preceding, easier situation before moving to a more difficult step or situation on the hierarchy. This is important in developing his skills and confidence in using these techniques. During regular therapy sessions, the clinician monitors the client's progress through this hierarchy, praises him when he is successful, encourages him when he is not, and makes suggestions when he has problems. In time, the client will report to the clinician that his speech is becoming much better in his everyday encounters.

By now, the client will be speaking more fluently or with easier stuttering in most situations. Although he is not yet out of the woods, he is well on his way.

OTHER APPROACHES

Camperdown

Sue O'Brian, Mark Onslow, Angela Cream, and Ann Packman (2003) developed the Camperdown program for adults. It is based on earlier prolonged speech treatments (e.g., Ingham & Andrews, 1973) but requires less treatment time and gives clients more self-reliance in the establishment, transfer, and maintenance of their controlled fluency.

The program has four stages. First are the individual teaching sessions, in which clients learn prolonged speech and practice using two 1-to-9 scales to track their progress. One is the *stuttering severity* scale (1, no stuttering; 9, extremely severe stuttering), and the other is the *speech naturalness* scale (1, extremely natural speech; 9, extremely unnatural speech). Unlike traditional methods of teaching prolonged speech via detailed instruction in slow rate, gentle onsets, light contacts, and continuous airflow, the Camperdown approach uses an exemplar video of a clinician speaking with prolonged speech at approximately 70 syllables per minute (or a 7 on the naturalness scale). Clients are coached by the clinician to imitate the model and to continue to practice using the model with the clinician's feedback until they can maintain 100 percent fluent prolonged speech in the clinic setting. This involves frequent self-evaluation of their naturalness and severity ratings during multiple monologues to achieve consistently fluent speech.

After clients can produce the monologue fluently with prolonged speech, they complete a group practice day, in which they learn to speak at gradually faster rates, fluently and naturally, and to assess their speech on the severity scale as well as a nine-point naturalness scale. Subsequently, they begin individual problem-solving sessions, consisting of weekly individual meetings with a clinician to facilitate generalizing fluent speech to everyday situations. These sessions involve the clinician mentoring clients' planning and carrying out generalization activities, as well as further practice of fluent speech. Clients' speech has to meet two criteria for three consecutive weeks at this stage. Both within-clinic and beyond-clinic conversations must show low levels of stuttering severity (ratings of 1–2) and normal levels of speech naturalness (ratings of 1–3).

The final stage of the program, performance-contingent maintenance, lasts about a year and involves repeated clinic maintenance visits by clients. During these visits, stuttering severity and speech naturalness levels are expected to be equivalent to those required previously. If these severity and naturalness criteria are met, clinic visits are scheduled at fading intervals: 2 weeks, 2 weeks, 4 weeks, 8 weeks, and 24 weeks. If the criteria are not met at any visit, that visit is repeated, and progress is momentarily stalled until it is met.

The authors of the program indicate that this approach is an important advance over previous stuttering treatments because it requires relatively little treatment time (i.e., 20 hours to establish fluency). Because the program doesn't involve extensive teaching and measurement of prolonged speech targets, the authors believe that it can be used by generalist clinicians rather than just stuttering specialists. A more detailed description of the program and the latest references are available online.[4] More information can also

[4]https://adultstutteringtreatment.wordpress.com

be obtained from the Australian Stuttering Research Centre that was previously at the University of Sydney and is now at the University of Technology Sydney.

Several studies have been carried out to assess the long-term outcome of this approach. O'Brian and colleagues (2003) reported on 30 adults who reduced stuttering from a pretreatment mean of 7.9 %SS to a mean of 0.4 %SS at the end of treatment and maintained that same reduction when measured a year after treatment ended. O'Brian, Packman, and Onslow (2008) designed a telehealth model of the Camperdown program, conducted entirely by e-mail and telephone consultation, reporting a 75 percent reduction in stuttering from before treatment to 6 months after. Carey et al. (2010) conducted a randomized control comparison of Camperdown done via telehealth with Camperdown done face-to-face. The telehealth group had a mean pretreatment %SS of 6.86 and reduced it to 2.58 one year after treatment had ended; the face-to-face group had a mean pretreatment %SS of 5.44 and reduced to 2.5 one year after treatment had ended. This suggests the telehealth version is as effective as the face-to-face version.

Avoidance Reduction Therapy

Vivian Sisskin (2018) has written an excellent chapter on her avoidance reduction approach, which is based on the work of Joseph and Vivian Sheehan (e.g., 1984), with whom she worked and practiced avoidance reduction therapy. The heart of the therapy is to help clients reduce the struggle behaviors that create the most noticeable features of stuttering beyond early childhood. One of the "mantras" of this approach is that clients are taught to do less, rather than more. This means that clients are taught to go ahead and stutter openly without trying to hold their stuttering back or conceal it or feel ashamed of it. Many of the elements of Sisskin's therapy are similar to the integrated approach described in this textbook—which is pleasing for us both—but her approach discourages efforts to *control* stuttering. In other words, she believes clients should just let their stuttering out, but do it without struggle, fear, and shame. In my approach, the feeling of control, achieved by holding onto a moment of stuttering openly and ending the stutter slowly and loosely, is celebrated. But overall, the approaches are quite similar because they are focused on reducing struggle and the negative emotions associated with stuttering. In addition to her fine chapter, Sisskin (2017) describes and demonstrates her approach in a DVD titled "Avoidance Reduction Therapy in a Group Setting," available from the Stuttering Foundation.

Pharmacological Approaches

Because the use of drugs in the treatment for stuttering has a long history but until recently has been short on scientific evidence, this section will be more of a review than a recommendation. Complaints and concerns about the lack of tightly controlled drug studies go back at least as far as Van Riper (1973), who noted that a valid drug study would involve at least two groups of people who stutter: one group would receive the drug and the other group would receive a placebo that had the same side effects. Another critically important aspect of a good study is "double-blinding": neither the experimenter nor the participant knows whether the participant was given the drug or the placebo. A third characteristic is that the experimenter should make multiple measures of the drugs' effects on the frequency and severity of stuttering, as well as measures of how the people who stuttered perceived their speech. Finally, in a good study, authors will report the drop-out rate or attrition that occurred over the course of the study given that dropping out of a study may indicate dissatisfaction with results, with the demands placed on participants, or on side effects that weren't necessarily tracked by the authors.

Van Riper pointed out that the few early studies that used placebos and were double blind had mixed results, although tranquilizers and sedatives seemed to reduce the severity of stuttering and make subjects feel better about their speech. At one time, there was some hope that an antipsychotic drug called haloperidol, which blocked receptors for the neurotransmitter dopamine, might prove to be effective.

In a later review of pharmacological approaches to stuttering, Brady (1991) reported that improved studies indicated that tranquilizers and sedatives reduced the severity of stuttering compared to placebos, and he also discussed a number of studies on haloperidol. Several authors (Prins, Mandelkorn, & Cerf, 1980; Rosenberger, 1980; Swift, Swift, & Arellano, 1975) who studied haloperidol suggested that its effectiveness might result from diminishing the uptake of dopamine, which could interfere with fluency if it were produced in excess. Although haloperidol seemed to work directly on stuttering symptoms, rather than through overall sedative or tranquilizing mechanisms, major side effects contraindicated its use. Its side effects included drowsiness, sexual dysfunction, excess movement of limbs, and the risk of a permanent, neurologically based movement disorder, tardive dyskinesia. When I worked in Australia, I participated in a haloperidol trial and found that it reduced the tension in my stuttering, allowing blocks to seemingly melt in my mouth, but the side effects were hard to bear. I was always on the verge of falling asleep, and my legs were uncontrollably wiggling.

A research review by Maguire, Yu, Franklin, and Riley (2004) presented the evidence that medications that reduce the uptake of dopamine can be effective in reducing stuttering. These authors recently completed a study of olanzapine, a dopamine antagonist, which doesn't have the same side effects as other drugs that reduce dopamine, such as haloperidol or its replacements risperidone and pimozide. In a double-blind study, 5 mg/d of olanzapine was reported to significantly ($p < .05$) reduce stuttering compared with the placebo on each of the following three measures: the SSI-3, the clinician's global impression, and the participant's self-rating of stuttering. The only side effect noted was a tendency for weight gain, but that was minimized via counseling about diet and exercise. Maguire, Riley, Franklin, and Gumusaneli (2010) described their model of the action of the neurotransmitter dopamine in the etiology of stuttering and presented an update on the effect of a new drug called pagoclone. In a separate publication, Maguire et al. (2010) showed that pagoclone reduced stuttering in 88 patients by 19.4 percent, whereas a placebo group of 44 patients reduced stuttering by only 5.1 percent in an 8-week trial. When this trial was over and all patients were offered and continued to use pagoclone, the entire group showed a reduction of 40 percent after a year of treatment. The only significant side effect was headache, experienced by about 12 percent of the pagoclone patients.

Maguire, Yeh, and Ito (2012) included the above study in their more recent review of the treatment of stuttering using pharmacological approaches, but did not report on any more recent studies of the effect of pharmacological agents on stuttering.

In summary, although case studies appearing in the literature (e.g., Brady & Ali, 2000) frequently report the success of a variety of medications, large-scale double-blind studies most frequently support drugs that interfere with the uptake of dopamine, especially olanzapine and pagoclone. It appears, however, that at this time and for most individuals who stutter, medication for stuttering has not proven any more effective than traditional treatment.

Treatment and Support Groups

My description of treatment groups will largely draw on my own experience as a client in one of Van Riper's stuttering modification treatment groups (see Van Riper (1958) for a description of his group therapy) and as a clinician in fluency-shaping therapy groups (Guitar, 1976). Manning and DiLollo (2018) provide a good description of group stuttering therapy in their chapter on treatment of adolescents and adults.

Among the benefits of group therapy is the mutual support that its members experience as they face the challenges of confronting and changing their stuttering. An effective group leader will facilitate extensive interaction among group members so that they encourage each other, share hopes and fears, and provide a safe haven for trying out new behaviors. Many of us in Van Riper's group paired up to do some of our beyond-clinic assignments together. We were able to give each other helpful feedback, both in our group sessions and when we went out together to work on our speech in shopping areas and restaurants. Seeing each other's stuttering made ours more bearable, and vying with each other to bring back "trophies" of successful changes in our speech was healthy competition. The techniques we were taught and the changes we made in our behaviors, feelings, and attitudes were, I suspect, much the same as would have occurred in individual therapy, but the group made the road we had to travel less lonely. Van Riper measured the outcome of his treatment 5 years after the end of therapy, using the following five criteria: (1) the client's speech must be at or below 0.5 on the Iowa Scale of Severity of Stuttering (Sherman, 1952; this scale is a 1–7 scale requiring perceptual judgments of severity); (2) the client must not be avoiding words or situations; (3) stuttering must not be interfering with the client's social or vocational adjustment; (4) the client's word and situation fears must be close to zero; and (5) the client's stuttering must present no concern to himself or others (Van Riper, 1958). The seven members of our group have had our ups and downs, and several of us have had some additional therapy, but most of us did fairly well, but not perfectly, in terms of Van Riper's criteria.

The fluency-shaping groups I worked with in Australia as a clinician (Guitar, 1976; Howie & Andrews, 1984) focused first on learning a prolonged speech pattern to replace stuttering and shaping conversational speech to sound essentially normal. Group members then generalized their fluency to their natural environments. In this approach, the group functioned primarily as a setting in which conversational speech could be practiced, with only minor attention to the support that group members provided each other. Treatment in a group promoted an efficient use of the clinician's time as well as opportunities for members to practice using fluent speech in the give-and-take of a conversation among six people. Results of treatment varied widely for individuals (Guitar, 1976), but the overall group mean of percent syllables stuttered went from 14 percent before treatment to 3.9 percent a year after treatment, with essentially normal mean speech rates (Howie & Andrews, 1984). Subsequent modifications of the program brought follow-up percentages to even lower levels (1–2 %SS) (Andrews & Craig, 1982).

Support or self-help groups differ from treatment groups because their main function is to provide an atmosphere in which members can freely share their feelings and develop a sense of connectedness to others who stutter, and they can provide an excellent opportunity for maintenance of improvement made in formal therapy. In my experience, getting together with others who stutter and sharing experiences, especially triumphs and frustrations, gives us a great opportunity to continue working on strategies that we have found helpful, as well as feel the support and encouragement of others. Probably the most important part of the group experience is sharing and mutual support, rather than specific work on techniques. Our group at the University of Vermont, which has been running for almost 40 years, is a mix of support and therapy. Participants share their experiences; comment supportively on each other's techniques; give themselves speech assignments, both for that meeting and for the 2 weeks in between meetings; and tell funny stories. There is much therapeutic humor, directed both at stuttering and at difficult listeners.

Ramig (1993) surveyed 62 self-help participants and found that 49 of them believed that their fluency had improved "at least somewhat" as a result of attending meetings regularly.

The majority of respondents felt that the group experience improved their feelings about themselves, as well as their comfort in their personal and work environments. Information about the return rate of the survey was not available. Ramig did note that there is a paucity of research on the impact of self-help groups on the lives of people who stutter, and he gave 17 suggestions for designing studies on self-help groups.

An excellent review of self-help groups as a supplement to traditional therapy was presented in a chapter by Yaruss et al. (2007). This chapter lists several national self-help groups for stuttering organizations and provides evidence of benefit to participants gathered by self-report studies. More recently, a chapter by Trichon and Raj (2018) gives a history of the stuttering self-help movement and an update on national self-help meetings, international self-help organizations, and Internet-based peer support for stuttering. The National Stuttering Association provides excellent mentoring for people who want to start their own self-help groups, including assistance in setting up a Web site. For an example, see the University of Vermont stuttering group's Web site.[5]

Assistive Devices

For hundreds of years, practitioners have offered people who stutter an incredible array of devices to help them speak more fluently. These devices have included ivory forks placed under the tongue, auditory feedback–delaying devices inserted in the ear, respiration-monitoring belts snugged around the chest, and masking noise generators triggered by sensors wrapped around the throat (Van Riper, 1982). Some have been used alone, and others have been used as an adjunct to therapy. Several devices have helped those who stutter who have not been able to find relief through traditional therapy, but too often, false hopes for a miracle cure have been raised.

Merson (2003) presented a brief overview of devices such as the Edinburgh Masker, the Fluency Master, the Casa Futura DAF, and the SpeechEasy. He reported that he only uses such devices with clients who seem to not be helped by other therapy procedures alone, using these devices only as an adjunct to more traditional stuttering modification and fluency-shaping therapy techniques. Of the 10 patients who have used the Fluency Master (masking triggered by phonation) for 12 to 24 months, five reported that their stuttering was 100 percent reduced, two reported a 50 percent reduction, one stopped using it, and two more could not be contacted. Of the 37 patients who had used the SpeechEasy for 3 to 5 months, 55 percent reported that its effectiveness was retained, 53 percent reported less frequent stuttering, 52 percent reported less tense stuttering, and 28 percent reported that their speech was more fluent *without* the SpeechEasy. These data are not objective measures of fluency but are the subjective reports of clients who were surveyed and may be unreliable.

Another "soft" source of information about the use of assistive devices is a survey conducted by the Stuttering Foundation (Fraser, 2004; Trautman, 2003). The Foundation contacted 800 adults who had requested information about electronic devices from its Web site. Just over 100 individuals returned the survey, and of these, only 22 had actually bought a device. Most of those who didn't buy a device cited high costs and the absence of evidence of long-term benefit. Of those who bought devices, 12 bought a SpeechEasy, 6 bought a Casa Futura DAF, 3 bought a Fluency Master, and 1 bought an unspecified device. Initial reports suggested that 14 of the 22 purchasers were happy with their devices. A later follow-up survey to learn how they felt after having used their device for a year was able to reach 8 of these 14 individuals. Of those eight individuals, three were still happy with their device, three were not happy, and two reported mixed reactions. Some of those who were no longer happy with their device reported that it didn't work when their stutters were those that stop phonation; others reported that their device didn't work well in noisy environments.

Ramig (personal communication, March 8, 2005) reported that he and his private practice colleagues had evaluated over 60 stuttering patients over a 2-year period, fitting over 40 of them with a SpeechEasy device. Only a few of those patients were able to receive supplemental traditional therapy. He indicated that the device helped one-third of the clients significantly, one-third were helped marginally, and one-third were not helped at all. For some of his clients, it was the only effective treatment they have experienced. Ramig further noted that for the device to be useful for most clients, the clients must have been able to initiate appropriate voicing during their stuttering blocks, and they must have paid attention to the auditory feedback from the device. He emphasized that he only dispenses the device for adults, teens, and children over 11 years old, believing that younger children can be helped by other therapeutic approaches. His reluctance to fit very young children stems primarily from the thought that their auditory cortex is not yet fully developed and the fact that the effect of prolonged exposure to DAF and frequency altered pitch is unknown at this time.

Ramig, Ellis, and Pollard (2010) have written a comprehensive chapter on the SpeechEasy, including video clips of clients using it and talking about their experiences with it. It is a thorough account of his and other's experiences using the SpeechEasy with clients. Another interesting take on the SpeechEasy is available from a YouTube video titled "SpeechEasy Revisited." In 2003, the Oprah Winfrey show had a "miracle cure" demonstration of a young man using the SpeechEasy appearing to cure his stuttering in an instant, sending his family into tearful gratitude. The YouTube clip contains the original 2003 miracle cure show followed by a 2010 interview with same young man whose stuttering has returned.

[5]www.burlingtonstutters.org

SUMMARY

- Advanced stuttering is characterized by repetitions, prolongations, and blocks, accompanied by over-learned patterns of tension, struggle, and escape and avoidance behaviors. Clients will also typically have negative attitudes, feelings, and beliefs about stuttering and about speaking.
- I believe that because these behaviors are so well-learned, treatment must focus on teaching people who stutter new stuttering management skills as responses to old cues that would otherwise still tend to elicit struggle and avoidance behaviors.
- Treatment begins by helping the client confront and understand his stuttering and, in the process, decreasing fear and shame. Then, the clinician teaches stuttering management skills (going directly into stutters, holding onto them with voicing and/or airflow, and, as fear and tension decrease, finishing the word slowly and loosely). When these skills are done well on real feared words, they are termed "high-quality stutters."
- The client first learns stuttering management skills in the clinic and then generalizes them into his daily life. He practices them in many situations with the clinician's support and then on his own. He also learns to voluntarily stutter and be open about his stuttering to other people.
- For many clients, continued work is needed on increasing approach behaviors and decreasing avoidance behaviors. For all clients, the responsibility for managing their own speech is gradually transferred to them over the course of treatment.
- A variety of other treatments are available for advanced stuttering, including controlled fluency, individual and group approaches, intensive and non-intensive treatment, medication, and assistive devices. Knowing about these options can give you a wider range of options to offer your clients, especially those who need something more or something different from the integrated approach offered in this chapter.

STUDY QUESTIONS

1. Summarize the main differences between *intermediate stuttering in school-age children* and *advanced stuttering in adolescents and adults* and the treatment approaches used for them.
2. How does "exploring stuttering" help a client decrease his fear and shame associated with stuttering? What role the clinician play in this process?
3. Do you think it is a treatment failure if a client has mild stuttering after treatment? Explain the reasoning behind your answer.
4. How does "catch and release" help extinguish fear of stuttering.
5. If a client has kept his stuttering a hidden secret all his life, how do you motivate him to be more open about it?
6. Many clients are reluctant to use voluntary stuttering. What are some reasons you could give them as to why it may be helpful? Are there any clients with whom you would not use it?
7. In my approach to teaching controlled fluency, I advocate teaching clients four separate components of this skill before they combine them. In contrast, clinicians using the Camperdown program prefer to teach clients a variant of controlled fluency using a video model of someone speaking with all the components already combined (speaking with prolonged speech at 70 syllables per minute). What are the advantages and disadvantages of each approach?
8. Imagine yourself being an individual who stutters who is in search of a place to share your experiences and get support. How do you look for one in your town or city? Does National Stuttering Association or Stuttering Home Page or the Stuttering Foundation have suggestions to find a group near you?
9. Which clients would be most suited for treatment with a pharmacological approach? Which clients would be most suited for an assistive device?
10. What do you think are the most valid measures of the benefits of a treatment approach?

SUGGESTED PROJECTS

1. Choose a behavior of yours that you would like to change, and develop a self-therapy plan to explore your present behavior, identify the change you would like to make, and develop a hierarchy to practice the new behavior. Report on your success.

2. Write out a talk that you could have with a new adult client to describe the possible course of treatment (see the section on "Beginning Therapy"). Make your talk both challenging and inspirational.
3. If you are someone who doesn't stutter, your biggest fear in doing voluntary stuttering is probably that you will be unable to stutter convincingly, and a listener will unmask you. Confront that fear by stuttering to several listeners, and see if that decreases your fear.
4. After you have learned controlled fluency, see if you can use it on just single words ("slide-outs") 20 times before noon. In trying to do this, see if you can develop a novel way to remind yourself.
5. Watch a session of the Van Riper videos (e.g., the session on desensitization), and see if you can determine what made him so effective as a stuttering therapist.

SUGGESTED READINGS

Fraser, M. (2010). *Self-therapy for the stutterer* (11th ed.). Memphis, TN: Stuttering Foundation.

This self-help book contains a sequenced program for an adult who stutters to use, either on his own or with the help of a clinician or supportive friend. It describes many of the techniques you have been reading about in this book. In addition, it contains many personal and inspirational messages for the reader. I recommend it not only to individuals who stutter but also to clinicians so that they may get another perspective on adult stuttering therapy.

Guitar, B., & Guitar, C. (2005). *If you stutter: Advice for adults (DVD).* Memphis, TN: Stuttering Foundation.

This video presents a broad spectrum of treatment approaches, and many of them are demonstrated by adults who have benefited from stuttering therapy.

Guitar, B., & McCauley, R. (Eds.) (2010). *Treatment of stuttering: Established and emerging interventions.* Baltimore, MD: Lippincott Williams & Wilkins.

This book has four approaches for adults and adolescents who stutter: two behavioral treatments, one involving the SpeechEasy device, and one on pharmacological therapy. Each chapter is illustrated with a video that depicts the treatment process as well as before- and after-therapy interviews with clients.

Manning, W., & DiLollo, A. (2018). *Clinical decision making in fluency disorders* (4th ed.). San Diego, CA: Plural Publishing.

An excellent and sensible book about stuttering therapy by knowledgeable clinicians. It has the added benefit of being written by individuals who stutter and who have largely recovered. Their clinical experiences are shared throughout the book, putting readers in the shoes of the authors' many clients.

National Stuttering Association Web site: www.westutter.org

This site contains a wealth of information for adolescents and adults who stutter, including basic information about the nature of stuttering and treatment opportunities. A DVD, Transcending Stuttering, about the struggle and triumph of many individuals who stutter, is among NSA's recent offerings.

Shapiro, D. (2011) *Stuttering intervention: A collaborative journey to fluency freedom.* Austin, TX: Pro-Ed.

This book is a thoughtful account of working with people who stutter, written by an experienced clinician who stutters himself. Shapiro is particularly eloquent on the feelings that affect people who stutter.

Stuttering Foundation Web site: www.stutteringhelp.org

Background information on stuttering and its treatment, books, videos, and lists of clinicians who specialize in stuttering are offered on this site.

Stuttering Home Page: www.mnsu.edu/comdis/kuster/stutter.html

Developed by Judy Kuster at Mankato University, the Stuttering Home Page offers a wide variety of helpful pages and links. On this site, the user can connect to chat rooms and access an annual online conference and its archives, the latest research, and commentary by people who stutter. Links to stuttering sites in other countries are also provided.

Van Riper, C. (1975b). *Therapy in action (DVD).* Memphis, TN: Stuttering Foundation.

This nine-session DVD shows a master clinician conducting stuttering modification treatment with an adult who stutters. Van Riper takes this young man from the assessment to the final treatment meeting in seven sessions. There are then 1-year and 20-year follow-up interviews. Van Riper introduces each session describing what he has planned for the session and then follows the session with a commentary on what was accomplished.

15

Related Disorders of Fluency

Chapter Objectives

After studying this chapter, readers should be able to:

- Describe the multiple possible etiologies and speech characteristics associated with neurogenic stuttering
- Describe the evaluation and treatment of neurogenic stuttering
- Describe the conditions that may give rise to psychogenic stuttering, particularly in regard to information that may be obtained from the case history and interview
- Describe the speech characteristics of psychogenic stuttering
- Describe methods to differentiate between psychogenic and neurogenic stuttering
- Describe trial therapy for psychogenic stuttering and how that may be continued beyond the initial trial
- Describe the characteristics of cluttering including concomitant problems
- Describe the evaluation of cluttering and concomitant problems

- Describe why motivation is a major issue in the treatment of cluttering
- Describe the treatment of cluttering

Key Terms

Delayed auditory feedback (DAF): Hearing one's own voice a half-second or so after speaking. This is usually done via a computer program, with the client speaking into a microphone and hearing himself through headphones. It typically forces a client to speak more slowly and reduces stuttering dramatically.

Fluency-inducing or fluency-enhancing conditions: Stimuli that usually cause a person who stutters to speak much more fluently. Examples are speaking in a rhythmic or staccato manner, speaking under loud masking noise so the client can't hear his own voice, and speaking while very relaxed.

Mazing: A disorder of spoken language characterized by false starts, hesitations, and revisions that make the speaker's message difficult to understand

Pacing: A treatment technique in which each individual syllable is spoken separately, sometimes accompanied by physical movement such as tapping a finger as each syllable is spoken

Posttraumatic stress disorder (PTSD): An anxiety disorder that occurs after a person has experienced a traumatic event

Prolonged speech: A treatment for stuttering that induces the client to stretch out sounds, start words with a gentle onset of phonation, and touch the articulators lightly when producing consonants

Traumatic brain injury (TBI): An injury to the brain from an external force. This may be either an injury that penetrates the skull (such as a bullet shot into the head) or a closed-head injury (such as a bomb concussion close to a person) where penetration does not occur.

Trial therapy: A brief treatment of stuttering carried out during the evaluation to determine which treatment techniques are most effective

This chapter discusses three fluency disorders that are related to "developmental" stuttering that was discussed in the first 14 chapters. These disorders—neurogenic stuttering, psychogenic stuttering, and cluttering—are similar to developmental stuttering in some ways, but are generally distinctly different in etiology, symptoms, and treatment. Figure 15.1 gives an overview of the chapter.

NEUROGENIC ACQUIRED STUTTERING

Nature

The term "neurogenic acquired stuttering" denotes stuttering that appears to be caused or exacerbated by neurological disease or damage. It is typically acquired after childhood, and its etiology may be stroke, head trauma, tumor, disease processes such as Parkinson's, or drug toxicity. Additional, though rare, causes are dialysis dementia, seizure disorders, bilateral thalamotomy, or thalamic stimulation (Duffy, 2013). Demyelination of the corpus callosum has recently been identified as a cause of stuttering (Decker, Guitar, & Solomon, 2018). Stuttering has also been seen in active duty service members with combat-related brain injury and co-occurring posttraumatic stress disorder (PTSD).[1]

Understanding neurogenic stuttering may help us understand some aspects of typical or "developmental" stuttering. Moreover, neurogenic stuttering in patients may be an early diagnostic sign of a neurological problem. Helm-Estabrooks (1999) describes this eloquently: "Fluent speaking is, perhaps, the most refined motor act performed by humans, requiring complex coordination of many different muscle groups. It can be sensitive, therefore, to even small changes in neurological status, which may be why stuttering occurs in a wide range of neurological disorders, from Parkinson's disease to closed head injury. If this fact is ignored, clinicians may be overlooking an important early indicator of neurological disease" (p. 265).

Some writers prefer to use the term "neurogenic disfluency," because they don't consider neurogenic stuttering to be true stuttering. Such usage may, however, blur the distinction between two different phenomena that may occur with neurological insults. One is an increase in normal types of disfluencies (e.g., whole-word and phrase repetitions, revisions, interjections, and pauses); the other is a speech disorder presenting stutter-like disfluencies (i.e., part-word repetitions, prolongations, and blocks), sometimes accompanied by tension, struggle, escape, and avoidance behaviors.

Although much of the literature on neurogenic stuttering consists of single-case studies (e.g., Bijleveld, Lebrun, & van Dongen, 1994), there have been several attempts by

[1]This etiology is discussed in the section on psychogenic stuttering when I talk about differential diagnosis between neurogenic and psychogenic stuttering.

I-I recently-ly had a st-st-stroke
Neurogenic Stuttering

I've j....(silent block)...j ust ex-ex-ex-experienced an e....(silent block) ..... e motionally upsetting event
Psychogenic Stuttering

Why-why uh does everyone...you know..uh...tell me ... ask me ..uh...to...uh...to repeat....well.... to repeat what I've....what I've....uh....just said?
Cluttering

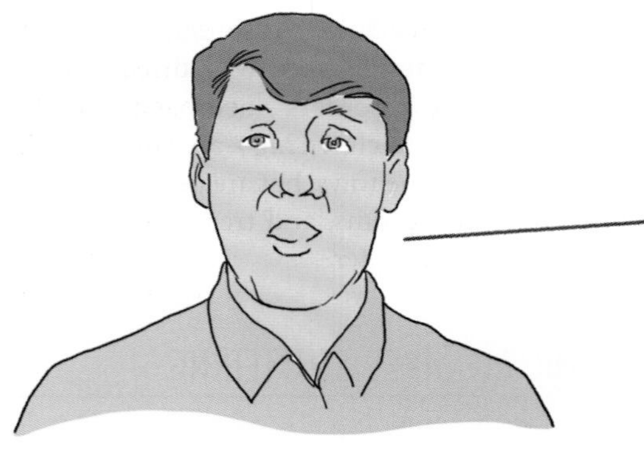

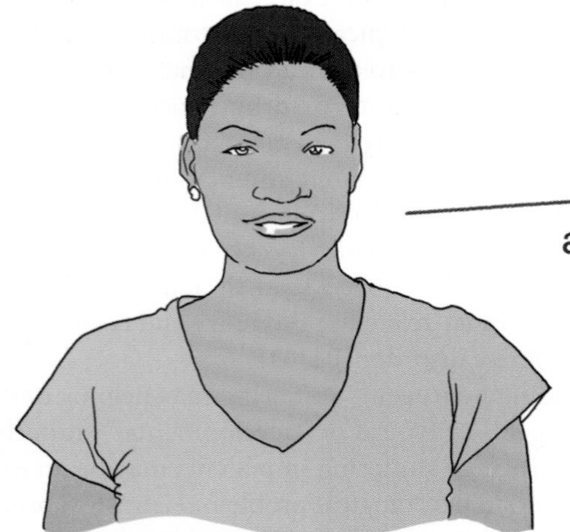

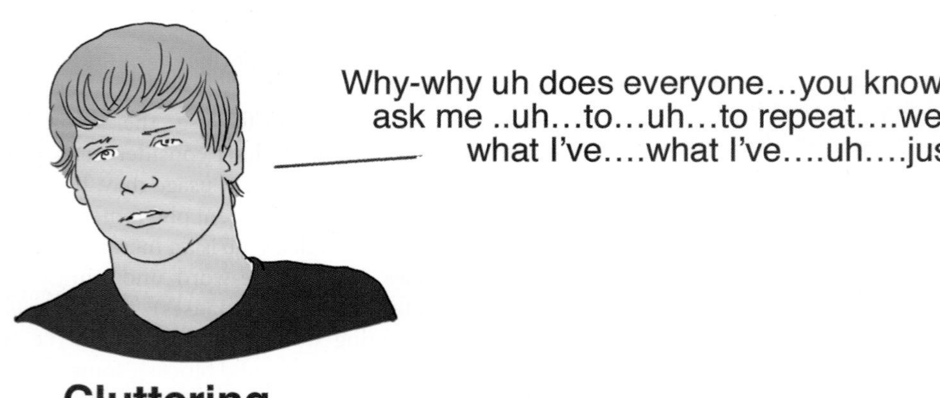

Figure 15.1 Overview of the chapter.

clinician-researchers to summarize their findings on multiple cases and thereby develop a clearer picture of the disorder. Canter (1971) wrote a seminal article that went beyond case studies to suggest a possible way of categorizing types of neurogenic stuttering. He proposed three subgroups. One is dysarthric stuttering—seen, for example, in individuals who have Parkinson's disease or have a cerebellar lesion—in which stuttering appears to emerge from the same lack of neuromotor control as the primary dysarthric disorder. The second is apraxic stuttering, in which stuttering may arise from a basic problem in motor planning. Both silent blocks and repetitions occur as the speaker struggles to sequence the appropriate speech movements. The third subgroup is dysnomic stuttering, which sometimes accompanies aphasia. Stuttering symptoms occur as an individual searches for the word he is having trouble retrieving. Canter speculated that there may be a parallel to this type of stuttering in children who have word-retrieval problems and who develop stuttering as a result of their emotional reactions to the word-retrieval difficulty. Canter seems to believe that acquired stuttering following neurological disease or insult is closely related to, or is caused by, the neuropathologies underlying dysarthria, apraxia of speech, or difficulty remembering names (dysnomia). Later studies take a different view—that neurogenic stuttering may often be a separate disorder, related to deficits in the neural circuitry underlying developmental stuttering.

Rosenbek (1984) also summarized findings from multiple cases. He made the point that neurogenic stuttering should be distinguished from other disfluent behaviors that are associated with neurological problems, such as palilalia (word and phrase repetitions produced with increasing rate and decreasing loudness). It should also be distinguished from repetitions that some patients make as they try to correct their motor speech or linguistic errors. Observations of his own patients led Rosenbek to suggest that stuttering following nervous system damage is characterized primarily by involuntary repetitions of correct sounds and syllables, not those produced in error that occur at any place in a word (initial, medial, final). In other words, his view differed from that of Canter (1971). But Rosenbeck was distressed by the lack of detail in clinicians' descriptions of patients with this disorder and called for a moratorium on the use of the term "neurogenic stuttering" until more is known about it. Despite his call for a moratorium, case studies of "neurogenic stuttering" have continued to flow forth in the literature.

More recently, Theys, De Nil, Thijs, van Wieringen, and Sunaert (2013) studied a relatively large group of stroke patients with neurogenic stuttering, distinguishing between those with a substantial number of stuttering-like disfluencies (n = 20) and those with more typical disfluencies (n = 17). Using statistical analysis of brain scans made soon after the strokes, they found differences in the two groups in both gray and white matter areas. Specifically, they identified nine affected areas of the left hemisphere cortico-basal ganglia-cortex neural network that distinguished patients who had numerous stuttering-like disfluencies from the control group. Affected areas included inferior frontal cortex, superior temporal cortex, infraparietal cortex, basal ganglia, superior longitudinal fasciculus, and internal capsule. This circuitry is thought to have important sensory and motor functions in typical speech production, including articulatory planning, auditory monitoring of speech, and internal timing (e.g., Guenther, 2007; Guenther, Ghosh, & Tourville, 2006). Citing a number of brain imaging studies of developmental stuttering, the authors suggest that both developmental and neurogenic stuttering may have their origins in deficits in the cortico-basal ganglia-cortical circuitry. They go on to suggest that these deficits may also give rise to concomitant problems (such as auditory processing difficulties) in both developmental and neurogenic stuttering.

Diagnosis and Evaluation

Helm-Estabrooks (1999) and Ringo and Dietrich (1995) provided a framework for assessing neurogenic stuttering and distinguishing it from other disorders. These authors suggested that the following procedures are important not only for evaluating individual cases but also for gathering data that may make a contribution to the literature.

1. A complete case history reflecting:
   - Onset of stuttering and its association with other neurological or psychological signs
   - The client's level of concern, anxiety, or fear about his stuttering
   - Extent to which stuttering interferes with communication
   - Changes in stuttering since onset
   - The client's history and family history of speech, language, or learning problems
   - The client's and relatives' handedness
   - Neurological and psychological health history
   - This information can be gathered initially through a case history and then supplemented during the interview.
2. Direct assessment of speech:
   - The Stuttering Severity Instrument (Riley, 2009) should be administered, and speech should be video recorded during conversation and reading samples.
   - Stuttering in speech samples should be analyzed for:
     - ☐ Proportion of stuttering on function (grammatical) words versus content (substantive) words (more stuttering on function words suggests neurogenic)
     - ☐ Presence of stuttering on noninitial syllables, such as in these words "exciteme-me-ment," "cowb-b-b-oy," and "canister-er-er" (more stuttering on noninitial syllables suggests neurogenic)
   - Absence of secondary (i.e., escape and avoidance) behaviors such as eye blinks, head nods, and use of "um" to get a word started. (Absence of secondary behaviors suggests neurogenic)
     - ☐ The same short passage should be read aloud six times to determine if stuttering is reduced progressively through the repeated readings. See Chapter 1 for more information and references for this *adaptation* procedure. (Lack of adaptation suggests neurogenic.)

  - ☐ Speaking in a variety of fluency-inducing conditions should be explored, especially speaking in a rhythm while swinging an arm, speaking while listening to loud masking noise, and speaking slowly under **delayed auditory feedback (DAF)** set at a maximum delay. (If fluency-inducing conditions do not increase fluency, this suggests neurogenic.)

3. Other assessment components:
   - Helm-Estabrooks (1999) recommended using the Aphasia Diagnostic Profiles (Helm-Estabrooks, 1992) to exclude the possibility that the stuttering actually reflects language formulation problems.
   - Helm-Estabrooks (1999) also recommended that if other neurological problems are present and might interfere with treatment, neuropsychological testing would be important for assessing the client's capabilities.
   - De Nil, Jokel, and Rochon (2007) also strongly suggested testing for other disorders that may affect communication or treatment. These include dysarthria, aphasia, motor disorders, cognitive disorders, and chronic pain. These authors also provide an assessment battery that includes measures of attitudes about stuttering, including the S-24 (Andrews & Cutler, 1974) and the Locus of Control for Behavior (Craig, Franklin, & Andrews, 1984).
   - I would add to this list of assessment targets the distinction between stuttering-like disfluencies (repetitions of sounds, syllables and monosyllabic words, prolongations, or blocks) and typical disfluencies (multisyllable word repetitions, phrase repetitions, interjections, revision-incomplete phrases) that was used by Theys et al. (2013).

The information gathered from the above procedures can be used to improve our understanding of neurogenic stuttering, to differentially diagnose neurogenic stuttering (i.e., distinguish it from other fluency disorders), and to help in planning treatment. The data on the client's and relatives' handedness and history of speech, language, or learning problems are primarily used to determine if a client might have a predisposition for stuttering. Left-handedness or ambidexterity as well as a history of speech or language problems in a family may predispose an individual for stuttering (Geschwind & Galaburda, 1985). If a client began to stutter or if previous stuttering recurred or worsened in association with the occurrence of neurological problems, neurogenic stuttering should be suspected. On the other hand, stuttering that appeared in conjunction with the onset of psychological problems may be of psychogenic origin. Sometimes these etiologies are difficult to sort out and are discussed further in the section on psychogenic stuttering.

It is difficult to be *certain* that an individual has neurogenic stuttering rather than disfluencies caused by other impairments. A diagnosis of neurogenic stuttering can be more certain if other signs of neuropathology are shown. As indicated earlier, every effort needs to be made to rule out memory problems, language formulation problems (such as in aphasia), and emotional distress as the *source* of a client's disfluencies. Sometimes a combination of neurogenic and psychogenic issues may contribute to disfluencies, as I describe in a section on stuttering related to military experience later in this chapter.

Considerations for Treatment

Helm-Estabrooks (1999) suggested several criteria for determining which clients have the potential to benefit from treatment. She noted that some neurogenic stuttering is quite mild and may not result in a handicap that warrants treatment. Other individuals, whose stuttering may be a serious handicap, may have other health problems that are far more serious, such as a progressive neurological disorder. A third consideration is the extent to which other neurological problems, such as dementia, may interfere with treatment. If a client does have severe and persistent stuttering, is motivated to undergo treatment, and has adequate cognitive and linguistic abilities to benefit from treatment, then several treatment options are available.

Treatment Approaches

Because individuals with neurogenic stuttering do not usually have the cognitive and emotional involvement (e.g., fear, shame, and negative feeling about self) that characterize developmental stuttering in adults, treatment is often entirely behavioral. An exception is when the neurological etiology of the stuttering is known and can be treated by surgery or drugs. De Nil et al. (2007) noted that not all patients with neurogenic stuttering need treatment because, as Helm, Butler, and Cantor (1980) have indicated, neurogenic stuttering may appear and then gradually improve without treatment.

1. **Behavioral treatments.** Many of the treatments (or components thereof) that are used for developmental stuttering have also been used for neurogenic stuttering with some success.
   - ***Pacing***. This is essentially a technique of speaking one syllable at a time, so that each syllable is spoken separately, without the usual coarticulation across syllables. As a result, speech is produced more slowly and with a strong, staccato rhythm. This treatment was developed by Helm (1979) for patients with palilalia (i.e., rapid repetition of whole words and phrases), but has been used for neurogenic stuttering as well (Helm-Estabrooks, 1999). To facilitate pacing, especially in those patients who have difficulty slowing their speech, pacing devices can be used. One example is a pacing board (Helm-Estabrooks & Kaplan, 1989); another is a molded form that fits over the patient's index finger and makes tapping more distinct (Rentschler,

Driver, & Callaway, 1984). With either of these devices, the patient moves a finger from place to place, timing each syllable with a finger movement. Helm-Estabrooks (1999) suggested that pacing could begin with a device and progress to simply tapping rhythmically on the thigh to produce fluent speech. My own experience with individuals with developmental stuttering who have used syllable-timed speech to become fluent is that this treatment does not easily generalize to normal-sounding (nonstaccato) speech.

- *Auditory masking and delayed auditory feedback (DAF).* Rentschler et al. (1984), Marshall and Starch (1984), and Helm-Estabrooks (1999) reported that masking and DAF can be used as therapeutic tools to induce fluency in neurogenic stuttering, and in some cases, fluency can then be generalized.
- *Slow rate and easy onset.* Market, Montague, Buffalo, and Drummond (1990) conducted a survey of clinicians who had worked with acquired neurogenic stuttering and found that many of them reported success with fluency-shaping tools, such as slow rate and easy onset.
- *Stuttering modification.* Only a modest percentage of the clinicians surveyed by Market and colleagues (1990) reported that they had used such stuttering modification tools as light contacts, preparatory sets, cancellations, and pullouts.
- *Electromyographic biofeedback for tension reduction.* Reports by Helm-Estabrooks (1986) and Rubow, Rosenbek, and Schumaker (1986) suggested that training patients to relax muscles with the help of biofeedback can be effective in reducing neurogenic stuttering.

2. **Neurosurgery.** Sometimes when a neurological problem requires surgical intervention, the surgery resolves or improves stuttering. Cases reported by Donnan (1979) and Jones (1966) suggested that for whatever reason, surgery that resolved a neurological problem may also resolve stuttering. Andy and Bhatnagar (1992) reported on four patients who were improved by surgical implantations of electrodes to stimulate the thalamus for other neurological conditions. The implication is that some disturbance in neurological functioning can result in stuttering, and when the neurosurgery changes this neurological functioning, stuttering can be resolved. This finding is consistent with recent evidence suggesting that brain structure and function may be aberrant in developmental stuttering (e.g., Chang, 2014; Chang et al., 2015, 2017; Cykowski, Fox, Ingham, Ingham, & Robin, 2010).
3. **Medications.** As I described in Chapter 14, a number of drugs such as haloperidol, olanzapine, and pagoclone have been tried with varying degrees of success with developmental stuttering. These medications have not been tried, as far as I know, with neurogenic stuttering. Rather, case studies have reported that drugs for seizure disorders, schizophrenia, depression, anxiety, Parkinson's disease, and asthma can *precipitate* stuttering in individuals who have not stuttered previously (Baratz & Mesulam, 1981; Duffy, 2013; Elliott & Thomas, 1985; McClean & McClean, 1985; Nurnberg & Greenwald, 1981; Quader, 1977). In most of these cases, stuttering is reduced or eliminated when drug dosage is adjusted or an alternative drug is used. In other studies, drugs have been given for other symptoms and have relieved stuttering (Perino, Famularo, & Tarroni, 2000; Turgut, Utku, & Balci, 2002).

Overall, there is no clear consensus about effective treatments for neurogenic stuttering, and few studies present evidence of the long-term effectiveness of treatment. In part, this may be because the many different etiologies of neurogenic stuttering and the relative rarity of this disorder make long-term group studies of treatment of neurogenic stuttering perhaps impossibly challenging.

Summary and Conclusions

Acquired neurogenic stuttering differs from developmental stuttering in a number of ways. Neurogenic stuttering usually has a sudden onset in adulthood, stuttering may occur with similar frequency on function and content words, stuttering is less restricted to the initial syllables of words, repeated readings of the same passage have less of an effect on neurogenic stuttering, many fluency-inducing conditions do not reduce stuttering, and often there is little fear, shame, and few secondary behaviors. Effective therapy may include behavioral approaches—such as pacing or slowing speech—surgery, and adjustments in dosages for drugs taken to address the underlying neurological problem.

Having highlighted the differences between developmental and neurogenic stuttering in this brief summary, I would also like to consider their similarities by asking this question: what does acquired neurogenic stuttering tell us about developmental stuttering? First, I will assume that both developmental and acquired neurogenic stuttering have neurological deficits at their cores. The evidence regarding acquired neurogenic stuttering suggests that insults to the brain in most regions—left hemisphere, right hemisphere, and subcortical areas—can result in at least temporary disfluencies (Duffy, 2013). The study by Theys et al. (2013) suggests deficits in the cortico-basal ganglia-cortical network may be operating in both developmental stuttering and stroke-induced neurogenic stuttering. This finding highlights the need for brain imaging studies of groups of patients with neurogenic stuttering with other etiologies.

The evidence that acquired neurogenic stuttering is often *not* accompanied by fear or secondary symptoms suggests that they are independent of the core symptoms, which supports the belief that these aspects of stuttering are reactions that develop as a child experiences more and more negative responses to his difficulty, by listeners and himself.

TABLE 15.1 Comparative Characteristics of Neurogenic Stuttering Compared with Developmental Stuttering

Characteristic	Developmental Stuttering	Neurogenic Stuttering
Etiology	Deficits in the speech production areas of the brain	Specific injuries or disease processes in neural pathways for speech
Onset	Usually in early childhood between ages 2 and 5 years	Often in adulthood, after brain injury or disease process
Development or change over time	If it does not disappear in early childhood, stuttering usually gets gradually more severe during childhood and adolescence	Stuttering usually remains similar to what it was like on onset
Types of stuttering behavior	Repetitions, prolongations, and blocks	Most often repetitions, but sometimes also prolongations or blocks
Frequency of stuttering	Almost always below 45 percent syllables stuttered	Similar to frequency of developmental stuttering
Secondary behaviors	Beyond early childhood, tension and struggle often observed, along with escape and avoidance behaviors	Typically, very few secondary behaviors or none
Emotional response to stuttering	Beyond early childhood, frequently notable emotional reactions such as struggle, embarrassment, and shame	Usually little emotional response to stuttering, except occasional frustration
Locus of stutters	Stutters tend to occur on syllables at beginnings of words and at beginnings of phrases More stuttering on content words than function words	Stutters occur at many locations in words and phrases Stutters may occur just as often on function as on content words
Response to fluency-inducing conditions such as swinging arm or choral reading	Stuttering markedly reduced in fluency-inducing conditions	Sometimes no improvement with fluency-inducing conditions
Adaptation effect: repeated reading of a passage	Adaptation frequently seen—stuttering frequency and severity decrease with repeated reading of passage	Adaptation often does not change the frequency or severity of stuttering
Treatment	Stuttering modification or fluency-shaping treatments can make substantial improvements	Pacing (speaking one syllable at a time) can be helpful, as can slowing speech rate

In conclusion, professionals working with clients having acquired neurogenic stuttering should be encouraged to develop systematic ways of collecting and sharing data (see Appendix B of Ringo & Dietrich, 1995) so that this infrequently occurring disorder can be better understood. As a consequence, we may better understand stuttering of all kinds.

A comparison of the characteristics of neurogenic stuttering compared with developmental stuttering is given in Table 15.1.

PSYCHOGENIC ACQUIRED STUTTERING

Nature

Psychogenic stuttering, like neurogenic stuttering, is often but not always a late-onset disorder. Its major identifying feature is that it typically begins after a prolonged period of stress or after a traumatic event. It has sometimes been characterized as a conversion symptom (i.e., a physical or behavioral expression of a psychological conflict) (Lazare, 1981). Unlike malingering or faking, this type of stuttering is not conscious, volitional behavior by the client but is involuntary. Several authors (Baumgartner, 1999; Duffy, 2013; Mahr & Leith, 1992; Roth, Aronson, & Davis, 1989) have described its manifestations, diagnosis, and treatment, and this section borrows a good deal from them.

The stuttering pattern of this disorder resembles developmental stuttering in terms of core behaviors (i.e., repetitions, prolongations, and blocks), but in some cases, secondary behaviors may be unusual and occur independently of attempts to produce stuttered words (Baumgartner, 1999). Psychogenic stuttering may occur alone or together with other signs of psychological or neurological involvement. Strict definitions of psychogenic stuttering exclude cases in which childhood stuttering had been resolved but then reappeared under prolonged or sudden stress. Nonetheless, these cases may respond to treatment as readily as do many cases of true psychogenic stuttering.

When I conducted intensive group stuttering therapy in Australia, I treated a young man whose stutter had started in his late teens. He had never stuttered as a child, nor did he have a family history of stuttering. The onset of his stuttering occurred when, unable to afford graduate education in his preferred area, geology, he went into a teacher training program, which included a practicum experience. During this classroom training, he began to stutter, was required to leave teacher education, and was then able to attend graduate school in geology. He came to our intensive group stuttering therapy stuttering rather severely, with secondary characteristics, but quite socially confident. After 3 weeks, he was completely fluent (as were the other members of the group), and he continued to maintain his fluency (unlike some of the group members) for as long as I was able to follow him, 18 months following the end of treatment.

I have no evidence of this, but I would speculate that for this young man, the anxiety of teaching for the first time created some initial disfluency when he spoke to his classes. Perhaps, anxiety interferes with fine motor control in many people. After this initial loss of speech-motor control, his natural self-consciousness, combined with a desire to find a way out of the teaching profession, somehow turned a spontaneous and momentary disfluency into a full-blown stutter. Because it had become conditioned to many stimuli associated with speaking, the stuttering persisted even though he had left teaching and returned to his first love, geology. Speculating further, his treatment may have been successful because the stuttering had begun within the past few years, and he was ripe for relearning his natural fluent speech pattern. If my speculation is correct, then some cases of psychogenic stuttering may resolve if they are treated promptly with an intensive speech retraining program and if the conflict that triggered the stuttering is alleviated.

Diagnosis and Evaluation

Roth et al. (1989) pointed out that adult-onset stuttering can have several etiologies that need to be considered: purely neurogenic, purely psychogenic, psychogenic accompanied by psychogenically based neurologic signs, and psychogenic with coexisting (but unrelated) neurologic disease or disorder. Thus, one of the first aims of an evaluation is to rule out a neurological etiology, particularly since adult-onset stuttering is sometimes the first sign of a neurologic disorder. A multidisciplinary approach, involving neurology, psychiatry, and speech-language pathology (SLP), may be best, especially if a client has neurological signs, such as headache, dizziness, or numbness of extremities. If the speech-language pathologist suspects there may be psychological or neurological causes for the stuttering, referral for further evaluation to specialists in these areas is appropriate.

The evaluation should include the following:

1. A complete case history obtained either exclusively in an interview or via a questionnaire followed up with an interview. The case history should obtain information concerning:
   - Onset of stuttering, including circumstances surrounding onset, such as whether it occurred during prolonged or acute stress and the nature and pattern of the stuttering when it began
   - Changes in stuttering since onset and whether there have been times of complete fluency
   - Current pattern of stuttering, its situational variability, and its impact on the client's life
   - Whether the individual stuttered previously at any time and if so, its nature and pattern and the extent of recovery
   - Family history of stuttering and other speech, language, or learning problems

   If the clinician can maintain an interested, accepting attitude, the client is more likely to reveal vital information about the emotions associated with the stuttering. Baumgartner (1999) noted that clients' expression of feelings may be accompanied by increased fluency, which is a sign of psychogenic basis for the stuttering.
2. Baumgartner (1999) suggests giving adult-onset clients a motor speech exam (Duffy, 2013) to rule out such motor speech disorders as apraxia or Parkinson's disease that might underlie stuttering. He also suggests that if clients show signs of language or cognitive problems, these should be further tested.
3. As with neurological stuttering, clients should be asked to speak under traditional **fluency-inducing or fluency-enhancing conditions** that were listed in the evaluation procedures for suspected neurogenic stuttering. If a client stutters even more frequently or severely while speaking under these conditions, psychogenic stuttering should be suspected (Baumgartner, 1999).

4. **Trial therapy** should be carried out, and the clinician should model what is expected of the client and liberally provide praise and support to encourage him. More specific steps include the following:
   - Have the client try to stay in a moment of stuttering. The clinician first models this, then instructs the client, and may even need to use a cue to help the client "catch" a moment of stuttering and hold on to it. In this and subsequent steps, the client may stop holding onto a stutter because he has run out of breath or for other reasons. The clinician should accept this and instruct him to "get the stutter going again," even though at this point, it may be a voluntary behavior rather than a true stutter.
   - While the client is holding onto a stutter, have him touch places on his face or throat where he appears to be tensing or "holding back" the word that is being stuttered.
   - While the client is holding onto a stutter, have him change the tension, the speeding up, or other elements of the stutter, so that the sound becomes prolonged voluntarily.
   - When the client has changed the "holding back" behaviors, the clinician should then coach him to slowly finish the stuttered word, making a slow transition from the stutter into the remainder of the word.
   - Following this, the clinician should guide the client through all of the steps just described for trial therapy on his own while reading aloud or conversing.

   If the trial therapy suggested does not seem to be working, a different trial therapy should be tried. One example of a different trial therapy is described in the section on stuttering as a result of stress and injuries while in the military. This involves manipulation of the thyrohyoid area of the neck to produce relaxation, accompanied by strong suggestion that this will relieve stuttering. Alternatively, **prolonged speech** can be used (see the Controlled Fluency section in Chapter 14). In any case, the point of trial therapy with psychogenic stuttering is to see if the client becomes dramatically more fluent during trial therapy—another sign of psychogenicity. Whatever approach works should be used as a complete approach to treatment, with steps for generalization.
5. Analysis of stuttering. Samples should be obtained of the client's conversational speech and reading aloud so that baseline measures of stuttering severity can be made with the SSI-4, and the patterns of stuttering can be examined. As mentioned above, unusual struggle behaviors, especially if they are independent of moments of stuttering, are signs of possible psychogenicity of stuttering.

Diagnosis of psychogenic stuttering is usually tentative. The clinician must weigh multiple factors, and even then, a conclusive diagnosis might never be reached. The most clear-cut pieces of evidence for this diagnosis are (1) adult onset during psychological stress and (2) the absence of neurological factors associated with the client's stuttering. Two other factors can help support the diagnosis—(3) dramatic improvement with trial therapy and (4) unusual or bizarre struggle behaviors.

Considerations for Treatment

Individuals who are able to decrease their stuttering in trial therapy and whose psychological adjustment is adequate are often good candidates for stuttering therapy. Even though they may need psychotherapy eventually, speech therapy may start immediately. On the other hand, clients who are unable to improve fluency during trial therapy and/or who are dysfunctional because of psychological issues may benefit from receiving psychotherapy concurrently with (or prior to) stuttering therapy. Individuals who resist the idea that their stuttering may have a stress-related basis and who do not improve with trial therapy may not be good candidates for treatment or may need extended treatment.

Treatment Approaches

Several published reports on psychogenic stuttering suggest that speech therapy can be very effective with this group of clients (Baumgartner, 1999; Duffy, 2013; Mahr & Leith, 1992; Roth et al., 1989). Baumgartner emphasized that clients benefit from an understanding that their stuttering is not the result of neurological problems and from the clinician's continuing encouragement about their progress.

Most treatments used with developmental stuttering have been reported to be effective with psychogenic stuttering (Roth et al., 1989). In my own experience, a fluency-shaping approach (specifically, prolonged speech) was very beneficial for the young adult, described earlier in this section, who had developed stuttering suddenly when he did not want to pursue a career in classroom teaching but was required to do so because of the financial support he'd received for his education. Roth et al. (1989) suggested that approaches such as easy onset, light contact, and easy repetitions can be effective. Baumgartner (1999) worked with clients to diminish extra motor behaviors and reduce the physical tension associated with their efforts to speak. Duffy (2013) provided a seven-step procedure in which the clinician helps the client reduce tension and change repetitive stutters into more normal-sounding prolongations while giving support and reassurance for gradual progress. Weiner (1981) employed desensitization combined with vocal control therapy that emphasized adequate respiratory support, gentle onsets, and optimal vocal resonance. Transfer was carried out using a hierarchy of easy-to-difficult situations. Unfortunately, no long-term treatment outcomes for therapy with psychogenic stuttering have been reported.

There are still many mysteries to be solved about psychogenic stuttering. One is whether the anomalies in brain activity patterns seen in developmental stuttering (Chapters 2 and 3) are present in this disorder. Another is whether psychological stress produces mistimings and discoordinations that result in the disorder or whether psychological factors actually result in highly coordinated struggle behaviors that reflect the speaker's efforts to speak despite primitive reflexes holding back speech. It is appropriate to ask what, if anything, psychogenic stuttering teaches us about developmental stuttering. Some electromyographic studies of developmental stuttering have shown cocontraction of speech production muscles in a fashion that impedes speech flow (Freeman & Ushijima, 1975; Guitar, Guitar, Neilson, O'Dwyer, & Andrews, 1988). If the same cocontractions are evident in psychogenic stuttering, it may suggest that these muscle activities in developmental stuttering are perhaps nonconscious learned, emotionally based "holding back" responses rather than evidence of discoordination.

Stuttering as a Result of Stress and Injuries While in the Military

This is a special section for those readers who will be working with active duty military service members or veterans whose stuttering appeared as the result of stress or injuries while in combat. The information comes from a presentation at the 2011 ASHA Convention about this topic presented by Roth, Manning, and Duffy (2011).[2]

Sudden-onset stuttering not infrequently appears in military personnel who have been in combat and who have sustained **traumatic brain injury (TBI)** and/or **posttraumatic stress disorder (PTSD)**. Such stuttering presents a challenge in terms of differential diagnosis (neurogenic, psychogenic stuttering, or a combination) and treatment. The combined experiences of Carole Roth, Kevin Manning, and Joe Duffy provide some guidelines for assessing and treating these clients. Their stuttering-like behaviors can include initial syllable or whole-word repetitions, prolongations, tension with facial grimaces, posturing of articulators or whispering before starting speech, hesitations, and/or blocking before initial sounds. These speech behaviors may be accompanied (and exacerbated) by attention problems, slow speed of processing, and word-retrieval problems. Other signs of TBI/PTSD may be present such as problems sleeping, nightmares, or difficulty concentrating.

Differential diagnosis is not always possible and may not be absolutely necessary. Signs of neurogenic stuttering, as indicated in the earlier section, include stuttering on both content and function words, lack of secondary symptoms such as tension and struggle, no reduction of stuttering during repeated reading of a passage, and little fear and anxiety about speech (e.g., De Nil et al., 2007). Signs of psychogenic stuttering, as indicated, include onset during psychological stress (which may include experience of combat injury), dramatic improvement during trial therapy, and absence of verified neurological impairment.

In the initial evaluation, and subsequently in treatment, it is important to listen carefully to the client's complaints and take them seriously. Moreover, the clinician should help the client understand why combat stress may produce stuttering. For example, the clinician can describe how all speakers may become disfluent if they are under the stress of hurry, confusion, or indecision. Combat stress can be thought of as an extreme and prolonged instance of this. A key part of the evaluation is trial therapy, which should be carried out with a positive, confident manner. Duffy (in Roth et al., 2011) suggests the clinician put her hands on the thyrohyoid area, feel for tension, and have the speaker talk while the clinician pulls the thyroid cartilage down to a more relaxed position. The client can be told that he is maintaining excessive tension in this area; the clinician can then guide him through a hierarchy of producing vowels, single words, sentences, and conversation in a very relaxed and slow style. A psychological basis of the stuttering is supported if the client becomes very fluent in this trial treatment. While individuals with developmental stuttering can be noticeably helped by trial therapy, it will usually not generalize to fluency during the remainder of the session. The clinician should be careful to explain the client's fluency to him, relating it to the relaxation that counteracts the excess tension developed as a response to stress.

If fluency is not obtained through muscle relaxation, then a fluency-shaping technique, such as slow, prolonged speech, should be used. Whichever technique is effective should be explained to the client and taught in subsequent sessions, with appropriate generalization to the client's everyday life. In many cases, group stuttering therapy or group psychotherapy (led by a psychologist) can be an effective adjunct to individual treatment, especially if some focus is made on other aspects of PTSD.

Summary and Conclusions

In the past 10 years, there has been an increasing acceptance of the idea that disfluencies associated with psychological trauma and stress may actually be a type of stuttering. The main diagnostic markers are (1) stuttering onset that occurs in late adolescence or adulthood, (2) stuttering onset that is associated with prolonged or acute stress, (3) unusual struggle behaviors that may not always be associated with moments of stuttering, (4) stuttering that increases in fluency-inducing conditions, and (5) dramatically improved fluency during trial treatment. Compared with neurogenic stuttering, there is relatively little known about the speech characteristics observed in psychogenic stuttering (such as the linguistic loci of stutters), nor is there consensus on the common types of core behaviors associated with this disorder.

Characteristics of psychogenic stuttering compared with developmental stuttering are summarized in Table 15.2.

[2]https://www.asha.org/Events/convention/handouts/2011/Duffy-Manning-Roth/

TABLE 15.2 Comparative Characteristics of Psychogenic Stuttering Compared with Developmental Stuttering

Characteristic	Developmental Stuttering	Psychogenic Stuttering
Etiology	Deficits in the speech production areas of the brain	Response to emotional stress
Onset	Usually in early childhood between ages 2 and 5 years	Late childhood or adulthood, soon after emotional stress
Development or change over time	If it does not disappear in early childhood, stuttering usually gets gradually more severe during childhood and adolescence	Stuttering usually remains similar to what it was like at onset
Types of stuttering behavior	Repetitions, prolongations, and blocks	May be similar to developmental stuttering. Alternatively, may consist of very rapid repetitions. Unusually steady eye contact is sometimes evident
Frequency of stuttering	From mild to severe. Almost always below 45 percent syllables stuttered	Usually high frequency
Secondary behaviors	Beyond early childhood, tension and struggle often observed, along with escape and avoidance behaviors	May consist of unusual or severe blocks
Emotional response to stuttering	Beyond early childhood, frequently notable emotional reactions such as struggle, embarrassment, and shame	Usually little emotional response to stuttering. In some cases, client may smile during stuttering
Locus of stutters	Stutters tend to occur on syllables at beginnings of words and at beginnings of phrases More stuttering on content words than function words	Stutters occur at many locations in words and phrases Stutters may occur just as often on function as on content words
Response to fluency-inducing conditions such as swinging arm or choral reading	Stuttering markedly reduced in fluency-inducing conditions	Sometimes, no improvement with fluency-inducing conditions. In some cases, stuttering becomes more severe
Adaptation effect: repeated reading of a passage	Adaptation frequently seen—stuttering frequency and severity decrease with repeated reading of passage	Adaptation often does not change the frequency or severity of stuttering
Treatment	Stuttering modification or fluency-shaping treatments can make substantial improvements	Treatment should be accompanied by strong suggestion that it will help. Intensive fluency-shaping (such as prolonged speech) may be immediately beneficial

MALINGERING

Although malingering (faking a disorder to receive some benefit) is not technically psychogenic, I think it would be helpful for me to describe this manifestation of stuttering in close proximity to my discussion of neurogenic and psychogenic stuttering since all three of these will occur with adult onset, which makes it important to differentially diagnose them. Also, who knows? You may someday be asked to testify in court if malingering stuttering is suspected.

Case reports by Shirkey (1987) and Seery (2005) describe protocols that they used to attempt to distinguish between developmental, neurogenic, or psychogenic stuttering, versus malingering. In each case, the person in question had been accused of a crime during which he spoke fluently, but claimed he was innocent because he stuttered so severely that he could not have been that individual. Their approaches were similar and the suggestions given here combine their reports. An additional report by the neuropsychologists Binder, Spector, and Youngjohn (2012) detailed three cases of possible malingered, neurogenic, or psychogenic stuttering that were evaluated after mild brain injury resulted in lawsuits or workers' compensation claims. Seery's protocol was used, along with other neuropsychological assessment procedures, to evaluate the claims of these clients.

The following diagnostic procedures may be helpful for differentiating malingering from developmental stuttering, although evidence gained in this way may not be foolproof. I use term "client" here for the individual who may or may not be malingering.

Develop a good working relationship with the client and elicit a speech sample to later analyze while, at the same time, gathering information about the client's history and experience as someone who stutters. Questions about the onset and development of the stuttering may help determine if—as in typical developmental stuttering—the client's stuttering onset was in childhood, the client experienced negative listener reactions, and the client was self-conscious about his stuttering.

The speech sample should be analyzed to determine the frequency of stuttering, secondary behaviors, the types of stutters, the variability of stuttering, and the loci of stutters. In malingering, the frequency may be more than 45 percent that would be above the range expected for developmental stuttering and suggestive of malingering (Seery, 2005). Other aspects of the stuttering that may indicate malingering are stereotyped and very severe types of stuttering, lack of secondary behaviors, and presence of good eye contact throughout the sample.

In the client's description of his stuttering onset and development, the time of onset may be unusual in cases of malingering, with onset typically in adulthood and a high level of consistency over time, but neurogenic and psychogenic stuttering may also show such features as onset in adulthood and little change in stuttering over a long period of time.

The clinician should have the client speak under fluency-inducing conditions, such as speaking in time to an arm swing or finger tapping, reading in unison with the clinician, and speaking in a slow, prolonged manner, either in response to DAF or in following the clinician's model of slow, prolonged speech. An individual who is malingering is likely to improve little or less than expected in these conditions that will usually create fluency in those with typical developmental stuttering. However, clients with neurogenic or psychogenic stuttering may also show less improvement than expected.

Obtain testimony from the client's friends and relatives about whether the client is typically more fluent than he has been in this interview. If someone is malingering by showing very severe and consistent stuttering in the interview, it is likely that friends and relatives will report less severe and less consistent stuttering in their interactions with him.

Readers who are tasked with evaluating a client suspected of malingered stuttering should consult the articles referred to in this section, especially Seery's report (2005) and her Table 1 that summarizes the characteristics of developmental, neurogenic, psychogenic, and malingered stuttering.

Characteristics of malingered stuttering—compared with developmental stuttering—are given in Table 15.3.

CLUTTERING

Nature

Many years ago, cluttering was described as "...a torrent of half-articulated words, following each other like peas running out of a spout" (Van Riper, 1954, p. 25). The essence of cluttering, as this quote suggests, is rapid speaking that is difficult to understand. Words may be collapsed, syllables may be omitted, or sounds may be slurred. Cluttering is often accompanied by disfluencies that differ from those typically heard in stuttering; instead of blocks, prolongations, and repetitions, individuals who clutter may produce fillers, incomplete phrases, word and phrase repetitions, revisions, and hesitations—all usually without tension. The speaking rate of a person who clutters is not continuously rapid, however, but gives the impression of coming in sudden impulsive bursts that are filled with misarticulations and disfluencies. In contrast to people who stutter, individuals who clutter become more fluent—as well as slower and more intelligible—when they make an effort to control their disorder. This rarely happens, unfortunately, because most people who clutter are often not aware they are "cluttering" unless someone brings it to their attention.

Several excellent publications on cluttering have described the disorder as manifesting the above speech characteristics but also as being characterized by, in many cases, language and learning problems (St. Louis, 1996; St. Louis, Myers, Bakker, & Raphael, 2007; St. Louis, Raphael, Myers, & Bakker, 2003; Ward & Scott, 2011). The language problems were first recognized by Weiss (1964), who described cluttering as a problem of "central language imbalance" that may reflect a disorganized formulation process. If he used the current parlance, Weiss would say it's a language disorder. The person who clutters seems to be unable to put his thoughts into coherent sentences and link them together in a logical way. Such language behavior is sometimes termed "**mazing**," a metaphor for repeated false starts, hesitations, and revisions that leave listeners puzzled about a speaker's verbal destination. The concomitant problems of people with cluttering may include distractibility, hyperactivity, learning difficulties, articulation problems, and auditory processing problems. Cluttering is sometimes accompanied by stuttering.

TABLE 15.3 Comparative Characteristics of Malingering Compared with Developmental Stuttering

Characteristic	Developmental Stuttering	Malingering
Etiology	Deficits in the speech production areas of the brain	Attempt to gain benefit by appearing to stutter. May fake more severe stuttering than is actually the case
Onset	Usually in early childhood between ages 2 and 5 years	Adulthood, sometimes after an accident to claim compensation or after a crime to claim innocence
Development or change over time	If it does not disappear in early childhood, stuttering usually gets gradually more severe during childhood and adolescence	Stuttering usually remains similar to what it was like on onset
Types of stuttering behavior	Repetitions, prolongations, and blocks	May be similar to developmental stuttering, but also may have unusual symptoms
Frequency of stuttering	From mild to severe. Almost always below 45 percent syllables stuttered	Sometimes, high frequency of stuttering
Secondary behaviors	Beyond early childhood, tension and struggle often observed, along with escape and avoidance behaviors	May appear like developmental, but also may be very rote, with the same type of stutter in each instance
Emotional response to stuttering	Beyond early childhood, frequently notable emotional reactions such as struggle, embarrassment, and shame	Typically little emotional response to stuttering. No shame or embarrassment
Locus of stutters	Stutters tend to occur on syllables at beginnings of words and at beginnings of phrases More stuttering on content words than function words	Stutters occur at many locations in words and phrases Stutters may occur just as often on function as on content words
Response to fluency-inducing conditions such as swinging arm or choral reading	Stuttering markedly reduced in fluency-inducing conditions	Usually, no improvement with fluency-inducing conditions
Adaptation effect: repeated reading of a passage	Adaptation frequently seen—stuttering frequency and severity decrease with repeated reading of passage	Adaptation often does not change the frequency or severity of stuttering
Treatment	Stuttering modification or fluency-shaping treatments can make substantial improvements	Treatment inappropriate

Cluttering, then, seems to be a disorder whose core signs or symptoms are rapid and irregular speech rate that is often unintelligible and replete with typical non–stuttering-like disfluencies. Language is often disorganized and the individual often lacks awareness of his difficulty and of listener cues signaling lack of understanding. Neuropsychological problems may or may not be present. Speculation about the neurophysiological basis of the disorder suggests abnormalities in the basal ganglia (Alm, 2004; Kent, 2000). More precise information was reported by Ward, Connally, Pliatsikas, Bretherton-Furness, and Watkins (2015), who conducted a functional MRI study of 17 individuals with cluttering and 17 matched controls. They found that the group with cluttering had the following characteristics compared with controls: greater activity in premotor cortex bilaterally and pre-supplementary motor area (SMA), greater activity in caudate nucleus and putamen of the basal ganglia, and reduced activity in lateral anterior cerebellum. No abnormal activity was seen in higher language areas. They surmised that these findings suggest that the major problem in cluttering is difficulty with both planning and execution in speech-motor control.

Diagnosis and Evaluation

The process of evaluating a client for possible cluttering differs for different ages (school age vs. adult) and will vary depending on the setting in which the evaluation takes place (e.g., school vs. university or hospital clinic). In many cases, especially with school-age children, a multidisciplinary approach to evaluation is important and may involve the SLP, classroom teacher, special educator, psychologist, and audiologist. In the following section, I give some general guidelines that reflect information gleaned from several sources, including Myers and St. Louis (1986, 2007), St. Louis (1996), St. Louis and colleagues (2003), and van Zaalen, Wijnen, and Dejonckere (2011).

Case History and Interview

The case history can be filled out by a client (or parent) beforehand and used as a guideline for the interview. Among the important areas to be covered in the case history and interview are the following:

- *The client's, parents', and/or teachers' perceptions of the problem.* What aspects of the cluttering "syndrome" are the presenting problem (from the viewpoint of the person completing the form and participating in the interview)? Because the individual who clutters is himself often unaware of his own speech, an adult or adolescent may report that his problem is that people say he's sometimes hard to understand. It should be ascertained, however, how cluttering affects him. For example, does he have a hard time in school, social situations, or his job because people don't always understand him?
- *How long the problem has existed.* In some cases, cluttering might have begun in preschool years, but it is usually not until the school years when listeners tell him that he's mumbling or talking too fast, or that they simply can't understand him. Nonetheless, it is useful to gather information about the individual's speech and language development—whether it was delayed, advanced, or atypical.
- *When and where the problem appears.* Cluttering can be variable, so it's important to understand which situations are particularly troublesome. This may depend on the listeners and the demands of the situation. Some children may do well when they are reading or giving one-word answers, but may lose intelligibility during narratives. Adults who clutter may be fluent and intelligible when speaking to close friends, but their intelligibility may suffer when speaking in more demanding situations.
- *Background on the individual and his family.* It is helpful in understanding a client's cluttering to view it in a larger perspective, including whether other members of the client's extended family clutter or have other communication or learning problems; whether the client has other problems, such as stuttering, that interfere with communication; and whether the client has received treatment for his communication problem(s) and how successful treatment has been.
- *Reasons for seeking treatment at this time.* A major determinant of success in cluttering therapy is the client's motivation. It is important to find out from the case history or interview whether the client is aware of his cluttering and whether it bothers him enough to undertake the hard work that successful therapy will require.
- *Other problems.* The case history and interview should determine if the client has any of the other problems that often accompany cluttering, such as receptive or expressive language difficulties, articulation problems, central auditory processing deficits, attention deficit/hyperactivity, reading problems, or learning disabilities.

Direct Assessment of Speech

The client's speech should be examined on a variety of tasks in a variety of situations. Cluttering, like stuttering, varies a great deal so it is easy to gain a false impression from a small sample of speech gathered in the clinic. The Web site for the International Cluttering Association (http://associations.missouristate.edu/ICA/) contains a link to software for evaluating cluttering. This Web site, frequently updated, also contains many helpful links for both clinicians and individuals who clutter.

Recording of Speech

The client should be digitally audio or video recorded for 15 or 20 minutes while performing a number of speaking tasks, including:

- A narrative about a topic not related to his speech, such as describing what he did on his last vacation or a favorite movie. This should be done in a way that really engages the client in talking so that a natural, unguarded sample can be obtained.
- Reading a passage appropriate for his reading level
- A conversation in which the client talks about something that really interests him
- For clients who report that their cluttering is situational, a sample should be recorded in the relevant environments.
- van Zaalen et al. (2011) also recommend that older clients should be asked to produce words that may be difficult, such as "statistical" or "chrysanthemum," as well as words with differing stress patterns such as "apply," "application," and "applicable" to assess their ability to handle complex phonological sequences and changing linguistic stress patterns. These authors also recommend retelling a story.

Analysis of Speech

After the recording has been made, the speech samples should be analyzed to assess speech rate in syllables per minute using the procedures described in Chapter 8. Many individuals who clutter can reduce their overly fast rate when they try; therefore, the narrative and reading samples may show slower rates than do conversation samples. If it is the clinician's impression during the evaluation that the client's speech rate was not slower during narrative or reading compared to conversation (as would be expected for most speakers), she should ask the client to engage in a narrative task and try to speak at a slow, normal rate. The client's ability to slow his speaking rate may be a good prognostic sign, because much of cluttering therapy is focused on slowing a client's speaking rate. The various samples can be compared to the speech rate norms for different ages that were given in Chapter 9.

Many individuals who clutter don't speak at a consistently fast rate, but at a relatively normal rate with sudden bursts of rapid speech. Assessment, therefore, should include measures of speech rate during these bursts and how frequently they occur. A comparison may be made between the client's articulatory rate (i.e., syllables per second with pauses excluded) during fast bursts of speech and during regular speech. The articulatory rates of typical adults in conversation are six to seven syllables per second (St. Louis et al., 2003).

Analysis of Cluttering

When seeing a client with suspected cluttering (or suspected stuttering, for that matter), analysis of speech samples should also include separate counts of normal-type disfluencies and stuttering-like disfluencies (see Chapters 7 and 9 for this distinction). The number of syllables that are normally disfluent and the number that are stuttered can be expressed as a proportion of the total number of syllables spoken in the sample. These measures will reflect the proportions of stuttering and cluttering in the client's speech. Some clients have both stuttering and cluttering in their speech, but one usually predominates. It has been suggested that when stuttering is mixed with cluttering, a client's cluttering may not be noticed until his stuttering is substantially reduced by therapy (Bakker, 2002; St. Louis et al., 2003).

Analysis of Meaningful versus Extraneous Syllables

When I evaluate a client with cluttering, I find it useful to calculate the ratio of the number of syllables spoken that are part of the intended message, if that can be reliably discerned, to the number of syllables spoken that are extraneous to the message. For example, in the utterance, "Well, you see, I think, I think the, the, the sky is well is blue" (15 syllables), we can assume that the speaker meant to convey "I think the sky is blue" (six syllables). Thus, 6 syllables, or 60 percent of the utterance, are extraneous, which undoubtedly detracts from the speaker's communicative effectiveness. This measure may be helpful also in assessing a client's progress in therapy.

Analysis of Intelligibility

The intelligibility of a sample should be assessed by having one or more listeners unfamiliar with the client gloss (i.e., interpret) each word and each utterance. The percentage of words and of utterances that are understood can be calculated, providing pretherapy measures of a client's intelligibility.

Language Assessment

The language skills of clients who clutter are likely to be affected by the disorder. In fact, Weiss (1964) described cluttering as a central language imbalance, suggesting that language deficits are at its core.

Wiig (2002) suggested that many aspects of the language of people with cluttering can be effectively tested using the Clinical Evaluation of Language Fundamentals (CELF-3) (Semel, Wiig, & Secord, 1995). Almost certainly this applies to the CELF-5 (Wiig, Semel, & Secord, 2013) which is appropriate for individuals from 5 to 21 years old. This test assesses "the relationships among semantics, syntax/morphology, and pragmatics, and the interrelated domains of receptive and expressive language." Wiig suggested that it be administered in such a way that a client's responses could be timed, because under time pressure, which simulates everyday conversational situations, the scores of a client who clutters might well be lower.

It may also be helpful to assess a client's pragmatic behaviors in the videotaped conversational sample described above. Pragmatic skills that may be lacking include appropriate turn taking, supplying complete information to the listener, and repairing communication when it breaks down.

Other aspects of language assessment are described in van Zaalen et al. (2011) and Myers and St. Louis (2007).

Assessment of Cluttering Characteristics

Clients may exhibit a variety of traits that are part of the cluttering syndrome. The clinician may find it helpful to use Daly's Predictive Cluttering Inventory (2006).[3] This checklist evaluates a client in four areas: pragmatics, speech-motor control, language cognition, and motor coordination for writing. It can be used for assessing areas of deficit as well as for treatment planning. These ratings help the clinician determine which cluttering characteristics are most salient and are therefore most in need of treatment.

---

[3]This is available in seven languages from http://associations.missouristate.edu/ICA/Resources/Resources%20and%20Links%20pages/clinical_materials.htm/

Assessment of Coexisting Disorders in Domains Other Than Communication

In the process of gathering information about a client, the clinician may become aware of challenges that affect communication but are not the province of only the SLP. These may include auditory processing disorders, attention-deficit disorder, hyperactivity, reading difficulties, social adjustment problems, illegible handwriting, and learning disabilities (Ward & Scott, 2011). These challenges may best be assessed with the help of other specialists, such as an audiologist, psychologist, learning specialist, reading specialist, and the classroom teacher.

Considerations for Treatment

Because clients who clutter are usually not aware of their problem and are often surprised when listeners don't understand them, they rarely seek treatment. Indeed, those who do seek treatment are often referred by someone else. Some individuals who clutter, however, can be motivated to work hard in therapy and can make good progress. Two positive prognostic signs are the ability to speak without cluttering if asked to do so and a specific reason for improving, such as getting or keeping a job or receiving a promotion at work. Children who clutter can often be engaged in games and activities that will create motivation for their work in treatment.

Treatment Approaches

The evaluation procedures described above should suggest the areas that are particular challenges for each client. Treatment can then focus on these areas of need. Lanouette (2011), Myers (2002, 2011), and Myers and St. Louis (2007) outlined several cluttering therapy strategies that they have explored in their work with cluttering over several years. I describe them in the following section with some minor changes:

1. Increase the client's awareness of his speech rate and his ability to decrease rate.
   - Simulate various speaking rates by having the client move his arm or walk at slow, medium, and fast tempos. Then, teach the client to attend to his sensory feedback while he is doing this so that he learns the feeling of these rates.
   - Alternate between speaking and moving various body parts or walking at various rates while attending to sensory feedback.
   - Use movements and walking paced by fast and slow music.
   - With children, engage in activities in which they can get speeding tickets or give speeding tickets to the clinician for speaking too fast.
   - Teach clients to attend to various verbal and nonverbal cues from a listener that indicates they are speaking too quickly or cannot be understood. For example, listeners may frown or show puzzlement on their faces or repeatedly ask the speaker to repeat himself.
   - For readers, put symbols at periods and commas, such as red or yellow lights, to help them slow their speech rate at relevant places in a text.
   - Teach phrasing and pausing in conversational speech.
   - Use the concept of a speedometer for children and ask them to speak at 75 miles per hour and then at 35 miles per hour.
   - Teach clients to speak with strong stress patterns by reciting poetry, for example.
2. Improve linguistic skills.
   - Teach clients to chunk and sequence their thoughts by having them write a story or narrative on cards, sequence them, and then tell the story aloud using the cards.
   - Involve clients in skits and plays so that they learn to follow a script and use turn taking.
   - Teach them such pragmatic skills as turn taking in conversation and staying on topic in conversation.
   - Teach them how to use complex sentences with subordinate clauses.
3. Facilitate fluency.
   - Use DAF to help clients learn to speak in a slower, more fluent manner.
   - Use DAF to teach proprioception, by having clients speak at a normal rate under maximal delay (i.e., 250 ms) by ignoring auditory feedback.
4. Increase the client's knowledge and awareness of cluttering.
   - Teach clients about the disorder of cluttering using Daly and Burnett-Stolnack's (1995) checklist to help the client learn which cluttering behaviors he has.
   - Have the client transcribe and analyze a recording of his cluttered speech.
   - Help the client become aware of his thought processes when he is talking in fast bursts of disorganized speech.

Further suggestions for treatment were presented by St. Louis and colleagues (2003), which included:

1. Rather than admonish the client to "slow down," have him match the clinician's speech rate using a computer-based program to display the clinician's and client's utterances. I have used Visi Pitch® for this, but there may be computer apps available for playing the clinician's model and the client's speech simultaneously.
2. To help clients achieve their potential to use normal speech, have them imagine themselves (i.e., in their mind's eye and ear) speaking effectively and have them use positive self-talk to strengthen their visual and auditory images. It may help also for the client and clinician to video record the client's best and worst speech and play these samples back to him to remind him of the range of his options.

3. When working on intelligibility and organization, begin with short utterances that are spoken clearly, and then gradually increase length and complexity while ensuring high quality of fluency, articulation, rate, and organization. Video recording and replaying them can help clients establish an auditory-visual image for what they are aiming.

In his chapter on treatment of cluttering, Daly (1986) provides his own guidelines for many of the treatment strategies described earlier. He believes that video feedback and analysis of audio samples are crucial for increasing a client's self-awareness. He also advocates helping clients learn to use relaxation exercises, mental imagery, and positive self-talk. His chapter has many references, which can help clinicians learn more about these activities.

There are very few studies of the treatment outcomes of cluttering therapy, and the ones that do exist consist of only one or two cases. A special edition of the *Journal of Fluency Disorders* (vol. 21, nos. 3–4, September–December 1996) on cluttering has a number of case studies. For example, data on a person who both cluttered and stuttered treated in a 3-week intensive smooth speech program indicated that the client's stuttering and speech rate were reduced to near-normal limits and that the gains appeared to be retained 10 months after treatment.

A report on a case study of the treatment of a teen who cluttered suggested two possible strategies to reduce overcoarticulation—the condensing of syllables so much that they become unintelligible (Healey, Nelson, & Scaler Scott, 2015). The two strategies were (1) having the client overarticulate his speech so that syllables were produced much more precisely and clearly and (2) having the client pause at natural places as he talked to slow his overall speech rate. Both strategies worked initially to reduce overcoarticulation, but only the pausing was used by the teen outside of the clinic.

One of the clients who was seen in our university clinic was treated for cluttering. Here are some details of his treatment. This young man, whom I shall call Alex, was an undergraduate who was referred to us by the Office of Student Services and Support. Alex had been diagnosed with—in addition to cluttering—attention deficit hyperactivity disorder (ADHD), as well as problems in visual acuity, organizational skills, and handwriting. His scores on the Predictive Cluttering Inventory (Daly, 2006) were 85/198 where any score between 80 and 120 indicates a mix of stuttering and cluttering. His score on the Overall Assessment of the Speaker's Experience of Stuttering (OASES) was 3.11, which indicated moderate/severe impairment.

Many aspects of treatment focused on helping Alex increase his awareness of his speech and his cluttering. He did not recognize how his rate of speech, omission of sounds and syllables, and narrative disorganization made him substantially unintelligible to listeners. He also did not pick up cues from listeners that they did not understand something he said, nor did he notice when listeners were signaling him that they were very busy or were frustrated that he wasn't giving them a turn to talk.

Early in the semester, his clinician used playback of audio/video recordings to teach Alex to self-evaluate his intelligibility. As he improved, the clinician brought in unfamiliar listeners to increase stress and generalize Alex's increasing ability to evaluate and self-correct his speech. At times, his clinician would make transcripts (in large font, because of his visual acuity problem) of his retelling a story he read, to have him "see" the extra sounds and irrelevancies he inserted. He then retold the story, correcting errors, and the clinician would replay the recorded improved sample, which she would praise and they would discuss. Another step in Alex's hierarchy was to go to a room with strangers who had been primed to occasionally nonverbally convey that they didn't understand something he said or that, after a period, they were too busy to talk or they wished to talk. With the clinician's guidance, Alex began to recognize listener cues and respond appropriately. Going further up the generalization hierarchy, Alex visited classes in which he talked, learned self-advocacy strategies (saying "give me a second to think about that"), talked with strangers around campus, and practiced job interviews. When he decided to stop therapy, Alex was gainfully employed and had become much more able to communicate effectively. At the end of his first semester in therapy, his scores on the OASES had improved from 3.11 to 2.72, which showed only moderate impairment.

Summary and Conclusions

Cluttering is a disorder with a probable neurological etiology. It is characterized by an excess of disfluencies, rapid rates of speech that often occur in momentary bursts, and lack of intelligibility, especially during bursts of increased rate. Although there is relatively little research on the nature and treatment of cluttering, there is some consensus that it isn't viewed as a problem until a child has reached school age. Evaluation procedures include (1) obtaining background information to determine, among other things, whether or not the client is aware of the problem and is motivated to undergo therapy; (2) direct assessment of speech on several different tasks to measure (i) frequency and type of disfluencies and (ii) speech rate and intelligibility overall as well as during fast bursts of speech; (3) language testing, particularly pragmatics and other aspects of expressive language; and (4) assessment of other possible concomitant disorders. Treatment should address the interdependent qualities of speech rate, fluency, intelligibility, and expressive language. Although many clinicians report success with motivated clients, there are essentially no outcome data on a particular treatment approach for cluttering.

Because cluttering most often co-occurs with stuttering, the disorders appear to be related in some as yet

TABLE 15.4 Comparison of Developmental Stuttering with Cluttering

Etiology	Developmental Stuttering	Cluttering
Etiology	Probably neurophysiological (anomalies in left hemisphere) exacerbated by temperament and environment	Neurological anomalies appear to consist of overactivity in premotor cortex pre-SMA and basal ganglia. These suggest a problem in planning and execution of speech-motor control
Typical onset	Usually ages 2–5, with some onsets in school years	May be present in preschool years, but often not diagnosed until problem interferes with school performance
Speech characteristics	Single-syllable whole-word repetitions, part-word repetitions, prolongations, and blocks. Frequency is usually more than 3 percent syllables stuttered. Secondary behaviors (escape and avoidance) common. Pattern varies somewhat	Excess of normal disfluencies, lack of intelligibility, especially during rapid bursts of speech. May slur syllables and leave out others entirely
Client's level of concern	Client typically shows frustration and embarrassment about stuttering, as well as fear of speaking	Frequently unaware of problem, except when listeners tell him they can't understand what he's said
Other diagnostic information	Frequency and severity are often variable from day to day and situation to situation	Often accompanied by stuttering, as well as language, attention, auditory processing, writing, and reading problems, and other learning disabilities
Treatment	School-age children and adults benefit from integration of behavioral, affective, and cognitive focus of stuttering therapy	Increase awareness of cluttering, particularly fast speech rate. Help client self-regulate speech rate and fluency. Improve awareness of listener cues and language skills such as narrative organization and pragmatics

undetermined way. Given the strong effect of slow speaking on stuttering and cluttering alike, it is possible that subgroups of individuals who stutter and those who clutter have difficulty maintaining a slow enough speech rate to match their capacity to synchronize the elements of language and speech output. Perhaps each disorder has a particular level of processing at which such dyssynchrony occurs.

The characteristics that distinguish cluttering from typical speech are summarized in Table 15.4.

STUDY QUESTIONS

1. If you had only one activity you could do with a client to differentiate neurogenic from psychogenic stuttering, which activity would you choose and why?
2. After reading about neurogenic stuttering, do you think that Canter's three categories of neurogenic stuttering are adequate? Why or why not?
3. Name four characteristics of stuttering behavior that appear to distinguish neurogenic stuttering from developmental stuttering.
4. What are contraindications (if any) for treatment of neurogenic stuttering?
5. If an adult-onset client had evidence of a neurological disorder, would you rule out psychogenic stuttering? Why or why not?
6. Compare the reported treatment success of psychogenic stuttering and neurogenic stuttering.
7. What are the contraindications (if any) for treatment of psychogenic stuttering?
8. What are the two most salient problems in cluttering?
9. Why might language and learning problems be related to the speech problems of cluttering?
10. What are the contraindications (if any) for treatment of cluttering?

SUGGESTED READINGS

Neurogenic Stuttering

De Nil, L., Jokel, R., & Rochon, E. (2007). Etiology, symptomatology, and treatment of neurogenic stuttering. In E. Conture, & R. F. Curlee (Eds.), *Stuttering and related disorders of fluency* (2nd ed., pp. 326–343). New York, NY: Thieme Medical Publishers.

This chapter covers prevalence and incidence of neurogenic stuttering in detail not seen elsewhere. The authors also present a critical review of the reported speech characteristics of neurogenic stuttering and indicate how different etiologies (e.g., stroke vs. head wound) may produce different speech characteristics.

Duffy, J. (2013). *Motor speech disorders* (3rd ed.). St. Louis, MO: Elsevier, Mosby.

Chapters 13, 14, 19, and 20 provide excellent coverage of the nature of neurogenic and psychogenic stuttering as well as their management. Duffy is particularly good at describing etiologies of these disorders and the other conditions with which they may be associated. His sections on management reflect his extensive clinical experience.

Ringo, C. C., & Dietrich, S. (1995). Neurogenic stuttering: An analysis and critique. *Journal of Medical Speech-Language Pathology, 3*, 111–122.

This article is particularly useful in that it critically examines characteristics of neurogenic stuttering that have been proposed by various authors since Canter's (1971) seminal publication about differential diagnosis of neurogenic stuttering. Each of seven characteristics is examined in light of evidence that it is present in neurogenic stuttering in a way that is different from its manifestation in developmental stuttering. Suggestions are made to standardize the data to be collected and reported on individual cases.

Psychogenic Stuttering

Baumgartner, J. (1999). Acquired psychogenic stuttering. In R. F. Curlee (Ed.), *Stuttering and related disorders of fluency* (2nd ed., pp. 269–288). New York, NY: Thieme Medical Publishers.

This chapter is an excellent starting place for anyone interested in learning about psychogenic stuttering. Baumgartner has been writing about this topic for several years and has firsthand clinical experience with individuals who have psychogenic stuttering, thus making the chapter a solid source for information.

Roth, C. R., Aronson, A. E., & Davis, L. J. (1989). Clinical studies in psychogenic stuttering of adult onset. *Journal of Speech and Hearing Disorders, 54*, 634–646.

This journal article examines the records of 12 patients who were evaluated and treated for psychogenic stuttering. Because the subjects were patients at the Mayo Clinic, they were examined thoroughly for psychological/psychiatric and neurological functioning in a standardized way, providing substantial evidence of the psychogenic nature of the stuttering. A case study is given to illustrate how stuttering can appear as a conversion reaction to emotional conflict. Clinical recommendations are given.

Van Riper, C. (1974). A handful of nuts. *WMU Journal of Speech Therapy, 11*(2), 1–3. Retrieved from http://www.mnsu.edu/comdis/kuster/vanriper/articles/nuts.html

This article describes several of Van Riper's clients who stuttered and were, he believed, psychotic.

Malingering

Seery, C. (2005). Differential diagnosis of stuttering for forensic purposes. *American Journal of Speech-Language Pathology, 14*, 284–297.

Although this article appears to be a case study, the background and protocols for evaluation are thorough and insightful. It is a must read for anyone who will be evaluating a case of suspected malingering of stuttering.

Cluttering

Kuster, J. *Online resources on cluttering: The other fluency disorder.* Retrieved from http://www.mnsu.edu/comdis/kuster/cluttering.html

This Web page is a treasure trove of useful resources on cluttering. Among them are videos, assessment techniques, computer-assisted cluttering instruments, treatment suggestions, links to support groups, and an extensive section on research.

Myers, F. L., & St. Louis, K. O. (2007). *Cluttering [DVD]*. Memphis, TN: The Stuttering Foundation.

This video provides excellent examples of cluttering in several young adults, as well as clear guidelines for evaluation and treatment.

Myers, F. L., & St. Louis, K. O. (Eds.) (1986). *Cluttering: A clinical perspective.* San Diego, CA: Singular Publishing Group, Inc.

This book, with an interesting forward by Charles Van Riper, is the first text on cluttering since the classic text on cluttering by Deso Weiss (1964). Chapters by the authors and other clinicians working with cluttering provide an overview of the disorder as well as practical suggestions for evaluation and treatment.

St. Louis, K. O., Raphael, L. J., Myers, F. L., & Bakker, K. (2003, Nov 18). Cluttering updated. *The ASHA Leader, 4–5*, 20–22.

This article, which is available online at www.asha.org, provides a clear synopsis of how to identify and evaluate cluttering, as well as specific suggestions for treating the core behaviors. For those who know little about cluttering, this publication is an excellent place to begin.

St. Louis, K. O. (Ed.) (1996). Research and opinion on cluttering: State of the art and science (Special issue). *Journal of Fluency Disorders, 21*(3–4), 171–374.

This special issue of JFD is rich with case studies of evaluations and treatments of individuals who clutter. It is therefore one of the few sources with data on treatment outcome, although the heterogeneity of the cases and the manner in which they are studied highlight the fact that research on cluttering is in its infancy. The cases studies are bracketed by overviews of the disorder at the beginning and critical reviews at the end that summarize the case studies and call attention to the poverty of credible data. A chapter by Myers is particularly valuable for its annotated list of publications on cluttering between 1964 and 1996.

Ward, D. (2017). *Stuttering and cluttering: Frameworks for understanding and treatment* (2nd ed.). Abingdon, UK: Taylor and Francis.

This is the second edition of a scholarly and clinical book on the nature and treatment of both cluttering and stuttering.

Ward, D., & Scott, K. S. (Eds.) (2011). *Cluttering: A handbook of research, intervention and education*. Hove, UK: Psychology Press.

This is a rich compendium of international authors discussing the nature of cluttering, as well as assessment and treatment. The two chapters on treatment have excellent overall organization as well as many ideas for specific activities. There are several chapters that describe clients with cluttering who also have other disorders such as Down's syndrome, learning disabilities, and autism spectrum disorders.

References

Abbiati, C., Guitar, B., & Hutchins, T. (2013, November). The development of an instrument to measure the speech attitudes of preschoolers who stutter. Paper presented at the Annual Meeting of the American Speech-Language-Hearing Association, Chicago.

Abbs, J. H. (1996). Mechanisms of speech motor execution and control. In N. Lass (Ed.), *Principles of experimental phonetics* (pp. 93–111). St. Louis, MO: Mosby.

Achenbach, T. M. (1988). *Child behavior checklist for ages 2–3*. Burlington, VT: University of Vermont.

Adams, M. (1977). A clinical strategy for differentiating the normally non-fluent child and the incipient stutterer. *Journal of Fluency Disorders, 2*(2), 141–148.

Adams, M. (1990). The demands and capacities model I: Theoretical elaborations. *Journal of Fluency Disorders, 15*, 135–141.

Adams, M., & Hayden, P. (1976). The ability of stutterers and nonstutterers to initiate and terminate phonation during production of an isolated vowel. *Journal of Speech and Hearing Research, 19*, 290–296.

Adams, M., & Runyan, C. M. (1981). Stuttering and fluency: Exclusive events or points on a continuum? *Journal of Fluency Disorders, 6*, 197–218.

Ahern, G. L., & Schwartz, G. E. (1985). Differential lateralization for positive and negative emotion in the human brain: EEG spectral analysis. *Neuropsychologia, 236*, 745–755.

Ainsworth, S., & Fraser, J. (2010). *If your child stutters: A guide for parents* (8th ed.). Memphis, TN: Stuttering Foundation.

Alfonso, P. J., Story, R. S., & Watson, B. C. (1987). The organization of supralaryngeal articulation in stutterers' fluent speech production: A second report. *Annual Bulletin Research Institute of Logopedics and Phoniatrics, 21*, 117–129.

Allen, G. D., & Hawkins, S. (1980). Phonological rhythm: Definition and development. In G. H. Yeni-Komshian, J. F. Kavanagh, & C. A. Ferguson (Eds.), *Child phonology* (Vol. 1, pp. 227–256). New York: Academic Press.

Allen, S. (1988). *Durations of segments in repetitive disfluencies in stuttering and nonstuttering children*. Unpublished manuscript, University of Vermont.

Allman, J. M., Hakeem, A., Erwin, J. M., Nimchinsky, E., & Hof, P. (2001). The anterior cingulate cortex: The evolution of an interface between emotion and cognition. *Annals of the New York Academy of Sciences, 935*, 107–117.

Alm, P. A. (2004). Stuttering and the basal ganglia circuits: A critical review of possible relations. *Journal of Communication Disorders, 37*, 325–396.

Alm, P. A., & Risberg, J. (2007). Stuttering in adults: The acoustic startle response, temperamental traits, and biological factors. *Journal of Communication Disorders, 40*, 1–41.

Ambrose, N., Cox, N., & Yairi, E. (1997). The genetic basis of persistence and recovery in stuttering. *Journal of Speech, Language, and Hearing Research, 40*, 556–566.

Ambrose, N., & Yairi, E. (1995). The role of repetition units in the differential diagnosis of early childhood incipient stuttering. *American Journal of Speech-Language Pathology, 4*, 82–88.

Ambrose, N., Yairi, E., & Cox, N. (1993). Genetic aspects of early childhood stuttering. *Journal of Speech and Hearing Research, 36*, 701–706.

Ambrose, N. G., & Yairi, E. (1999). Normative data for early childhood stuttering. *Journal of Speech, Language, and Hearing Research, 42*, 895–909.

Ambrose, N. G., Yairi, E., Loucks, T., Seery, C., & Throneburg, R. (2015). Relation of motor, linguistic and temperament factors in epidemiologic subtypes of persistent and recovered stuttering: Initial findings. *Journal of Fluency Disorders, 45*, 12–26.

Amster, B., & Klein, E. (2018). *More than fluency: The social, emotional, and cognitive dimensions of stuttering*. San Diego, CA: Plural Publishing.

Anderson, J., & Conture, E. G. (2000). Language abilities of children who stutter: A preliminary study. *Journal of Fluency Disorders, 25*(4), 283–304.

Anderson, J., Pellowski, M., & Conture, E. G. (2001, November). Temperament characteristics of children who stutter. Paper presented at the Annual meeting of the American Speech-Language Hearing Association, New Orleans, LA.

Anderson, J., Pellowski, M., Conture, E. G., & Kelly, E. (2003). Temperamental characteristics of young children who stutter. *Journal of Speech, Language, and Hearing Research, 46*, 1221–1233.

Anderson, J. D., Pellowski, M. W., & Conture, E. G. (2005). Childhood stuttering and disassociations across linguistic domains. *Journal of Fluency Disorders, 30*, 219–253.

Andrews, G., & Craig, A. (1982). Stuttering: Overt and covert measurement of the speech of treated subjects. *Journal of Speech and Hearing Disorders, 47*, 96–99.

Andrews, G., & Craig, A. (1988). Prediction of outcome after treatment for stuttering. *British Journal of Disorders of Psychiatry, 153,* 236–240.

Andrews, G., & Cutler, J. (1974). Stuttering therapy: The relation between changes in symptom level and attitudes. *Journal of Speech and Hearing Disorders, 39,* 312–319.

Andrews, G., & Harris, M. (1964). *The syndrome of stuttering.* London: Spastics Society Medical Education and Information Unit in association with W. Heinemann Medical Books.

Andrews, G., Hoddinott, S., Craig, A., Howie, P., Feyer, A-M., & Neilson, M. (1983). Stuttering: A review of research findings and theories circa 1982. *Journal of Speech and Hearing Disorders, 48,* 226–246.

Andrews, G., Howie, P., Dozsa, M., & Guitar, B. (1982). Stuttering: Speech pattern characteristics under fluency-inducing conditions. *Journal of Speech and Hearing Research, 25,* 208–216.

Andrews, G., & Ingham, R. (1971). Stuttering: Considerations in the evaluation of treatment. *British Journal of Communication Disorders, 6,* 129–138.

Andrews, G., Morris-Yates, A., Howie, P., & Martin, N. (1991). Genetic factors in stuttering confirmed. *Archives of General Psychiatry, 48*(11), 1034–1035.

Andrews, G., & Tanner, S. (1982). Stuttering treatment: An attempt to replicate the regulated-breathing method. *Journal of Speech and Hearing Disorders, 47,* 138–140.

Andy, O. J., & Bhatnager, S. C. (1992). Stuttering acquired from subcortical pathologies and its alleviation from thalamic pertubation. *Brain and Language, 42*(4), 385–401.

Arenas, R., & Zebrowski, P. (2013). The effects of autonomic arousal on speech production in adults who stutter: A preliminary study. *Speech, Language and Hearing, 16*(3), 176–185.

Arnott, S., Onslow, M., O'Brian, S., Packman, A., Jones, M., & Block, S. (2014). Group Lidcombe Program treatment of early stuttering: A randomized controlled trial. *Journal of Speech, Language, and Hearing Research, 57,* 1606–1618.

Arthur, G. (1952). *Arthur adaptation of the Leiter International Performance Test.* Los Angeles, CA: Western Psychological Services.

Ayres, J. J. B. (1998). Fear conditioning and avoidance. In W. O'Donohue (Ed.), *Learning and behavior therapy.* Boston, MA: Allyn and Bacon.

Azrin, N., & Nunn, R. (1974). A rapid method of eliminating stuttering by a regulated breathing approach. *Behavior Research and Therapy, 124,* 279–286.

Baker, D. J. (1967). The amount of information in the Oral Identification of Forms by normal speakers and selected speech-defective groups. In J. F. Bosma (Ed.), *Symposium of oral sensation and perception* (pp. 287–293). Springfield, IL: Thomas.

Bakker, K. (2002, November). Putting cluttering on the map: Looking back/Looking ahead. Paper presented at the Annual meeting of the American Speech Language Hearing Association, Atlanta.

Barasch, C. T., Guitar, B., McCauley, R. J., & Absher, R. G. (2000). Disfluency and time perception. *Journal of Speech, Language, and Hearing Research, 43,* 1429–1439.

Baratz, R., & Mesulam, M. (1981). Adult-onset stuttering treated with anticonvulsants. *Archives of Neurology, 38,* 132–133.

Bates, E., Appelbaum, M., Salcedo, J., Saygin, A. P., & Pizzamiglio, L. (2003). Quantifying dissociations in neuropsychological research. *Journal of Clinical and Experimental Neuropsychology, 25,* 1128–1153.

Battle, D. E. (2012). *Communication disorders in multicultural and international populations* (4th ed.). St. Louis, MO: Elsevier/Mosby.

Baumgartner, J. M. (1999). Acquired psychogenic stuttering. In R. Curlee (Ed.), *Stuttering and related disorders of fluency* (2nd ed., pp. 269–288). New York: Thieme.

Beal, D. S., Gracco, V. L., Lafaille, S. J., & De Nil, L. F. (2007). Voxel-based morphometry of auditory and speech-related cortex in stutterers. *Neuroreport, 18*(2), 1257–1260.

Beck, J. S. (1995). *Cognitive therapy: Basics and beyond.* New York: Guilford Press.

Beilby, J., Brynes, M. L., & Yaruss, J. S. (2012). Acceptance and Commitment Therapy for adults who stutter: Psychosocial adjustment and speech fluency. *Journal of Fluency Disorders, 37*(4), 289–299.

Beilby, J., & Yaruss, J. S. (2018). Acceptance and commitment therapy for stuttering disorder. In B. Amster, & E. Klein (Eds.), *More than fluency: The social, emotional, and cognitive dimensions of stuttering.* San Diego, CA: Plural Publishing.

Beitchman, J., Nair, R., Clegg, M., & Patel, P. (1986). Prevalence of speech and language in 5-year-old kindergarten children in Ottawa-Carleton region. *Journal of Speech and Hearing Disorders, 51,* 98–110.

Berk, L. E. (1991). *Child development* (2nd ed.). Boston, MA: Allyn & Bacon.

Bernstein Ratner, N. (1981). Are there constraints on childhood disfluency? *Journal of Fluency Disorders, 6,* 341–350.

Bernstein Ratner, N. (1995). Treating the child who stutters with concomitant language and phonological impairment. *Language, Speech, and Hearing Services in Schools, 26*(2), 180–186.

Bernstein Ratner, N. (1997). Stuttering: A psycholinguistic perspective. In R. F. Curlee, & G. M. Siegel (Eds.), *Nature and treatment of stuttering: New directions* (2nd ed., pp. 99–127). Needham Heights, MA: Allyn & Bacon.

Bernstein Ratner, N. (2005). Evidence-based practice in stuttering: Some questions to consider. *Journal of Fluency Disorders, 30*(3), 163–168.

Bernstein Ratner, N., & MacWhinney, B. (2018). Fluency Bank: A new resource for fluency research and practice. *Journal of Fluency Disorders, 56,* 69–80.

Bernstein Ratner, N., & Sih, C. C. (1987). Effects of gradual increases in sentence length and complexity on children's dysfluency. *Journal of Speech and Hearing Disorders, 52,* 278–287.

Bernthal, J., Bankson, N., & Flipsen, P. (2017). *Articulation and phonological disorders: Speech sound disorders in children* (8th ed.). London: Pearson.

Berry, R. C., & Silverman, F. H. (1972). Equality of intervals on the Lewis-Sherman-scale of stuttering severity. *Journal of Speech and Hearing Research, 15,* 185–188.

Beurskens, R., Helmich, I., Rein, R., & Boch, O. (2014). Age-related changes in prefrontal activity during walking and dual-task situations: A fNIRS study. *International Journal of Psychophysiology, 92*(3), 122–128.

Biederman, J., Rosenbaum, J. F., Chaloff, J., & Kagan, J. (1995). Behavioral inhibition as a risk factor for anxiety disorders. In J. Biederman, J. F. Rosenbaum, J. Chaloff, & J. Kagan (Eds.), *Anxiety disorders in children* (pp. 61–81). New York: Guildford Press.

Bijleveld, H., Lebrun, Y., & van Dongen, H. (1994). A case of acquired stuttering. *Folia Phoniatrica et Logopedica, 46,* 250–253.

Binder, L., Spector, J., & Youngjohn, J. (2012). Psychogenic stuttering and other acquired nonorganic speech and language abnormalities. *Archives of Clinical Neuropsychology, 27*(5), 557–568.

Black, J. W. (1951). The effects of delayed sidetone on vocal rate and intensity. *Journal of Speech and Hearing Disorders, 16*, 56–60.

Blood, G. W. (1985). Laterality differences in child stutterers: Heterogeneity, severity levels, and statistical treatment. *Journal of Speech and Hearing Disorders, 50*, 66–72.

Blood, G. W., & Blood, I. M. (1989). Multiple data analysis of dichotic listening advantages of stutterers. *Journal of Fluency Disorders, 14*, 97–107.

Blood, G. W., Blood, I., Tellis, G., & Gabel, R. (2001). Communication apprehension and self-perceived communication competence in adolescents who stutter. *Journal of Fluency Disorders, 263*, 161–178.

Bloodstein, O. (1944). Studies in the psychology of stuttering: XIX. The relationship between oral reading rate and severity of stuttering. *Journal of Speech Disorders, 9*, 161–173.

Bloodstein, O. (1948). *Conditions under which stuttering is reduced or absent*. Unpublished doctoral dissertation, University of Iowa, Iowa City.

Bloodstein, O. (1950). Hypothetical conditions under which stuttering is reduced or absent. *Journal of Speech and Hearing Disorders, 15*, 142–153.

Bloodstein, O. (1958). Stuttering as an anticipatory struggle reaction. In J. Eisenson (Ed.), *Stuttering: A symposium* (pp. 3–69). New York: Harper & Row.

Bloodstein, O. (1960a). The development of stuttering: I. Changes in nine basic features. *Journal of Speech and Hearing Disorders, 25*, 219–237.

Bloodstein, O. (1960b). The development of stuttering: II. Developmental phases. *Journal of Speech and Hearing Disorders, 25*, 366–376.

Bloodstein, O. (1961a). Stuttering in families of adopted stutterers. *Journal of Speech and Hearing Disorders, 26*, 395–396.

Bloodstein, O. (1961b). The development of stuttering: III. Theoretical and clinical implications. *Journal of Speech and Hearing Disorders, 26*, 67–82.

Bloodstein, O. (1974). The rules of early stuttering. *Journal of Speech and Hearing Disorders, 39*, 379–394.

Bloodstein, O. (1975). Stuttering as tension and fragmentation. In J. Eisenson (Ed.), *Stuttering: A second symposium* (pp. 1–95). New York: Harper & Row.

Bloodstein, O. (1987). *A handbook on stuttering* (4th ed.). Chicago, IL: National Easter Seal Society.

Bloodstein, O. (1993). *Stuttering: The search for a cause and a cure*. Boston, MA: Allyn & Bacon.

Bloodstein, O. (1995). *A handbook on stuttering* (5th ed.). San Diego, CA: Singular.

Bloodstein, O. (1997). Stuttering as an anticipatory struggle reaction. In R. F. Curlee, & G. M. Siegel (Eds.), *The nature and treatment of stuttering: New directions* (2nd ed., pp. 169–181). Boston, MA: Allyn & Bacon.

Bloodstein, O. (2001). Incipient and developed stuttering as two distinct disorders: Resolving a dilemma. *Journal of Fluency Disorders, 26*, 67–73.

Bloodstein, O. (2002). Early stuttering as a type of language difficulty. *Journal of Fluency Disorders, 27*, 163–167.

Bloodstein, O., & Gantwerk, B. (1967). Grammatical function in relation to stuttering in young children. *Journal of Speech and Hearing Research, 10*, 786–789.

Bloodstein, O., & Ratner, N. B. (1997). Inferences and conclusions. In O. Bloodstein (Ed.), *A handbook on stuttering* (6th ed.). Clifton Park, NY: Thompson-Delmar Learning.

Bloodstein, O., & Ratner, N. B. (2008). *A handbook on stuttering* (6th ed.). Clifton Park, NY: Thomson Delmar Learning.

Bluemel, C. S. (1932). Primary and secondary stuttering. *Quarterly Journal of Speech, 18*, 187–200.

Bluemel, C. S. (1957). *The riddle of stuttering*. Danville, IL: Interstate Publishing Co.

Boberg, E., Yeudall, L., Schopflocher, D., & Bo-Lassen, P. (1983). The effect of an intensive behavioral program on the distribution of EEG alpha power in stutterers during the processing of verbal and visuospatial information. *Journal of Fluency Disorders, 8*, 245–263.

Böhme, G. (1968). Stammering and cerebral lesions in early childhood: Examinations of 802 children and adults with cerebral lesions. *Folia Phoniatrica, 20*, 239–249.

Boey, R., Van de Heyning, P., Wuyts, F., Heylen, L., Stroap, R., & De Bodt, M. (2009). Awareness and reactions of young stuttering children aged 2–7 years old towards their speech disfluency. *Journal of Communication Disorders, 42*(5), 334–346.

Boey, R., Wuyts, F., Van de Heyning, P., De Bodt, M., & Heylen, L. (2007). Characteristics of stuttering-type disfluencies in Dutch-speaking children. *Journal of Fluency Disorders, 32*(4), 310–329.

Bolles, R. C. (1970). Speech-specific defense reactions and avoidance learning. *Psychological Review, 77*, 32–48.

Boone, D., McFarlane, S., Von Berg, S., & Zraick, R. (2014). *The voice and voice therapy*. New York: Pearson Education.

Borden, G. J. (1983). Initiation versus execution time during manual and oral counting by stutterers. *Journal of Speech and Hearing Research, 26*, 389–396.

Bosshardt, H-G. (1999). Effects of concurrent mental calculation on stuttering, inhalation and speech timing. *Journal of Fluency Disorders, 24*, 43–72.

Bosshardt, H-G. (2002). Effects of concurrent cognitive processing on the fluency of word repetition: Comparison between persons who do and do not stutter. *Journal of Fluency Disorders, 27*, 93–113.

Bosshardt, H-G. (2006). Cognitive processing load as a determinant of stuttering: Summary of a research programme. *Clinical Linguistics and Phonetics, 20*, 371–385.

Boswell, J. (1819). *The Life of Samuel Johnson*. London: R. Edwards and J. Offor.

Botterill, W., & Kelman, E. (2010). Palin parent–child interaction. In B. Guitar, & R. J. McCauley (Eds.), *Treatment of stuttering: Established and emerging interventions* (pp. 63–90). Baltimore, MD: Wolters Kluwer/Lippincott Williams & Wilkins.

Bouton, M. (2016). *Learning and behavior: A contemporary synthesis* (2nd ed.). Sunderland, MA: Sinauer Associates, Inc.

Boyce, W. T., Chesney, M., Alkon-Leonard, A., Tschann, J., Adams, S., Chesterman, B., et al. (1995). Psychobiologic reactivity to stress and childhood respiratory illness: Results of two prospective studies. *Psychosomatic Medicine, 57*, 411–422.

Brady, J. P. (1991). The pharmacology of stuttering: A critical review. *American Journal of Psychiatry, 148*, 1309–1316.

Brady, J. P., & Ali, Z. (2000). Alprazolam, citalopram, and clomipramine for stuttering. *Journal of Clinical Psychopharmacology, 20*, 287.

Brady, J. P., & Berson, J. (1975). Stuttering, dichotic listening, and cerebral dominance. *Archives of General Psychiatry, 32*, 1449–1452.

Branigan, G. (1979). Some reasons why successive single word utterances are not. *Journal of Child Language, 6*, 411–421.

Braun, A. R., Varga, M., Stager, S., Schulz, G., Selbie, S., Maisog, J., et al. (1997a). Altered patterns of cerebral activity during speech and language production in developmental stuttering: An H2(15)O positron emission tomography study. *Brain, 120*, 761–784.

Braun, A. R., Varga, M., Stager, S., Schulz, G., Selbie, S., Maisog, J. M., et al. (1997b). A typical lateralization of hemispherical activity in developmental stuttering: An H2(15)O positron emission tomography study. In W. Hulstijn, H. F. M. Peters, & P. H. H. M. van Lieshout (Eds.), *Speech production: Motor control, brain research and fluency disorders* (pp. 279–292). Amsterdam, The Netherlands: Elsevier.

Brayton, E., & Conture, E. (1978). Effects of noise and rhythmic stimulation on the speech of stutterers. *Journal of Speech and Hearing Research, 21*, 285–294.

Brosch, S., Haege, A., & Johannsen, H. (2002). Prognostic indicators for stuttering: The value of computer-based speech analysis. *Brain and Language, 82*, 75–87.

Brosch, S., Haege, A., Kalehne, P., & Johannsen, S. (1999). Stuttering children and the probability of remission: The role of cerebral dominance and speech production. *International Journal of Pediatric Otorhinolaryngology, 47*, 71–76.

Brown, J., & Jacobs, A. (1949). The role of fear in the motivation and acquisition of responses. *Journal of Experimental Psychology, 39*(6), 747–759.

Brown, S. F. (1937). The influence of grammatical function on the incidence of stuttering. *Journal of Speech Disorders, 2*, 207–215.

Brown, S. F. (1938a). A further study of stuttering in relation to various speech sounds. *Quarterly Journal of Speech, 24*, 390–397.

Brown, S. F. (1938b). Stuttering with relation to word accent and word position. *Journal of Abnormal Social Psychology, 33*, 112–120.

Brown, S. F. (1938c). The theoretical importance of certain factors influencing the incidence of stuttering. *Journal of Speech Disorders, 3*, 223–230.

Brown, S. F. (1943). An analysis of certain data concerning loci of "stutterings" from the viewpoint of general semantics. *Papers from the Second American Congress of General Semantics, 2*, 194–199.

Brown, S. F. (1945). The loci of stutterings in the speech sequence. *Journal of Speech Disorders, 10*, 181–192.

Brown, S. F., & Moren, A. (1942). The frequency of stuttering in relation to word length during oral reading. *Journal of Speech Disorders, 7*, 153–159.

Brown, S., Ingham, R. J., Ingham, J., Laird, A. R., & Fox, P. T. (2005). Stuttered and fluent speech production: An ALE meta-analysis of functional neuroimaging studies. *Human Brain Mapping, 25*(1), 105–117.

Brundage, S., & Bernstein Ratner, N. (1989). The measurement of stuttering frequency in children's speech. *Journal of Fluency Disorders, 14*, 351–358.

Brutten, G. J. (1986). Two-factor theory. In G. H. Shames, & H. Rubin (Eds.), *Stuttering then and now*. Columbus, OH: Charles C. Merrill.

Brutten, G. J., & Dunham, S. (1989). The Communication Attitude Test: A normative study of grade school children. *Journal of Fluency Disorders, 14*, 371–377.

Brutten, G. J., & Shoemaker, D. J. (1967). *The modification of stuttering*. Englewood Cliffs, NJ: Prentice-Hall.

Brutten, G. J., & Shoemaker, D. J. (1969). Stuttering: the disintegration of speech due to conditioned negative emotion. In B. B. Gray, & G. England (Eds.), *Stuttering and the conditioning therapies*. Monterey, CA: Monterey Institute for Speech & Hearing.

Brutten, G. J., & Vanryckeghem, M. (2007). *Behavior Assessment Battery for school-age children who stutter*. San Diego, CA: Plural Publishing.

Bryngelson, B. (1935). Sideness as an etiological factor in stuttering. *Journal of Genetic Psychology, 47*, 204–217.

Buck, S., Lees, R., & Cook, F. (2002). The influence of family history of stuttering on the onset of stuttering in young children. *Folia Phoniatrica et Logopedica, 54*, 117–124.

Budde, K. S., Barron, D. S., & Fox, P. T. (2014). Stuttering, induced fluency, and natural fluency: A hierarchical series of activation likelihood estimation meta-analysis. *Brain and Language, 139*, 99–107.

Burman, D. D., Bitan, T., & Booth, J. R. (2008). Sex differences in neural processing of language among children. *Neuropsychologia, 46*(5), 1349–1362.

Byrd, C. T., Wolk, I., & Davis, B. L. (2007). Role of phonology in childhood stuttering and its treatment. In E. Conture, & R. Curlee (Eds.), *Stuttering and related disorders of fluency* (3rd ed., pp. 168–182). New York: Thieme.

Calkins, S. D. (1994). Origins and outcomes of individual differences in emotion regulation. In N. A. Fox, & J. Campos (Eds.), *The development of emotional regulation: Biological and behavioral considerations*. Chicago, IL: Society for Research Child Development.

Calkins, S. D., & Fox, N. A. (1994). Individual differences in the biological aspects of temperament. In J. E. Bates, & T. D. Wachs (Eds.), *Temperament: Individual differences at the interface of biology and behavior* (pp. 199–217). Washington, DC: American Psychological Association.

Callan, D. E., Kent, R. D., Guenther, F. H., & Vorperian, H. K. (2000). An auditory-feedback based neural network model of speech production that is robust to developmental changes in the size and shape of the articulatory system. *Journal of Speech, Language, and Hearing Research, 43*, 721–736.

Canter, G. (1971). Observations on neurogenic stuttering: A contribution to differential diagnosis. *British Journal of Communication Disorders, 6*, 139–143.

Caplan, D. (1987). *Neurolinguistics and linguistic aphasiology*. Cambridge, UK: Cambridge University Press.

Carey, B., O'Brian, S., Onslow, M., Block, S., Jones, M., & Packman, A. (2010). Randomized controlled non-inferiority trial of a telehealth treatment for chronic stuttering: The Camperdown Program. *International Journal of Language and Communication Disorders, 45*(1), 108–120.

Caruso, A. J., Abbs, J. H., & Gracco, V. L. (1988). Kinematic analysis of multiple movement coordination during speech in stutterers. *Brain, 111*, 439–455.

Caruso, A. J., Chodzko-Zajko, W., Bidinger, D., & Sommers, R. (1994). Adults who stutter: Responses to cognitive stress. *Journal of Speech and Hearing Research, 37*, 746–754.

Caruso, A. J., Chodzko-Zajko, W., & McClowry, M. (1995). Emotional arousal and stuttering: The impact of cognitive stress. In C. W. Starkweather, & H. F. M. Peters (Eds.), *Stuttering: Proceedings of the first world congress on fluency disorders*. Nijmegen, The Netherlands: International Fluency Association.

Chang, S-E. (2010). Similarities in speech and white matter characteristics in idiopathic developmental stuttering and adult-onset stuttering. *Journal of Neurolinguistics, 23*(5), 455–469.

Chang, S-E. (2014). Research update in neuroimaging studies of children who stutter. *Seminars in Speech and Language, 35*, 67–79.

Chang, S-E., Angstadt, M., Chow, H., Etchell, A., Garnett, E., Choo, A. L., et al. (2017). Anomalous network architecture of the resting brain in children who stutter. *Journal of Fluency Disorders, 55*, 46–67.

Chang, S-E., Erickson, K., Ambrose, N. G., Hasegawa-Johnson, M., & Ludlow, C. L. (2008). Brain anatomy differences in childhood stuttering. *NeuroImage, 39*(3), 1333–1344.

Chang, S-E., Horowitz, B., Ostuni, J., Reynolds, R., & Ludlow, C. L. (2011). Evidence of left inferior frontal-premotor structural and functional connectivity deficits in adults who stutter. *Cerebral Cortex, 21*(11), 2507–2518.

Chang, S-E., Kenny, M., Loucks, T., & Ludlow, C. L. (2009). Brain activation abnormalities during speech and non-speech in stuttering speakers. *NeuroImage, 46*(1), 201–212.

Chang, S-E., & Zhu, D. (2013). Neural network connectivity difference in children who stutter. *Brain, 136*(12), 3709–3726.

Chang, S-E., Zhu, D. C., Choo, A. L., & Angstadt, M. (2015). White matter neuroanatomical differences in young children who stutter. *Brain, 138*(Part 3), 694–711.

Chase, C. H. (1996). Neurobiology of learning disabilities. *Seminars in Speech, Language and Hearing, 17*(3), 173–181.

Chen, H., Xu, J., Zhou, Y., Gao, Y., Wang, G., Xia, J., et al. (2015). Association study of stuttering candidate genes GNPTAB, GNPTG and NAGPA with dyslexia in Chinese population. *BMC Genetics, 6*(7), 1–7.

Chmela, K. A., & Reardon, N. A. (2001). *The school-aged child who stutters: Working effectively with attitudes and emotions: A workbook.* Memphis, TN: Stuttering Foundation of America.

Choi, D., Conture, E. G., Walden, T. A., Jones, R., & Kim, H. (2016). Emotional diathesis, emotional stress, and childhood stuttering. *Journal of Speech, Language, and Hearing Research, 59*, 616–630.

Choo, A. L., Burnham, E., Hicks, K., & Chang, S-E. (2016). Disassociations among linguistic, cognitive, and auditory-motor neuroanatomical domains in children who stutter. *Journal of Communication Disorders, 61*, 29–47.

Chow, H., & Chang, S-E. (2017). White matter developmental trajectories associated with persistence and recovery of childhood stuttering. *Human Brain Mapping, 38*(7), 3345–3359.

Chuang, C. K., Fromm, D. S., Ewanowski, S. J., & Abbs, J. H. (1980, November). Nonspeech articulatory sensori-motor control differences between stutterers and nonstutterers. Paper presented at the Annual Conference of the American Speech and Hearing Association, Detroit, MI.

Clarke-Stewart, A., & Friedman, S. (1987). *Child development: Infancy through adolescence.* New York: John Wiley & Sons.

Cohen, M. S., & Hanson, M. L. (1975). Intersensory processing efficiency of fluent speakers and stutterers. *British Journal of Disorders of Communication, 102*, 111–122.

Colburn, N., & Mysak, E. D. (1982a). Developmental disfluency and emerging grammar. I. Disfluency characteristics in early syntactic utterances. *Journal of Speech and Hearing Research, 25*, 414–420.

Colburn, N., & Mysak, E. D. (1982b). Developmental disfluency and emerging grammar. II. Co-occurrence of disfluency with specified semantic-syntactic structures. *Journal of Speech and Hearing Research, 25*, 421–427.

Colcord, R. D., & Adams, M. R. (1979). Voicing duration and vocal SLP changes associated with stuttering reduction during singing. *Journal of Speech and Hearing Research, 22*, 468–479.

Coleman, T. J. (2000). *Clinical management of communication disorders in culturally diverse children.* Boston, MA: Allyn & Bacon.

Conrad, C. (1996). Fluency in multicultural populations. In L. Cole, & V. R. Deal (Eds.), *Communication disorders in multicultural populations.* Rockville, MD: American Speech-Language-Hearing Association.

Conture, E. G. (1982). *Stuttering.* Englewood Cliffs, NJ: Prentice-Hall.

Conture, E. G. (1990). *Stuttering* (2nd ed.). Englewood Cliffs, NJ: Prentice-Hall.

Conture, E. G. (2001). *Stuttering: Its nature, diagnosis, and treatment.* Boston, MA: Allyn & Bacon.

Conture, E. G., Louko, L., & Edwards, M. L. (1993). Simultaneously treating stuttering and disordered phonology in children. *American Journal of Speech-Language Pathology, 2*, 72–81.

Conture, E. G., McCall, G. N., & Brewer, D. W. (1977). Laryngeal behavior during stuttering. *Journal of Speech and Hearing Research, 20*, 661–668.

Conture, E. G., & Melnick, K. (1999). Parent–child group approach to stuttering in preschool and school-age children. In M. Onslow, & A. Packman (Eds.), *Early stuttering: A handbook of intervention strategies* (pp. 17–51). San Diego, CA: Singular.

Conture, E. G., & Walden, T. A. (2012). Dual diathesis-stressor model of stuttering. In L. Bellakova, & Y. Filatova (Eds.), *Theoretical issues of fluency disorders* (pp. 94–127). Moscow: National Book Center.

Cooper, E. B., & Cooper, C. S. (1993). Fluency disorders. In D. E. Battle (Ed.), *Communication disorders in multicultural organizations* (pp. 189–211). Boston, MA: Andover Medical Publishers.

Cordes, A. K. (1994). The reliability of observational data: I. Theories and methods for speech-language pathology. *Journal of Speech and Hearing Research, 37*, 264–278.

Cordes, A. K., & Ingham, R. J. (1999). Effects of time-interval judgment training on real-time measurement of stuttering. *Journal of Speech, Language, and Hearing Research, 42*, 862–879.

Coster, W. (1986). *Aspects of voice and conversation in behaviorally inhibited and uninhibited children.* Unpublished doctoral dissertation, Harvard University, Cambridge, MA.

Coulter, C., Anderson, J., & Conture, E. G. (2009). Childhood stuttering and dissociations across linguistic domains: A replication and extension. *Journal of Fluency Disorders, 34*(4), 257–278.

Cox, N., & Yairi, E. (2000, November). Genetics of stuttering: insights and recent advances. Paper presented at the Annual Meeting of the American Speech-Language-Hearing Association, Washington, DC.

Craig, A., & Andrews, G. (1985). The prediction and prevention of relapse in stuttering. *Behavior Modification, 9*, 427–442.

Craig, A., Franklin, J., & Andrews, G. (1984). A scale to measure locus of control of behavior. *British Journal of Medical Psychology, 57*, 173–180.

Craig, A., Hancock, K., Tran, Y., Craig, M., & Peters, M. (2002). Epidemiology of stuttering in the community across the entire life span. *Journal of Speech, Language, and Hearing Research, 45*, 1097–1105.

Craske, M. G., Treanor, M., Conway, C. C., Zbozinek, T., & Vervliet, B. (2014). Maximizing exposure therapy: An inhibitory learning approach. *Behaviour Research and Therapy, 58*, 10–23.

Cross, D. E., & Cooke, P. (1979). Vocal and manual reaction times of adult stutterers and nonstutterers (Abstract). *American Speech-Language and Hearing Association*, *21*, 693.

Cross, D. E., & Luper, H. L. (1979). Voice reaction time of stuttering and nonstuttering children and adults. *Journal of Fluency Disorders*, *4*, 58–77.

Cross, D. E., & Luper, H. L. (1983). Relation between finger reaction time and voice reaction time in stuttering and nonstuttering children and adults. *Journal of Speech and Hearing Research*, *26*, 356–361.

Cross, D. E., Sweet, J., & Bates, D. (1985, November). Mental imagery and stuttering: Electroencephalographic and physiological characteristics. Paper presented at the Annual Conference of the American Speech and Hearing Association, Washington, DC.

Crystal, D. (1987). Towards a bucket theory of language disability: Taking account of interaction between linguistic levels. *Clinical Linguistics and Phonetics*, *1*, 7–22.

Culatta, R., & Goldberg, S. (1995). *Stuttering therapy: An integrated approach to theory and practice*. Boston, MA: Allyn & Bacon.

Cullinan, W. L., & Springer, M. T. (1980). Voice initiation times in stuttering and nonstuttering children. *Journal of Speech and Hearing Research*, *23*, 344–360.

Curlee, R. (1984). Stuttering disorders: An overview. In J. M. Costello (Ed.), *Speech disorders in children* (pp. 227–260). San Diego, CA: College-Hill Press.

Curlee, R. (1993). Identification and management of beginning stuttering. In R. Curlee (Ed.), *Stuttering and related disorders of fluency* (pp. 1–22). New York: Thieme Medical Publishers.

Curry, F., & Gregory, H. H. (1969). The performance of stutterers on dichotic listening tasks thought to reflect cerebral dominance. *Journal of Speech and Hearing Research*, *12*, 73–82.

Cykowski, M. D., Fox, P. T., Ingham, R. J., Ingham, J. C., & Robin, D. A. (2010). A study of the reproducibility and etiology of diffusion anisotropy differences in developmental stuttering: A potential role for impaired myelination. *NeuroImage*, *52*(4), 1495–1504.

Dalton, P., & Hardcastle, W. J. (1977). *Disorders of fluency*. New York: Elsevier.

Daly, D. A. (1986). The clutterer. In K. S. Louis (Ed.), *The atypical stutterer*. New York: Academic Press.

Daly, D. A. (2006). Predictive cluttering inventory. Available at http://associations.missouristate.edu/ICA

Daly, D. A., & Burnett-Stolnack, M. L. (1995). Identification of and treatment planning for stuttering clients: Two practical tools. *The Clinical Connection*, *8*, 15.

Damian, S. (2014). *Voice: A stutterer's odyssey*. North Fayette, PA: Behler Publications.

Daniels, D. E. (2008). Working with people who stutter of diverse cultural backgrounds: Some ideas to consider. *Perspectives on Fluency and Fluency Disorders*, *18*, 95–100.

Daniels, D. E., Gabel, R., & Hughes, S. (2012). Recounting the K-12 school experiences of adults who stutter: A qualitative analysis. *Journal of Fluency Disorders*, *37*(2), 71–82.

Darley, F. L., & Spriestersbach, D. (1978). *Diagnostic methods in speech pathology* (2nd ed.). New York: Harper & Row.

Davenport, R. W. (1977). *Dichotic ear preferences of stuttering adults*. Unpublished doctoral dissertation, Iowa State University, Ames, Iowa.

Davidson, R. J. (1984). Affect, cognition, and hemispheric specialization. In C. E. Izard, J. Kagan, & R. Zajonc (Eds.), *Emotion, cognition and behavior*. Cambridge, UK and New York: Cambridge University Press.

Davidson, R. J. (1995). Cerebral asymmetry, emotion, and affective style. In R. J. Davidson, & K. Hugdahl (Eds.), *Brain asymmetry* (pp. 361–387). Cambridge, MA: MIT press.

Davis, D. M. (1940). The relation of repetitions in the speech of young children to certain measures of language maturity and situational factors: Parts II & III. *Journal of Speech Disorders*, *5*, 235–246.

Davis, M., & Guitar, B. (1976). *Speech rate of elementary school children in Vermont*. Graduate student research paper, University of Vermont, Burlington, VT.

De Nil, L. F. (1995, November). Linguistic and motor approaches to stuttering: Exploring unification. Paper presented at the Annual Conference of the American Speech-Language-Hearing Association, Orlando, FL.

De Nil, L. F., & Abbs, J. H. (1991). Kinaesthetic acuity of stutterers and nonstutterers for oral and non-oral movements. *Brain*, *114*, 2145–2158.

De Nil, L. F., & Bosshardt, H-G. (2001). Studying stuttering from a neurological and cognitive information processing perspective. In H-G. Bosshardt, J. S. Yaruss, & H. F. M. Peters (Eds.), *Stuttering research: Research, therapy and self-help: Proceedings of the 3rd World Congress on Fluency Disorders* (pp. 53–58). Nijmegen: Nijmegen University Press.

De Nil, L. F., & Brutten, G. J. (1991). Speech-associated attitudes of stuttering and normally fluent children. *Journal of Speech and Hearing Research*, *34*, 60–66.

De Nil, L. F., Jokel, R., & Rochon, E. (2007). Etiology, symptomatology, and treatment of neurogenic stuttering. In E. Conture, & R. Curlee (Eds.), *Stuttering and related disorders of fluency* (3rd ed., pp. 326–343). New York: Thieme.

De Nil, L. F., Kroll, R. M., & Houle, S. (1998, November). A PET study of neural activation changes following stuttering treatment. Paper presented at the Annual Conference of the American Speech-Language-Hearing Association, San Antonio.

De Nil, L. F., Kroll, R. M., & Houle, S. (2001). Functional neuroimaging of cerebellar activation during single word reading and verb generation in stuttering and nonstuttering adults. *Neuroscience Letters*, *302*, 77–80.

De Nil, L. F., Kroll, R. M., Houle, S., Ludlow, C. L., Braun, A. R., Ingham, R. J., et al. (1995, November). Advances in stuttering research using positron emission tomography brain imaging. Paper presented at the Annual meeting of the American Speech-Language-Hearing Association, Orlando, FL.

De Nil, L. F., Kroll, R. M., Kapur, S., & Houle, S. (1995, November). Silent and oral reading in stuttering and non-stuttering adults: A positron emission tomography study. Paper presented at the Annual Meeting of the American Speech-Language-Hearing Association, Orlando.

De Nil, L. F., Kroll, R. M., Kapur, S., & Houle, S. (2000). A positron emission tomography study of silent and oral single word reading in stuttering and nonstuttering adults. *Journal of Speech, Language, and Hearing Research*, *43*, 1038–1053.

De Nil, L. F., Kroll, R. M., Lafaille, S. J., & Houle, S. (2003). A positron emission tomography study of short- and long-term treatment effects on functional brain activation in adults who stutter. *Journal of Fluency Disorders*, *28*, 357–380.

de Sonneville-Koedoot, C., Stolk, E., Rietveld, T., & Franken, M. C. (2015). Direct versus indirect treatment for preschool children who stutter: The RESTART randomized trial. *PLoS ONE*, *10*(7), e0133758.

Decker, B., Guitar, B., & Solomon, A. (2018). Corpus callosum demylenination associated with acquired stuttering. *BMJ Case Reports, 2018.* doi:10.1136/bcr-2017-223486

Dehqan, A., Bakhtiar, M., Panahi, S., & Ashayeri, H. (2008). Relationship between stuttering severity in children and their mothers speaking rate. *São Paulo Medical Journal, 126*(1), 29–33.

DeJoy, D. A., & Gregory, H. H. (1973). The relationship of children's disfluencies to the syntax, length, and vocabulary of their sentences. Abstract. *ASHA, 15*, 472.

DeJoy, D. A., & Gregory, H. H. (1985). The relationship between age and frequency of disfluency in preschool children. *Journal of Fluency Disorders, 10*, 107–122.

Dietrich, S., Barry, S. J., & Parker, D. E. (1995). Middle latency auditory responses in males who stutter. *Journal of Speech and Hearing Research, 38*, 5–17.

DiSimoni, F. G. (1974). Preliminary study of certain timing relationships in the speech of stutterers. *Journal of the Acoustical Society of America, 56*, 695–696.

Dolcos, F., & McCarthy, G. (2006). Brain systems mediating cognitive interference by emotional distraction. *Journal of Neuroscience, 26*(7), 2072–2079.

Donnan, G. A. (1979). Stuttering as a manifestation of stroke. *Medical Journal of Australia, 1*, 44–45.

Douglass, L. C. (1943). A study of bilaterally recorded electroencephalograms of adult stutterers. *Journal of Experimental Psychology, 32*, 247–265.

Dowling, M. (2014). *Young children's personal, social and emotional development* (4th ed.). Thousand Oaks, CA: Sage Publications.

Drayna, D. (1997). Genetic linkage studies of stuttering: Ready for prime time? *Journal of Fluency Disorders, 22*, 237–241.

Duffy, J. (2013). *Motor speech disorders: Substrates, differential diagnosis and management* (3rd ed.). St. Louis, MO: Elsevier.

Dunn, D. (2018). *Peabody picture vocabulary test* (5th ed.). New York: Pearson.

Dworzynski, K., Remington, A., Rijsdijk, F., Howell, P., & Plomin, R. (2007). Genetic etiology in cases of recovered and persistent stuttering in an unselected, longitudinal sample of young twins. *American Journal of Speech-Language Pathology, 6*(2), 169–178.

Edelman, G. (1992). *Bright air, brilliant fire: On the matter of mind.* New York: Basic Books.

Eggers, K. (2012). *Temperamental characteristics of children with developmental stuttering.* Tilburg, Netherlands: Tilburg University.

Elliott, R. L., & Thomas, B. J. (1985). A case report of alprazolam-induced stuttering. *Journal of Clinical Psychopharmacology, 5*, 159–160.

Ellis, B. J., & Boyce, W. T. (2008). Biological sensitivity to context. *Current Directions in Psychological Science, 5*, 183–187.

Ellis, J. B., Finan, D., & Ramig, P. R. (2008). The influence of stuttering severity on acoustic startle response. *Journal of Speech, Language, and Hearing Research, 51*(4), 836–850.

Embrechts, M., & Ebben, H. (1999). A comparison between the interactions of stuttering and nonstuttering children and their parents. In K. L. Baker, L. Rustin, & F. Cook (Eds.), *Proceedings of the Fifth Oxford Dysfluency Conference, 7th-10th July, 1999* (pp. 125–133). Oxford: Kevin Baker.

Erickson, R. (1969). Assessing communication attitudes among stutterers. *Journal of Speech and Hearing Research, 12*, 711–724.

Ezrati-Vinacour, R., Platzky, R., & Yairi, E. (2001). The young child's awareness of stuttering-like disfluency. *Journal of Speech, Language, and Hearing Research, 44*, 368.

Faber, A., & Mazlish, E. (2016). *How to talk so kids will listen and listen so kids will talk.* New York: Scribner.

Fagan, M. K. (2002). *Stuttering, social-cognitive, and emotional development.* Unpublished manuscript, Columbia, MO.

Fagnani, C., Fibiger, S., Skytthe, A., & Hjelmborg, J. (2011). Heritability and environmental effects for self-reported periods with stuttering: A twin study from Denmark. *Logopedics, Phoniatrics, Vocology, 36*(3), 114–120.

Fanselow, M. (1994). Neural organization of the defensive behavior system responsible for fear. *Psychonomic Bulletin & Review, 1*(4), 429–438.

Felsenfeld, S. (1997). Epidemiology and genetics of stuttering. In R. Curlee, & G. Siegel (Eds.), *The nature and treatment of stuttering: New directions* (2nd ed., pp. 3–23). Boston, MA: Allyn & Bacon.

Felsenfeld, S., Kirk, K., Zhu, G., Statham, D., Neale, M., & Martin, N. (2000). A study of the genetic and environmental etiology of stuttering in a selected twin sample. *Behavior Genetics, 305*, 359–366.

Femrell, L., Avall, M., & Lindstrom, E. (2012). Two-year follow-up of the Lidcombe Program in ten Swedish-speaking children. *Folia Phoniatrica et Logopedica, 64*, 248–253.

Fibiger, S. (1971). Stuttering explained as a physiological tremor. *Quarterly Progress and Status Report: Speech Transmission Laboratory, 12*, 2–3.

Fibiger, S. (1972). Further discussion on stuttering explained as a physiological tremor. *Quarterly Progress and Status Report: Speech Transmission Laboratory.*

Findlay, K., & Shenker, R. (2014, November). Establishing benchmarks for linguistically diverse populations: Treatment time for the Lidcombe Program. Paper presented at the Annual meeting of the American Speech-Language and Hearing Association, Orlando, FL.

Finn, P. (2003). Self-regulation and the management of stuttering. *Seminars in Speech and Language, 24*, 27–32.

Finn, P. (2007). Self-control and the treatment of stuttering. In E. Conture, & R. Curlee (Eds.), *Stuttering and related disorders of fluency* (3rd ed., pp. 344–359). New York: Thieme.

Flechsig, P. (1927). *Meine myelogenetische Hirnlehre.* Berlin: Julius Springer.

Foundas, A. L., Bollich, A. M., Corey, D. M., Hurley, M., & Heilman, K. M. (2001). Anomalous anatomy of speech-language areas in adults with persistent developmental stuttering. *Neurology, 57*, 207–215.

Foundas, A. L., Bollich, A. M., Feldman, S., Corey, D. M., Hurley, M., Lemen, L. C., & Heilman, K. M. (2004). Aberrant auditory processing and atypical planum temporale in developmental stuttering. *Neurology, 63*(9), 1640–1646.

Fowlie, G. M., & Cooper, E. B. (1978). Traits attributed to stuttering and nonstuttering children by their mothers. *Journal of Fluency Disorders, 34*, 233–246.

Fox, N., & Davidson, R. (1984). Hemispheric substrates of affect: Developmental model. In N. Fox, & R. Davidson (Eds.), *The psychobiology of affective development.* Hillsdale, NJ: Lawrence Erlbaum Associates.

Fox, P. T. (2003). Brain imaging in stuttering: Where next? *Journal of Fluency Disorders, 284*, 265–272.

Fox, P. T., Ingham, R. J., Ingham, J. C., Hirsch, T. B., Downs, J. H., Martin, C., et al. (1996). A PET study of the neural systems of stuttering. *Nature, 382,* 158–162.

Fox, P. T., Ingham, R. J., Ingham, J. C., Zamarripa, F., Xiong, J-H., & Lancaster, J. L. (2000). Brain correlates of stuttering and syllable production: A PET performance-correlation analysis. *Brain, 123,* 1985–2004.

Franken, M. C. J., Kielstra-van der Schalk, C. J., & Boelens, H. H. (2005). Experimental treatment of early stuttering: A preliminary study. *Journal of Fluency Disorders, 30,* 189–199.

Frankenburg, W., & Dodds, J. (1967). The Denver Developmental Screening Test. *Journal of Pediatrics, 71*(2), 181–191.

Fraser, J. (2004). Results of survey on electronic devices. *Stuttering Foundation Newsletter, 3,* 7.

Frattali, C. (1998). *Measuring Outcomes in Speech-Language Pathology.* New York: Thieme.

Freeman, F. J., & Ushijima, T. (1975). Laryngeal activity accompanying the moment of stuttering: A preliminary report of EMG investigations. *Journal of Fluency Disorders, 1,* 36–45.

Freeman, F. J., & Ushijima, T. (1978). Laryngeal muscle activity during stuttering. *Journal of Speech and Hearing Research, 21,* 538–562.

Gabbard, C. (2016). *Lifelong motor development.* Philadelphia, PA: Wolters Kluwer.

Gaines, N. D., Runyan, C. M., & Meyers, S. C. (1991). A comparison of young stutterers' fluent versus stuttered utterances on measures of length and complexity. *Journal of Speech and Hearing Research, 34,* 37–42.

Garfinkel, H. A. (1995). Why did Moses stammer? and, was Moses left-handed? *Journal of the Royal Society of Medicine, 88,* 256–257.

Geschwind, N., & Galaburda, A. (1985). Cerebral lateralization: Biological mechanisms, associations, and pathology: I. A hypothesis and a program for research. *Archives of Neurology, 42,* 429–459.

Gibson, E. (1972). Reading for some purpose. In J. F. Kavanaugh, & I. Mattingly (Eds.), *Language by ear and by eye.* Cambridge, MA: MIT Press.

Gildston, P. (1967). Stutterers' self-acceptance and perceived parental acceptance. *Journal of Abnormal Psychology, 721,* 59–64.

Gillam, R. B., Logan, K. J., & Pearson, N. A. (2009). *TOCS: Test of childhood stuttering.* Austin, TX: Pro-Ed.

Goldman, R., & Fristoe, M. (2015). *GFTA-3: Goldman-Fristoe Test of Articulation.* Minneapolis, MN: Pearson Assessment.

Goldman-Eisler, F. (1968). *Psycholinguistics: Experiments in spontaneous speech.* New York: Academic Press.

Goldstein, B. (2000). *Cultural and linguistic diversity resource guide for speech-language pathologists.* San Diego, CA: Singular Publishing Group.

Gordon, P. A., Luper, H. L., & Peterson, H. A. (1986). The effects of syntactic complexity on the occurrence of disfluencies in 5 year old stutterers. *Journal of Fluency Disorders, 11,* 151–164.

Gottwald, S. (2010). Stuttering prevention and early intervention: A multidimensional approach. In B. Guitar, & R. J. McCauley (Eds.), *Treatment of stuttering: Established and emerging interventions* (pp. 91–117). Baltimore, MD: Lippincott Williams & Wilkins.

Gottwald, S., & Starkweather, C. W. (1984, November). Stuttering prevention: Rationale and method. Paper presented at the Annual meeting of the American Speech and Hearing Association, San Francisco, CA.

Gottwald, S., & Starkweather, C. W. (1985, November). The prognosis of stuttering. Paper presented at the Annual meeting of the American Speech and Hearing Association, Washington, DC.

Gottwald, S., & Starkweather, C. W. (1999). Stuttering prevention and early intervention: A multiprocess approach. In M. Onslow, & A. Packman (Eds.), *Handbook of early stuttering intervention* (pp. 53–82). San Diego, CA: Singular.

Gray, J. A. (1987). *The psychology of fear and stress* (2nd ed.). Cambridge, UK: Cambridge University Press.

Greenspan, S. I. (1993). Making time for your child. *Parents,* (August), 111–114.

Guenther, F. H. (1994). A neural network model of speech acquisition and motor equivalent speech production. *Biological Cybernetics, 72*(1), 43–53.

Guenther, F. H. (2007). Neuroimaging of normal speech production. In R. J. Ingham (Ed.), *Neuroimaging in communication sciences and disorders* (pp. 1–51). San Diego, CA: Plural Publications.

Guenther, F. H., Ghosh, S. S., & Tourville, J. A. (2006). Neural modeling and imaging of the cortical interactions underlying syllable production. *Brain and Language, 96*(3), 280–301.

Guitar, B. (1976). Pretreatment factors associated with the outcome of stuttering therapy. *Journal of Speech and Hearing Research, 19,* 590–600.

Guitar, B. (1978). Between parent and stuttering child. *WMU Journal of Speech, Language and Hearing, 14.*

Guitar, B. (1997). Therapy for children's stuttering and emotions. In R. F. Curlee, & G. M. Siegel (Eds.), *Nature and treatment of stuttering: New directions* (2nd ed., pp. 280–291). Boston, MA: Allyn & Bacon.

Guitar, B. (1998). *Stuttering: An integrated approach to its nature and treatment* (2nd ed.). Philadelphia, PA: Lippincott Williams & Wilkins.

Guitar, B. (2000). Emotion, temperament and stuttering: Some possible relationships. In K. L. Baker, L. Rustin, & F. Cook (Eds.), *Proceedings of the Fifth Oxford Dysfluency Conference, 7th-10th July, 1999* (pp. 1–6). Berkshire, UK: K. L. Baker.

Guitar, B. (2003). Acoustic startle responses and temperament in individuals who stutter. *Journal of Speech, Language, and Hearing Research, 461,* 233–240.

Guitar, B. (2004). Burn your textbooks! Evidence-based practice in stuttering treatment. In A. Packman, A. Meltzer, & H. F. M. Peters (Eds.), *Theory, research and therapy in fluency disorders: Proceedings of the Fourth World Congress in Fluency Disorders* (pp. 21–27). Nijmegen, the Netherlands: Nijmegen University Press.

Guitar, B., & Bass, C. (1978). Stuttering therapy: The relation between attitude change and long-term outcome. *Journal of Speech and Hearing Disorders, 43,* 392–400.

Guitar, B., & Fraser, J. (2007). *Stuttering: Basic clinical skills* [DVD]. Memphis, TN: Stuttering Foundation.

Guitar, B., & Grims, S. (1977, November). Developing a scale to assess communication attitudes in children who stutter. Paper presented at the Annual meeting of the American Speech-Language-Hearing Association, Atlanta.

Guitar, B., & Guitar, C. (2003). *Stuttering and your child: Help for parents.* Memphis, TN: Stuttering Foundation.

Guitar, B., Guitar, C., & Fraser, J. (2010). *Stuttering and your child: Help for families [DVD].* Memphis, TN: Stuttering Foundation.

Guitar, B., Guitar, C., Neilson, P. D., O'Dwyer, N. J., & Andrews, G. (1988). Onset sequencing of selected lip muscles in stutterers and nonstutterers. *Journal of Speech and Hearing Research, 31*, 28–35.

Guitar, B., Kazenski, D., Howard, A., Cousins, F., Fader, E., & Haskell, P. (2015). Predicting treatment time and long-term outcome of the Lidcombe Program: A replication and reanalysis. *American Journal of Speech-Language Pathology, 24*, 533–544.

Guitar, B., Kopff-Schaefer, H., Donahue-Kilburg, G., & Bond, L. (1992). Parent verbal interaction and speech rate. *Journal of Speech and Hearing Research, 35*, 742–754.

Guitar, B., & Marchinkowski, L. (2001). Influence of mothers' slower speech rate on their children's speech rate. *Journal of Speech, Language, and Hearing Research, 44*(4), 853–861.

Guitar, B., & McCauley, R. J. (2010). *Treatment of stuttering: Established and emerging interventions*. Baltimore, MD: Lippincott Williams & Wilkins.

Guitar, B., & Reville, J. (1997). *Easy talker: A fluency workbook for school-age children*. Austin, TX: Pro-Ed Publishers.

Guttormsen, L., Kefalianos, E., & Naess, K-A. (2015). Communication attitudes in children who stutter: A meta-analytic review. *Journal of Fluency Disorders, 46*, 1–14.

Habib, M., Daquin, G., Milandre, L., Royere, M. L., Rey, M., Lanteri, A., et al. (1995). Mutism and auditory agnosia due to bilateral insular damage: Role of the insula in human communication. *Neuropsychologia, 333*, 327–339.

Hadders-Algra, M., & Forssberg, H. (2002). Development of motor function in health and disease. In H. Lagercrantz, M. L. Hanson, P. Evrard, & C. H. Rodeck (Eds.), *The newborn brain: Neuroscience and clinical applications*. Cambridge, UK: Cambridge University Press.

Hakim, H. B., & Bernstein Ratner, N. (2004). Nonword repetitions abilities of children who stutter: An exploratory study. *Journal of Fluency Disorders, 29*, 179–199.

Hall, J. W., & Jerger, J. (1978). Central auditory function in stutterers. *Journal of Speech and Hearing Research, 21*, 324–337.

Hall, N., Wagovich, S., & Bernstein Ratner, N. (2007). Language consideration in childhood stuttering. In R. Curlee, & E. G. Conture (Eds.), *Stuttering and related disorders of fluency* (3rd ed., pp. 153–167). New York: Thieme.

Hampton, A., & Weber-Fox, C. (2008). Non-linguistic auditory processing in stuttering: Evidence from behavior and event-related brain potentials. *Journal of Fluency Disorders, 33*(4), 253–273.

Han, T-U., Park, J., Domingues, C., Moretti-Ferreira, D., Paris, E., Sainz, E., et al. (2014). A study of the role of the FOXP2 and CNTNAP2 genes in persistent developmental stuttering. *Neurobiology of Disease, 69*, 23–31.

Hannley, M., & Dorman, M. F. (1982). Some observations on auditory function and stuttering. *Journal of Fluency Disorders, 7*, 93–108.

Harrison, E., Bruce, M., Shenker, R., & Koushik, S. (2010). The Lidcombe Program for school-age children who stutter. In B. Guitar, & R. J. McCauley (Eds.), *Treatment of stuttering: Established and emerging interventions* (pp. 150–166). Baltimore, MD: Lippincott Williams & Wilkins.

Harrison, E., & Onslow, M. (2010). The Lidcombe Program for preschool children who stutter. In B. Guitar, & R. J. McCauley (Eds.), *Treatment of stuttering: Established and emerging interventions* (pp. 118–149). Baltimore, MD: Lippincott Williams & Wilkins.

Haynes, W. O., & Hood, S. B. (1978). Disfluency changes in children as a function of the systematic modification of linguistic complexity. *Journal of Communication Disorders, 11*, 79–33.

Healey, K. T., Nelson, S., & Scaler Scott, K. (2015). A case study of cluttering treatment outcomes in a teen. *Procedia-Social and Behavioral Sciences, 193*, 141–146.

Helliesen, G. G. (2002). *Forty years after therapy: One man's story*. Newport News, VA: Apollo Press.

Helm, N. A. (1979). Management of palilalia with a pacing board. *Journal of Speech and Hearing Disorders, 44*, 350–353.

Helm, N. A., Butler, R. B., & Canter, G. (1980). Neurogenic acquired stuttering. *Journal of Fluency Disorders, 5*, 269–279.

Helm-Estabrooks, N. (1986). Diagnosis and management of neurogenic stuttering in adults. In K. S. Louis (Ed.), *The atypical stutterer*. New York: Academic Press.

Helm-Estabrooks, N. (1992). *Aphasia diagnostic profiles*. Chicago, IL: Applied Symbolix.

Helm-Estabrooks, N. (1999). Stuttering associated with acquired neurological disorders. In R. Curlee (Ed.), *Stuttering and related disorders of fluency* (2nd ed., pp. 255–268). New York: Thieme.

Helm-Estabrooks, N., & Kaplan, E. (1989). *Boston stimulus boards*. Chicago, IL: Applied Symbolix.

Hennessey, N., Dourado, E., & Beilby, J. (2014). Anxiety and speaking in people who stutter: An investigation using the emotional Stroop Task. *Journal of Fluency Disorders, 40*, 44–57.

Hernandez, L. M. (2001). *A normative investigation of the speech-associated attitude of preschool and kindergarten children*. Masters thesis, University of Central Florida, Orlando.

Herndon, G. (1967). A study of the time discrimination abilities of stutterers and nonstutterers. *Speech Monographs, 34*, 303–304.

Hertsberg, N. (2010). *Differences in pitch variation in preschool-age children who do and do not stutter*. B. S. Unpublished undergraduate honors thesis, University of Vermont, Burlington, VT.

Hickok, G., Houde, J., & Rong, F. (2011). Sensorimotor integration in speech processing: Computational basis and neural organization. *Neuron, 69*(3), 407–422.

Hickok, G., & Poeppel, D. (2007). The cortical organization of speech processing. *Nature Reviews Neuroscience, 8*, 393–402.

Hilger, A., Zelaznik, H. N., & Smith, A. (2016). Evidence that bimanual motor timing performance is not a significant factor in developmental stuttering. *Journal of Speech, Language, and Hearing Research, 59*, 674–685.

Hill, D. (2003). Differential treatment of stuttering in the early stages of development. In H. H. Gregory, J. Campbell, C. Gregory, & D. Hill (Eds.), *Stuttering therapy: Rationale and procedures* (pp. 142–185). Boston, MA: Allyn & Bacon.

Hill, H. (1954). An experimental study of disorganization of speech and manual responses in normal subjects. *Journal of Speech and Hearing Disorders, 19*, 295–305.

Hillman, R. E., & Gilbert, H. R. (1977). Voice onset time for voiceless stop consonants in the fluent reading of stutterers and nonstutterers. *Journal of the Acoustical Society of America, 61*, 610–611.

Hiscock, M., & Kinsbourne, M. (1977). Selective listening asymmetry in preschool children. *Developmental Psychology, 133*, 217–224.

Hiscock, M., & Kinsbourne, M. (1980). Asymmetry of verbal-manual time sharing in children: a follow-up study. *Neuropsychologia, 18*, 151–162.

Hodson, B. W. (2004). *Hodson assessment of phonological patterns (HAPP-3)* (3rd ed.). East Moline, IL: LinguiSystems.

Hodson, B. W., & Paden, E. P. (1991). *A phonological approach to remediation: Targeting intelligible speech.* Austin, TX: Pro-Ed.

Hollister, J., Van Horne, A., & Zebrowski, P. (2017). The relationship between grammatical development and disfluencies in preschool children who stutter and those who recover. *American Journal of Speech-Language Pathology, 26*(1), 1–13.

Holloway, J. L., Allen, M. T., Myers, C. E., & Servatius, R. J. (2014). Behaviorally inhibited individuals demonstrate significantly enhanced conditioned response acquisition under non-optimal learning conditions. *Behavioural Brain Research, 261*, 49–55.

Hood, L. (1987, November). Middle latency responses in stutterers. Paper presented at the Annual meeting of the American Speech-Language-Hearing Association, New Orleans, LA.

Horovitz, L. J., Johnson, S. B., Pearlman, R. C., Schaffer, E. J., & Hedin, A. K. (1978). Stapedial reflex and anxiety in fluent and disfluent speakers. *Journal of Speech and Hearing Research, 214*, 762–767.

Horvath, A. T., Misra, K., Epner, A., & Cooper, G. (2016, August 31). *Social learning theory and addiction.* Available at http://MentalHelp.net

Howell, P., El-Yaniv, N., & Powell, D. J. (1987). Factors affecting fluency in stutterers when speaking under altered auditory feedback. In H. F. M. Peters, & W. Hulstijn (Eds.), *Speech motor dynamics in stuttering* (pp. 361–369). New York: Springer.

Howell, P., & Van Borsel, J. (2011). *Multilingual aspects of fluency disorders.* Tonawanda, NY: Multicultural Matters.

Howie, P. M. (1981). Concordance for stuttering in monozygotic and dizygotic twin pairs. *Journal of Speech and Hearing Research, 24*, 317–321.

Howie, P. M., & Andrews, G. (1984). Treatment of adult stutterers: Managing fluency. In R. Curlee, & W. Perkins (Eds.), *Nature and treatment of stuttering: New directions* (pp. 425–445). San Diego, CA: College-Hill Press.

Hubbard, C. P., & Yairi, E. (1988). Clustering of disfluencies in the speech of stuttering and nonstuttering preschool children. *Journal of Speech and Hearing Research, 312*, 228–233.

Humphrey, D. R., & Reed, D. J. (1983). Separate cortical systems for control of joint movement and joint stiffness: Reciprocal activation and coactivation of antagonist muscles. *Advances in Neurology, 39*, 347–372.

Ingham, R. J. (1979). Comment on Stuttering therapy: The relation between attitude change and long-term outcome. *Journal of Speech and Hearing Disorders, 44*, 397–400.

Ingham, R. J. (2001). Brain imaging studies of developmental stuttering. *Journal of Communication Disorders, 34*, 493–516.

Ingham, R. J. (2003). Brain imaging and stuttering: Some reflection on current and future developments. *Journal of Fluency Disorders, 284*, 411–420.

Ingham, R. J., & Andrews, G. (1973). Details of a token economy stuttering therapy programme for adults. *Australian Journal of Human Communication Disorders, 1*, 13–20.

Ingham, R. J., Cordes, A. K., & Finn, P. (1993). Time-interval measurement of stuttering: Systematic replication of Ingham, Cordes & Gow (1993). *Journal of Speech and Hearing Research, 36*, 503–515.

Ingham, R. J., Cordes, A. K., & Gow, M. (1993). Time-interval measurement of stuttering: Modifying interjudge agreement. *Journal of Speech and Hearing Research, 36*, 503–515.

Ingham, R. J., Fox, P. T., & Ingham, J. C. (1995, November). A report on a functional-activation and functional-lesion PET study of stuttering in adults. Paper presented at the Annual Conference of the American Speech-Language-Hearing Association, Orlando, FL.

Ingham, R. J., Gow, M., & Costello, J. M. (1985). Stuttering and speech naturalness: Some additional data. *Journal of Speech and Hearing Disorders, 502*, 217–219.

Ingham, R. J., Ingham, J. C., Bothe, A., Wang, Y., & Kilgo, M. (2015). Efficacy of the Modifying Phonation Intervals (MPI) stuttering treatment program with adults who stutter. *American Journal of Speech-Language Pathology, 24*, 256–271.

Ingham, R. J., Ingham, J. C., Euler, H. A., & Neumann, K. (2017). Stuttering treatment and brain research in adults: A still unfolding relationship. *Journal of Fluency Disorders, 55*, 106–119.

Ingham, R. J., Ingham, J. C., Finn, P., & Fox, P. T. (2003). Towards a functional neural systems model of developmental stuttering. *Journal of Fluency Disorders, 284*, 297–318.

Ingham, R. J., Wang, Y., Ingham, J., Bothe, A., & Grafton, S. (2013). Regional brain activity change predicts responsiveness to treatment for stuttering in adults. *Brain and Language, 127*(3), 510–519.

International Classification of Functioning, Disability, and Health: ICF. (2001). *Geneva*, Switzerland: World Health Organization.

Ito, T. (1986). Speech dysfluency and the acquisition of syntax in children 2–6 years old. *Folia Phoniatrica, 38*, 310 Abstract.

Jaffe, J., & Anderson, S. W. (1979). Prescript to Chapter 1: Communication rhythms and the evolution of language. In A. W. Siegman, & S. Feldman (Eds.), *Of speech and time: Temporal speech patterns, interpersonal contexts.* Hillsdale, NJ: Lawrence Erlbaum Associates.

James, W. (1890). *The principles of psychology.* New York: Holt & Co.

Jancke, L., Hanggi, J., & Steinmetz, H. (2004). Morphological brain differences between adult stutterers and non-stutterers. *BMC Neurology, 4*, 23.

Janssen, P., Kraaimaat, F., & Brutten, G. (1990). Relationship between stutterers' genetic history and speech associated variables. *Journal of Fluency Disorders, 8*, 39–48.

Jensen, P. J., Sheehan, J. G., Williams, W. M., & LaPointe, L. L. (1975). Oral-sensory-perceptual integrity of stutterers. *Folia Phoniatrica, 272*, 106–115.

Johnson, K. N., Walden, T. A., Conture, E. G., & Karrass, J. (2010). Spontaneous regulation of emotions in pre-school children who stutter: Preliminary findings. *Journal of Speech, Language, and Hearing Research, 53*(6), 1478–1495.

Johnson, W. (1938). The role of evaluation in stuttering behavior. *Journal of Speech Disorders, 3*, 85–89.

Johnson, W. (1955). A study of the onset and development of stuttering. In W. Johnson, & R. R. Leutenegger (Eds.), *Stuttering children and adults.* Minneapolis, MN: University of Minnesota Press.

Johnson, W. (1942). A study of the onset and development of stuttering. *Journal of Speech Disorders, 7*, 251–257.

Johnson, W., & Associates. (1959). *The onset of stuttering.* Minneapolis, MN: University of Minnesota Press.

Johnson, W., & Brown, S. (1935). Stuttering in relation to various speech sounds. *Quarterly Journal of Speech, 21*, 481–496.

Johnson, W., Darley, F., & Spriestersbach, D. (1952). *Diagnostic manual in speech correction: A professional training workbook.* New York: Harper & Brothers.

Johnson, W., & Inness, M. (1939). Studies in the psychology of stuttering: XIII. A statistical analysis of the adaptation and consistency effects in relation to stuttering. *Journal of Speech Disorders, 4*, 79–86.

Johnson, W., & Knott, J. R. (1937). Studies in the psychology of stuttering: I. The distribution of moments of stuttering in successive readings of the same material. *Journal of Speech Disorders, 2*, 17–19.

Johnson, W., & Rosen, L. (1937). Studies in the psychology of stuttering: VII. Effects of certain changes in speech pattern upon frequency of stuttering. *Journal of Speech Disorders, 2*, 105–109.

Johnson, W., & Solomon, A. (1937). Studies in the psychology of stuttering: IV. A quantitative study of expectation of stuttering as a process involving a low degree of consciousness. *Journal of Speech Disorders, 2*, 95–97.

Jokel, R., De Nil, L. F., & Sharpe, K. (2007). Speech disfluencies in adults with neurogenic stuttering associated with stroke and traumatic brain injury. *Journal of Medical Speech-Language Pathology, 15*(3), 243–261.

Jones, R. K. (1966). Observations on stammering after localized cerebral injury. *Journal of Neurology, Neurosurgery and Psychiatry, 29*, 192–195.

Jones, J. E., & Niven, P. (1993). *Voices and silences.* New York: Charles Scribner's Sons.

Jones, M., Onslow, M., Harrison, E., & Packman, A. (2000). Treating stuttering in young children: Predicting treatment time in the Lidcombe Program. *Journal of Speech, Language, and Hearing Research, 43*, 1440–1450.

Jones, M., Onslow, M., Packman, A., Williams, S., & Ormond, T. (2005). Randomized control trial of the Lidcombe programme of early stuttering intervention. *BMJ, 331*, 659.

Jones, R., Choi, D., Conture, E. G., & Walden, T. A. (2014). Temperament, emotion, and childhood stuttering. *Seminars in Speech and Language, 35*(2), 114–131.

Jurgens, U. (1979). Vocalization as an emotional indicator. *Behavior, 69*(1), 88–117.

Jurgens, U. (1994). The role of the periaqueductal grey in vocal behaviour. *Behavioural Brain Research, 62*(2), 107–117.

Juste, F. S., & Furquim de Andrade, C. R. (2011). Speech disfluency types of fluent and stuttering individuals: Age effects. *Folia Phoniatrica et Logopedica, 63*(2), 57–64.

Kagan, J. (1981). *The second year: The emergence of self-awareness.* Cambridge, MA: Harvard University Press.

Kagan, J. (1989). Temperamental contributions to social behavior. *American Psychologist, 44*, 668–674.

Kagan, J. (1994a). The realistic view of biology and behavior. *The Chronicle of Higher Education, 5*, A64.

Kagan, J. (1994b). *Galen's prophecy: Temperament in human nature.* New York: Basic Books.

Kagan, J., Reznick, J. S., & Snidman, N. (1987). The physiology and psychology of behavioral inhibition in children. *Child Development, 58*, 1459–1473.

Kagan, J., & Snidman, N. (1991). Temperamental factors in human development. *American Psychologist, 468*, 856–862.

Kang, C., Riazuddin, S., Mundorf, J., Krasnewich, D., Friedman, P., Mulliken, J., & Drayna, D. (2010). Mutations in the lysosomal enzyme-targeting pathway and persistent stuttering. *New England Journal of Medicine, 362*(8), 677–685.

Karlin, I. W. (1947). A psychosomatic theory of stuttering. *Journal of Speech Disorders, 12*(3), 319–322.

Karniol, R. (1992). Stuttering out of bilingualism. *First Language, 12*(38), 255–283.

Karrass, J., Walden, T. A., Conture, E. G., Graham, C. G., Arnold, H. S., & Hartfield, K. N. (2006). Relation of emotional reactivity and regulation to childhood stuttering. *Journal of Communication Disorders, 32*, 402–423.

Kasprisin-Burrelli, A., Egolf, D., & Shames, G. (1972). A comparison of parental verbal behavior with stuttering and nonstuttering children. *Journal of Communication Disorders, 5*, 335–346.

Kay, D. (1964). The genetics of stuttering. In G. Andrew, & M. Harris (Eds.), *The syndrome of stuttering* (pp. 132–143). London: The Spastics Society Medical Education and Information Unit.

Kell, C., Neumann, K., von Kriegstein, K., Posenenske, C., von Gudenberg, A., Euler, H. A., & Giraud, A-L. (2009). How the brain repairs stuttering. *Brain, 132*(10), 2747–2760.

Kelly, E. (1994). Speech rates and turn-taking behaviors of children who stutter and their fathers. *Journal of Speech and Hearing Research, 37*, 1284–1267.

Kelly, E., & Conture, E. G. (1992). Speaking rates, response time latencies, and interrupting behaviors of young stutterers, nonstutterers, and their mothers. *Journal of Speech and Hearing Research, 35*, 1256–1267.

Kelly, E., Smith, A., & Goffman, L. (1995). Orofacial muscle activity of children who stutter. *Journal of Speech and Hearing Research, 38*, 1025–1036.

Kelman, E., & Nicholas, A. (2008). *Practical intervention for early childhood stammering: Palin PCI.* Milton Keynes, UK: Speechmark.

Kent, R. D. (1981). Sensorimotor aspects of speech development. In R. D. Alberts, & M. R. Peterson (Eds.), *The development of perception: Psycho-biological perspectives.* New York: Academic Press.

Kent, R. D. (1984). Stuttering as a temporal programming disorder. In R. F. Curlee, & W. H. Perkins (Eds.), *Nature and treatment of stuttering: New directions* (pp. 283–301). San Diego, CA: College-Hill Press.

Kent, R. D. (1985). Developing and disordered speech: Strategies for organization. *ASHA Reports, 15*, 29–37.

Kent, R. D. (1993). Speech intelligibility and communicative competence in children. In A. P. Kiser & D. B. Gray (Eds.), *Enhancing children's communication: Research foundations for intervention* (Vol. 2, pp. 223–229*)*. Baltimore, MD: Brooks Publishing.

Kent, R. D. (1997). *The speech sciences.* San Diego, CA: Singular Publishing Company.

Kent, R. D. (2000). Research on speech motor control and its disorders: A review and prospective. *Journal of Communication Disorders, 33*, 391–428.

Kent, R. D., & Perkins, W. (1984). *Oral-verbal fluency: Aspects of verbal formulation, speech motor control and underlying neural systems.* Unpublished manuscript.

Kent, R. D., & Vorperian, H. K. (1995). Anatomic development of the craniofacial-oral-laryngeal systems: A review. *Journal of Medical Speech-Language Pathology, 3*, 145–190.

Kent, R. D., & Vorperian, H. K. (2007). In the mouths of babes: Anatomic motor and sensory foundations of speech development. In R. Paul (Ed.), *Language disorders from a developmental perspective: Essays in honor of Robin Chapman`* (pp. 56–80). Mahwah, NJ: Lawrence Erlbaum.

Kent, R. D., & Vorperian, H. K. (2013). Speech impairment in Down Syndrome: A review. *Journal of Speech, Language, and Hearing Research, 56*, 178–210.

Kenyon, E. L. (1942). The etiology of stammering: Fundamentally a wrong psychophysiologic habit in control of the vocal cords for the production of an individual speech sound. *Journal of Speech Disorders, 7*, 97–104.

Kidd, K. K. (1977). A genetic perspective on stuttering. *Journal of Fluency Disorders, 2*, 259–269.

Kidd, K. K. (1984). Stuttering as a genetic disorder. In R. F. Curlee, & W. H. Perkins (Eds.), *Nature and treatment of stuttering: New directions* (pp. 149–169). San Diego, CA: College-Hill Press.

Kidd, K. K., Heimbuch, R. C., Records, M. A., Oehlert, G., & Webster, R. L. (1980). Familial stuttering patterns are not related to one measure of severity. *Journal of Speech and Hearing Research, 23*, 539–545.

Kidd, K. K., Kidd, J. R., & Records, M. A. (1978). The possible causes of the sex ratio in stuttering and its implications. *Journal of Fluency Disorders, 3*, 13–23.

Kidd, K. K., Reich, T., & Kessler, S. (1973). A genetic analysis of stuttering suggesting a single major locus. *Genetics, 742*(Pt 2), S92.

Kinsbourne, M. (1989). A model of adaptive behavior related to cerebral participation in emotional control. In G. Gianotti, & C. Caltagirone (Eds.), *Emotions and the dual brain*. New York: Springer-Verlag.

Kinsbourne, M. B., & Bemporad, E. (1984). Lateralization of emotion: A model and the evidence. In N. A. Fox, & R. J. Davidson (Eds.), *The psychology of affective development*. Hillsdale, NJ: Lawrence Erlbaum Associates.

Kinsbourne, M., & Hicks, R. (1978). Functional cerebral space: A model for overflow, transfer and interference effects in human performance: A tutorial review. In M. Kinsbourne (Ed.), *Asymmetrical function of the brain* (pp. 345–362). Cambridge, UK: Cambridge University Press.

Kleinow, J., & Smith, A. (2000). Influences of length and syntactic complexity on the speech motor stability of the fluent speech of adults who stutter. *Journal of Speech, Language, and Hearing Research, 432*, 548–559.

Kloth, S., Janssen, P., Kraaimaat, F., & Brutten, G. (1995). Speech-motor and linguistic skills of young stutterers prior to onset. *Journal of Fluency Disorders, 20*, 157–170.

Kloth, S., Janssen, P., Kraaimaat, F., & Brutten, G. (1998). Child and mother variables in the development of stuttering among high-risk children: A longitudinal study. *Journal of Fluency Disorders, 23*, 217–230.

Kloth, S. A. M., Kraaimaat, F. W., Janssen, P., & Brutten, G. J. (1999). Persistence and remission of incipient stuttering among high-risk children. *Journal of Fluency Disorders, 244*, 253–265.

Knott, J. R., Johnson, W., & Webster, M. J. (1937). Studies in the psychology of stuttering: II. A quantitative evaluation of expectation of stuttering in relation to the occurrence of stuttering. *Journal of Speech Disorders, 2*, 20–22.

Kolk, H., & Postma, A. (1997). Stuttering as a covert repair phenomenon. In R. F. Curlee, & G. M. Siegel (Eds.), *Nature and treatment of stuttering: New directions* (2nd ed., pp. 182–203). Boston, MA: Allyn & Bacon.

Kraft, S. J. (2010). *Genome-wide association study of persistent developmental stuttering*. PhD Thesis, University of Illinois, Urbana-Champaign, IL.

Kraft, S. J., & Yairi, E. (2012). Genetic basis of stuttering: State of the art, 2011. *Folia Phoniatrica et Logopedica, 64*, 34–47.

Kramer, M., Green, D., & Guitar, B. (1987). A comparison of stutterers and nonstutterers on masking level differences and synthetic sentence identification tasks. *Journal of Communication Disorders, 20*, 379–390.

Kroll, R. M., De Nil, L. F., & Houle, S. (1999, November). Towards an scientific understanding of stuttering and treatment: PET scan studies. Paper presented at the Annual Conference of the American Speech-Language-Hearing Association, San Francisco.

Kroll, R. M., De Nil, L. F., Kapur, S., & Houle, S. (1997). A positron emission tomography investigation of post-treatment brain activation in stutterers. In W. Hulstijn, H. F. M. Peters, & P. H. H. M. van Lieshout (Eds.), *Speech production: Motor control, brain research and fluency disorders* (pp. 307–319). Amsterdam, The Netherlands: Elsevier.

Kroll, R. M., & Scott-Sulsky, L. (2010). The Fluency Plus Program: An integration of fluency shaping and cognitive restructuring procedures for adolescents and adults who stutter. In B. Guitar, & R. J. McCauley (Eds.), *Treatment of stuttering: Established and emerging interventions* (pp. 277–311). Baltimore, MD: Lippincott Williams & Wilkins.

Langevin, M., Huinck, W. J., Kully, D., Peters, H. F. M., Lomheim, H., & Tellers, M. (2006). A cross-cultural, long-term outcome evaluation of the ISTAR Comprehensive Stuttering Program across Dutch and Canadian adults who stutter. *Journal of Fluency Disorders, 31*(4), 229–256.

Langevin, M., Packman, A., & Onslow, M. (2010). Parent perceptions of the impact of stuttering on their preschoolers and themselves. *Journal of Communication Disorders, 43*(5), 407–423.

Langlois, A., Hanrahan, L. L., & Inouye, L. L. (1986). A comparison of interactions between stuttering children, nonstuttering children, and their mothers. *Journal of Fluency Disorders, 11*, 263–273.

Langlois, A., & Long, S. H. (1988). A model for teaching parents to facilitate fluent speech. *Journal of Fluency Disorders, 13*, 163–172.

Lanouette, E. B. (2011). Intervention strategies for cluttering disorders. In D. Ward, & K. S. Scott (Eds.), *Cluttering: A handbook of research, intervention and education* (pp. 175–197). Hove, UK: Psychology Press.

LaSalle, L. R. (1999, November). Temperament in preschoolers who stutter: A preliminary investigation. Paper presented at the Annual meeting of the American Speech-Language-Hearing Association, San Francisco.

LaSalle, L. R., & Conture, E. G. (1995). Disfluency clusters of children who stutter: Relation of stutterings to self-repairs. *Journal of Speech and Hearing Research, 38*, 965–977.

Latterman, C., Euler, H. A., & Neumann, K. (2008). A randomized control trial to investigate the impact of the Lidcombe Program on early stuttering in German-speaking preschoolers. *Journal of Fluency Disorders, 33*, 52–65.

Lauter, J. L. (1995). Visions of speech and language: Noninvasive imaging techniques and their applications to the study of human communication. In H. Winitz (Ed.), *Current approaches to the study of language development and disorders* (pp. 277–390). Timonium, MD: York Press.

Lauter, J. L. (1997). Noninvasive brain imaging in speech motor control and stuttering: Choices and challenges. In W. Hulstijn, H. F. M. Peters, & P. H. H. M. van Lieshout (Eds.), *Speech production: Motor control, brain research, and fluency disorders* (pp. 233–258). Amsterdam, The Netherlands: Elsevier.

Lazare, A. (1981). Current concepts in psychiatry: Conversion symptoms. *New England Journal of Medicine, 305*, 745.

LeDoux, J. E. (2002). *Synaptic self: How our brains become who we are*. New York: Viking.

LeDoux, J. E. (2015). *Anxious: Using the brain to understand and treat fear and anxiety*. New York: Viking.

Lee, B. S. (1951). Artificial stutter. *Journal of Speech and Hearing Disorders, 16*, 53–55.

Lee, W-S., Kang, C., Drayna, D., & Kornfield, S. (2011). Analysis of mannose 6-phosphate uncovering enzyme mutations associated with persistent stuttering. *Journal of Biological Chemistry, 286*, 39786–39793.

Levitin, D., & Menon, V. (2003). Musical structure is processed in "language" areas of the brain: A possible role for Brodmann Area 47 in temporal coherence. *NeuroImage, 20*(4), 2142–2152.

Lewis, M. (2000). Self-conscious emotions: Embarrassment, pride, shame and guilt. In M. Lewis, & J. M. Haviland-Jones (Eds.), *Handbook of emotions* (2nd ed.). New York: Guilford Press.

Lidz, T. (1968). *The person: His development throughout the life cycle*. New York: Basic Books.

Lieberman, A. (2018). Counseling issues: Addressing behavioral and emotional considerations in the treatment of communication disorders. *American Journal of Speech-Language Pathology, 27*, 13–23.

Liebetrau, R., & Daly, D. A. (1981). Auditory processing and perceptual abilities of organic and functional stutterers. *Journal of Fluency Disorders, 6*, 219–231.

Lincoln, M., & Onslow, M. (1997). Long-term outcome of an early intervention for stuttering. *American Journal of Speech-Language Pathology, 6*, 51–58.

Lindsay, J. S. (1989). Relationship of developmental disfluency and episodes of stuttering to the emergence of cognitive stages in children. *Journal of Fluency Disorders, 14*, 271–284.

Livingston, L. A., Flowers, Y. E., Hodor, B. A., & Ryan, B. P. (2000). The experimental analysis of interruption during conversation for three children who stutter. *Journal of Developmental and Physical Disabilities, 12*, 235–266.

Logan, K., & Conture, E. G. (1995). Length, grammatical complexity, and rate differences in stuttered and fluent conversational utterances of children who stutter. *Journal of Fluency Disorders, 20*, 35–61.

Luchsinger, R. (1944). Biological studies on monozygotic and dizigotic twins relative to size and form of the larynx. *Archiv Julius Klaus-Stiftung fur Verergungsforchung, 19*, 3–4.

MacKinnon, S., Hall, S., & MacIntyre, P. (2007). Origins of the stuttering stereotype: Stereotype formation through anchoring-adjustment. *Journal of Fluency Disorders, 32*(4), 297–309.

MacPhereson, M. K., & Smith, A. (2013). Influences of sentence length and syntactic complexity on the speech motor control of children who stutter. *Journal of Speech, Language, and Hearing Research, 56*, 89–102.

Maguire, G., Franklin, D., Vatakis, N. G., Morgenshtern, E., Denko, T., Yaruss, J. S., et al. (2010). Exploratory randomized clinical study of pagoclone in persistent developmental stuttering: The Examining Pagoclone for Persistent Stuttering Study. *Journal of Clinical Psychopharmacology, 30*(1), 48–56.

Maguire, G., Riley, G., Franklin, D., & Gumusaneli, E. (2010). The physiological basis and pharmacological treatment of stuttering. In B. Guitar, & R. J. McCauley (Eds.), *Treatment of stuttering: Established and emerging interventions* (pp. 329–354). Baltimore, MD: Lippincott Williams & Wilkins.

Maguire, G., Yeh, C., & Ito, B. (2012). Review article: Overview of the diagnosis and treatment of stuttering. *Journal of Experimental & Clinical Medicine, 4*(2), 92–97.

Maguire, G., Yu, B., Franklin, D., & Riley, G. (2004). Alleviating stuttering with pharmacological interventions. *Expert Opinion in Pharmacotherapy, 5*, 1565–1571.

Mahr, G., & Leith, W. (1992). Psychogenic stuttering of adult onset. *Journal of Speech and Hearing Research, 35*, 283–286.

Mahurin-Smith, J., & Ambrose, N. G. (2013). Breastfeeding may protect against persistent stuttering. *Journal of Communication Disorders, 46*(4), 351–360.

Malecot, A., Johnston, R., & Kizziar, P-A. (1972). Syllabic rate and utterance length in French. *Phonetica, 26*, 235–251.

Manning, W. H., & DiLollo, A. (2018). *Clinical decision making in fluency disorders* (4th ed.). San Diego, CA: Plural Publishing.

Mansson, H. (2000). Childhood stuttering: Incidence and development. *Journal of Fluency Disorders, 25*(1), 47–57.

Mansson, H. (2005). Stammens kompleksitet og diversitet. *Dansk Audiologopaedi, 41*, 13–33.

Market, K. E., Montague, J. C., Buffalo, M. D., & Drummond, S. A. (1990). Acquired stuttering: Descriptive data and treatment outcomes. *Journal of Fluency Disorders, 15*, 21–33.

Marshall, R. C., & Starch, S. A. (1984). Behavioral treatment of acquired stuttering. *Australian Journal of Human Communication Disorders, 12*, 87–92.

Martin, R., Haroldson, S., & Triden, K. (1984). Stuttering and speech naturalness. *Journal of Speech and Hearing Disorders, 27*, 53–58.

Maske-Cash, W., & Curlee, R. (1995). Effect of utterance length and meaningfulness on the speech initiation times of children who stutter and children who do not stutter. *Journal of Speech and Hearing Research, 38*, 18–25.

Mattes, L. J., & Omack, D. R. (1991). *Speech and language assessment for the bilingually handicapped*. Oceanside, CA: Academic Communication Associates.

Matthews, S., Williams, R., & Pring, T. (2010). Parent–child interaction therapy and dysfluency: A single-case study. *International Journal of Language and Communication Disorders, 32*(3), 346–357.

Max, L., Guenther, F. H., Gracco, V. L., Ghosh, S. S., & Wallace, M. E. (2004). Unstable or insufficiently activated internal models and feedback-biased motor-control as sources of dysfluency: A theoretical model of stuttering. *Contemporary Issues in Communication Science and Disorders, 31*, 105–122.

McCall, G. N., & Rabuzzi, D. D. (1973). Reflex contraction of middle-ear muscles secondary to stimulation of laryngeal nerves. *Journal of Speech and Hearing Research, 16*, 56–61.

McCauley, R. J. (1996). Familiar strangers: Criterion-referenced measures in communication disorders. *Language, Speech, and Hearing Services in Schools, 27*, 122–131.

McClean, M. D. (1990). Neuromotor aspects of stuttering: Levels of impairment and disability. In J. Cooper (Ed.), *Research needs in stuttering: Roadblocks and future directions (ASHA Reports, 18)* (pp. 64–71). Rockville, MD: American Speech-Language-Hearing Association.

McClean, M. D., & McClean, A. (1985). Case report of stuttering acquired in association with phenytoin use for post-head-injury seizures. *Journal of Fluency Disorders, 10*, 241–255.

McClean, M. D., Kroll, R. M., & Loftus, N. S. (1990). Kinematic analysis of lip closure in stutterers' fluent speech. *Journal of Speech and Hearing Research*, *33*, 755–760.

McDearmon, J. R. (1968). Primary stuttering at the onset of stuttering: A reexamination of data. *Journal of Speech and Hearing Research*, *11*, 631–637.

McDevitt, S. C., & Carey, W. B. (1978). The measurement of temperament in 3 7-year-old children. *Journal of Child Psychology and Psychiatry, and Allied Disciplines*, *19*, 245–253.

McDevitt, S. C., & Carey, W. B. (1995). *Behavioral style questionnaire*. West Chester, PA: TemperaMetrics.

McFarlane, S. C., & Prins, D. (1978). Neural response time of stutterers and nonstutterers in selected oral motor tasks. *Journal of Speech and Hearing Research*, *21*, 768–778.

Merits-Patterson, R., & Reed, C. G. (1981). Disfluencies in the speech of language-delayed children. *Journal of Speech, Language, and Hearing Research*, *24*, 55–58.

Merson, R. M. (2003). Audiotory sidetone and the management of stuttering: From Wollensack to SpeechEasy. Paper presented at the International Stuttering Awareness Day Online Conference.

Meyers, S. C., & Freeman, F. J. (1985a). Interruptions as a variable in stuttering and disfluency. *Journal of Speech and Hearing Research*, *28*, 428–425.

Meyers, S. C., & Freeman, F. J. (1985b). Mother and child speech rate as a variable in stuttering and disfluency. *Journal of Speech and Hearing Research*, *28*, 436–444.

Miles, S., & Ratner, N. B. (2001). Parental language input to children at stuttering onset. *Journal of Speech, Language, and Hearing Research*, *44*, 1116–1130.

Milisen, R. (1938). Frequency of stuttering with anticipation of stuttering controlled. *Journal of Speech Disorders*, *3*, 207–214.

Milisen, R., & Johnson, W. (1936). A comparative study of stutterers, former stutterers and normal speakers whose handedness has been changed. *Archives of Speech*, *1*, 61–68.

Millard, S. R., Edwards, S., & Cook, F. (2009). Parent–child interaction therapy: Adding to the evidence. *International Journal of Speech-Language Pathology*, *11*(1), 61–76.

Millard, S. R., Nicholas, A., & Cook, F. M. (2008). Is parent–child interaction therapy effective in reducing stuttering? *Journal of Speech, Language, and Hearing Research*, *51*, 636–650.

Millard, S. R., Zebrowski, P., & Kelman, E. (2018). Palin parent–child interaction therapy: The bigger picture. *American Journal of Speech-Language Pathology*. doi:10.1044/2018_AJSLP-ODC11-17-0199

Miller, B., & Guitar, B. (2009). Long-term outcomes of the Lidcombe Program for early stuttering intervention. *American Journal of Speech-Language Pathology*, *18*, 42–49.

Miller, N. E. (1948). Studies of fear as an acquirable drive: 1. Fear as motivation and fear-reduction as reinforcement in the learning of new responses. *Journal of Experimental Psychology*, *38*, 89–101.

Miller, S. (1993). *Multiple measures of anxiety and psychophysiologic arousal in stutterers and nonstutterers during nonspeech and speech tasks of increasing complexity*. Unpublished doctoral dissertation, University of Texas, Dallas, TX.

Mineka, S. (1985). Animal models of anxiety-based disorders: Their usefulness and limitations. In A. H. Tuma, & J. Mase (Eds.), *Anxiety and the anxiety disorders*. Hillsdale, NJ: Lawrence Erlbaum Associates.

Mineka, S., & Oehlberg, K. (2008). The relevance of recent developments in classical conditioning to understanding the etiology and maintenance of anxiety disorders. *Acta Psychologica*, *127*(3), 567–580.

Minifie, F. D., & Cooker, H. S. (1964). A disfluency index. *Journal of Speech and Hearing Disorders*, *29*, 189–192.

Mogenson, G., Jones, D., & Yim, C. (1980). From motivation to action: Functional interface between the limbic system and the motor system. *Progress in Neurobiology*, *14*(2–3), 69–97.

Mohan, R., & Weber, C. M. (2015). Neural systems mediating processing of sound units of language distinguish recovery vs. persistence in stuttering. *Journal of Neurodevelopmental Disorders*, *7*(1), 28.

Molt, L. F. (1997). Event-related cortical potentials and language processing in stutterers. Paper presented at the 2nd World Congress on Fluency Disorders, San Francisco, CA.

Molt, L. F., & Guilford, A. M. (1979). Auditory processing and anxiety in stutterers. *Journal of Fluency Disorders*, *4*, 255–267.

Moore, W. H. (1984). Hemispheric alpha asymmetries during an electromyographic biofeedback procedure for stuttering: A single subject experimental design. *Journal of Fluency Disorders*, *9*(2), 143–162.

Moore, W. H., & Haynes, W. O. (1980). Alpha hemispheric asymmetry and stuttering: Some support for a segmentation dysfunction hypothesis. *Journal of Speech and Hearing Research*, *23*, 229–247.

Mowrer, O. H. (1939). A stimulus–response analysis of anxiety and its role as a reinforcing agent. *Psychological Review*, *46*(6), 553–565.

Mowrer, O. H., & Lamoreaux, R. (1942). Avoidance conditioning and signal duration—a study of secondary motivation and reward. *Psychological Monographs*, *54*(5), 1–34.

Murphy, W. P., Quesal, R. W., Reardon-Reeves, N., & Yaruss, J. S. (2013). *Minimizing bullying for children who stutter*. McKinney, TX: Stuttering Therapy Resources.

Myers, F. L. (1978). Relationship between eight physiological variables and severity of stuttering. *Journal of Fluency Disorders*, *3*, 181–191.

Myers, F. L. (2002, November). Putting cluttering on the map: Looking back/looking ahead. Paper presented at the Annual meeting of the American Speech Language and Hearing Association, Atlanta.

Myers, F. L. (2011). Treatment of cluttering: A cognitive-behavioral approach centered on rate control. In D. Ward, & K. S. Scott (Eds.), *Cluttering: A handbook of research, intervention and education* (pp. 152–174). Hove, UK: Psychology Press.

Myers, F. L., & St. Louis, K. (1986). *Cluttering: A clinical perspective*. San Diego, CA: Singular.

Myers, F. L., & St. Louis, K. (2007). *Cluttering* [DVD]. Memphis, TN: Stuttering Foundation.

Namasivayam, A. K., & van Lieshout, P. (2011). Speech motor skill and stuttering. *Journal of Motor Behavior*, *43*(6), 477–489.

Namasivayam, A. K., van Lieshout, P., McIlroy, W. E., & De Nil, L. F. (2009). Sensory feedback dependence hypothesis in persons who stutter. *Human Movement Science*, *28*(6), 688–707.

National Institute of Neurological Disorders and Stroke. (2011). *Mucolipidoses fact sheet*. Available at http://www.ninds.nih.gov/disorders/mucolipidoses/detail_mucolipidoses.htm

Navon, D. (1984). Resources—a theoretical stone soup. *Psychological Review*, *912*, 216–234.

Neef, N., Butfering, C., Auer, T., Metzger, F. L., Euler, H. A., Frahm, J., et al. (2017). Altered morphology of the nucleus accumbens in persistent developmental stuttering. *Journal of Fluency Disorders, 55*, 84–93.

Neilson, M. D. (1980). *Stuttering and the control of speech: A systems analysis approach*. Unpublished doctoral dissertation. Kensington, NSW: University of New South Wales, Kensington, NSW, Australia.

Neilson, M. D., Howie, P. M., & Andrews, G. (1987, August). Does foetal testosterone play a role in the aetiology of stuttering?. Paper presented at the Fifth International Australasian Winter Conference on Brain Research, Queenstown, NZ.

Neilson, M. D., & Neilson, P. D. (1987). Speech motor control and stuttering: A computational model of adaptive sensory-motor processing. *Speech Communication, 6*, 325–333.

Neilson, M. D., & Neilson, P. D. (1988). Sensory-motor integration capacity of stutterers and nonstutterers. Paper presented at the Second Australian International Conference on Speech Science and Technology, Sydney, Australia.

Neilson, P. D., & Neilson, M. D. (2005a). An overview of adaptive model theory: Solving the problems of redundancy, resources, and nonlinear interactions in human movement control. *Journal of Neural Engineering, 2*, S279–S312.

Neilson, P. D., & Neilson, M. D. (2005b). Motor maps and synergies. *Human Movement Science, 24*, 774–797.

Neilson, P. D., Neilson, M. D., & O'Dwyer, N. J. (1992). Adaptive model theory: Application to disorders of motor control. In J. J. Summers (Ed.), *Approaches to the study of motor control and learning*. Amsterdam, The Netherlands: Elsevier Science Publishers.

Neilson, P. D., Quinn, P. T., & Neilson, M. D. (1976). Auditory tracking measures of hemispheric asymmetry in normals and stutterers. *Australian Journal of Human Communication, 4*, 121–126.

Nelson, N. (2010). *Language and literacy disorders: Infancy through adolescence*. New York: Pearson.

Netsell, R. (1981). The acquisition of speech motor control: A perspective with direction for research. In R. Stark (Ed.), *Language behavior in infancy and early childhood*. New York: Elsevier-North Holland.

Neumann, K., & Euler, H. A. (2010). Neuroimaging and stuttering. In B. Guitar, & R. McCauley (Eds.), *Stuttering treatment: Established and emerging approaches* (pp. 355–377). Baltimore, MD: Lippincott Williams & Wilkins.

Neumann, K., Euler, H. A., Wolff von Gudenberg, A., Giraud, A-L., Lanfermann, H., Gall, V., Preibisch, C. (2003). The nature and treatment of stuttering as revealed by fMRI: A within- and between-group comparison. *Journal of Fluency Disorders, 28*, 381–410.

Neumann, K., Preibisch, C., Euler, H. A., Wolff von Gudenberg, A., Lanfermann, H., Gall, V., Giraud, A-L. (2005). Cortical plasticity associated with stuttering therapy. *Journal of Fluency Disorders, 30*, 23–29.

Newman, L., & Smit, A. (1989). Some effects of variations in response time latency on speech rate, interruptions, and fluency in children's speech. *Journal of Speech, Language, and Hearing Research, 32*, 635–644.

Nippold, M. A. (2012). Stuttering and language ability in children: questioning the connection. *American Journal of Speech-Language Pathology, 21*, 183–196.

Nippold, M. A. (2016). *Later language development: School-aged children, adolescents, and young adults* (4th ed.). Austin, TX: Pro-Ed.

Nittrouer, S., Studdert-Kennedy, M., & McGowan, R. S. (1989). The emergence of phonetic segments: Evidence from the spectral structure of fricative-vowel syllables spoken by children and adults. *Journal of Speech and Hearing Research, 32*, 120–132.

Ntourou, K., Conture, E. G., & Lipsey, M. W. (2011). Language abilities of children who stutter: A meta-analytical review. *Journal of Speech-Language Pathology, 20*(3), 163–179.

Ntourou, K., Conture, E. G., & Walden, T. A. (2013). Emotional reactivity and regulation in pre-school age children who stutter. *Journal of Fluency Disorders, 38*(3), 260–274.

Ntourou, K., DeFranco, E., Conture, E. G., & Waldon, T. (in review). Short Behavioral Inhibition Scale: A parent-report measure of behavioral inhibition for young children. *American Journal of Speech-Language Pathology.*

Nudelman, H. B., Herbrich, K. E., Hess, K. R., Hoyt, B. D., & Rosenfield, D. B. (1992). A model of the phonation response time of stutterers and fluent speakers to frequency-modulated tones. *Journal of the Acoustical Society of America, 92*(4 Pt 1), 1882–1888.

Nudelman, H. B., Herbrich, K. E., Hoyt, B. D., & Rosenfield, D. B. (1987). Dynamic characteristics of vocal frequency tracking in stutterers and nonstutterers. In H. F. M. Peters, & W. Hulstijn (Eds.), *Speech motor dynamics in stuttering*. Wien, Austria: Springer-Verlag.

Nudelman, H. B., Herbrich, K. E., Hoyt, B. D., & Rosenfield, D. B. (1989). A neuro-science model of stuttering. *Journal of Fluency Disorders, 14*, 399–427.

Nurnberg, H., & Greenwald, B. (1981). Stuttering: An unusual side effect of phenothiazines. *American Journal of Psychiatry, 138*, 386–387.

O'Brian, S., Carey, S., Lowe, R., Onslow, M., Packman, A., & Cream, A. (2017). *Camperdown Program: Stuttering treatment guide*. Sydney, Australia: Australian Stuttering Research Centre.

O'Brian, S., Packman, A., & Onslow, M. (2008). Telehealth delivery of the Camperdown program for adults who stutter: A Phase I trial. *Journal of Speech, Language, and Hearing Research, 51*, 184–195.

O'Brian, S., Smith, K., & Onslow, M. (2014). Webcam delivery of the Lidcombe Program for early stuttering: A Phase 1 clinical trial. *Journal of Speech, Language, and Hearing Research, 57*, 825–830.

O'Brien, S., Onslow, M., Cream, A., & Packman, A. (2003). The Camperdown Program: Outcomes of a new prolonged-speech treatment model. *Journal of Speech, Language, and Hearing Research, 464*, 933–946.

O'Brien, S., Packman, A., & Onslow, M. (2004). Self-rating of stuttering severity as a clinical tool. *American Journal of Speech-Language Pathology, 133*, 219–226.

Olander, L., Smith, A., & Zelaznik, H. N. (2010). Evidence that a motor timing deficit is a factor in the development of stuttering. *Journal of Speech and Hearing Research, 53*, 876–886.

Onslow, M., Andrews, C., & Costa, L. (1990). Parental severity scaling of early stuttered speech: Four case studies. *Australian Journal of Human Communication, 18*, 47–61.

Onslow, M., Andrews, C., & Lincoln, M. (1994). A control/experimental trial of an operant treatment for early stuttering. *Journal of Speech and Hearing Research, 37*, 1244–1259.

Onslow, M., Costa, L., & Rue, S. (1990). Direct early intervention with stuttering: Some preliminary data. *Journal of Speech and Hearing Disorders, 55*, 405–416.

Onslow, M., Harrison, E., Jones, M., & Packman, A. (2002). Beyond-clinic speech measures during the Lidcombe Program of early stuttering intervention. *ACQuiring Knowledge in Speech, Language, and Hearing, 4*, 82–85.

Onslow, M., Jones, M., O'Brian, S., Packman, A., Menzies, R., Lowe, R., et al. (2018). Comparison of percentage syllables stuttered with parent-reported severity ratings as a primary outcome measure in clinical trials of early stuttering treatment. *Journal of Speech, Language, and Hearing Research, 61*, 811–819.

Onslow, M., Packman, A., & Harrison, E. (2003). *The Lidcombe program of early stuttering intervention: A clinician's guide.* Austin, TX: Pro-Ed.

Onslow, M., Webber, M., Harrison, E., Arnott, S., Bridgman, K., & Carey, B., et al. (2017, December). *The Lidcombe Treatment Guide.* Retrieved from http://lidcombeprogram.org

Ooki, S. (2005). Genetic and environmental influences on stuttering and tics in Japanese twins. *Twin Research and Human Genetics, 8*, 529–575.

Orton, S. (1927). Studies in stuttering. *Archives of Neurology and Psychiatry, 18*, 671–672.

Orton, S., & Travis, L. (1929). Studies in stuttering: IV. Studies of action currents in stuttering. *Archives of Neurology and Psychiatry, 21*, 61–68.

Oyler, M. E. (1992, November). Self perception and sensitivity in stuttering adults. Paper presented at the Annual meeting of the American Speech-Language-Hearing Association, San Antonio, TX.

Oyler, M. E. (1996). *Vulnerability in stuttering children.* Doctoral Dissertation, University of Colorado, Boulder, CO.

Oyler, M. E., & Ramig, P. R. (1995, November). Vulnerability in stuttering children. Paper presented at the Annual meeting of the American Speech-Language-Hearing Association, Orlando, FL.

Packman, A., & Attanasio, J. (2010, November). A model of the mechanisms underpinning early intervention for stuttering. Paper presented at the Annual conference of the American Speech-Language and Hearing Association, Philadelphia.

Packman, A., Code, C., & Onslow, M. (2007). On the causes of stuttering: Integrating theory with brain and behavioral research. *Journal of Neurolinguistics, 20*(5), 353–362.

Paul, R., & Norbury, C. (2012). *Language disorders: From infancy through adolescence.* St. Louis, MO: Elsevier.

Paulesu, E., Frith, C., & Frackowiak, R. (1993). The neural correlates of the verbal component of working memory. *Nature, 362*(6418), 342–345.

Pavuluri, M. N., & Passaroti, A. (2008). Neural bases of emotional processing in pediatric bipolar disorder. *Expert Review of Neurotherapeutics, 8*(9), 1381–1387.

Pearl, S. Z., & Bernthal, J. E. (1980). The effect of grammatical complexity upon disfluency behavior of nonstuttering preschool children. *Journal of Fluency Disorders, 5*, 55–68.

Perino, M., Famularo, G., & Tarroni, P. (2000). Acquired transient stuttering during a migraine attack. *Headache, 40*, 170–172.

Perkins, W. H., Kent, R. D., & Curlee, R. F. (1991). A theory of neuropsycholinguistic function in stuttering. *Journal of Speech and Hearing Research, 34*, 734–752.

Peters, H. F. M., & Hulstijn, W. (1984). Stuttering and anxiety: The difference between stutterers and nonstutterers in verbal apprehension and physiologic arousal during the anticipation of speech and non-speech tasks. *Journal of Fluency Disorders, 9*, 67–84.

Peters, T. J., & Guitar, B. (1991). *Stuttering: An integrated approach to its nature and treatment.* Baltimore, MD: Lippincott Williams & Wilkins.

Pierson, S. M. (2004). *Evaluating validity and reliability of the Teacher Assessment of Student Communicative Competence (TASCC) by comparing students who do and do not stutter.* Masters Thesis, University of Vermont, Burlington, VT.

Pietranton, A. A. (2012). An evidence-based practice primer: Implication and challenges for the treatment of fluency disorders. In N. Bernstein Ratner & J. Tetnowski (Eds.), *Current issues in stuttering research and practice* (pp. 47–60). Mahway, NJ: Lawrence Erlbaum Associates, Inc.

Pindzola, R., Jenkins, M., & Lokken, K. (1989). Speaking rates of young children. *Language, Speech, and Hearing Services in Schools, 20*, 133–138.

Platt, J., & Basili, A. (1973). Jaw tremor during stuttering block: An electromyographic study. *Journal of Communication Disorders, 6*, 102–109.

Ponsford, R., Brown, W., Marsh, J., & Travis, L. (1975). Proceedings: Evoked potential correlates of cerebral dominance for speech perception in stutterers and non-stutterers. *Electroencephalography and Clinical Neurophysiology, 39*, 434.

Pool, K. D., Devous, M. D., Freeman, F. J., Watson, B. C., & Finitzo, T. (1991). Regional cerebral blood flow in developmental stutterers. *Archives of Neurology, 48*, 509–512.

Poulos, M. G., & Webster, W. G. (1991). Family history as a basis for subgrouping people who stutter. *Journal of Speech and Hearing Research, 34*, 5–10.

Prather, E., Breecher, S. V., Stafford, M., & Wallace, E. (1980). *Screening test of adolescent language.* Los Angeles, CA: Western Psychological Services.

Prelock, P. A., & Hutchins, T. L. (Eds.). (2018). *Essential clinical guide to communication disorders.* New York: Springer.

Preus, A. (1981). *Identifying subgroups of stutterers.* Oslo, Norway: Universitetsforlaget.

Prins, D. (Ed.) (1991). *Theories of stuttering as event and disorder: Speech production processes.* Amsterdam, The Netherlands: Elsevier Science Publishers.

Prins, D. (1999). Describing the consequences of disorders: Comment on Yaruss (1998). *Journal of Speech, Language, and Hearing Research, 42*, 1395–1397.

Prins, D., Mandelkorn, T., & Cerf, F. A. (1980). Principal and differential effects of haloperidol and placebo treatments upon speech disfluencies in stutterers. *Journal of Speech and Hearing Research, 23*, 614–629.

Quader, S. (1977). Dysarthria: An unusual side effect of tricyclic antidepressants. *British Medical Journal, 9*, 97.

Quinn, P. (1972). Stuttering, cerebral dominance, and the dichotic word test. *Medical Journal of Australia, 2*, 639–642.

Rahman, P. (1956). *The self-concept and ideal self-concept of stutterers as compared to nonstutterers.* Unpublished masters thesis, Brooklyn College, Brooklyn, NY.

Ramig, P. (1993). The impact of self-help groups on persons who stutter: A call for research. *Journal of Fluency Disorders, 18*, 351–361.

Ramig, P. R., Ellis, J. B., & Polland, R. (2010). Application of the SpeechEasy to stuttering treatment: Introduction, background and preliminary observations. In B. Guitar, & R. J. McCauley (Eds.), *Treatment of stuttering: Established and emerging interventions* (pp. 312–328). Baltimore, MD: Lippincott Williams & Wilkins.

Rautakoski, P., Hannus, T., Simberg, S., Sandnabba, N. K., & Santilla, P. (2012). Genetic and environmental effects on stuttering: A twin study from Finland. *Journal of Fluency Disorders, 37*, 202–210.

Raza, M., Amjad, R., Riazuddin, S., & Drayna, D. (2012). Studies in a consanguineous family reveal a novel locus for stuttering on chromosome 16q. *Human Genetics, 131*(2), 311–313.

Raza, M., Domingues, C., Webster, R., Sainz, E., Paris, E., Rahn, R., et al. (2016). Mucolipidosis types II and III and non-syndromic stuttering are associated with different variants in the same genes. *European Journal of Human Genetics, 24*, 529–534.

Raza, M., Mattera, R., Morell, R., Sainz, E., Rahn, R., Gutierrez, J., et al. (2015). Association between rare variants in AP4E1, a component of intra-cellular trafficking, and persistent stuttering. *American Journal of Human Genetics, 97*(5), 715–725.

Raza, M., Riazuddin, S., & Drayna, D. (2010). Identification of an autosomal recessive stuttering locus on chromosome 3q13.2-3q13.33. *Human Genetics, 128*(4), 461–463.

Reilly, S., Onslow, M., Packman, A., Cini, E., Conway, L., Ukoumunne, O., et al. (2013). Natural history of stuttering to 4 years of age: A prospective community-based study. *Pediatrics, 132*(3), 460–467.

Reilly, S., Onslow, M., Packman, A., Wake, M., Bavin, E., & Prior, M. (2009). Predicting stuttering onset by the age of 3: A prospective, community cohort study. *Pediatrics, 123*, 270–277.

Rentschler, G., Driver, L., & Callaway, E. (1984). The onset of stuttering following drug overdose. *Journal of Fluency Disorders, 9*, 265–284.

Riaz, N., Steinberg, S., Ahmad, J., Pluzhnikov, A., Riazuddin, S., Cox, N., & Drayna, D. (2005). Genomewide significant linkage to stuttering on chromosome 12. *American Journal of Human Genetics, 76*(4), 647–651.

Richels, C. G., & Conture, E. (2007). An indirect approach for early intervention for childhood stuttering. In E. Conture, & R. Curlee (Eds.), *Stuttering and related disorders of fluency*. New York: Thieme Medical Publishers.

Richels, C. G., & Conture, E. G. (2010). Indirect treatment of childhood stuttering: Diagnostic predictors of treatment outcome. In B. Guitar, & R. J. McCauley (Eds.), *Treatment of stuttering: Established and emerging interventions* (pp. 18–55). Baltimore, MD: Lippincott Williams & Wilkins.

Riley, G. (1972). A stuttering severity instrument for children and adults. *Journal of Speech and Hearing Disorders, 37*, 314–322.

Riley, G. (1994). *Stuttering severity instrument for children and adults* (3rd ed.). Austin, TX: Pro-Ed.

Riley, G. (2009). *Stuttering Severity Instrument* (4th ed.). Greenville, SC: Super Duper Publications.

Riley, G., & Riley, J. (1979). A component model for diagnosing and treating children who stutter. *Journal of Fluency Disorders, 4*(4), 279–293.

Ringo, C. C., & Dietrich, S. (1995). Neurogenic stuttering: An analysis and critique. *Journal of Medical Speech-Language Pathology, 32*, 111–122.

Ripley, A. (2005, May 2). How to get out alive: From hurricanes to 9/11: What the science of evacuation reveals about how humans behave in the worst of times. *Time, 165*, 58–62.

Ripley, A. (2008). *Unthinkable: Who survives when disaster strikes and why?* New York: Crown Publishers.

Roberts, P., & Shenker, R. (2007). Assessment and treatment of stuttering in bilingual speakers. In E. G. Conture, & R. Curlee (Eds.), *Stuttering and related disorders of fluency* (3rd ed., pp. 183–210). New York: Thieme.

Roessler, R., & Bolton, B. (1978). *Psychosocial adjustment to disability*. Baltimore, MD: University Park Press.

Rogers, C. (1942). *Counseling and psychotherapy*. Cambridge, MA: Riverside Press.

Rogers, C. (1957). The necessary and sufficient conditions of therapeutic personality change. *Journal of Consulting Psychology, 21*, 95–103.

Rogers, C. (1961). *On Becoming a Person*. Boston, MA: Houghton Mifflin.

Rommel, D., Hage, P., Kalehne, P., & Johannsen, H. (2000). Development, maintenance, and recovery of childhood stuttering: Prospective longitudinal data 3 years after first contact. In K. L. Baker, L. Rustin, & F. Cook (Eds.), Proceedings of the Fifth Oxford Disfluency Conference, 7th-10th July, 1999 (pp. 168–182). Berkshire, UK: Kevin L. Baker.

Rosenbek, J. C. (1984). Stuttering secondary to nervous system damage. In R. F. Curlee, & W. H. Perkins (Eds.), *Nature and treatment of stuttering: New directions* (pp. 31–48). San Diego, CA: College-Hill Press.

Rosenberger, P. B. (1980). Dopaminergic systems and speech fluency. *Journal of Fluency Disorders, 5*(3), 255–267.

Rosenfield, D., & Goodglass, H. (1980). Dichotic testing of cerebral dominance in stutterers. *Brain and Language, 11*, 170–180.

Roth, C., Manning, K., & Duffy, J. (2011, November). *Acquired stuttering in post-deployed. Paper presented at the Annual Meeting of the American Speech-Language-Hearing Association Convention*, San Diego, CA.

Roth, C., Aronson, A., & Davis, L. (1989). Clinical studies in psychogenic stuttering of adult onset. *Journal of Speech and Hearing Disorders, 54*, 634–646.

Rothbart, M. K. (2011). *Becoming who we are: Temperament and personality in development*. New York: Guilford Press.

Rothbart, M. K., Ahadi, S. A., Hershey, K. L., & Fisher, P. (2001). Investigation of temperament at three to seven years: The Children's Behavior Questionnaire. *Child Development, 72*, 1394–1408.

Rousseau, I., Packman, A., Onslow, M., Harrison, E., & Jones, M. (2007). An investigation of language and phonological development and the responsiveness of preschool age children in the Lidcombe Program. *Journal of Communication Disorders, 40*(5), 382–397.

Rubow, R., Rosenbek, J., & Schumaker, J. (1986). Stress management in the treatment of neurogenic stuttering. *Biofeedback and Self Regulation, 11*, 77–78.

Rustin, L. (1991). *Parents, families, and the stuttering child*. London: Whurr.

Sackett, D., Straus, S., Richardson, W., Rosenberg, W., & Haynes, R. (2000). *Evidence-based medicine: How to practice and teach EBM*. New York: Churchill Livingstone.

Schiavetti, N., & Metz, D. E. (1997). Stuttering and the measurement of speech naturalness. In R. F. Curlee, & G. M. Siegel (Eds.), *Nature and treatment of stuttering: New directions* (2nd ed., pp. 398–412). Boston, MA: Allyn & Bacon.

Schmahmann, J. D., & Caplan, D. (2006). Cognition, emotion and the cerebellum. *Brain, 129*(Pt 2), 290–292.

Schwartz, M. F. (1974). The core of the stuttering block. *Journal of Speech and Hearing Disorders, 39*, 169–177.

Scott, L. (undated). *Implementing cognitive behavior therapy with school-age children* [DVD No. 6500]. Memphis, TN: Stuttering Foundation.

Scott, L., & Guitar, C. (2004). *Stuttering: For kids, by kids* [DVD]. Memphis, TN: Stuttering Foundation.

Scott, L., & Guitar, C. (2012). *Stuttering: Straight talk for teachers* [DVD]. Memphis, TN: Stuttering Foundation.

Seeman, M. (1937). The significance of twin pathology for the investigation of speech disorders. *Archive gesamte Phonetik 1, Part II*, 88–92.

Seery, C. (2005). Differential diagnosis of stuttering for forensic purposes. *American Journal of Speech-Language Pathology, 14*, 284–297.

Segalowitz, S. J., & Brown, D. (1991). Mild head injury as a source of developmental disabilities. *Journal of Learning Disabilities, 24*(9), 551–559.

Semel, E., Wiig, E., & Secord, W. (1995). *Clinical evaluation of language fundamentals—3*. San Antonio, TX: Psychological Corporation.

Shafir, R. Z. (2000). *The zen of listening: Mindful communication in the age of distraction*. Wheaton, IL: Theosophical Publishing House.

Shapely, K., & Guyette, T. (2010). Review of "TOCS: Test of childhood stuttering". *Mental Measurements Yearbook, 18*, 138.

Shapiro, A. I. (1980). An electromyographic analysis of the fluent and dysfluent utterances of several types of stutterers. *Journal of Fluency Disorders, 5*, 203–231.

Shapiro, A. I., & DeCicco, B. A. (1982). The relationship between normal dysfluency and stuttering: An old question revisited. *Journal of Fluency Disorders, 7*, 109–121.

Shapiro, D. A. (1999). *Stuttering intervention: A collaborative journey to fluency freedom*. Austin, TX: Pro-Ed.

Shapiro, D. A. (2011). *Stuttering intervention: A collaborative journey to fluency freedom* (2nd ed.). Austin, TX: Pro-Ed.

Shaywitz, B. A., Shaywitz, S. E., Pugh, K. R., Constable, R. T., Skudlarski, P., Fulbright, R. K., et al. (1995). Sex differences in the functional organization of the brain for language. *Nature, 373*, 607–609.

Sheehan, J. G. (1970). *Stuttering: Research and therapy*. New York: Harper & Row.

Sheehan, J. G. (1974). Stuttering behavior: A phonetic analysis. *Journal of Communication Disorders, 7*, 193–212.

Sheehan, J. G. (1975). Conflict theory and avoidance-reduction therapy. In J. Eisenson (Ed.), *Stuttering: A second symposium*. New York: Harper & Row.

Sherman, D. (1952). Clinical and experimental use of the Iowa scale of severity of stuttering. *Journal of Speech and Hearing Disorders, 17*, 316–320.

Shirkey, E. (1987). Forensic verification of stuttering. *Journal of Fluency Disorders, 12*, 197–203.

Shors, T. J., Weiss, C., & Thompson, R. F. (1992). Stress-induced facilitation of classical conditioning. *Science, 257*(5069), 537–539.

Shugart, Y. Y., Mundorff, J., Kilshaw, J., Doheny, K., Doan, B., Wanyee, J., et al. (2004). Results of a genome-wide linkage scan for stuttering. *American Journal of Medical Genetics, 124A*, 133–135.

Siegel, G. M. (2007, December). Random observations. *ASHA Leader*.

Silverman, E-M. (1974). Word position and grammatical function in relation to preschoolers' speech disfluency. *Perceptual and Motor Skills, 39*, 267–272.

Silverman, F. H. (1988). The monster study. *Journal of Fluency Disorders, 13*, 225–231.

Simonyan, K., & Horowitz, B. (2011). Laryngeal motor cortex and control of speech in humans. *The Neuroscientist, 17*(2), 197–208.

Sisskin, V. (2017). *Avoidance reduction therapy in a group setting* [DVD]. Memphis, TN: Stuttering Foundation.

Sisskin, V. (2018). Avoidance reduction therapy for stuttering. In B. J. Amster, & E. R. Klein (Eds.), *More than fluency: The social, emotional, and cognitive dimensions of stuttering* (pp. 157–186). San Diego, CA: Plural Publishing.

Sisskin, V. (2018). Avoidance reduction therapy for stuttering (ARTS). In B. Amster, & E. Klein (Eds.), *More than fluency: The social, emotional, and cognitive dimensions of stuttering*. San Diego, CA: Plural Publishing.

Skinner, E., & McKeehan, A. (1996). *Preventing stuttering in the preschool child: A video program for parents [Videotape]*. San Antonio, TX: Communication Skill Builders.

Smith, A. (1989). Neural drive to muscles in stuttering. *Journal of Speech and Hearing Research, 32*, 252–264.

Smith, A. (1999). Stuttering: A unified approach to a multifactorial, dynamic disorder. In N. Bernstein Ratner, & E. C. Healey (Eds.), *Stuttering research and practice: Bridging the gap*. Mahwah, NJ: Lawrence Erlbaum Associates.

Smith, A., Denny, M., Shaffer, L., Kelly, E., & Hirano, M. (1996). Activity of intrinsic laryngeal muscles in fluent and disfluent speech. *Journal of Speech and Hearing Research, 39*(2), 329–348.

Smith, A., & Goffman, L. (2004). Interaction of motor and language factors in the development of speech production. In B. Maasen, R. D. Kent, H. F. M. Peters, P. H. H. M. van Lieshout, & W. Hulstijn (Eds.), *Speech motor control in normal and disordered speech* (pp. 227–252). Oxford: Oxford University Press.

Smith, A., Goffman, L., Sasiekaran, J., & Weber-Fox, C. (2012). Language and motor abilities of preschool children who stutter: Evidence from behavioral and kinematic indices of non-word repetition performance. *Journal of Fluency Disorders, 37*(4), 344–358.

Smith, K., Iverach, L., O'Brian, S., Kefalianos, E., & Reilly, S. (2014). Anxiety of children and adolescents who stutter: A review. *Journal of Fluency Disorders, 40*, 22–34.

Smith, A., & Kelly, E. (1997). Stuttering: A dynamic, multifactorial model. In R. F. Curlee, & G. Siegel (Eds.), *Nature and treatment of Stuttering: New directions* (2nd ed., pp. 204–217). Boston, MA: Allyn & Bacon.

Smith, A., McCauley, R., & Guitar, B. (2000). Development of the Teacher Assessment of Student Communicative Competence (TASCC) in grades 1 through 5. *Communication Disorders Quarterly, 221*, 3–11.

Smith, A., Sadagopan, N., Walsh, B., & Weber-Fox, C. (2010). Phonological complexity affects speech motor dynamics in adults who stutter. *Journal of Fluency Disorders, 35*, 1–18.

Smith, A., & Weber, C. (2017). How stuttering develops: The Multifactorial Dynamic Pathways Theory. *Journal of Speech, Language, and Hearing Research, 60*, 2483–2505.

Snidman, N., & Kagan, J. (1994). The contribution of infant temperamental differences to the acoustic startle response. *Psychophysiology, 31* Supplement 1 [abstract], S92.

Sommer, M., Koch, M. A., Paulus, W., Weiller, C., & Buchel, C. (2002). Disconnection of speech-relevant brain areas in persistent developmental stuttering. *Lancet, 360*, 380–383.

Sommers, R., Brady, W. A., & Moore, W. H., Jr. (1975). Dichotic ear preferences of stuttering children and adults. *Perceptual and Motor Skills, 41*, 931–938.

Spencer, C., & Weber-Fox, C. (2014). Preschool speech articulation and nonword repetition abilities may help predict eventual recovery or persistence of stuttering. *Journal of Fluency Disorders, 41*, 32–46.

St. Louis, K. (1996). Research and opinion on cluttering. [Special issue]. *Journal of Fluency Disorders, 21*, 171–374.

St. Louis, K. (2001). *Living with stuttering: Stories, basics, resources, and hope*. Morgantown, WV: Populore Publishing Company.

St. Louis, K., Myers, F. L., Bakker, K., & Raphael, L. J. (2007). Understanding and treating cluttering. In E. Conture, & R. Curlee (Eds.), *Stuttering and related disorders of fluency* (3rd ed., pp. 297–322). New York: Thieme.

St. Louis, K., Raphael, L., Myers, F., & Bakker, K. (2003, November 18). Cluttering updated. *ASHA Leader, 8*, 20–22.

St. Onge, K. (1963). The stuttering syndrome. *Journal of Speech and Hearing Research, 6*, 195–197.

Stager, S., Jeffries, K. J., & Braun, A. R. (2003). Common features of fluency-evoking conditions studied in stuttering subjects and controls: An H(2)15O PET study. *Journal of Fluency Disorders, 284*, 319–336.

Starkweather, C. W. (1980). A multiprocess behavioral approach to stuttering therapy. *Seminars in Speech, Language and Hearing, 1*, 327–337.

Starkweather, C. W. (1985). The development of fluency in normal children. In *Stuttering therapy: Prevention and intervention with children*. Memphis, TN: Stuttering Foundation of America.

Starkweather, C. W. (1987). *Fluency and stuttering*. Englewood Cliffs, NJ: Prentice-Hall.

Starkweather, C. W. (1991). Stuttering: The motor-language interface. In H. F. M. Peters, W. Hulstijn, & C. W. Starkweather (Eds.), *Speech motor control and fluency*. Amsterdam, The Netherlands: Excerpta Medica.

Starkweather, C. W., & Gottwald, S. (1990). The demands and capacities model II: Clinical application. *Journal of Fluency Disorders, 15*, 143–157.

Starkweather, C. W., Gottwald, S., & Halfond, M. H. (1990). *Stuttering prevention: A clinical method*. Englewood Cliffs, NJ: Prentice-Hall.

Starkweather, C. W., Hirschman, P., & Tannenbaum, R. S. (1976). Latency of vocalization onset: Stutterers versus nonstutterers. *Journal of Speech and Hearing Research, 19*, 481–492.

Starkweather, C. W., & Myers, M. (1979). Duration of subsegments within the intervocalic interval in stutterers and nonstutterers. *Journal of Fluency Disorders, 4*, 205–214.

Stephenson-Opsal, D., & Bernstein Ratner, N. (1988). Maternal speech rate modification and childhood stuttering. *Journal of Fluency Disorders, 13*, 49–56.

Sternberger, J. P. (1982). The nature of segments in the lexicon: Evidence from speech errors. *Lingua, 56*, 235–259.

Stocker, B., & Usprich, C. (1976). Stuttering in young children and level of demand. *Journal of Childhood Communication Disorders, 1*, 116–131.

Strasberg, S., Johnson, E., & Perry, T. (2016). "Stuttering" after minor head trauma. *American Journal of Emergency Medicine, 34*(3), 685.

Strong, J. C. (1977). *Dichotic speech perception: A comparison between stutterers and nonstutterers ages five to nine*. Unpublished doctoral dissertation, Pennsylvania State University, University Park, PA.

Studdert-Kennedy, M. (1987). The phoneme as a perceptuomotor structure. In A. Allport, D. McKay, D. Prinz, & E. Scheerer (Eds.), *Language perception and production*. London: Academic Press.

Subramanian, A., & Yairi, E. (2006). Identification of traits associated with stuttering. *Journal of Communication Disorders, 39*(3), 200–216.

Sussman, H. (2016). Why the left hemisphere is dominant for speech production: Connecting the dots. *Biolinguistics, 9*, 116–123.

Sussman, H., & MacNeilage, P. (1975). Hemispheric specialization for speech production and perception in stutterers. *Neuropsychologia, 13*, 19–26.

Swift, W. J., Swift, E. W., & Arellano, M. (1975). Haloperidol as a treatment for adult stuttering. *Comprehensive Psychiatry, 16*, 61–67.

Tanoue, Y., & Oda, S. (1989). Weaning time of children with infantile autism. *Journal of Autism and Developmental Disorders, 19*(3), 425–434.

Taylor, G. (1937). *An observational study of the nature of stuttering at onset*. Master's Thesis, State University of Iowa, Iowa City.

Taylor, O. (1986). *Treatment of communication disorders in culturally and linguistically diverse populations*. San Diego, CA: College-Hill Press.

Taylor, O. (1994). *Communication and communication disorders in a multicultural society*. San Diego, CA: Singular Publishing Group.

Taylor, R. M., & Morrison, L. P. (1996). *Taylor-Johnson Temperament Analysis Manual*. Thousand Oaks, CA: Psychological Publications, Inc.

Tellis, G. (2008). Multicultural considerations in assessing and treating Hispanic Americans who stutter. *Perspectives on Fluency and Fluency Disorders, 18*, 101–110.

Tellis, G., & Tellis, C. (2003). Multicultural issues in school settings. *Seminars in Speech and Language, 24*(1), 21–26.

Theys, C., De Nil, L. F., Thijs, V., Van Wieringen, A., & Sunaert, S. (2013). A crucial role for the cortico-strieto-cortical loop in the pathogenesis of stroke-related neurogenic stuttering. *Human Brain Mapping, 34*(9), 2103–2112.

Theys, C., van Wieringen, A., & De Nil, L. F. (2008). A clinician survey of speech and non-speech characteristics of neurogenic stuttering. *Journal of Fluency Disorders, 33*(1), 1–23.

Thomas, A., & Chess, S. (1977). *Temperament and development*. New York: Brunner/Mazel, Inc.

Thomson, K. S. (2009). *Young Charles Darwin*. New Haven, CT: Yale University Press.

Throneburg, R., & Yairi, E. (1994). Temporal dynamics of repetitions during the early stage of childhood stuttering: An acoustic study. *Journal of Speech and Hearing Research, 37*, 1067–1075.

Till, J. A., Reich, A., Dickey, S., & Sieber, J. (1983). Phonatory and manual reaction times of stuttering and nonstuttering children. *Journal of Speech and Hearing Research, 26*, 171–180.

Tilsen, S. (2016). Selection and coordination: The articulatory basis for the emergence of phonological structure. *Journal of Phonetics, 55*, 53–77.

Toscher, M. M., & Rupp, R. R. (1978). A study of the central auditory processes in stutterers using the Synthetic Sentence Identification SSI test battery. *Journal of Speech and Hearing Research, 21*, 779–792.

Toyomura, A., Fujii, T., & Kuriki, S. (2011). Effect of external auditory pacing on the neural activity of stuttering speakers. *NeuroImage, 57*(4), 1507–1516.

Trajkovski, N., Andrews, C., Onslow, M., Packman, A., O'Brian, S., & Menzies, R. (2009). Using syllable-timed speech to treat preschool children who stutter: A multiple baseline experiment. *Journal of Fluency Disorders, 34*(1), 1–10.

Trautman, L. S. (2003). SFA conducts survey on satisfaction with electronic devices. *Stuttering Foundation Newsletter, Fall, 6.*

Travis, L. (1925). Muscular fixation of the stutterer's voice under emotion. *Science, 62,* 207–208.

Travis, L. (1931). *Speech pathology.* New York: Appleton-Century.

Travis, L. E., & Knott, J. R. (1937). Bilaterally recorded brain potentials from normal speakers and stutterers. *Journal of Speech Disorders, 2,* 239–241.

Trichon, M., & Raj, E. (2018). Peer support for people who stutter: History, benefits, and accessibility. In B. J. Amster, & E. R. Klein (Eds.), *More than fluency: The social, emotional, and cognitive dimensions of stuttering* (pp. 187–214). San Diego, CA: Plural Publishing.

Tudor, M. (1939). *An experimental study of the effect of evaluative labeling on speech fluency.* Unpublished master's thesis, University of Iowa, Iowa City.

Tumanova, V., Conture, E. G., Lambert, E. W., & Walden, T. A. (2014). Speech disfluencies of preschool-age children who do and do not stutter. *Journal of Communication Disorders, 49,* 25–41.

Turgut, N., Utku, U., & Balci, K. (2002). A case of acquired stuttering resulting from left parietal infarction. *Acta Neurologica Scandinavica, 105,* 408.

Turnbaugh, K. R., Guitar, B. E., & Hoffman, P. R. (1979). Speech clinicians' attribution of personality traits as a function of stuttering severity. *Journal of Speech and Hearing Research, 22,* 37–45.

Usler, E., & Weber-Fox, C. (2015). Neurodevelopment for syntactic processing distinguishes childhood stuttering recovery vs. persistence. *Journal of Neurodevelopmental Disorders, 7*(1), 3–4.

van Beijsterveldt, C. E., Felsenfeld, S., & Boomsma, D. I. (2010). Bivariate genetic analyses of stuttering and nonfluency in a large sample of 5-year-old twins. *Journal of Speech, Language, and Hearing Research, 53*(3), 609–619.

Van Borsel, J., Maes, E., & Foulon, S. (2001). Stuttering and bilingualism: A review. *Journal of Fluency Disorders, 26,* 179–205.

Van Borsel, J., Moeyaert, J., Mostaert, C., Rosseel, R., van Loo, E., & van Renterghem, T. (2006). Prevalence of stuttering in regular and special school populations in Belgium based on teacher perceptions. *Folia Phoniatrica et Logopedica, 58,* 289–302.

van Lieshout, P., Ben-David, B., Lipski, M., & Namasivayam, A. K. (2014). The impact of threat and cognitive stress on speech motor control in people who stutter. *Journal of Fluency Disorders, 40,* 93–109.

van Lieshout, P., Hulstijn, W., & Peters, H. F. M. (2004). Searching for the weak link in the speech production chain of people who stutter. In B. Maassen, R. D. Kent, H. F. M. Peters, P. H. H. M. van Lieshout, & W. E. Hulstijn (Eds.), *Speech motor control in normal and disordered speech* (pp. 313–356). Oxford, UK: Oxford University Press.

Van Riper, C. (1936). Study of the thoracic breathing of stutterers during expectancy and occurrence of stuttering spasm. *Journal of Speech Disorders, 1,* 61–72.

Van Riper, C. (1954). *Speech correction: Principles and methods* (3rd ed.). Englewood Cliffs, NJ: Prentice-Hall.

Van Riper, C. (1958). Experiments in stuttering therapy. In J. Eisenson (Ed.), *Stuttering: A symposium* (pp. 273–390). New York: Harper & Row.

Van Riper, C. (1971). *The nature of stuttering.* Englewood Cliffs, NJ: Prentice-Hall.

Van Riper, C. (1973). *The treatment of stuttering.* Englewood Cliffs, NJ: Prentice-Hall.

Van Riper, C. (1974). The alauf problem in stuttering. *Journal of Fluency Disorders, 1*(1), 2–9.

Van Riper, C. (1975a). The stutterer's clinician. In J. Eisenson (Ed.), *Stuttering: A second symposium* (pp. 453–492). New York: Harper & Row.

Van Riper, C. (1975b). *Therapy in action.* Memphis, TN: Stuttering Foundation.

Van Riper, C. (1982). *The nature of stuttering* (2nd ed.). Englewood Cliffs, NJ: Prentice Hall.

Van Riper, C. (1990). Final thoughts about stuttering. *Journal of Fluency Disorders, 155*(6), 317–318.

Van Riper, C., & Hull, C. J. (1955). The quantitive measurement of the effect of certain situations on stuttering. In W. Johnson, & R. R. Leutenegger (Eds.), *Stuttering children and adults.* Minneapolis, MN: University of Minnesota Press.

van Zaalen, Y., Wijnen, F., & Dejonckere, P. (2011). Cluttering and learning disabilities. In D. Ward, & K. S. Scott (Eds.), *Cluttering: A handbook of research, intervention and education* (pp. 100–114). Hove, UK: Psychology Press.

Vanryckeghem, M., & Brutten, G. (1993). The Communication Attitude Test: A test-retest reliability investigation. *Journal of Fluency Disorders, 17,* 177–190.

Vanryckeghem, M., & Brutten, G. (1997). The speech-associated attitude of children who do and do not stutter and the differential effect of age. *American Journal of Speech-Language Pathology, 6,* 67–73.

Vanryckeghem, M., Brutten, G., & Hernandez, L. (2005). A comparative investigation of the speech-associated attitude of preschool and kindergarten children who do and do not stutter. *Journal of Fluency Disorders, 30*(4), 307–318.

Vanryckeghem, M., Hernandez, L., & Brutten, G. (2001, November). The KiddyCAT: A measurement of speech-associated attitude of preschoolers. Paper presented at the Annual Meeting of the American Speech-Language and Hearing Association, New Orleans.

Vanryckeghem, M., Hylebos, C., Brutten, G., & Peleman, M. (2001). The relationship between communication attitude and emotion of children who stutter. *Journal of Fluency Disorders, 26*(1), 1.

Vanryckeghem, M., Vanrobayes, S., & De Niels, T. (2015). The KittyCAT: A test-retest reliability investigation. *Cross Cultural Communication, 11*(4), 10–16.

Velleman, S. L. (2015). *Speech sound disorders in children.* Baltimore, MD: Wolters Kluwer Health.

Veneziano, E. (2013). A Cognitive-Pragmatic Model for the change from single-word to multiword speech: A constructivist approach. *Journal of Pragmatics, 56,* 133–150.

Verdolini, K., & Lee, T. D. (2004). Optimizing motor learning in speech interventions: Theory and practice. In C. Sapienza & J. Casper (Eds.), *Voice rehabilitation in medical speech-language pathology: For clinicians, by clinicians.* Austin, TX: Pro-Ed.

Viswanath, N. S., Lee, H. S., & Chakraborty, R. (2004). Evidence for a minor gene influence on persistent developmental stuttering. *Human Biology, 76,* 401–412.

Vrana, S. R., Spence, E. L., & Lang, P. J. (1988). The startle probe: A new measure of emotion? *Journal of Abnormal Psychology, 97,* 487–491.

Wakaba, Y. (1998). Research on temperament of stuttering children with early onset. Paper presented at the 2nd World Conference on Fluency Disorders, San Francisco.

Walden, T. A., Frankel, C. B., Buhr, A. P., Johnson, K. N., Conture, E. G., & Karrass, J. M. (2012). Dual diathesis-stressor model of emotional and linguistic contributions to developmental stuttering. *Journal of Abnormal Child Psychology, 40*(4), 633–644.

Wall, M., & Myers, F. (1995). *Clinical management of childhood stuttering* (2nd ed.). Austin, TX: Pro-Ed.

Wallen, V. (1960). A Q-technique study of the self-concepts of adolescent stutterers and nonstutterers. *Speech Monographs [Abstract], 27*, 257–258.

Walsh, B., Mettel, K. M., & Smith, A. (2015). Speech motor planning and execution deficits in early childhood stuttering. *Journal of Neurodevelopmental Disorders, 7*(1), 27.

Walsh, B., & Smith, A. (2013). Oral electromyography activation patterns for speech are similar in preschoolers who do and do not stutter. *Journal of Speech, Language, and Hearing Research, 56*, 1441–1454.

Walton, P. (2012). *Fun with fluency: For the school-age child*. Austin, TX: Pro-Ed.

Wampold, B. E. (2015). How important are the common factors in psychotherapy? An update. *World Psychiatry, 14*, 270–277.

Ward, D., Connally, E. L., Pliatsikas, C., Bretherton-Furness, J., & Watkins, K. E. (2015). Some neurological underpinnings of cluttering: Some initial findings. *Journal of Fluency Disorders, 43*, 1–16.

Ward, D., & Scott, K. S. (2011). *Cluttering: A handbook of research, intervention and education*. Hove, UK: Psychology Press.

Waters, E. (1995). Appendix A: The Attachment Q-Set (version 3.0). *Monographs of the Society for Research in Child Development, 60*, 234–246.

Watkins, K., Smith, S., Davis, S., & Howell, P. (2008). Structural and functional abnormalities of the motor system in developmental stuttering. *Brain, 131*(1), 50–59.

Watkins, R. V., Yairi, E., & Ambrose, N. G. (1999). Early childhood stuttering III: Initial status of expressive language abilities. *Journal of Speech, Language, and Hearing Research, 42*(5), 1125–1135.

Watson, B. C., & Alfonso, P. J. (1987). Physiological bases of acoustic LRT in nonstutterers, mild stutterers, and severe stutterers. *Journal of Speech and Hearing Research, 30*, 434–447.

Watson, J. B., & Kayser, H. (1994). Assessment of bilingual/bicultural children and adults who stutter. *Seminars in Speech, Language and Hearing, 15*, 149–163.

Watts, A., Eadie, P., Block, S., Mensah, F., & Reilly, S. (2014). Language ability of children with and without a history of stuttering: A longitudinal cohort study. *International Journal of Speech-Language Pathology, 17*(1), 86–95.

Weber, C. M., & Smith, A. (1990). Autonomic correlates of stuttering and speech assessed in a range of experimental tasks. *Journal of Speech and Hearing Research, 33*, 690–706.

Webster, W. G. (1993a). Evidence in bimanual finger tapping of an attentional component to stuttering. *Behavioural Brain Research, 37*, 93–100.

Webster, W. G. (1993b). Hurried hands and tangled tongues: Implications of current research for the management of stuttering. In E. Boberg (Ed.), *Neuropsychology of stuttering* (pp. 73–111). Edmonton, Alberta, Canada: University of Alberta Press.

Webster, W. G. (1997). Principles of human brain organization related to lateralization of language and speech motor functions in normal speakers and stutterers. In W. Hulstijn, H. F. M. Peters, & P. H. H. M. van Lieshout (Eds.), *Speech production: Motor control, brain research and fluency disorders* (pp. 119–139). Amsterdam, The Netherlands: Elsevier.

Weiller, C., Isensee, C., Rijntjes, M., Huber, W., Müller, S., Bier, D., et al. (1995). Recovery from Wernicke's aphasia: A positron emission tomographic study. *Annals of Neurology, 376*, 723–732.

Weiner, A. E. (1981). A case of adult onset of stuttering. *Journal of Fluency Disorders, 6*, 181–186.

Weiss, A. L., & Zebrowski, P. M. (1992). Disfluencies in the conversations of young children who stutter: Some answers about questions. *Journal of Speech and Hearing Research, 356*, 1230–1238.

Weiss, D. A. (1964). *Cluttering*. Englewood Cliffs, NJ: Prentice-Hall.

Welch, J., & Byrne, J. A. (2001). *Jack: Straight from the Gut*. New York: Warner Books.

West, R. (1931). The phenomenology of stuttering. In R. West (Ed.), *A symposium on stuttering*. Madison, WI: College Typing Company.

West, R., Nelson, S., & Berry, M. (1939). The heredity of stuttering. *Quarterly Journal of Speech, 25*, 23–30.

Wexler, K., & Mysack, E. (1982). Disfluency characteristics of 2-, 4- and 6-year old males. *Journal of Fluency Disorders, 7*, 37–46.

Wiig, E. (2002, November). Putting cluttering on the map: Looking back/looking ahead. Paper presented at the Annual meeting of the American Speech Language and Hearing Association, Atlanta.

Wiig, E., Secord, W., & Semel, E. (2013). *Clinical Evaluation of Language Fundamentals—5: Screening Test*. New York: Pearson.

Wijnen, F. (1990). The development of sentence planning. *Journal of Child Language, 173*, 651–675.

Wilkenfeld, J. R., & Curlee, R. F. (1997). The relative effects of questions and comments on children's stuttering. *American Journal of Speech-Language Pathology, 63*, 79–89.

Williams, D. E. (1978). The problem of stuttering. In F. Darley, & D. Spriestersbach (Eds.), *Diagnostic methods in speech pathology* (pp. 284–321). New York: Harper & Row.

Williams, D. (2004). *The genius of Dean Williams*. Memphis, TN: Stuttering Foundation of America.

Williams, K. (2007). *Expressive Vocabulary Test—2*. New York: Pearson.

Williams, D., Darley, F., & Spriestersbach, D. (1978). Appraisal of rate and fluency. In F. Darley, & D. Spriestersbach (Eds.), *Diagnostic methods in speech pathology* (2nd ed., pp. 256–283). New York: Harper & Row.

Williams, D. E., Silverman, F. H., & Kools, J. A. (1968). Disfluency behavior of elementary-school stutterers and nonstutterers: The adaptation effect. *Journal of Speech and Hearing Research, 11*, 622–630.

Wingate, M. E. (1964). Recovery from stuttering. *Journal of Speech and Hearing Disorders, 29*, 312–321.

Wingate, M. E. (1976). *Stuttering: Theory and treatment*. New York: Irvington.

Wingate, M. E. (1983). Speaking unassisted: Comments on a paper by Andrews et al. *Journal of Speech and Hearing Disorders, 48*, 255–263.

Wingate, M. E. (1988). *The structure of stuttering: A psycholinguistic approach*. New York: Springer-Verlag.

Winnicott, D. W. (1971). *Playing and reality*. New York: Routledge.

Winslow, M., & Guitar, B. (1994). The effect of turn-taking on disfluencies: A case study. *Language, Speech, and Hearing Services in Schools*, *25*, 251–257.

Wischner, G. J. (1950). Stuttering behavior and learning: A preliminary theoretical formulation. *Journal of Speech and Hearing Disorders*, *15*, 324–325.

Witz, B. (2018, July 29). Remembering a pioneer of baseball's mental side. *New York Times*. Available at https://www.nytimes.com/2018/07/25/sports/ken-ravizza-sports-psychologist.html

Wood, F., Stump, D., McKeehan, A., Sheldon, S., & Proctor, J. (1980). Patterns of regional cerebral blood flow during attempted reading aloud by stutterers both on and off haloperidol medication: Evidence for inadequate left frontal activation during stuttering. *Brain and Language*, *9*, 141–144.

Woods, S., Shearsby, J., Onslow, M., & Burnham, D. (2002). Psychological impact of the Lidcombe Program of early stuttering intervention. *International Journal of Language and Communication Disorders*, *37*(1), 31–40.

Woods, C. L., & Williams, D. E. (1976). Traits attributed to stuttering and normally fluent males. *Journal of Speech and Hearing Research*, *19*, 267–278.

Woolf, G. (1967). The assessment of stuttering as struggle, avoidance, and expectancy. *British Journal of Disorders of Communication*, *2*, 158–171.

World Health Organization. (1980). *International classification of impairments, disabilities, and handicaps: A manual of classification relating to the consequences of disease*. Geneva, Switzerland: World Health Organization.

Wu, J., Maguire, G., Riley, G., Fallon, J., LaCasse, L., Chin, S., et al. (1995). A positron emission tomography [18F]deoxyglucose study of developmental stuttering. *Neuroreport*, *63*, 501–505.

Wynne, M. K., & Boehmler, R. M. (1982). Central auditory function in fluent and disfluent normal speakers. *Journal of Speech and Hearing Research*, *25*, 54–57.

Yairi, E. (1981). Disfluencies of normally speaking two-year old children. *Journal of Speech and Hearing Research*, *24*, 490–495.

Yairi, E. (1982). Longitudinal studies of disfluencies in two-year old children. *Journal of Speech and Hearing Research*, *25*, 155–160.

Yairi, E. (1983). The onset of stuttering in two- and three-year old children: A preliminary report. *Journal of Speech and Hearing Disorders*, *48*, 171–178.

Yairi, E. (1997a). Early stuttering. In R. F. Curlee, & G. M. Siegel (Eds.), *Nature and treatment of stuttering: New directions* (2nd ed.). Boston, MA: Allyn & Bacon.

Yairi, E. (1997b). Home environment and parent–child interaction in childhood stuttering. In R. F. Curlee, & G. M. Siegel (Eds.), *Nature and treatment of stuttering: New directions* (2nd ed., pp. 24–48). Boston, MA: Allyn & Bacon.

Yairi, E. (2007). Subtyping stuttering. I. A review. *Journal of Fluency Disorders*, *32*, 165–196.

Yairi, E., & Ambrose, N. (1992a). A longitudinal study of stuttering in children: A preliminary report. *Journal of Speech and Hearing Research*, *35*, 755–760.

Yairi, E., & Ambrose, N. (1992b). Onset of stuttering in preschool children: Selected factors. *Journal of Speech and Hearing Research*, *35*, 782–788.

Yairi, E., & Ambrose, N. (1996). *Disfluent speech in early childhood stuttering*. Unpublished manuscript, University of Illinois.

Yairi, E., & Ambrose, N. (1999). Early childhood stuttering I: Persistency and recovery rates. *Journal of Speech, Language, and Hearing Research*, *42*(5), 1097–1112.

Yairi, E., & Ambrose, N. (2005). *Early childhood stuttering: For clinicians by clinicians*. Austin, TX: Pro-Ed.

Yairi, E., & Ambrose, N. G. (2013). Epidemiology of stuttering: 21st century advances. *Journal of Fluency Disorders*, *38*(2), 66–87.

Yairi, E., Ambrose, N., & Cox, N. (1996). Genetics of stuttering: A critical review. *Journal of Speech and Hearing Research*, *394*, 771–784.

Yairi, E., Ambrose, N. G., Paden, E., & Throneburg, R. (1996). Predictive factors of persistence and recovery: Pathways of childhood stuttering. *Journal of Communication Disorders*, *29*, 51–77.

Yairi, E., & Lewis, B. (1984). Disfluencies at the onset of stuttering. *Journal of Speech and Hearing Research*, *27*, 154–159.

Yaruss, J. S. (1998). Describing the consequences of disorders: Stuttering and the International Classification of Impairments, Disabilities, and Handicaps. *Journal of Speech, Language, and Hearing Research*, *41*, 249–257.

Yaruss, J. S. (1999). Utterance length, syntactic complexity, and childhood stuttering. *Journal of Speech, Language, and Hearing Research*, *422*, 329–344.

Yaruss, J. S. (2002). Facing the challenge of treating stuttering in the schools: Part 1. Selecting goals and strategies for success. *Seminars in Speech and Language*, *23*, 153–159.

Yaruss, J. S. (2003). Facing the challenge of treating stuttering in schools. Part 2: Selecting goals and strategies for success. *Seminars in Speech and Language*, *24*(2), entire issue.

Yaruss, J. S. (2012). What does it mean to say that a person "accepts" stuttering? In P. Reitzes, & D. Reitzes (Eds.), *Stuttering: Inspiring stories and professional wisdom* (pp. 97–101). Chapel Hill, NC: StutterTalk, Inc.

Yaruss, J. S., & Conture, E. G. (1995). Mother and child speaking rates and utterance lengths in adjacent fluent utterances: Preliminary observations. *Journal of Fluency Disorders, 20*, 257–278.

Yaruss, J. S., Newman, R. M., & Flora, T. (1999). Language and disfluency in nonstuttering children's conversational speech. *Journal of Fluency Disorders*, *24*, 185–207.

Yaruss, J. S., Pelczarski, K., & Quesal, R. W. (2010). Comprehensive treatment for school-age children who stutter: Treating the entire disorder. In B. Guitar, & R. J. McCauley (Eds.), *Treatment of stuttering: Established and emerging interventions* (pp. 215–244). Baltimore, MD: Lippincott Williams & Wilkins.

Yaruss, J. S., & Quesal, R. W. (2006). Overall assessment of the speaker's experience of stuttering (oases): documenting multiple outcomes in stuttering treatment. *Journal of fluency disorder, 31*, 90–115.

Yaruss, J. S., & Quesal, R. W. (2016). *The Overall Assessment of the Speaker's Experience of Stuttering*. McKinney, TX: Stuttering Therapy Resources.

Yaruss, J. S., Quesal, R. W., & Reeves, N. (2007). Self-help and mutual aid groups as an adjunct to stuttering therapy. In E. Conture, & R. Curlee (Eds.), *Stuttering and related disorders of fluency* (3rd ed., pp. 256–276). New York: Thieme.

Yaruss, J. S., Reeves, N., & Herring, C. (2018). How speech-language pathologists can minimize bullying in children who stutter. *Seminars in Speech and Language*, *39*, 342–355.

Young, M. A. (1961). Predicting ratings of severity of stuttering. *Journal of Speech and Hearing Disorders*, (Supplement 7), 31–54.

Young, M. A. (1981). A reanalysis of Stuttering therapy: The relation between attitude change and long-term outcome. *Journal of Speech and Hearing Disorders*, *46*, 221–222.

Young, M. A. (1984). Identification of stuttering and stutterers. In R. F. Curlee, & W. H. Perkins (Eds.), *The nature and treatment of stuttering: New directions* (pp. 13–30). San Diego, CA: College-Hill.

Zackheim, C., & Conture, E. G. (2003). Childhood stuttering and speech dysfluencies in relation to children's mean length of utterance: A preliminary study. *Journal of Fluency Disorders*, *28*(2), 115–142.

Zebrowski, P. (1991). Duration of the speech disfluencies of beginning stutterers. *Journal of Speech and Hearing Research*, *343*, 483–491.

Zebrowski, P. (2003). Developmental stuttering. *Pediatric Annals*, *32*(7), 453–458.

Zebrowski, P., & Kelly, E. (2002). *Manual of stuttering intervention*. Clifton Park, NY: Singular.

Zebrowski, P. M., Weiss, A. L., Savelkoul, E. M., & Hammer, C. S. (1996). The effect of maternal rate reduction on the stuttering, speech rates and linguistic productions of children who stutter: Evidence from individual dyads. *Clinical Linguistics and Phonetics*, *10*(3), 189–206.

Zengin-Bolatkale, H. (2016). *Cortical associates of emotional reactivity and regulation in children who stutter*. Doctoral dissertation, Vanderbilt University, Nashville, TN.

Zengin-Bolatkale, H. (2017, November). Cortical markers of emotion and stuttering frequency of young children. Paper presented at the Annual meeting of the American Speech-Language-Hearing Association, Los Angeles.

Zimmermann, G. N. (1980). Articulatory dynamics of fluent utterances of stutterers and nonstutterers. *Journal of Speech and Hearing Research*, *23*, 95–107.

Zimmermann, G. N., & Knott, J. R. (1974). Slow potentials of the brain related to speech processing in normal speakers and stutterers. *Electroencephalography and Clinical Neurophysiology*, *37*, 599–607.

Zimmermann, G. N., Smith, A., & Hanley, J. M. (1981). Stuttering: In need of a unifying conceptual framework. *Journal of Speech and Hearing Research*, *24*, 25–31.

Zolkoskia, S. M., & Bullock, L. M. (2012). Resilience in children and youth: A review. *Children and Youth Services Review*, *34*(12), 2295–2303.

Author Index

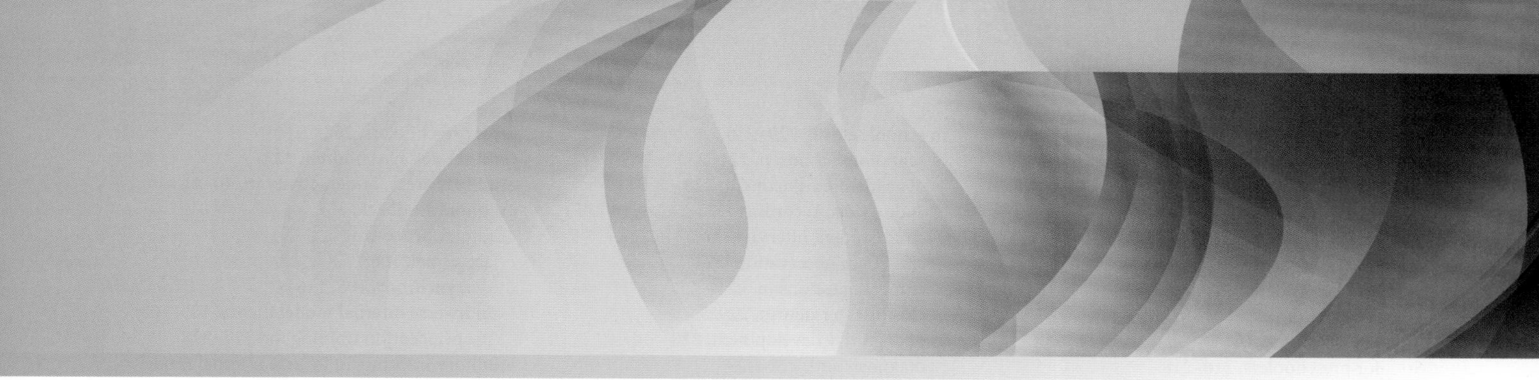

Subject Index

Note: Page numbers followed by "*f*" indicate figures; those followed by "*t*" indicate tables.

A

B

C

P

Q

R

S

CCS1218